Principles of Pathophysiology and Emergency Medical Care

To my wife, who faced extreme adversity and overcame it,
and to my daughter, who keeps reminding me of what is important in life.

Principles of Pathophysiology and Emergency Medical Care

Jeffrey W. Myers, D.O., NREMTP
Resident Physician
Department of Emergency Medicine
State University of New York at Buffalo
Buffalo, New York

Marianne Neighbors, EdD, RN
Professor
University of Arkansas
School of Nursing
Fayetteville, Arkansas

Ruth Tannehille-Jones, MS, RN
Divisional Chair
Nursing and Allied Health Programs
Northwest Technical Institute
Springdale, Arkansas

DELMAR
THOMSON LEARNING™

Australia Canada Mexico Singapore Spain United Kingdom United States

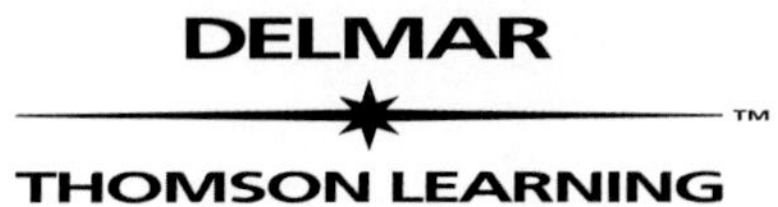

Principles of Pathophysiology and Emergency Medical Care
by Marianne Neighbors, Ruth Tannehill-Jones
edited by Jeffrey Myers

Health Care Publishing Director:
William Brottmiller

Executive Editor:
Cathy L. Esperti

Acquisitions Editor:
Cathy L. Esperti

Developmental Editor:
Darcy M. Scelsi

Editorial Assistant:
Matthew Thouin

Executive Marketing Manager:
Dawn F. Gerrain

Channel Manager:
Jennifer McAvey

Project Editor:
Mary Ellen Cox

Production Coordinator:
Anne Sherman

Art and Design Coordinator:
Jay Purcell

Printed in Canada
1 2 3 4 5 XXX 05 04 03 02 01

For more information, contact Delmar,
5 Maxwell Road, P.O. Box 8007
Clifton Park, NY 12065

Or you can visit our Internet site at http://www.delmar.com

Library of Congress Cataloging-in-Publication Data
Principles of pathophysiology and emergency medical care / edited by Jeffrey W. Myers, Marianne Neighbors, Ruth Tannehill-Jones.
p. cm.
Includes bibliographical references and index.
ISBN 0-7668-2548-5 (alk. paper)
1. Physiology, Pathological. 2. Medical emergencies. 3. Emergency medical services.
I. Myers, Jeffrey W. II. Neighbors, Marianne. III. Tannehill-Jones, Ruth.

RB113 .P75 2002
616.07—dc21 2001047339

NOTICE TO THE READER

Publisher does not warrant or guarantee any of the products described herein or perform any independent analysis in connection with any of the product information contained herein. Publisher does not assume, and expressly disclaims, any obligation to obtain and include information other than that provided to it by the manufacturer.

The reader is expressly warned to consider and adopt all safety precautions that might be indicated by the activities herein and to avoid all potential hazards. By following the instructions contained herein, the reader willingly assumes all risks in connection with such instructions.

The Publisher makes no representation or warranties of any kind, including but not limited to, the warranties of fitness for particular purpose or merchantability, nor are any such representations implied with respect to the material set forth herein, and the publisher takes no responsibility with respect to such material. The publisher shall not be liable for any special, consequential, or exemplary damages resulting, in whole or part, from the readers' use of, or reliance upon, this material.

Contents

Preface xi

Acknowledgments xii

Unit 1
Concepts of Human Disease 1

CHAPTER 1: INTRODUCTION TO HUMAN DISEASES 3

Disease, Disorder, and Syndrome .4
Pathology .4
Pathophysiology .5
Etiology .5
Predisposing Factors .6
- Age / 6
- Sex / 6
- Environment / 6
- Lifestyle / 7
- Heredity / 7

Analyzing Disease Risk .8
- Disease Rates / 8
- Risk Factor Analysis / 8

Assessment .8
Prognosis .9
Treatment .9

CHAPTER 2: THE CELLULAR ENVIRONMENT AND MECHANISMS OF DISEASE 13

Cellular Environment .14
- Cell Anatomy / 15
- Cell Reproduction and Genetics / 16
- Tissue Types / 20

Causes of Disease .21
- Hereditary / 21
- Traumatic / 22
- Inflammation/Infection / 22
- Hyperplasias/Neoplasms / 22
- Nutritional Imbalance / 23
- Impaired Immunity / 24

Aging .25
Death .25
- Cellular Injury / 25
- Cellular Adaptation / 26
- Cell and Tissue Death / 27
- Organism Death / 28

CHAPTER 3: NEOPLASMS 31

Terminology Related to Neoplasms and Tumors .32
Classification of Neoplasms .32
Benign and Malignant Neoplasms .34
Hyperplasias and Neoplasms .35
Development of Malignant Neoplasms (Cancer) .36
Invasion and Metastasis of Cancer .37
Grading and Staging of Cancer .37
Causes of Cancer .38
- Chemical Carcinogens / 38
- Hormones / 39
- Radiation / 39
- Viruses / 39
- Genetic Predisposition / 39
- Personal Risk Behaviors / 40

Cancer Prevention .40
Frequency of Cancer .41
Diagnosis of Cancer .42
Signs and Symptoms of Cancer .43
Cancer Treatment .44

CHAPTER 4: INFLAMMATION AND INFECTION 47

Defense Mechanisms .48
Inflammation .49
The Inflammatory Process .49
Chronic Inflammation .51
Inflammatory Exudates .51
Inflammatory Lesions .52
- Abscesses / 52
- Ulcer / 52
- Cellulitis / 52

Tissue Repair and Healing .53
- Tissue Repair / 53
- Tissue Healing / 54

Delayed Wound Healing / 55
Complications of Wound Healing / 55
Infection 56
Frequency and Types of Infection / 56
Testing for Infection / 58

CHAPTER 5: FLUID, ELECTROLYTE, AND ACID-BASE BALANCE 63

Physiology of Fluid and Acid-Base Balance 64
Fluid Compartments / 64
Body Fluid Distribution / 65
Electrolytes / 65
Movement of Body Fluids / 65
Regulators of Fluid Balance / 68
Acid-Base Balance / 69
Regulators of Acid-Base Balance / 69
Factors Affecting Fluid and Electrolyte Balance 70
Age / 70
Lifestyle / 70
Disturbances in Fluid, Electrolyte, and Acid-Base Balance 70
Fluid Distrubances / 70
Electrolyte Disturbances / 71
Acid-Base Disturbances / 78
Assessment 82
Health History / 82
Physical Examination / 82
Diagnostic and Laboratory Data / 83
Management 85
Parenteral Fluids / 85
Blood Transfusion / 85

CHAPTER 6: PATHOPHYSIOLOGY OF SHOCK 91

Classification of Shock 92
Hypovolemic Shock / 92
Cardiogenic Shock / 96
Neurogenic Shock / 96
Vasogenic Shock / 97
Assessment of Shock 99
Age-Related Differences in Shock 100

Unit II
Common Diseases and Disorders 103

CHAPTER 7: RESPIRATORY DISEASES AND DISORDERS 105

Anatomy and Physiology .106
Common Signs and Symptoms 109
Diagnostic Tests 111
Common Diseases of the Respiratory System 112
Diseases of the Upper Respiratory System / 112
Diseases of the Bronchi and Lungs / 114
Diseases of the Pleura and Chest / 118
Diseases of the Cardiovascular and Respiratory Systems / 120
Trauma 121
Rib Fracture / 121
Flail Chest / 121
Sternal Fracture / 121
Pneumothorax and Hemothorax / 122
Pulmonary Contusion / 123
Traumatic Asphyxia / 123
Diaphragmatic Injury / 123
Developmental and Genetic Disorders 123
Cystic Fibrosis / 124
Effects of Aging on the System 124

CHAPTER 8: CARDIOVASCULAR DISEASES AND DISORDERS 127

Anatomy and Physiology .128
Common Signs and Symptoms 132
Diagnostic Tests 133
Common Diseases of the Cardiovascular System . .134
Diseases of Arteries / 134
Diseases of the Heart / 139
Diseases of the Veins / 147
Trauma 147
Hemorrhage / 148
Pericardial Tamponade / 148
Blunt Cardiac Injury / 148
Great Vessel Injury / 149
Developmental Diseases and Disorders 149
Atrial Septal Defect / 149
Ventricular Septal Defect / 149
Patent Ductus Arteriosus / 149
Coarctation of the Aorta / 149
Tetralogy of Fallot / 149
Effects of Aging on the System 151

CHAPTER 9: NEUROLOGICAL DISEASES AND DISORDERS 155

Anatomy and Physiology 156
- The Central Nervous System (CNS) / 156
- The Peripheral Nervous System (PNS) / 158

Common Signs and Symptoms 159
Diagnostic Tests 160
Common Diseases of the Nervous System 161
- Infectious Diseases / 161
- Vascular Disorders / 163
- Functional Disorders / 165
- Dementia / 169
- Altered Mental Status / 171
- Tumors / 171

Trauma 171
- Skull Fractures / 171
- Diffuse Axonal Injury / 172
- Focal Brain Injuries / 173
- Spinal Cord Injury / 176

Genetic and Developmental Disorders 178
- Cerebral Palsy / 178
- Spina Bifida / 178

Effects of Aging on the System 179

CHAPTER 10: MUSCULOSKELETAL DISEASES AND DISORDERS 183

Anatomy and Physiology 184
Common Signs and Symptoms 185
Diagnostic Tests 186
Common Diseases of the Musculoskeletal System . .186
- Diseases of Bone / 187
- Diseases of Joints / 190
- Diseases of Muscle and Connective Tissue / 191
- Neoplasms / 192

Trauma 193
- Fracture / 193
- Strains and Sprains / 194
- Dislocations and Subluxations / 196
- Crush Injury / 197
- Compartment Syndrome / 197
- Low Back Pain (LBP) / 198
- Bursitis / 199
- Tendonitis / 199
- Torn Rotator Cuff / 199
- Torn Meniscus / 199
- Cruciate Ligament Tears / 199
- Shin Splints / 200

Genetic and Developmental Disorders 200
- Muscular Dystrophy (MD) / 200
- Osteogenesis Imperfecta / 200

Effects of Aging on the System 201

CHAPTER 11: ENDOCRINE DISEASES AND DISORDERS 205

Anatomy and Physiology 206
Common Signs and Symptoms 209
Diagnostic Tests 209
Common Diseases of the Endocrine System 209
- Thyroid Gland Diseases / 210
- Adrenal Gland Diseases / 211
- Disorders of Glucose and Metabolism / 212

Trauma 215
Effects of Aging on the System 215

CHAPTER 12: IMMUNE AND LYMPHATIC DISEASES AND DISORDERS 219

Anatomy and Physiology 220
Common Signs and Symptoms 223
Diagnostic Tests 223
Common Diseases of the Immune System 224
- Hypersensitivity Disorders / 224
- Immune Deficiency Disorders / 231

Common Diseases of the Lymphatic System 233
- Lymphadenitis / 234
- Lymphangitis / 234
- Lymphedema / 234
- Lymphoma / 235
- Mononucleosis / 235

Trauma 235
Effects of Aging on the Immune System 235

CHAPTER 13: GASTROENTEROLOGIC DISEASES AND DISORDERS 239

Anatomy and Physiology 240
Common Signs and Symptoms 242
Assessment 243
Common Diseases and Disorders 244
- Diseases of the Mouth / 245
- Diseases of the Throat and Esophagus / 245
- Diseases of the Stomach / 247
- Diseases of the Small Intestine / 248

Disease of the Colon / 250
Diseases of the Rectum / 253
Gastrointestinal Bleeding / 254
Diseases of the Liver / 254
Diseases of the Gallbladder / 258
Diseases of the Pancreas / 259
Trauma .259
Solid Organ Trauma / 259
Hollow Organ Trauma / 260
Evaluation of Abdominal Pain .260
Developmental and Genetic Disorders .260
Developmental Malformations / 261
Cleft Lip and Palate / 262
Pyloric Stenosis / 262
Hirschsprung's Disease / 263
Effects of Aging on the System .263

CHAPTER 14: RENAL AND UROLOGIC DISEASES AND DISORDERS 269

Anatomy and Physiology .270
Common Signs and Symptoms .271
Diagnostic Tests .271
Common Diseases of the Renal and Urologic System .272
Urinary Tract Infection (UTI) / 272
Diseases of the Kidney / 274
Diseases of the Bladder / 279
Trauma .280
Straddle Injuries / 280
Neurogenic Bladder / 280
Effects of Aging on the System .280

CHAPTER 15: TOXICOLOGIC EMERGENCIES 283

Routes of Entry .284
Ingestion / 285
Inhalation / 285
Injection / 285
Absorption / 286
General Management of Toxicologic Emergencies .286
Toxidromes .287
Cholinergic Toxidrome / 288
Anticholinergic Toxidrome / 289
Opioid Toxidrome / 289
Hallucinogenic Toxidrome / 290
Sympathomimetic Toxidrome / 290
Substances of Abuse .291
Alcohol / 291
Cocaine / 291
Narcotics / 292
Marijuana / 292
Mushrooms / 293
Chemical Agents .293
Caustic Agents / 293
Common Household Chemicals / 293
Carbon Monoxide / 294
Hydrocarbons / 295
Alcohols / 295
Organophosphates / 295
Metals / 295
Medications .297
Cardiovascular Medications / 297
Psychiatric Medications / 298
Sedative and Hypnotics / 299
Analgesics / 300
Xanthines / 302
Food Poisoning .302
Insect and Snake Bites .303

CHAPTER 16: HEMATOLOGIC SYSTEM DISEASES AND DISORDERS 309

Anatomy and Physiology .310
Common Signs and Symptoms .312
Diagnostic Tests .313
Common Diseases of the Hematologic System .315
Disorders of Red Blood Cells / 315
Disorders of White Blood Cells / 317
Disorders of Platelets / 318
Trauma .319
Developmental and Genetic Disorders .319
Effects of Aging on the System .319

CHAPTER 17: INTEGUMENTARY DISEASES AND DISORDERS 325

Anatomy and Physiology .326
Common Signs and Symptoms .327
Diagnostic Tests .327
Common Diseases of the Integumentary System .329
Infectious Diseases / 329
Trauma .334
Mechanical Skin Injury / 334
Thermal Skin Injury / 335

Electrical Injury / 336
Radiation Injury / 336
Pressure Injury / 336
Effects of Aging on the System 337

CHAPTER 18: EYE AND EAR DISEASES AND DISORDERS 341

Anatomy and Physiology 342
Eye / 342
Ear / 343
Common Signs and Symptoms 345
Diagnostic Tests of the Eye 345
Diagnostic Tests of the Ear 346
Common Diseases of the Eye 346
Refractive Errors / 347
Inflammation and Infection / 347
Cataract / 348
Glaucoma / 348
Nystagmus / 349
Common Diseases of the Ear 349
Infection / 349
Ménière's Disease / 351
Labyrinthitis / 351
Trauma 351
Corneal Abrasion / 351
Conjunctival Hemorrhage / 352
Hyphema / 352
Ruptured Globe / 352
Orbital Fracture / 352
Chemical Trauma / 352
Retinal Detachment / 352
Ruptured Tympanic Membrane / 353
Basilar Skull Fracture / 353
Separation of Ear Cartilage / 353
Effects of Aging on the System 353

CHAPTER 19: ENVIRONMENTAL DISEASES AND DISORDERS 357

Heat Emergencies 358
Physiology of the Thermoregulatory Mechanism / 358
Fever / 359
Heat Cramps / 360
Heat Exhaustion / 360
Heat Stroke / 360
Cold Emergencies 360
Hypothermia / 361
Frostbite / 363
Water Emergencies 363
Near Drowning / 364
Diving Emergencies / 364
Altitude Emergencies 366
Physiologic Response to Altitude / 367
Acute Mountain Sickness / 368
High Altitude Cerebral Edema / 369
High Altitude Pulmonary Edema / 369

CHAPTER 20: BEHAVIORAL DISEASES AND DISORDERS 373

Common Signs and Symptoms 374
Diagnostic Tests 374
Common Mental Health Disorders 374
Developmental Mental Health Disorders / 375
Substance Related Mental Disorders / 376
Organic Mental Disorders / 379
Psychosis / 380
Mood or Affective Disorders / 380
Dissociative Disorders / 381
Anxiety Disorders / 382
Somatoform Disorders / 383
Personality Disorders / 384
Trauma 384
Grief / 384
Suicide / 385
Mental Health Disorders in the Older Adult 385

CHAPTER 21: REPRODUCTIVE DISEASES AND DISORDERS 389

Anatomy and Physiology 390
Female Anatomy and Physiology / 390
Male Anatomy and Physiology / 391
Common Signs and Symptoms 391
Diagnostic Tests 392
Common Disease of the Reproductive System 394
Female Reproductive System Diseases / 394
Male Reproductive System Diseases / 397
Sexually Transmitted Diseases (STD) / 397
Trauma 401
Rape / 401
Effects of Aging on the System 401

CHAPTER 22: DISORDERS RELATED TO LABOR AND DELIVERY 405

Obstetric History 406

Physiology of Normal Pregnancy 407

- Reproductive System / 407
- Cardiovascular System / 407
- Respiratory System / 407
- Musculoskeletal System / 407
- Gastroenterologic (GI) System / 407
- Renal System / 407

Common Disorders of Pregnancy 407

- Hyperemesis Gravidarum / 408
- Abortion / 408
- Ectopic Pregnancy / 409
- Placenta Previa / 409
- Abruptio Placenta / 410
- Disseminated Intravascular Coagulation / 411
- Pregnancy-Induced Hypertension / 411
- Chronic Medical Problems / 412
- Hemolytic Diseases / 413
- Multiple Pregnancy / 414
- Substance Abuse / 415
- Preterm Labor / 415

Physiology of Normal Childbirth 415

- Onset Labor / 415
- Maternal Systemic Responses to Labor / 416
- Variables Affecting Labor / 418
- Stages of Labor / 421

Complications of Childbirth 423

- Preterm Labor and Birth / 424
- Premature Rupture of Membranes / 425
- Dystocia / 425
- Abnormal Duration of Labor / 427
- Prolapsed Cord / 427

Postpartum Care and Complications 428

- Care of Infant / 428
- Care of Mother / 429
- Newborn Physiological Changes / 430
- Maternal Physiologic Changes / 431
- Postpartum Complications / 433

Trauma in Pregnancy 436

CHAPTER 23: CHILDHOOD DISEASES AND DISORDERS 439

Infectious Diseases 440

- Viral Diseases / 440
- Bacterial Diseases / 443
- Fungal Diseases / 444
- Parasitic Diseases / 445

Respiratory Diseases 445

- Sudden Infant Death Syndrome / 445
- Croup / 446
- Asthma / 446
- Pneumonia / 446
- Respiratory Failure / 446

Digestive Diseases 447

- Fluid Imbalances / 447

Cardiovascular Diseases .448

Musculoskeletal Diseases 448

Hematologic Diseases 448

- Leukemia / 448

Neurologic Diseases 448

- Reye's Syndrome / 448

Eye and Ear Diseases 448

Trauma 449

- Child Abuse / 449
- Suicide / 449
- Poisoning / 450

GLOSSARY 455

INDEX 471

Preface

To the best of my knowledge, this is the first text on pathophysiology of disease that is geared specifically to the EMS provider. Others are intended for a broader audience. This text covers the conditions and diseases most pertinent to field emergency care or critical care transport, using the 1998 DOT EMT-Paramedic National Standard Curriculum as a guide. There are a number of conditions not covered in the paramedic curriculum that I chose to include because: (1) the presence of the condition potentially impacts field management; (2) exacerbations of the chronic disease are sometimes seen by EMS; or 3) the condition is common and it would be helpful to the EMS provider to have some exposure to its pathophysiology.

This text, written for the EMS provider, follows the 1998 DOT EMT-Paramedic National Standard Curriculum. This does not mean that it is not appropriate for a First Responder, EMT-Basic, or EMT-Intermediate. EMS providers at all levels should benefit from this text, especially if they are interested in advancing to the EMT-Paramedic level. However, a certain amount of medical knowledge and experience in EMS is assumed.

As the title suggests, this text explores the pathophysiology behind disease. While some aspects of patient management are discussed, such information is presented in a general manner. Specific information, such as medication dosages and in some cases specific agents, are omitted for two reasons. First, the focus is on the pathophysiology of disease, and not the treatment. Second, emergency medicine is a dynamic field and there are variations in protocols across the country and even within the same region. If there are any conflicts between the information presented in this text and your protocol, **follow your protocol**. Use your medical director, paramedic instructor, or regional medical authority as resources if differences exist between this text and your local protocol.

As a former quality engineer, I am always looking to improve what I do. I encourage the reader, regardless of training level, to provide feedback on this text, whether positive or negative, either directly to Delmar Thomson Learning (http://www.delmar.com) or to me at *myersj@alum.rpi.edu*.

Thank you for taking the time to read *Principles of Pathophysiology and Emergency Medical Care* and please enjoy the text.

Jeffrey W. Myers, D.O., NREMTP

Acknowledgments

I want to acknowledge Darcy Scelsi, my primary contact at Delmar, and the rest of the Delmar team for providing all the necessary materials, reviewing and correcting the manuscripts, and assembling the text into the final product. I also would like to thank the reviewers, who suggested better ways of presenting the material. Above all, I am thankful to have had the opportunity to pass along knowledge to others.

UNIT I

Concepts of Human Disease

CHAPTER

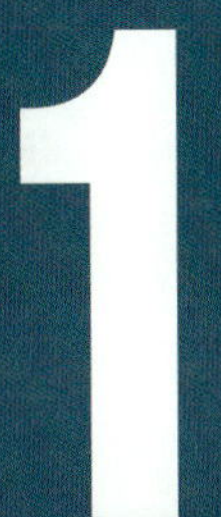

Introduction to Human Diseases

CONTENT OUTLINE

- Disease, Disorder, and Syndrome
- Pathology
- Pathophysiology
- Etiology
- Predisposing Factors
  - Age
  - Sex
  - Environment
  - Lifestyle
  - Heredity
- Analyzing Disease Risk
  - Disease Rates
  - Risk Factor Analysis
- Assessment
- Prognosis
- Treatment

KEY TERMS

Acute
Assessment
Auscultation
Causal risk factor
Chronic
Co-morbidity
Complication
Differential diagnosis
Disease
Disorder
Etiology
Exacerbation
Fatal
Holistic medicine
Homeostasis
Iatrogenic
Idiopathic
Incidence rate
Lethal
Morbidity
Mortality rate
Non-causal risk factor
Nosocomial
Palliative
Palpation
Pathogenesis
Pathogens
Pathologic
Pathologist
Pathology
Pathophysiology
Percussion
Predisposing factors
Prevalence rate
Prevalent
Preventive
Prognosis
Remission
Signs
Symptoms
Syndrome

LEARNING OBJECTIVES

Upon completion of the chapter, the student should be able to:

1. Define basic terminology used in the study of human diseases.
2. Define the pathophysiology and etiology of disease.
3. Describe the Standard Precaution guidelines for disease prevention.
4. Identify the predisposing factors to human diseases.
5. Discuss the factors involved in analyzing disease risk.
6. Explain the difference between the diagnosis and prognosis of a disease.
7. Describe some common tests used to diagnose disease states.

OVERVIEW

The study of human diseases is important to understanding a variety of other topics in the health care field. Diseases that affect the human can range from mild to severe, and may be acute (short-term) or chronic (long-term). Some diseases affect only one part of the body or a particular body system, while others affect several parts of the body or body systems at the same time. There are many factors that influence the body's ability to stay healthy or predispose the body to a disease process. Some of these factors are controllable, but some are strictly related to heredity. Diseases can be diagnosed by professional health care providers using a variety of techniques and tests.

DISEASE, DISORDER, AND SYNDROME

In the study of human disease, there are several terms used that are similar and often used interchangeably, but may not have the exact same definition. **Disease** may be defined in several ways. It may be called a change in structure or function within the body, which is considered to be abnormal, or it may be defined as any change from normal. It usually refers to a condition in which there are abnormal symptoms occurring, and a pathological state is present, such as in pneumonia or leukemia. Both of these definitions have one underlying concept. That concept is the alteration of **homeostasis** (HOME-ee-oh-**STAY**-sis). Homeostasis is the state of sameness or normalcy that the body strives to maintain. The body is remarkable in its ability to maintain homeostasis, but once this homeostasis is no longer maintained the body is diseased or "not at ease."

Disorder is defined as a derangement or abnormality of function. The term disorder can also refer to a pathological condition of the body or mind but more commonly is used to refer to a problem such as a vitamin deficiency (nutritional disorder). It is also used to refer to structural problems, such as a malformation of a joint (bone disorder) or a condition where the term disease does not seem to apply, such as dysphagia (swallowing disorder). Because disease and disorder are so closely related they are often used synonymously.

The term **syndrome** (SIN-drome) refers to a group of symptoms which may be caused by a specific disease but may also be caused by several interrelated problems. Examples include Tourette's syndrome, Down syndrome, and Acquired Immunodeficiency Syndrome (AIDS), which are discussed later in the text.

PATHOLOGY

Pathology (pah-THOL-oh-jee) can be broadly defined as the study of disease (patho = disease, ology = study). A **pathologist** (pah-THOL-oh-jist) is one who studies disease. There are many types of pathologists since there are numerous ways to study disease. A surgical pathologist inspects surgical tissue or biopsies for evidence of disease (Figure 1–1). The medical examiner or coroner is a pathologist who

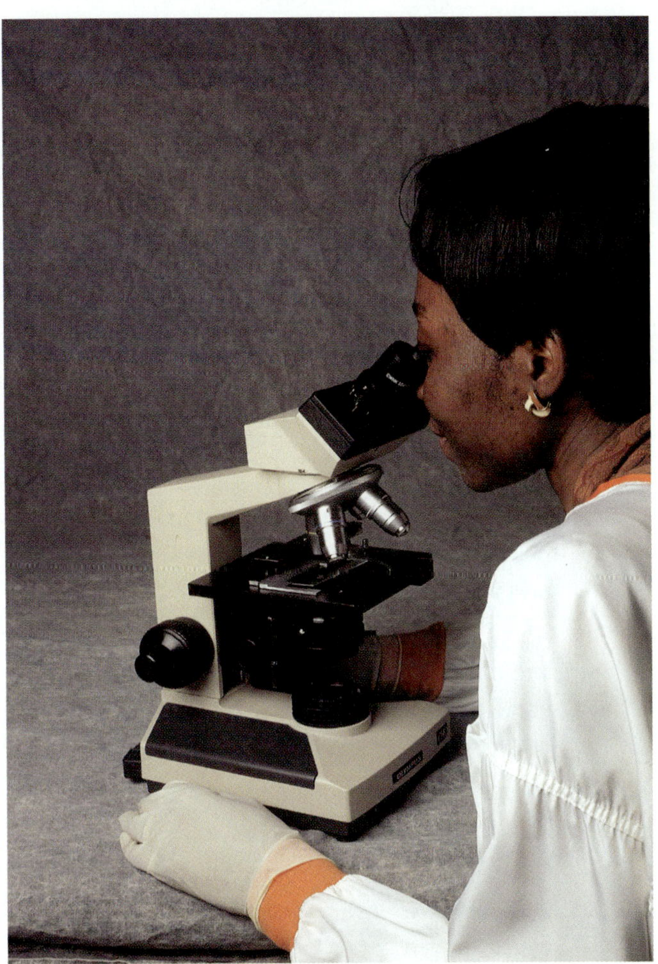

Figure 1–1 Pathologist examining pathogens through a microscope.

studies human tissue to determine the cause of death and to provide evidence of criminal involvement in a death. Other types of pathologists are outlined in Table 1–1.

TABLE 1–1 Types of Pathologists

Pathologist	Role or Subject
Experimental	Research
Academic	Teaching
Anatomic	Clinical Examinations
Autopsy	Postmortem
Surgical	Biopsies
Clinical	Laboratory Examinations
Hematology	Blood
Immunology	Antigen / Antibodies
Microbiology	Microorganisms

The prefix "patho" can be used in a variety of ways to describe disease processes or the disease itself. Microorganisms or agents that cause disease are called **pathogens** (PATH-oh-jens). These include bacteria, viruses, fungi, protozoans, and helminths (worms). All are pathogens that cause a pathogenic reaction. Fractures that are caused by a disease process that weakens the bone, such as osteoporosis, would be called **pathologic** (path-oh-LODGE-ick) fractures.

PATHOPHYSIOLOGY

Pathophysiology (PATH-oh-FIZ-ee-ol-oh-jee, patho = disease, physiology = study of) is the study of how and why a disease develops and progresses. Asthma is a very well-known condition, with almost everyone knowing someone who has asthma. An acute asthma attack is a cascade of events that begins with an exposure to something that causes an allergic reaction in the respiratory tree. This exposure initiates a cascade that results in narrowing of the smaller airways, limiting the amount of air allowed to provide gas exchange. Knowledge of the pathophysiology of a disease or condition allows treatments to be developed based upon the mechanism causing the disease. Knowledge of the pathophysiology of a disease also allows the EMS provider to alter a treatment approach (after discussion with the medical control physician) for patients that may not fit into a standard treatment protocol.

The pathophysiology of a disease may be explained in terms of time. An **acute** (a-CUTE) disease is short term, and usually has a sudden onset. If the disease lasts for an extended period of time or the healing process is progressing slowly, it is classified as a **chronic** (KRON-ick) condition. Many chronic conditions may undergo acute exacerbations of the chronic disease. Asthma is an excellent example of a disease that is chronic and undergoes acute exacerbations. Most patients with asthma are well controlled and do not have any problems with their disease. However, if the patient develops an upper respiratory infection or is exposed to an allergen, that patient may develop an acute asthma attack. EMS providers see many of these acute exacerbations of chronic disease in their practice. Table 1–2 lists several examples of acute and chronic diseases.

ETIOLOGY

The **etiology** (EE-tee-OL-oh-jee) of a disease describes the cause of a disease. Etiology is commonly used to simply mean "the cause." One may say that the cause is unknown or of "unknown etiology." The cause or etiology of pneumonia may be a virus or a bacterium. The etiology of

TABLE 1-2 Examples of Acute and Chronic Diseases

Acute	Chronic
Upper Respiratory Infections	Arthritis
Lacerations	Hypertension
Middle Ear Infection	Diabetes Mellitus
Gastroenteritis	Low Back Pain
Pneumonia	Heart Disease
Fractures	Asthma

athlete's foot is a fungus named *tinea pedis*. Another term used to mean the cause is unknown is **idiopathic** (ID-ee-oh-**PATH**-ick). If an individual is diagnosed as having idiopathic gastric pain, it means the cause of the pain in the stomach is unknown.

Other terms related to cause of disease are **iatrogenic** (eye-AT-roh-**JEN**-ick) and **nosocomial** (NOS-oh-**KOH**-me-al). Iatrogenic (iatro = medicine, physician, genic = arising from) means that the problem arose related to a prescribed treatment. An example of an iatrogenic problem is the development of anemia in a patient undergoing chemotherapy treatments for cancer. Nosocomial is a closely related term. Nosocomial implies that the disease was acquired from a hospital environment. An example would be a postoperative patient developing an incisional staphylococcal infection. The best way to prevent nosocomial infections is through the practice of good hand washing. A good hand washing technique is described in Healthy Highlight 1–1.

HEALTHY HIGHLIGHT 1–1

Hand Washing Technique

To prevent the spread of disease between oneself and others, good and frequent hand washing is the best prevention. Follow the good hand washing steps listed below:

- Use an antimicrobial soap when possible. Have paper towels available to use to dry hands and to turn off the water.
- Adjust water temperature and force. Wet hands and wrists, and use a fingernail cleaner (if available) to gently clean under the nails on both hands, while holding hands under the running water.
- Apply a small amount of liquid soap. Work into a lather on wrists and hands. Briskly rub hands together, being sure to wash areas between fingers and around each wrist.
- Rinse well from fingertips to wrists. Be careful not to touch the sides of the basin.
- Dry each hand from fingertips to wrist using a paper towel. When finished, turn off the water using a paper towel as a barrier between the hands and the faucet.
- Discard soiled towels into the trash basket.

PREDISPOSING FACTORS

Predisposing factors, also known as risk factors, make a person more susceptible to disease. Predisposing factors are not the cause of the disease, nor do people with predisposing factors always develop the disease. These factors include age, sex, environment, lifestyle, and heredity. Some risk factors are controllable, such as lifestyle behaviors, while others such as age are not.

Age

From the beginning of life until death our risk of disease follows our age. Newborns are at risk of disease because their immune systems are not fully developed. On the other hand, the elderly are at risk because their immune systems are degenerating or wearing out. Girls in their early teens are high risk for a difficult or problem pregnancy, while women over the age of thirty are also considered high risk. The older we become, the higher the risk for diseases such as cancer, heart disease, stroke, senile dementia, and Alzheimer's.

Sex

Some diseases are more **prevalent** (occurring more often) in one gender or the other. Men are more at risk for diseases such as lung cancer, gout, and parkinsonism. Other disorders or diseases occur more often in women, including osteoporosis, rheumatoid arthritis, and breast cancer.

Environment

Air and water pollution may lead to respiratory and gastrointestinal disease. Poor sanitation, excessive noise, and stress are also environmental risk factors. Occupational diseases, such as lung disease, are high among miners and persons working in areas where there are increased amounts of dust or other particles in the air. Farmers are considered to be at higher risk for diseases because of their increased exposure to dust, pesticides and other pollutants. Farmers also have an increased risk for trauma injuries caused by safety problems around farm machinery. People living in rural, remote areas and people living in impoverished, inner-city areas generally do not have health care available comparable to those in other areas. This increases their risk for developing chronic illnesses, and may increase the frequency of exacerbations of those illnesses.

Lifestyle

Lifestyle factors fall into a category over which the individual has some control. Choosing to improve health behaviors in these areas would lead to a reduction in risk, and thus a possibility of avoiding the occurrence of the disease. Such factors include smoking, drinking alcohol, poor nutrition (excessive fat, salt and sugar, and not enough fruits, vegetables and fiber), lack of exercise, and stress.

Practicing health behaviors to prevent contamination, and thus disease, is also an important lifestyle behavior. The Centers for Disease Control and Prevention recommend the use of Standard Precautions when caring for any individual where there is a chance of being contaminated with blood or body fluids (Healthy Highlight 1–2). This is an important measure to prevent transmission of any disease that can be passed between humans in blood or body fluids, such as hepatitis, *E. coli* infections, and acquired immunodeficiency syndrome (AIDS).

Heredity

Although one cannot change genetic makeup, being aware of hereditary risk factors may encourage the individual to change lifestyle behaviors to reduce the risk of disease. For example, coronary heart disease has been shown to have a high familial tendency. Persons with this family inheritance are compounding their chances if they smoke, have poor nutritional habits, and don't exercise routinely. Breast cancer and cervical cancer also have familial tendencies. Women with family members who have been diagnosed with breast cancer or cervical cancer are at a higher risk for developing these diseases. These women should routinely be screened for evidence of cancer and should complete monthly breast self-exams. With this knowledge about

HEALTHY HIGHLIGHT 1–2

Standard Precautions

The use of Standard Precautions is recommended by the Centers for Disease Control and Prevention for the care of all patients.

- Hand washing—after touching blood, body fluids, even if gloves are worn; use an antimicrobial soap.
- Gloves—wear gloves when touching blood or body fluids and contaminated items; change gloves after patient contact or contact with contaminated items; wash hands.
- Eye wear, mask and face shield—wear protection for the eyes, mouth, and face when doing procedures where there is a risk of splashing or spraying of blood or body secretions.
- Gown—wear a gown to protect the clothing from splashing or spraying of blood or body fluids.
- Equipment—wear gloves when handling equipment contaminated with blood or body fluids; clean equipment appropriately after use; discard disposable equipment in proper containers.
- Environment control—follow proper procedures for cleaning and disinfecting the patient's environment after use.
- Linen—use proper procedure for disposing of linen contaminated with blood or body fluids.
- Blood-borne pathogens—do not recap needles; dispose of used needles, and other sharp instruments in proper containers; use a mouthpiece for resuscitation; keep one available in areas where there is likelihood of need.

hereditary factors, individuals may choose to decrease their overall risk by improving their lifestyle health behaviors.

ANALYZING DISEASE RISK

When encountering a patient and developing a treatment plan, the EMS provider evaluates the likelihood of each possible disease. In many cases, the assessment is clear, but in some cases the assessment may not be as clear. The EMS provider can utilize his knowledge of pathophysiology and analyze the risk of certain conditions, utilizing this assessment to direct treatment.

Disease Rates

The **incidence rate** of disease describes the rate of new cases of a disease over a period of time. The American Cancer Society estimates that there will be almost 48,000 new cases of malignant melanoma in the year 2000; therefore, the incidence rate of melanoma is approximately 48,000 people per year. The **prevalence rate** is the number of people who have a certain disease at any given point in time. According to the Framingham study, which looked at long-term factors influencing cardiovascular disease, up to one-fifth of the people enrolled in the study had hypertension; therefore, the prevalence rate of hypertension in that population is one in five people. The **mortality rate** of a disease is the rate of death for a given disease. The American Cancer Society estimates that approximately 8,000 people will die from malignant melanoma in the year 2000; therefore, the mortality rate from melanoma is approximately 8,000 per year.

These rates can change over time. The incidence rate of a particular disease can increase because of an overall increase in the number of people who get that disease per year as well as improved screening for that disease. The incidence rate may decrease from improved preventative health activities. The prevalence rate can be affected by similar factors. The mortality rate can decrease by improved detection and treatment.

Risk Factor Analysis

A **causal risk factor** is a risk factor that directly contributes to development of a disease. For example, cigarette smoking is a causal risk factor for lung cancer because cigarette smoking directly contributes to the development of lung cancer. A **non-causal risk** factor is a risk factor that does not directly cause a disease, but still increases the risk for a person to develop a disease. For example, increasing age is a risk factor in many diseases, but does not directly cause those diseases.

ASSESSMENT

Assessment is the identification of signs and symptoms related to a disease or disorder. An assessment is made after a methodical study by the EMS provider utilizing data collected from a medical history, physical examination, and diagnostic tests (Figure 1–2).

A medical history is a systems review that may include such information as previous illnesses, family illness, predisposing factors, medication allergies, current illnesses and current **symptoms** (SIMP-tums; what patients report as their problem or problems). Examples of symptoms may include stomach pain, headache, and nausea.

The EMS provider proceeds with a head to toe physical examination of the patient looking for **signs** of the disease. Signs differ from symptoms in that signs are observable or measurable. Signs are what the EMS provider sees or measures. Examples of signs could include runny nose, vomiting, elevated blood pressure, and elevated temperature.

During the physical examination the EMS provider may utilize other skills, such as **auscultation** (AWS-kul-**TAY**-shun; using a stethoscope to listen to body cavities), **palpation** (pal-PAY-shun; feeling lightly or pressing firmly on internal organs or structures), and **percussion** (per-KUSH-un; tapping over various body areas to produce a vibrating sound). All the results are compared to a normal standard to identify problems.

A **differential diagnosis** is a list of possible diagnoses that is developed during the evaluation of every patient. The differential diagnosis consists of diseases and disorders that are most likely to be responsible for the patient's signs and symptoms. It may also include diseases and disorders that are not as likely, but are life threatening and must be ruled out or excluded, based upon signs, symptoms, and lab work. To illustrate this

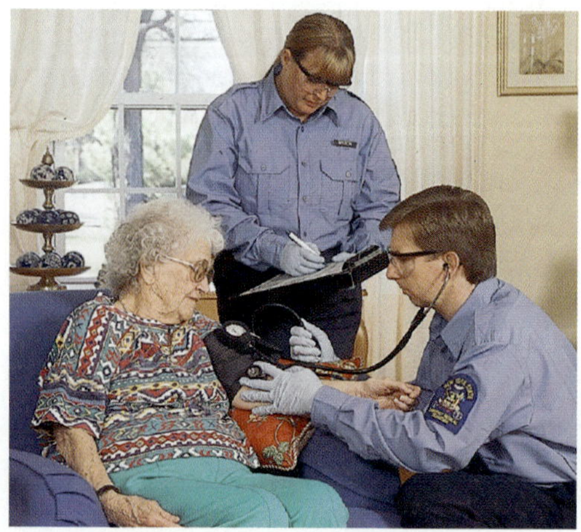

Figure 1–2 EMS provider checking a patient.

process, let's take a patient who is complaining of chest pain. A complaint of chest pain can have many etiologies, from those that are benign, such as musculoskeletal chest pain, to those that can be deadly, such as a heart attack or a rupturing thoracic aneurysm. Based upon the presenting signs and symptoms, the EMS provider may decide that the chest pain in this particular patient is *most likely* musculoskeletal in origin; however, certain symptoms and risk factors are present that may be indicative of a heart attack. The heart attack would have to be ruled out by a work-up at the Emergency Department and perhaps the hospital's chest pain unit before becoming more certain of the diagnosis of musculoskeletal chest pain. A *working diagnosis* is the mostly likely diagnosis that is used to guide further laboratory and procedural evaluation to arrive at the final diagnosis.

Diagnostic tests and procedures that are performed in the Emergency Department to assist in determining a diagnosis are numerable. The routine or most common include urinalysis, complete blood count (CBC), chest X-ray (CXR), and electrocardiography (ECG). See Table 1–3 for examples of common diagnostic tests and procedures.

PROGNOSIS

Prognosis (prawg-KNOW-sis) is the predicted or expected outcome of the disease. For example, the prognosis of the common cold would be that the individual should feel better in seven to ten days.

The duration of the disease may be described as acute in nature. An acute disease is one that usually has a sudden onset, and lasts a short amount of time, like days or weeks. Many acute diseases are related to the respiratory system. Again, the common cold would be a good example.

If the disease persists for a long time it is considered to be chronic. Chronic diseases may begin insidiously (slowly and without symptoms) and may last for the entire life of the individual. As one ages the occurrence of chronic disease increases. One of the most common chronic diseases is hypertension or high blood pressure.

Chronic diseases often go through periods of **remission** and **exacerbation** (x-AS-er-**BAY**-shun). Remission refers to a time when symptoms are diminished or temporarily resolved. Exacerbation refers to a time when symptoms flare up or become worse. Leukemia is a disease that progresses through periods of remission and exacerbation. Both acute and chronic diseases may range from mild to life threatening.

The prognosis may be altered or changed at times if the individual develops a **complication**. A complication is the onset of a second disease or disorder in an individual who is already affected with a disease. An individual with a fractured arm may have a prognosis of the arm healing in six to eight weeks. If the individual suffers the complication of bone infection, the prognosis may change drastically.

Diseases commonly leading to the death of an individual have a high mortality rate. Other terms the medical community uses to refer to a deadly disease include **fatal** and **lethal**.

The **morbidity** of disease refers to the residual effects of a given disease. For example, the morbidity of a significant pneumonia may include a long hospital stay and several weeks of medication use before a patient fully recovers from the illness. The term co-morbidity refers to chronic conditions that affect the complication rate or even mortality rate of a given disease. For example, an older patient with a chronic respiratory condition, such as poorly controlled asthma or emphysema will have a different complication rate and mortality rate than a younger patient without any co-morbid conditions who develops a pneumonia of a similar severity.

A physician's prognosis may also consider survival rate. Survival rate is the percentage of people with a particular disease who live for a set period of time. For example, the two-year survival rate of individuals with lung cancer would be the percentage of people alive two years after diagnosis.

TABLE 1–3 Examples of Common Diagnostic Tests and Procedures

CBC	Urinalysis	Chest X-ray
Electrocardiogram	Mammography	TB Skin Test
Occult Blood Test	PAP Smear	EGD
Serum Electrolytes	Blood Glucose	CT or CAT Scan
Arteriogram	Ultrasound	Upper GI Series

TREATMENT

The EMS provider initiates field treatment based upon his evaluation of the acute signs and symptoms. Once the patient is stabilized, the acute phase of the disease is controlled, and the final diagnosis is established, the patient's physician will work with the individual to explain or outline a plan of care. The physician may offer treatment options to the individual with expected outcomes or prognoses. The individual's entire being should be taken into consideration. The concept considering the whole person rather than just the physical being is called **holistic medicine**. From a holistic viewpoint there is interaction between the spiritual, cognitive, social, physical, and emotional being. These areas do not work independently, but have a dynamic interaction (Figure 1–3).

Treatment interventions may include (1) medications, (2) surgery, (3) exercise, (4) nutritional modifications, (5) physical therapy, (6) complementary therapies, and (7) education. Individuals and family members should be educated and involved in the treatment plan. Failure to involve the individual and family may decrease compliance and lead to failure in the plan.

After the treatment plan is implemented, the physician will follow up with the individual to determine effectiveness. The individual and physician should work together to modify the plan if it is found to be ineffective. Implementation of the plan usually requires an entire health care team. The team may include nurses, a physical therapist, social worker, clergy, and other health care professionals as needed.

The best treatment option is a **preventive** plan. In preventive treatment, care is given to prevent disease. Examples of preventive care are breast mammograms to screen for breast cancer, blood pressure screening for hypertension, routine dental care to prevent dental caries, and hemoccult stool test for colon cancer.

Other treatment plans may include **palliative** (**PAL**-ee-AY-tiv) treatment. Palliative treatment is aimed at preventing pain and discomfort, but does not seek to cure the disease. Treatment for end-term cancer and other serious chronic conditions may be palliative.

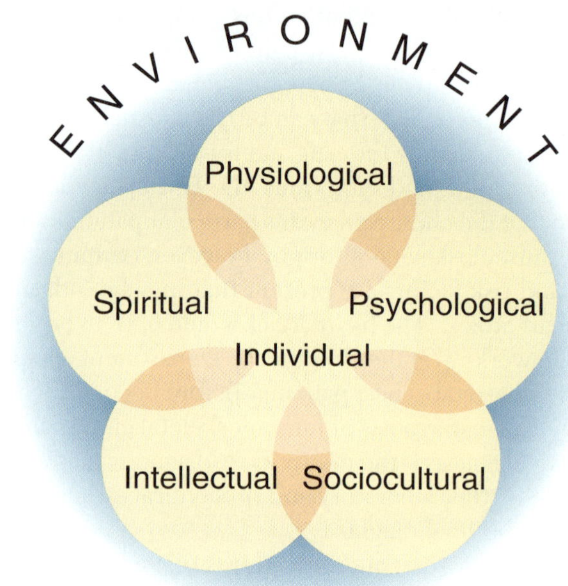

Figure 1–3 Holistic medicine.

SUMMARY

The study of human diseases is important to any EMS provider. Disease can affect any body system or organ and can range from mild to severe, depending on many factors. There are several risk factors for disease that can be controlled to some extent by one's lifestyle. Other diseases may not be prevented or controlled, but may need medical intervention for treatment or cure. Prehospital assessment and treatment of a disease is usually accomplished by a team of EMS providers under the direction of the medical control physician.

REVIEW QUESTIONS

Short Answer

1. Identify why it is important to study human diseases.

2. List the five predisposing factors for disease and one disease related to each factor.

Matching

3. Match the terms in the left column with the correct definition in the right column.

____ Pathophysiology
____ Prevalence rate
____ Differential diagnosis
____ Etiology
____ Prognosis
____ Treatment
____ Diagnosis

a. the cause of disease
b. interventions to cure or control a disease
c. study of how and why a disease progresses
d. the number of people diagnosed with a disease at a given time
e. the identification or naming of a disease
f. consists of diseases and disorders that are most likely to be responsible for the patient's signs and symptoms
g. the predicted or expected outcome of a disease

CASE STUDY

Stan Cotton was injured at a soccer game where you are coaching. He was accidentally tripped by another player while running down the field. He is able to walk to the sideline with assistance but has obvious bleeding on his legs and one arm. You grab the first aid box and go to his side. What do you do next? What equipment might you use to give aid to Stan? What Standard Precautions should apply to this case?

BIBLIOGRAPHY

Note: The books listed below can be used for further study in any chapter of this textbook. Thus, they are not listed in the bibliographies for each successive chapter but are only in this bibliography for Chapter 1.

Anderson, D. (1994). *Dorland's illustrated medical dictionary.* (28th ed.). Philadelphia: W. B. Saunders Co.
Dambro, M. (1997). *Griffith's 5 minute clinical consult.* Baltimore: Williams & Wilkins.
Damjanov, I. (1996). *Pathology for the health-related professions.* Philadelphia: W. B. Saunders Co.
Gould, B. E. (1997). *Pathophysiology for the health-related professions.* Philadelphia: W. B. Saunders Co.
Guyton, A. (1992). *Human physiology and mechanisms of disease* (5th ed.). Philadelphia: W. B. Saunders Co.
Huether, S., & McCance, K. L. (1996). *Understanding pathophysiology.* St Louis: Mosby-Year Book, Inc.
O'Toole, M. T., (Ed.) (1997). *Miller-Keene encyclopedia and dictionary of medicine, nursing, and allied health* (6th ed.). Philadelphia: W. B. Saunders Co.
Paradiso, C. (1995). *Lippincott's review series pathophysiology.* Philadelphia: J. B. Lippincott Co.
Stalheim-Smith, A., & Fitch, G. K. (1993). *Understanding human anatomy and physiology.* Minneapolis: West Publishing Co.
Thomas, C. L., (Ed.) (1997). *Taber's cyclopedic medical dictionary* (18th ed.). Philadelphia: F. A. Davis Co.

CHAPTER 2

The Cellular Environment and Mechanisms of Disease

CONTENT OUTLINE

- Cellular Environment
  - Cell Anatomy
  - Cell Reproduction
  - Tissue Types
- Causes of Disease
  - Hereditary
  - Traumatic
  - Inflammation/Infection
  - Hyperplasias/Neoplasms
  - Nutritional Imbalance
  - Impaired Immunity
- Aging
- Death
  - Cellular Injury
  - Cellular Adaptation
  - Cell and Tissue Death
  - Organism Death

KEY TERMS

AIDS
Alleles
Allergen
Allergy
Anomaly
Anoxia
Antibodies
Antigens
Apoptosis
Atrophy
Autoimmunity
Autolysis
Autosome
Benign
Cachexia
Cancer
Congenital
Cytoplasm
Degenerative
Dominant
Dysplasia
Encapsulated
Enteral
Eukaryotic
Gangrene
Genes
Genotype
Germ cells
Heterozygous
Homozygous
Hyperplasia
Hypertrophy
Hypoxia
Immunodeficiency
Infarct
Infection
Inflammation
Ischemia
Malignant
Meiosis
Metaplasia
Metastatic
Metastasize
Mitosis
Morbidity
MYC
Necrosis
Neoplasia
Neoplasms
Oncology
Organ rejection
Organelle
Parenteral
Phenotype
Prokaryotic
Protoplasm
Receptors
Recessive
Somatic
TPN
Trauma
Tumor

LEARNING OBJECTIVES

Upon completion of the chapter, the student should be able to:

1. Name the organelles contained within the typical animal cell.
2. Describe the basic structure, components, and function of these organelles.
3. Describe the difference between cell mitosis and cell meiosis.
4. List the two means of acquiring an abnormal gene.
5. List the four ways of transmitting genetic disorders to offspring.
6. Describe the features of the four main tissue classifications.
7. Identify important terminology related to the mechanisms of human disease.
8. Describe the causes of disease.
9. Identify disorders in each category of the causes of disease.
10. Compare the various types of impaired immunity.
11. Identify the basic changes in the body occurring in the aging process.
12. Describe the process of cell/tissue injury, adaptation, and death.

OVERVIEW

The cellular environment is an interesting mix of components that perform together to form the basic building blocks of the human body. Each cell has similar components; however, the number and size of some of the components are different based upon the specific purpose or function of the cell. Cells undergo a programmed death after aging. Each cell contains a complete set of genes that serves as the blueprint for its operations. Genes can be altered, resulting in genetic diseases that can be passed along to offspring in a variety of ways. In the uterus, cells differentiate into one of four basic tissue types and prepare to follow the instructions contained within the DNA.

The human body is a complex machine that normally runs in an efficient, balanced manner. When changes occur in the body caused by lifestyle behaviors, abnormal growths, nutritional problems, bacterial invasion, or any other factor that upsets the balance, the result may be a disease process. Human disease may be very minor or life-threatening. Diseases are caused by a variety of factors, some controllable and some not. Even normal changes in the body can make an individual more susceptible to disease. As the body ages, some changes put the individual at higher risk for developing disease. Many changes or alterations in cell and tissue structure may occur. Some of these changes are reversible, but some may cause cellular, tissue, organ, or system death.

CELLULAR ENVIRONMENT

The cell is the basic unit of biological organization of the human body. Our bodies are made up of trillions of cells. Although cells have different functions in the body, they all have certain common structural properties. All cells are composed of **protoplasm**, which is a solution of carbohydrates, proteins, lipids, nucleic acids, and inorganic salts surrounded by a limiting cell membrane. This protoplasm (proto first and plasm formed) is predominantly water with organic compounds in a colloidal suspension and inorganic compounds in solution. These compounds are the building blocks of structures within the protoplasm called **organelles**. Some organelles are common to most cells. Higher cells like those of the human boby are called **eukaryotic** cells (eu = true); cells that do not have membrane-bound organelles (e.g., bacteria) are called **prokaryotic** cells. Organelles that are common to all eukarytic cells are the nucleus, the mitochondria, the endoplasmic reticulum, ribosomes, the Golgi aparatus, and lysosomes. If a cell has a specialized function that other cells do not have, for example, movement, the cell will have specialized organelles. Cells in our bodies that move materials across their exposed or free surface will be covered with row on row of hundreds of cilia. (For instance, cells in our respiratory tract produce mucus to trap dust and microorganisms that get past the hairs in our nose then move the material to our throat to be swallowed and passed out through the digestive system.) The human sperm cell, which must travel up the uterus of the female to the upper one-third of the fallopian or uterine tube to fertilize an egg, has a flagellum to propel it along its journey.

Cell Anatomy

The basic animal cell contains several important structures and features. Cells that are specialized for a particular function, for example producing a hormone, will have more of a particular structure that allows it to perform its function more efficiently. Figure 2–1 is a three-dimensional representation of the typical animal cell, showing its components. We briefly discuss the components and their functions.

The feature that differentiates animal cells from plant cells is the existence of a cell wall in plant cells. Animal cells have a flexible cell membrane that is composed of a double layer of molecules. The cell membrane allows certain particles to pass freely into and out of the cell while blocking other molecules from crossing over the membrane. The cell membrane contains **receptors** that help the cell communicate with other cells. These receptors typically respond to molecules that are transported in the extracellular fluid and bind to particular receptors. Molecules that activate cells include hormones, neurotransmitters, and medications. Once activated, the receptor begins a cascade of events within the cell in response to the trigger. Some receptors are designed to transport specific materials, for example, electrolytes (see Chapter 5), across the cell membrane.

The liquid inside the cell called the cell **cytoplasm** is composed mainly of water and bathes the organelles, allowing materials to move around inside the cell. Cytoplasm is sometimes called the intracellular fluid when discussing the location of water within the body (see Chapter 5). The organelles are the structures within the cell that control activities within the cell.

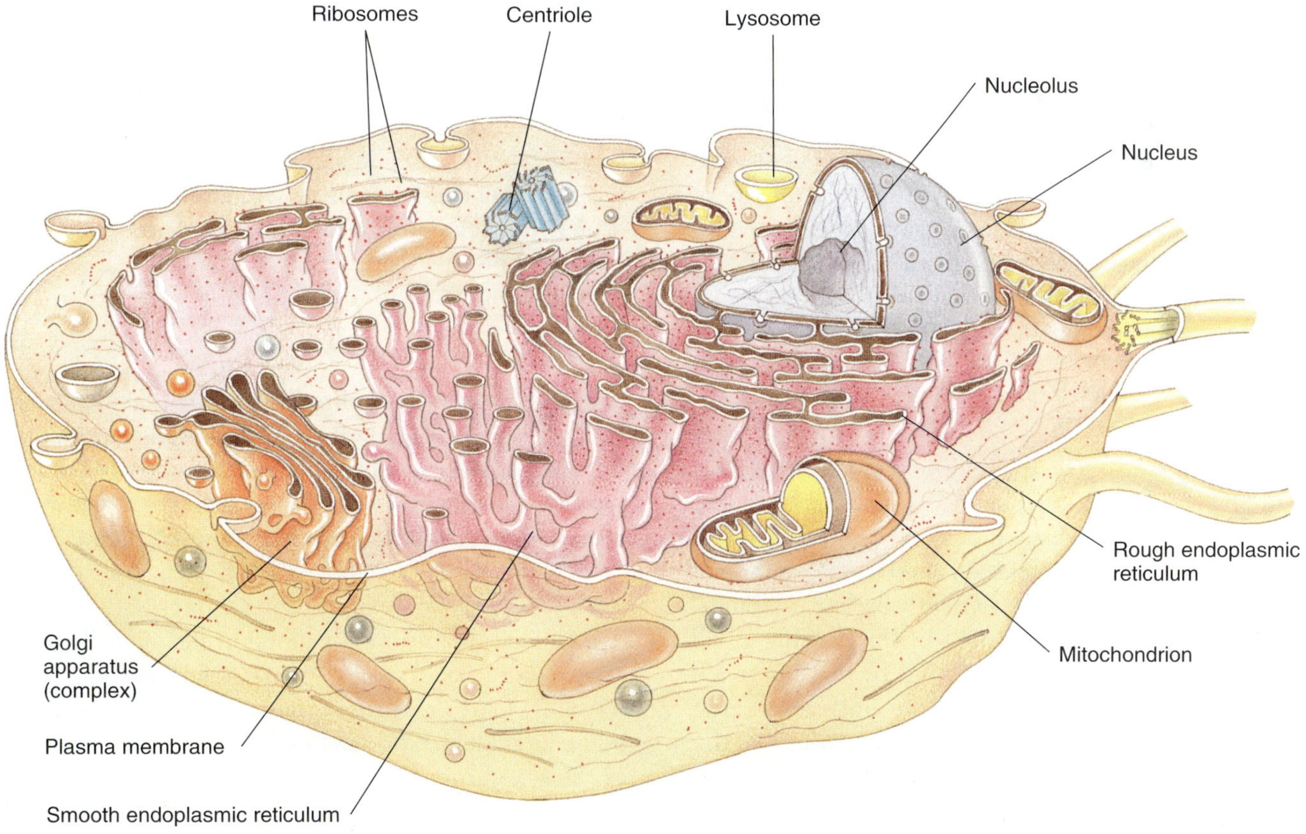

Figure 2–1 A diagram of a typical animal cell.

The cell nucleus is the command center for the cell. It contains the genetic material, in the form of DNA and RNA, which coordinates cell functions, directs the production and transportation of proteins, and responds to triggers that activate the cell receptors. The nucleus has its own membrane which is similar to the cell membrane. The DNA and RNA inside the nucleus are generally clumped together into the nucleolus, except when needed for cell reproduction or to provide the instructions for protein production.

Mitochondria are the organelles within the cell responsible for producing the energy used to perform its function. Food molecules (for example, glucose) combine with oxygen in an environment that causes the release of energy, water, and carbon dioxide. This energy is used to drive the other operations within the cell, for example, transporting molecules across the cell membrane or manufacturing a hormone.

Lysosomes are the organelles responsible for breaking down cellular components into smaller materials to feed the mitochondria. Lysosomes contain very powerful digestive agents that not only break down food, but also break down cell components that require repair. Lysosomes also act as a suicide agent in older cells, releasing the entire store of digestive enzymes at a programmed time to kill the cell. This process of self-digestion is called **autolysis** and the process of programmed cellular suicide is called **apoptosis**. It is believed that this preprogrammed cellular suicide fails in some cancers, allowing the cancer to spread quickly because the cells are not programmed to die and remain to spread the disease.

Ribosomes are tiny granules that serve as the site of protein production. Ribosomes are not bound by a membrane and are located throughout the cell. Messenger RNA from the nucleus attaches to the ribosome, thereby providing it with the genetic codes it requires to produce proteins.

The endoplasmic reticulum (ER) is a complex system of membranes that interconnect the cell and nuclear membranes. The ER is formed by the membrane folding over on itself, forming cavities. There are two types of ER, rough and smooth.

Rough ER has ribosomes attached to its membrane. These ribosomes cause the ER to take on a "rough" appearance. Proteins synthesized by the ribosomes will be collected into the pockets formed by the ER which are called vesicles. These vesicles store and transport the proteins until they are either required elsewhere in the cell or can be transported out of the cell.

Smooth ER, in contrast, does not have ribosomes attached to it. Additionally, smooth ER is located only in certain cells, for example, cells in the gonads that produce sex hormones (see Chapter 11) and certain cells in the intestine, suggesting that smooth ER may be involved in fat transportation.

The Golgi (GOHL-jee) apparatus is an organelle that consists of an assembly of flat sacks. They collect the compounds that are to be released or excreted from the cell and concentrate them into a smaller volume. The Golgi apparatus is also involved in synthesizing carbohydrates, which can be broken down and used for energy, and can store the digestive enzymes used by the lysosomes to break down food. The Golgi apparatus will vary in size and number based upon the individual cell's specific function.

Each cell contains two centrioles located near and on opposite sides of the cell nucleus. The centrioles function during cell division to lay the framework necessary to move the cellular components, including the DNA, to the proper location in the two daughter cells formed during cell reproduction.

Cell Reproduction and Genetics

The nucleus of each cell of the normal human body has forty-six chromosomes, or twenty-three pairs of chromosomes. Most **somatic** (body) cells have the ability to reproduce in a process called **mitosis** (mi-TOE-sis). During mitosis, the forty-six chromosomes duplicate and divide into two identical daughter cells, each containing forty-six chromosomes (Figure 2–2). **Germ** (sex) **cells**, specifically the ova and sperm, also have forty-six chromosomes but division in these cells is different. Germ cells do not duplicate before division. This process is called **meiosis** (mi-OH-sis) and results in each cell carrying only one half, or twenty-three chromosomes (see Figure 2–2). Meiosis is necessary to maintain the normal forty-six chromosomes in a newly formed individual. When an ovum (carrying twenty-three chromosomes) is fertilized with a sperm (carrying twenty-three chromosomes), the newly formed individual will have a combined total of the normal forty-six chromosomes. One half, or twenty-three chromosomes, will have come from each parent.

Of the forty-six chromosomes each individual cell possesses, forty-four chromosomes, or twenty-two pairs, determine somatic or body function and are called **autosomes** (auto = self, somes = body). One pair (or two chromosomes) are sex chromosomes and determine the sex of the individual. Normal females have XX chromosomes as the sex chromosome while males have XY. A female germ cell or ovum undergoes meiosis and divides into two separate X chromosomes; thus, the only chromosome a

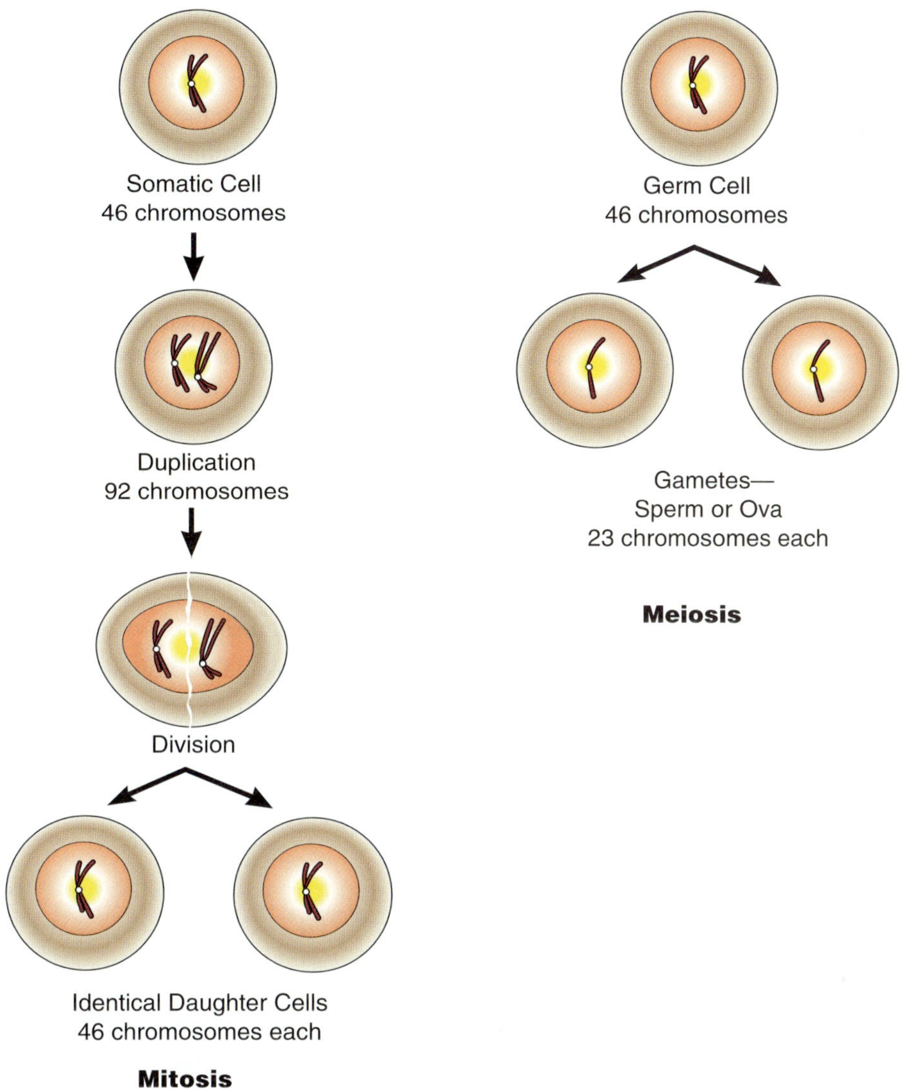

Figure 2-2 Cell division—mitosis and meiosis.

female may give is an X, or female, chromosome. Male germ cells or sperm undergo meiosis and divide into two separate chromosomes, one X and one Y, thus the male may give an X (female) or Y (male) chromosome. This explains why the male partner or sperm determines the sex of the fetus. If an X sperm combines with the ovum the result is XX and the fetus is female. If a Y sperm combines with the ovum the result is XY and the fetus is male. As each male germ cell division results in one X and one Y, there is a fifty/fifty chance of the fetus being male or female. These two chromosomes, the sex chromosomes, are in every cell of the body and are responsible for directing the activity of the cell specifically for a female or for a male.

Chromosomes are made of ultramicroscopic units of deoxyribonucleic acid (DNA) arranged in a specific order. Each ultramicroscopic unit of DNA is called a **gene**. Each chromosome is composed of thousands of genes located at specific positions in the chromosome. When the chromosomes (one from each parent) pair up during fertilization of the egg, the genes on the chromosomes align and are called **alleles** (ah-LEELS). This matched gene pair determines heredity, or, in other words, expresses those characteristics inherited from parents. When one thinks of genes and heredity, thoughts usually center on facial features such as hair and eye color, but genes also determine the entire physical makeup of the individual from the length of toes to the color and texture of skin. Heredity is thought to play a part in many other processes, such as the development of plaque in arteries and the occurrence of rheumatic fever, obesity, and alcoholism in families, to name only a few.

In order to understand basic heredity one must look at individual **genotypes**, or the genetic pattern of the individual. Each gene in an allele or matched pair of genes may be **dominant** (in control) or **recessive** (lacking control). Dominant genotypes are expressed with a capital letter (B, for example), while recessive genotypes are expressed with a small letter (b, for example). If the alleles or genes in a pair match, such as BB or bb, they are said to be **homozygous** (homo = one, zygo = yoked or paired). If the alleles do not match, such as Bb, they are **heterozygous** (hetero = different, zygo = yoked or paired). Expression of a trait such as brown hair or blue eyes is called **phenotype**. Generally speaking, homozygous alleles, whether dominant or recessive, will always express the trait. Heterozygous pairs will express the phenotype of the dominant gene only. Heterozygous pairs are often said to be carriers of recessive disorders as the recessive trait will not be expressed unless paired with another recessive gene (Figure 2–3).

Abnormalities may be caused by chromosomal, genetic, or environmental factors, or a combination of these. Chromosomal disorders are usually related to the number or placement of the chromosome. Chromosomes may fail to separate properly during cell division causing one daughter cell to have an extra chromosome while the other has no chromosomes. Abnormal number or structure of autosomal (or body) chromosomes is usually incompatible with life as these chromosomes carry a large number of essential genes. Major chromosomal abnormalities usually lead to spontaneous abortion of the fetus. The most common autosomal chromosomal disorder is Down syndrome. An abnormal number of chromosomes in the sex chromosomes is less serious but does lead to a number of abnormalities. Disorders due to abnormal sex chromosomes are not usually apparent until puberty when sexual characteristics are found to be abnormal.

There are two ways an individual may acquire an abnormal gene: (1) by mutation of the gene during meiosis affecting the newly formed fetus or (2) by passing of the abnormal gene from the parents (heredity). Genetic disorders are passed to offspring in four different ways: autosomal dominant, autosomal recessive, sex-linked dominant, and sex-linked recessive.

1. Autosomal dominant—dominant disorders are easily recognized because presence of the disorder identifies those individuals with the dominant gene. The line of inheritance is easily followed from one generation to another. Dominant genes

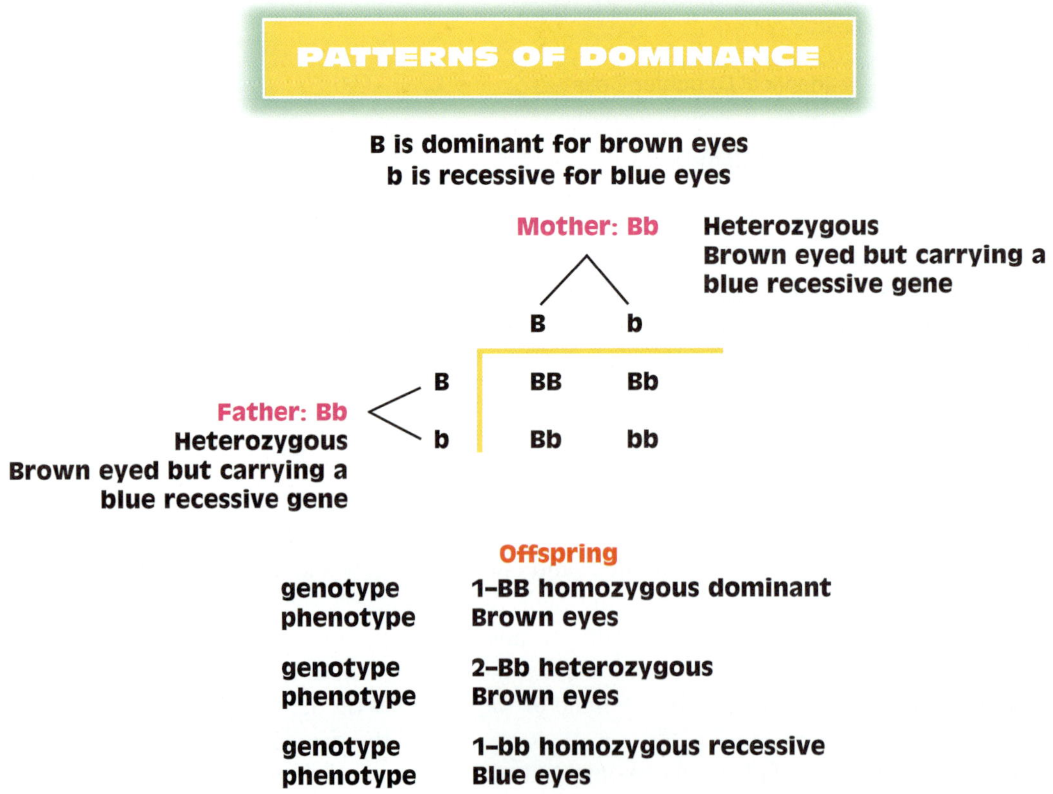

Figure 2–3 Patterns of dominance.

are always expressed whether homozygous (PP) or heterozygous (Pp). An example of an autosomal dominant disorder is polydactyly, having an excessive number of fingers or toes. Figure 2–4 demonstates how individuals carrying a dominant gene (P) would have polydactyly.

2. Autosomal recessive—recessive disorders are only seen when two recessive genes are paired (cc). Cystic fibrosis is an autosomal recessive disorder. Each parent may be phenotypically normal or without sign of the disorder but a heterozygous carrier (Cc) of the disorder. If each parent is heterozygous the chance of the offspring having the disorder is one in four (Figure 2–5A). If one parent has the disorder (cc), the chances increase to one in two (Figure 2–5B). If one parent is homozygous dominant (CC), none of the offspring will be affected (Figure 2–5C). The occurrence of recessive disorders are often very surprising to a family because this disorder may skip generations and hundreds of years before it may be paired with another recessive gene and expressed.
3. Sex-linked dominant—like autosomal dominant disorders, these are more rare than the recessive disorders and are easily recognized.
4. Sex-linked recessive—these disorders are typically carried by females and passed to males. The reason for this is that recessive gene disorders on the X chromosome of the female are overridden by the dominance of the normal gene on the other X chromosome. In males the X disorder is expressed because there is no corresponding gene on the Y chromosome. X-linked disorders usually appear every other generation because they are passed mother to son (Figure 2–6). The affected male (son) will pass this disorder to all his daughters, who then become carriers. The affected male is unable to pass this disorder to his sons because the male gives a Y chromosome to sons, not an X. All the carrier daughters may then pass the disorder to their sons. If the mother is a carrier (XX Hh) there is a possibility that some of her sons will not be affected. If the mother has the disorder (XX hh), which is very rare with X-linked disorders, then all her sons will have the disorder. Hemophilia and muscular dystrophy are both sex-linked recessive disorders.

Approximately two percent of all newborns have a significant birth defect or **congenital** (kon-JEN-ih-tahl; present at birth) **anomaly** (ah-NOM-ah-lee; abnormality). A high percentage of defects (65%) are caused by an unknown factor. Other causes are genetic (20%), chromosomal (5%), and environmental (10%). Chromosomal

AUTOSOMAL DOMINANT PATTERN

Polydactyly is dominant (P)
Normal finger number is recessive (p)

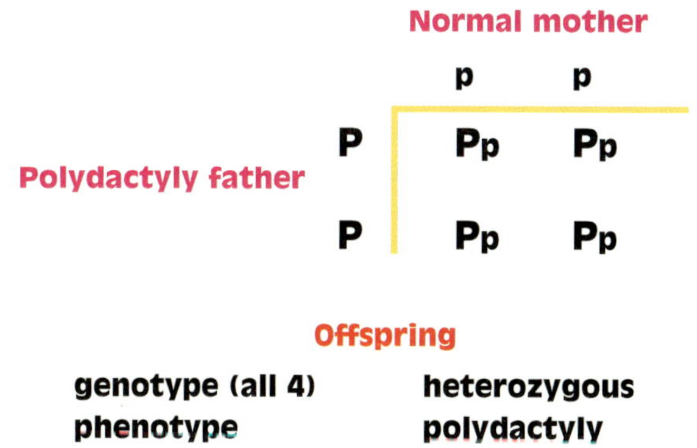

Figure 2–4 Autosomal dominant pattern.

AUTOSOMAL RECESSIVE PATTERN

Genotype	Phenotype
cc (affected)	cystic fibrosis
CC	normal
Cc (carrier)	normal

Mother
normal (carrier)

		C	c
Father **normal (carrier)**	C	CC	Cc
	c	Cc	cc

Offspring

genotype	**1–CC homozygous dominant**
phenotype	**normal**
genotype	**2–Cc heterozygous (carrier)**
phenotype	**normal**
genotype	**1–cc homozygous recessive**
phenotype	**cystic fibrosis**

If both parents are heterozygous, there is a 1 in 4 chance of having a child with cystic fibrosis.

(A)

Figure 2–5 Autosomal recessive pattern. *(continues)*

AUTOSOMAL RECESSIVE PATTERN

Genotype	Phenotype
cc (affected)	cystic fibrosis
CC	normal
Cc (carrier)	normal

Mother
normal (carrier)

		C	c
Father has cystic fibrosis	c	Cc	cc
	c	Cc	cc

Offspring

genotype 2–Cc heterozygous (carrier)
phenotype normal

genotype 2–cc homozygous recessive
phenotype cystic fibrosis

If one parent has the disorder, the chances of having a child with cystic fibrosis increase to 1 in 2.

(B)

AUTOSOMAL RECESSIVE PATTERN

Genotype	Phenotype
cc (affected)	cystic fibrosis
CC	normal
Cc (carrier)	normal

Mother
normal (carrier)

		C	c
Father normal (homozygous dominant)	C	CC	Cc
	C	CC	Cc

Offspring

genotype 2–CC homozygous dominant
phenotype normal

genotype 2–Cc heterozygous (carrier)
phenotype normal

If one parent is homozygous dominant, none of the offspring will be affected.

(C)

Figure 2-5 Autosomal recessive pattern. (Continued)

and genetic causes have been discussed. Environmental causes include maternal radiation, infection, metabolic disorders, drugs, and medications, to name only a few.

Tissue Types

As the human embryo is developing in the uterus, cells differentiate fairly early in the process, developing into specialized cells that form the framework for the body. Some cells differentiate into nerve cells, some into muscle, some into bone, and others into the organs. Tissue is defined as an organized arrangement of cells that cooperate in performing a particular function or functions. The four general classifications of tissue in the body are epithelium, connective tissue, nervous tissue, and muscle tissue. In the following paragraphs, we discuss the special features of each of these.

Epithelial tissue is the tissue that covers all body surfaces and organs. Epithelium also lines the body cavities and forms glands. It can be as thin as one layer of cells or can be several cells thick. Epithelium serves as a barrier between the organs and the external environment. The cells that make up the epithelium are tightly

SEX-LINKED RECESSIVE PATTERN

Hemophilia is recessive X-linked
X and Y are chromosomes
H and h are dominant and recessive genes found only on the X chromosome

Mother
normal (carrier)

		XH	Xh
Father normal	Yo	XYHo boy normal	XYho boy hemophiliac
	XH	XXHH girl normal	XXHh girl normal (carrier)

Figure 2-6 Sex-linked recessive pattern.

adhered to one another and can communicate directly with each other. Examples of epithelium include the skin and the lining of the gastrointestinal tract. Epithelium can be further classified by either the cell shape or function. A discussion of this classification is beyond the scope of this text.

Connective tissue cells, in contrast to epithelial cells, are not closely linked to one another. These cells produce a material that occupies the space between the cells. Connective tissue can have a variety of properties, from high elasticity to rigidity depending upon the proportions of different materials that make up the tissue. Some examples of connective tissue include bone, cartilage, and fascia. Connective tissue supports the other three types of tissue by forming a framework and making compartments for the other tissues.

Nerve tissue is a type of tissue that is specialized to transmit electrical impulses down the length of the cell and release chemicals from the ends to communicate with other cells and tissues close to the end of the nerve cell. Nerve tissue also gathers information from both inside and outside the body, and makes up the brain and spinal cord.

Muscle tissue, the fourth type of tissue, contains specialized structures within the cell that help the cell contract. Muscle tissue is highly organized into bundles with the cells oriented with their long axis in the direction of the bundles to allow the muscle to contract when signaled. There are three types of muscle tissue, smooth, skeletal, and cardiac. Smooth muscle is typically found within blood vessels and surrounding the digestive tract. This type of muscle is sometimes called involuntary muscle because it typically does not respond to voluntary control. These muscles are responsible for changing the diameter of blood vessels and propelling food and waste matter through the digestive tract. Skeletal muscle is sometimes called voluntary muscle because it typically requires thought to activate the muscle. Skeletal muscles are found linking bones together and allow us to move throughout our environment. Cardiac muscle, the third type of muscle tissue, is not under voluntary control but is different from smooth muscle in that some cells have the ability to transmit electrical impulses, much like nerve cells, and the cells have the ability to contract without any outside influence.

CAUSES OF DISEASE

To gain a better understanding of the different causes of diseases it is usually helpful to classify or divide them into smaller groups. This classification may be approached in several different yet logical ways. One commonly used approach is to divide the causes of disease into the following six categories:

1. Hereditary
2. Traumatic
3. Inflammation/Infection
4. Hyperplasias/Neoplasms
5. Nutritional Imbalance
6. Impaired Immunity

Hereditary

Hereditary diseases are caused by an alteration of an individual's genetic or chromosomal makeup. These diseases may or may not be apparent at birth. Hereditary diseases that are present at birth, even if not apparent, are called congenital (kon-JEN-ih-tahl) disorders. However, not all congenital disorders are inherited. Some other causes of congenital disorders include disease during pregnancy (fetal alcohol syndrome) or difficulty with delivery (cerebral palsy), to name only a few.

Hereditary diseases are classified in three basic ways. They are described as 1) a single gene abnormality, 2) an abnormality of several genes (polygenic), or 3) an abnormality of a chromosome, either entire absence of a chromosome or the presence of an additional chromosome. See Table 2–1 for the classification of hereditary diseases and examples.

Chromosomal and genetic abnormalities may or may not be compatible with life. Some abnormalities may be present, but cause no effect on the individual, while others may lead to the death and spontaneous abortion of the unborn child.

TABLE 2-1 Classification of Hereditary Disease with Examples

Single Gene	Polygenic	Chromosomal
Cystic Fibrosis	Gout	Klinefelter's Syndrome
Phenylketonuria	Hypertension	Turner's Syndrome
Sickle Cell Anemia	Congenital Heart Anomalies	Down Syndrome

More information related to hereditary diseases can be found in Unit Two under each specific body system.

Traumatic

Traumatic diseases are caused by a physical injury from an external force. Trauma is the leading cause of death in children and young adults. The type of **trauma** (TRAW-mah) or traumatic disease most commonly affecting individuals varies with age, race, and residence. For example, accidents, especially falls, are a common cause of traumatic disorders in older adults, while gunshot wounds are the most common cause of traumatic disease and even death in young adult black males living in urban areas. However, motor vehicle crashes (**MVC**s) are the most frequent cause of serious injury overall.

In general, classification of trauma includes:

1. motor vehicle crashes
2. falls
3. drowning
4. burns
5. ingested or inhaled objects
6. poisoning
7. penetrating injuries (such as a stab or gunshot wound)
8. physical abuse

Emergency management of trauma is often necessary to prevent the complications of shock, hemorrhage, and infection. Types of trauma commonly occurring in each body system are discussed in the specific system chapters.

Inflammation/Infection

Inflammation (IN-flah-**MAY**-shun) is a protective immune response that is triggered by any type of injury or irritant. Even the slightest trauma can initiate the inflammatory response. Signs of inflammation are redness, heat, swelling, pain, and loss of motion. **Infection** (in-FECT-shun) refers to the invasion of microorganisms into tissue that cause cell or tissue injury. Inflammation and infection are often used synonymously even though they are quite different. A tissue may be inflamed but not infected, but usually tissue that is infected will also be inflamed. An example of inflammation is a sunburn. The tissue is red, warm to the touch, swollen, painful, and uncomfortable when moving. Although this area is inflamed, it is usually not infected.

For tissue to be infected or for infection to occur, there has to be an invasion of microorganisms. Usually inflammation and infection go hand in hand. For example, when the skin is cut, the tissue around the cut will undergo a mild inflammation. As skin bacteria invade the cut tissue, the area becomes infected and usually the area becomes even more inflamed from the irritation to the tissue caused by the bacteria (Figure 2–7).

Diseases that are related to inflammation are identified with the suffix "itis." Examples include appendicitis (inflammation of the appendix), gastritis (inflammation of the stomach), colitis (inflammation of the colon), and encephalitis (inflammation of the brain). In many cases the inflammation will progress to an infection caused by the presence of bacteria in the region. For example, appendicitis may be caused by an obstruction of the appendix. Since the bacteria *Escherichia coli* (E. coli) are commonly found in the colon, the appendix becomes infected.

Hyperplasias/Neoplasms

Hyperplasias (HIGH-per-**PLAY**-zee-ahs; hyper = excessive, plasia = growth) and **neoplasms** (NEE-oh-plazms; neo = new, plasm = growth) are similar because in both there is an increase in cell number leading to an increase in tissue size. Hyperplasias differ from neoplasms, however, in terms of cause and growth limits. Hyperplasias are an overgrowth in response to some type of stimulus. An example of a hyperplasia would be enlargement of the thyroid gland (goiter) in response to a hormone deficiency.

Neoplasms (new growths) are commonly called **tumors**. The Latin word tumor means "swelling" and originally was used in the description of the swelling related to inflammation. The Greek term for swelling is

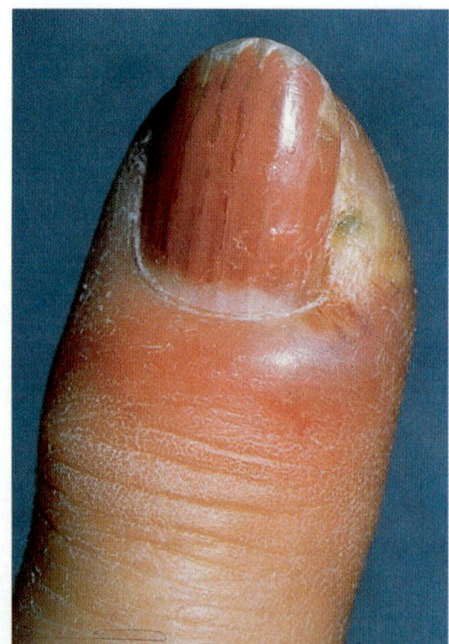

Figure 2–7 Inflammation of a finger.

onkos, which has been used to construct the word **oncology** (ong-KOL-oh-jee; onco = tumor, logy = study of) or the study of cancer. Although all tumors are not neoplasms, the words are often used synonymously.

Diseases with tumor involvement usually end with the suffix "oma." Examples include lipoma, carcinoma, melanoma, and sarcoma (Table 2–2). A hematoma is a "blood swelling" or a collection of blood in an area. A hematoma on the head due to a blunt blow would be an example.

Neoplasms or tumors (omas) may be classified as **benign** (beh-NINE) or **malignant** (mah-LIG-nant). Generally speaking benign tumors have a limited growth, are **encapsulated** (enclosed in a capsule) thus easily removed, and are not deadly. Malignant tumors are just the opposite. These tumors usually grow uncontrollably, have finger-like projections into surrounding tissue making removal very difficult, and are usually deadly. Malignant means deadly or progressing to death. With these definitions it is understandable why the terms tumor, malignancy, and cancer bring fear to an individual. Some "omas" or tumor diseases are commonly called **cancer**. Cancer is defined as any malignant tumor.

Malignant tumors invade surrounding tissue with finger-like or "crab like" projections. This explains why cancer comes from the Greek word *karkinos* meaning crab. This characteristic makes surgical removal of cancer quite difficult (Figure 2–8). Another characteristic of malignant neoplams is that they **metastasize** (meh-TAS-tah-sighz). Metastasize means to move to a different area of the body. **Metastatic** (MET-ah-**STAT**-ic) cancers move from a site of origin to another secondary site in the body. For example, lung cancer commonly metastasizes to the bone. More detailed information on hyperplasias and neoplasms is found in Chapter 3.

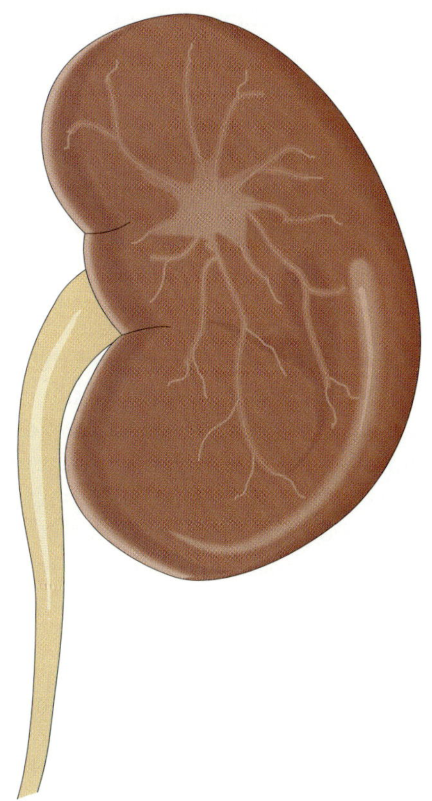

Figure 2–8 Crab-like appearance of cancer in a kidney.

Nutritional Imbalance

Good nutrition is important in maintaining good health and reducing the chance of disease. Nutritional disorders may cause problems with physical growth, mental and intellectual retardation, and even death in extreme cases. Most nutritional diseases are related to overconsumption or underconsumption of nutrients. Specific problems are

TABLE 2–2 Examples of Neoplasms or Tumors

Neoplasms/Tumors	Description
Adenoma	Usually benign tumor arising from glandular epithelial tissue
Carcinoma	Malignant tumor of epithelial tissue
Fibroma	Benign encapsulated tumor of connective tissue
Glioma	Malignant tumor of neurological cells
Lipoma	Benign fatty tumor
Melanoma	Malignant tumor of the skin
Sarcoma	Malignant tumor arising from connective tissue like muscle or bone

malnutrition, obesity, and excessive or deficient vitamins and/or minerals.

Malnutrition may be caused by inadequate nutrient intake or an intake of an adequate amount with poor nutritive value. Diseases that cause a problem with absorption of nutrients may also lead to malnutrition. Children and the elderly are the age groups most affected by malnutrition. Persons suffering with cancer often experience problems with malnutrition and become cachexia. **Cachexia** (ca-KECK-see-ah) is a term used to describe any individual who has an ill, thin, wasted appearance.

Persons who are unable to eat enough to maintain their body weight may have nutritional supplements provided in a liquid drink. Another way to supplement or provide for total nutritional intake is not through the alimentary canal or digestive system, but through a **parenteral** (pah-REN-ter-al; to administer by injection) route. Parenteral routes may include subcutaneous (sub = under, cutaneous = skin) or under the skin, intramuscular (intra = within, muscular = muscle) or in the muscle, or intravenous (intra = within, venous = vein) or in the vein administration. The intravenous route is the most common parenteral route utilized. Providing the total nutrition needed by giving nutritive liquid through a venous (vein) route is called total parenteral nutrition (**TPN**).

Nutrition may also be provided through an **enteral** (small intestine) route. A nasogastric (naso = nose, gastric = stomach) tube or a tube running through the nose and into the stomach may be utilized for feedings if the supplement is planned short-term. For longer-term enteral feeding, a gastrostomy (gastro = stomach, ostomy = opening; opening into the stomach) procedure is performed to place a tube through the abdominal and stomach wall. Enteral feeding, commonly called "tube feeding," is accomplished utilizing this method (Figure 2–9).

Although there are many individuals in the United States who have a nutritional deficiency, the most common problem is obesity. Obesity is primarily caused by overconsumption of nutrients and lack of exercise. Although obesity is difficult to define specifically for each individual, it is obvious that it is a major nutritional problem. Obesity shortens the life span of the individual by increasing the chance for arteriosclerosis leading to cardiovascular diseases. It also affects the individual's risk for developing bone/joint problems because of the increased pressure on the skeletal system.

Vitamin and mineral excesses and deficiencies are usually related to diet, metabolic disorders, and some medications. Hypervitaminosis may occur in individuals who consume large amounts of vitamins for an extended period of time.

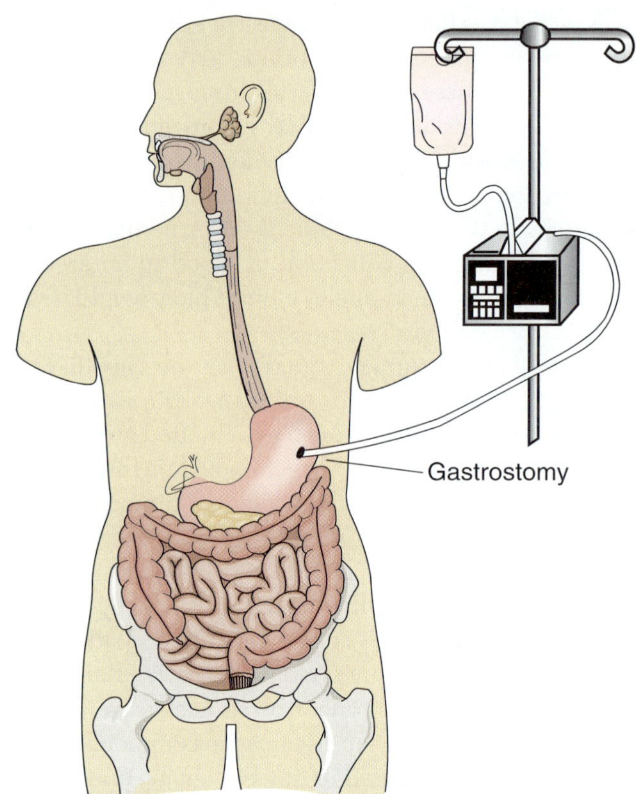

Figure 2–9 Gastrostomy feeding.

Nutritional guidelines for a healthy lifestyle are difficult to determine as they must cover a variety of ages and nutritional needs. Children, teens, and pregnant woman have very specific nutritional needs.

Impaired Immunity

The immune system of the body is a specialized group of cells, tissues, and organs that are designed to defend the body against pathogenic attacks. The body's first line of defense against pathogens is its normal structure and function, including an intact skin, mucous membranes, tears, and secretions. The immune system protects the body in basically two other ways through:

1. the inflammatory response in which leukocytes play a vital part in the killing of foreign invaders.
2. the specific antigen–antibody reaction in which the body responds to **antigens** (AN-tih-jens) by producing **antibodies**. Antigens are substances that cause the body some type of harm, thus setting off this specific reaction. Antibodies, also called immune bodies, are proteins that the body produces to react to and render the antigen harmless.

Impaired immunity occurs when some part of this system malfunctions. Common ways the system malfunctions include:

1. **Allergy**—the immune response is too intense or hypersensitive to an environmental substance. The **allergen** (environmental substance that causes a reaction) in an allergy may be such things as house dust, grass, pets, perfumes, or insect bites, to name a few. The allergens do not usually cause this type of reaction in most persons, but cause an allergic reaction in affected persons.
2. **Autoimmunity**—the immune response attacks its own self. In autoimmunity (auto = self) the body's lymphocytes (white blood cells that produce antibodies) cannot identify the body's own self-antigens, which are harmless. In response the lymphocytes form antibodies that then attack the body's own cells. Examples of autoimmunity diseases include rheumatoid arthritis and rheumatic fever.
3. **Immunodeficiency**—the immune response is unable to defend the body because of a decrease or absence of leukocytes, primarily lymphocytes. Persons with immunodeficiency are usually asymptomatic (without symptoms) except for recurrent infections. It is these recurrent infections that often lead to death. An example of an immunodeficiency disease is **AIDS** (Acquired Immunodeficiency Syndrome). Immunodeficiency may be caused by medications, chemotherapy, or radiation. Organ recipients are intentionally immunosuppressed or immunodeficient in order to save their transplanted organ. Without immunosuppressant medications the body's immune system would recognize the organ as foreign and attack it, leading to organ death. This process is called **organ rejection**. Cancer patients often undergo chemotherapy and radiation treatments that may cause immunodeficiency. Some medications also affect the system by depressing its ability to function properly. Chapter 12 discusses the immune system and related diseases in more detail.

AGING

There is no definite age in years when an individual becomes "aged." However, some statisticians consider the retirement age or age sixty-five as aged. An individual's body actually begins to age at physical maturity around age eighteen. The aging process is complicated, and not completely understood, but it is progressive and is not reversible. Diseases related to aging are often called **degenerative** diseases. Tissue degeneration is a change in functional activity to a lower or lesser level. Examples of degenerative diseases are degenerative joint disease and degenerative disc disease.

The mechanisms of aging are complex and thought to include such factors as heredity, lifestyle, stress, diet, and environment. One may slow the process of aging to some degree by living a healthy lifestyle, and controlling stress and environmental factors.

Hereditary factors may include increased life span related to an inherited ability to resist disease. Just as families have a history of disease patterns, they also appear to have a pattern of longevity. Thus, individuals who have relatives who live to be in their nineties may themselves live to that age. Individuals with a family history of members who have died of heart disease in their early years may also suffer the same problem. Although hereditary patterns cannot be controlled, longevity can be increased and disease decreased by controlling lifestyle behaviors that increase risk of chronic disease as previously mentioned.

The body replaces and repairs itself throughout its lifetime, but with aging, this process slows. As early as age forty there are changes in skin, endocrine function, vision, and muscle strength. Other changes in the aging process may include bone loss leading to osteoporosis; decreased melanin pigment production leading to graying of hair; decreased immunity leading to an increase in infections, and possible development of cancer; loss of brain and nerve cells, which may lead to senile dementia; and decrease in intestinal motility leading to constipation and possible diverticulosis.

DEATH

Humans are mortal, so eventually everyone will die. Even though we are unable to fully understand the aging process, cellular, tissue, and organ death is reviewed in an effort to understand the death of the organism as a whole.

Cellular Injury

Cellular injury and death may be caused by some type of trauma, **hypoxia** (HIGH-**POCK**-see-ah; not enough oxygen), **anoxia** (ah-NOCK-see-ah; no oxygen), drug or bacterial toxins, or viruses. Cells may undergo near death experiences and recuperate. This is considered to be reversible cell injury.

The ability of the cell to survive depends on several factors, including the amount of time the cell suffers and the type of cell injury that occurred. If the cause of the injury is short-term, the cell has a greater chance of survival.

The type of cell also plays a part in its ability to recuperate. The heart, brain, and nerve cells are easily injured and often suffer cell death. This is particularly important as these cells do not replace themselves. Even short-term injury may readily lead to death in these cells. Other cells are not as easily damaged. Connective and epithelial cells often recuperate, and even readily replace themselves by mitosis (cell division).

Cellular Adaptation

Cells that are exposed to adverse conditions often go through a process of adaptation. Once the condition is changed, these cells may have the ability to change back to their normal structure and function. However, some adaptations are permanent, so even if the condition improves, the cells are not able to return to normal. Types of adaptation include **atrophy** (AT-tro-fee), **hypertrophy** (HIGH-**PER**-tro-fee), hyperplasia (HIGH-per-PLAY-zee-ah), metaplasia (MET-ah-PLAY-zee-ah), **dysplasia** (dis-PLAY-zee-ah), and neoplasia (nee-oh-PLAY-zee-ah).

Atrophy (a = without, trophy = growth) is a decrease in cell size, which leads to a decrease in the size of the tissue and organ (Figure 2–10). Atrophy is often caused by the aging process itself or by disease. An example of atrophy related to aging would be the smaller size of the muscles and bones of the elderly. As the female ages the breasts and female reproductive organs atrophy, especially after menopause. Examples of disease or pathologic atrophy are usually related to decreased use of the organ, especially muscles. Spinal cord injuries lead to an inability to move muscles. Without use, muscle cells decrease in size and the muscle atrophies.

Hypertrophy (hyper = excessive, trophy = growth) is an increase in the size of the cell leading to an increase in tissue and organ size (Figure 2–11). Skeletal muscle and heart muscle cells do not increase in number by mitosis. Literally, what an individual has at birth is what the individual retains. This helps explain why some athletes may bulk up with exercise while others do not. The inherited number of muscle cells does not change with exercise, just the size of each cell. In order to adapt to an increased workload muscle cells increase in size. Increased workload on the skeletal muscles causes cellular hypertrophy and thus an increase in muscle size. Heart muscle hypertrophy is usually seen in the left ventricle of the heart (left ventricular hypertrophy). The left ventricle must work harder to pump blood through diseased valves and arteries. In order to adapt to this need, the cells increase in size and thus the left side of the heart enlarges.

Hyperplasia (hyper = increased, plasia = growth) is an increase in cell number that is commonly caused by hormonal stimulation (Figure 2–12). Hyperplasia is discussed in more detail in Chapter 3.

Metaplasia (meta = changed, plasia = growth) is a cellular adaptation in which the cell changes to another type of cell (Figure 2–13). An example is the columnar epithelial cells of the respiratory tree which often change to stratified squamous epithelial when exposed to the irritants of cigarette smoking. This protective adaptation may be reversible if the individual quits smoking.

Dysplasia (dys = bad or difficult, plasia = growth) usually follows metaplasia. It is an alteration in size, shape, and organization of cells (Figure 2–14). Dysplastic cells may change back to the normal cell structure if the irritant or stimulus is removed, but usually these cells progress to neoplasia.

Neoplasia (neo = new, plasia = growth) is the development of a new type of cell with an uncontrolled growth

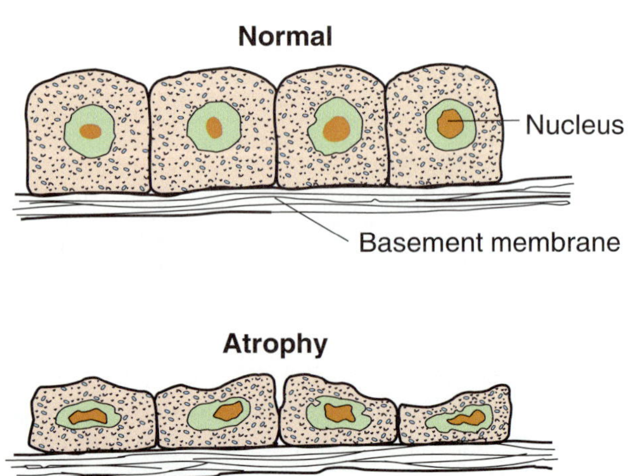

Figure 2–10 Normal cell versus atrophied cell.

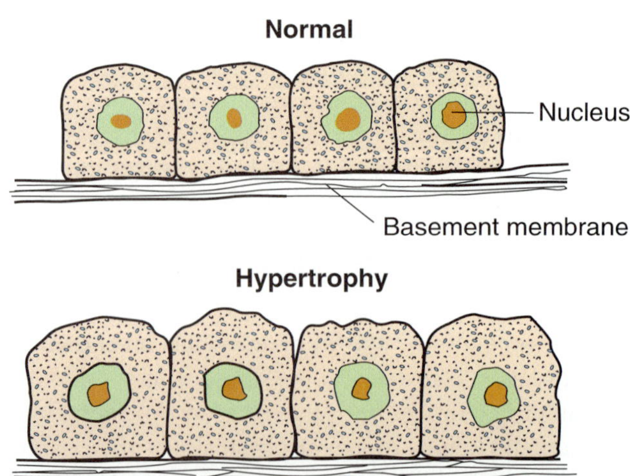

Figure 2–11 Normal cell versus hypertrophied cell.

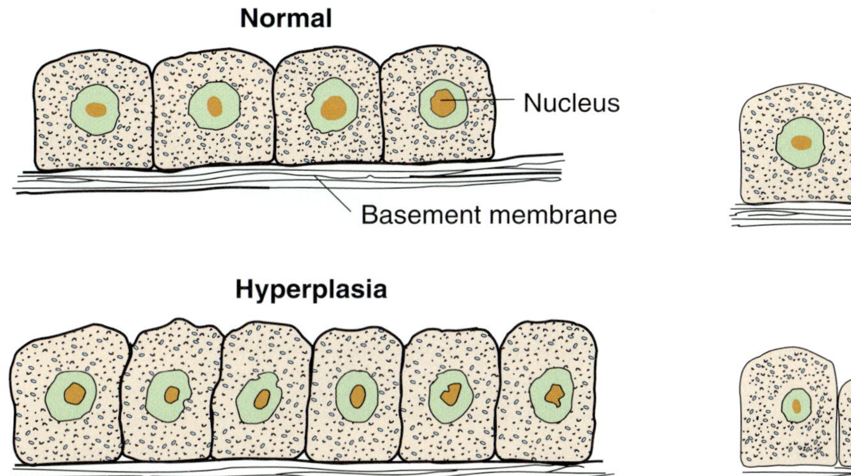

Figure 2–12 Normal tissue versus hyperplasia.

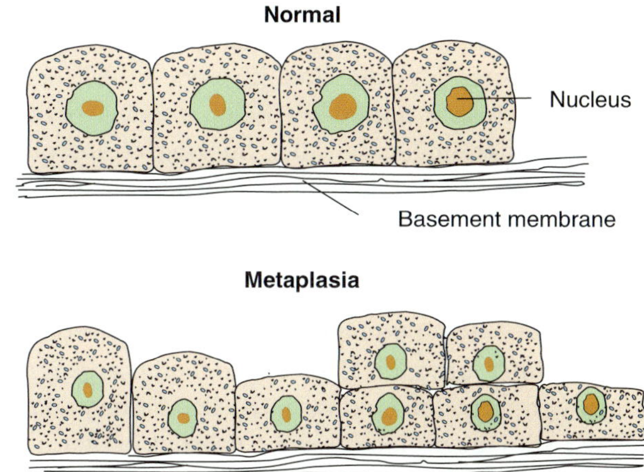

Figure 2–13 Normal tissue versus metaplasia.

pattern (Figure 2–15). Neoplasia is discussed in more detail in Chapter 3.

Cell and Tissue Death

Necrosis (nee-CROW-sis) is defined as cellular death. This cell death may involve a group of cells, and thus, tissue. When referring to dead cells or tissue one would describe the area as necrotic. Cell death, as previously mentioned, may be caused by trauma, hypoxia, anoxia, drug or bacterial toxins, or viruses. The most common causes of cell death are anoxia and hypoxia. Hypoxia caused by decreased blood flow is called **ischemia** (iss-KEE-me-ah; isch = hold back, emia = blood). When necrosis occurs because of ischemia, the area of dead cells (ischemic necrosis) is called an **infarct** (in-FARKT). Infarcts are commonly caused by of obstruction of arteries.

Cells that are injured and not able to recover eventually die. The cause of cell death may be determined by a pathologist as the gross and microscopic appearance of the tissue differs with the type of death. There are several types of necrosis primarily named by the microscopic appearance of the dead cells. The most common type of necrosis is called coagulation necrosis and is caused by cellular anoxia. A cell without oxygen cannot produce needed energy and eventually dies. Coagulation necrosis is the type of cell death experienced with myocardial infarction.

A common alteration in necrosis occurs when saprophytic (dead-tissue-loving) bacteria become involved in the necrotic tissue. With this occurrence, the necrotic

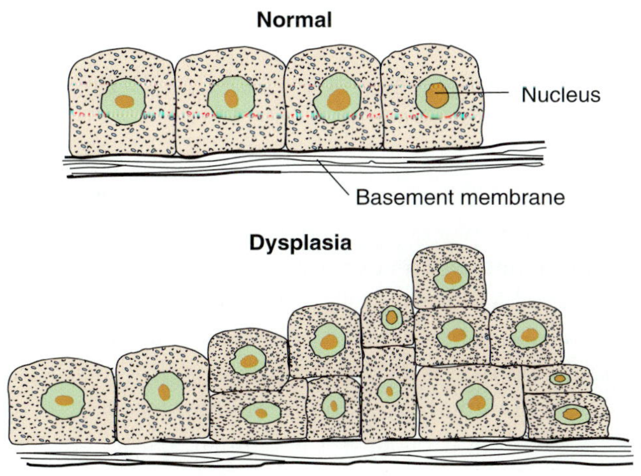

Figure 2–14 Normal tissue versus dysplasia.

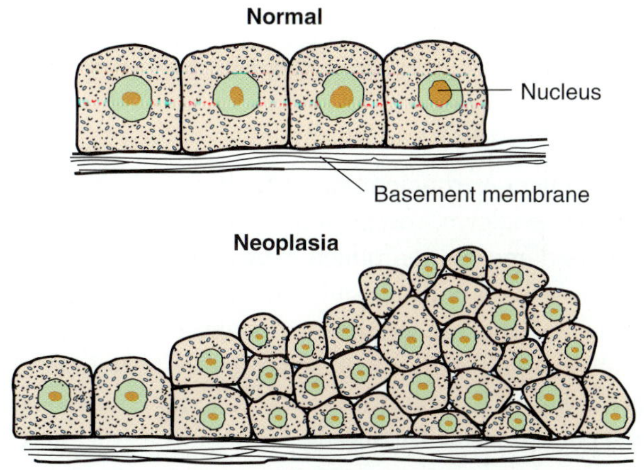

Figure 2–15 Normal tissue versus neoplasia.

tissue is now described as gangrenous or having the condition of **gangrene** (GANG-green). The type of gangrene may be wet, dry, or gas, depending on the appearance of the necrotic tissue. Wet gangrene usually occurs when the necrosis is caused by sudden stoppage of blood flow, as in the trauma of burning, freezing, or embolism. Dry gangrene occurs when blood flow has been slowed for a long period of time before necrosis occurred, as in the case of arteriosclerosis and advanced diabetes. With dry gangrene the tissue is black, shriveled, or mummified (Figure 2–16). This type of gangrene occurs only on the extremities, primarily the feet and toes. Gas gangrene occurs with dirty, infected wounds. The tissue becomes infected with anaerobic (growing without oxygen) bacteria that produce a toxic gas. This is an acute, painful, and often fatal type of gangrene.

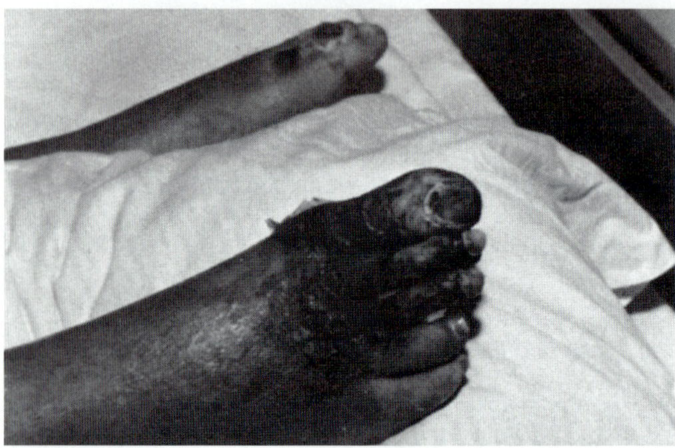

Figure 2–16 Gangrenous tissue of toes and foot.

Organism Death

Human death may be related to any of the aforementioned causes of disease. The aging process as we have discussed leads to death caused by a decrease in the ability to fight disease. Diseases that would not be lethal in our younger years, such as respiratory infections, may be the cause of death in an older individual. The most common cause of death in the United States is heart disease, followed by cancer and strokes (cerebrovascular accident). Heart disease is such a major cause of death that finding the cure for cancer would not produce as great an effect in human lives as decreasing heart disease. (See Chapter 8 for more information.)

Many times the human organism, like the cell, is not killed but may be disabled. Disability is called **morbidity** (state of being diseased). Oftentimes morbidity is so extreme that the individual's quality of life is severely limited. This is often seen in cases of severe brain injury or even some congenital disorders.

Prior to death, major organs such as the heart, lungs, and brain quit functioning. Once the brain ceases to function the individual is considered brain dead. Although death is difficult to define and determine in some cases, one guideline used is that of brain death. The criteria for determining brain death include:

1. a lack of response to stimuli
2. loss of all reflexes
3. absence of respirations or spontaneous breathing effort
4. lack of brain activity as shown by an EEG (electroencephalogram).

This issue of "death" and when an individual is actually dead is still controversial in the medical profession.

SUMMARY

The cellular environment forms the basic building blocks in the human body. The organelles have specific functions such as food breakdown, energy production, protein synthesis, and programmed cellular death. The male sperm and the female ovum undergo cell reproduction by meiosis, while all other cells undergo mitosis. Genes can be altered by mutation during cell division or can be inherited in a mutated state by one of four possible means. Cells differentiate into one of four basic types of tissue, epithelium, connective tissue, nervous tissue, and muscle tissue: each with its own properties.

Human diseases are caused by heredity, trauma, inflammation/infection, hyperplasias/neoplasms, nutritional imbalances, and/or impaired immunity. Lifestyle behaviors can also be contributing factors to disease development as can the aging process. Eventually all organisms die, and the process of death may occur at the cellular, tissue, or whole organism level.

REVIEW QUESTIONS

Matching

1. Match the cause of diseases in the left column with the example of a disease for that category in the right column.

_____	Hereditary	a. pneumonia
_____	Traumatic	b. motor vehicle accident
_____	Inflammation/infection	c. cancer
_____	Hyperplasias/neoplasms	d. obesity
_____	Nutritional imbalance	e. allergies
_____	Impaired immunity	f. cystic fibrosis

True or False

2. T F In autoimmunity the body's immune system attacks itself.
3. T F Some medications used to prevent or cure some diseases can cause immunodeficiency.
4. T F Diseases related to the aging process are called regenerative disorders.
5. T F Congenital disorders are easily recognized at birth.
6. T F Heart and brain cells are easily injured by hypoxia.
7. T F Heredity does not affect the aging process.
8. T F Cellular death occurs only in the event of hypoxia (lack of oxygen).

Short Answer

9. List the factors that affect a cell's ability to survive after injury.
10. How do cells adapt when exposed to adverse conditions?
11. What are the basic functions of the cellular components?
12. How many chromosomes are in the nucleus of each cell in the human body?
13. Which cells undergo meiosis instead of mitosis?
14. How does the process of meiosis differ from mitosis?
15. What is epithelium?

CASE STUDY

Cann Ragland, age twenty-nine, was seriously injured in a motorcycle accident. He is comatose and on life support equipment to maintain his breathing. He has not improved in two weeks with aggressive medical treatment. The family is questioning whether he is "alive or dead" at this time. What criteria can be used to determine this? What are the issues surrounding this determination?

BIBLIOGRAPHY

Bloodborne infections: A practical guide to OSHA compliance. (1992). Arlington, TX: Johnson & Johnson Medical, Inc.

Cotran, R.S., Kumar, V., & Robbins, S.L. (Eds.) (1994). *Pathologic basis of disease* (5th ed.). Philadelphia: W. B. Saunders Co.

Edlin, G., Golanty, E., & Brown, K.M. (1996). *Health and wellness* (5th ed.) Sudbury, MA: Jones and Bartlett Publishers.

Garner, J. S. and the Hospital Infection Control Practices Advisory Committee. (1996). Guideline for isolation precautions in hospitals. *American Journal of Infection Control, 24*, 24-52.

Mlot, C. (April 12, 1997). Insect-borne disease: Curing the carrier. *Science News, 151*, 223.

Rings on your fingers, germs on your hands. (1997). *American Journal of Nursing, 97*(5), 9.

Ross, M. H., Romrell, L. J. & Kay, G. I. (1995). Chapter 2: The cell, and Chapter 3: Tissues: Concept and classification. *Histology: a text and atlas* (3rd ed.) (pp. 18–57). Baltimore: Williams & Wilkins.

Stevens, W. K. (April 29, 1997). Disease is new suspect in ancient extinction. *New York Times*, C1+.

Verducci, T. (May 19, 1997). Staff infection. *Sports Illustrated, 86*, 84-86.

Wade, N. (May 6, 1997). Studies outline clever tricks of viruses. *New York Times*, C1+.

CHAPTER 3

Neoplasms

CONTENT OUTLINE

- Terminology Related to Neoplasms and Tumors
- Classification of Neoplasms
- Benign and Malignant Neoplasms
- Hyperplasias and Neoplasms
- Development of Malignant Neoplasms (Cancer)
- Invasion and Metastasis of Cancer
- Grading and Staging of Cancer
- Causes of Cancer
    - Chemical Carcinogens
    - Hormones
    - Radiation
    - Viruses
    - Genetic Predisposition
    - Personal Risk Behaviors
- Cancer Prevention
- Frequency of Cancer
- Diagnosis of Cancer
- Signs and Symptoms of Cancer
- Cancer Treatment

KEY TERMS

Anaplastic
Angiogenesis
Benign
Biopsy
Cachexia
Carcinogen
Carcinogenesis
Carcinoma
Carcinoma in situ
CAUTION
Chemotherapy
Curative
Cytology
Differentiation
Dysplasia
Frozen section
Grading
Hematoma
Hyperplasia(s)
Invasion
Leukemia
Lymphomas
Malignant
Metaplasia
Metastasis
Neoplasm(s)
Palliative
Pap test
Preventive
Radiation
Sarcoma
Staging
Tumor

LEARNING OBJECTIVES

Upon completion of the chapter, the student should be able to:

1. Define basic terminology used in the study of neoplasms.
2. Explain the system used to classify neoplasms.
3. Compare hyperplasias to neoplasms.
4. Identify the progression of cancer development.
5. State the signs and symptoms of cancer.
6. Identify some common carcinogenic substances.
7. Identify high risk behaviors for cancer development.
8. State the frequency of cancer development in the population.
9. Describe the curative, palliative, and preventive methods used in cancer treatment.

OVERVIEW

Thousands of individuals are diagnosed with neoplasms each year. The diagnostic statement "you have a tumor" often causes instant fear, dread, and tears for the individuals and families involved. Few statements in our society carry the emotional impact this one does. To most people this diagnosis is equivalent to a pronouncement of death. But not all tumors are malignant and thus not all are deadly. However, there are approximately 1.3 million individuals diagnosed with malignant neoplasms each year (American Cancer Society, 1999). This includes all types of cancers. Cancer can be diagnosed using a variety of diagnostic tests. Treatment of cancer is most successful when the cancer has been diagnosed early. Individuals can reduce their risk of developing some types of cancer by following preventive measures recommended by the American Cancer Society.

TERMINOLOGY RELATED TO NEOPLASMS AND TUMORS

The term **neoplasm** (NEE-oh-plazm; neo = new, plasm = growth) means a new growth. The term **tumor** may be simply defined as a swelling or as a neoplasm. Tumor is used as a sign of inflammation and in this instance it describes swelling. The term tumor as related to neoplasm means a new growth. Even though the terms tumor and neoplasm are used synonymously, not all neoplasms form tumors. **Leukemia** (loo-KEE-me-ah; leuk = white, emia = blood) is a malignant disease of the bone marrow that causes an increase in white blood cell production and may not form distinctive tumors. Similarly, not all tumors are neoplasms. A **hematoma** (HEM-ah-**TOH**-mah; hemat = blood, oma = tumor) is a large tumor or swelling filled with blood, commonly called a bruise or contusion (Figure 3–1).

CLASSIFICATION OF NEOPLASMS

Neoplasms may be classified in a variety of ways. Two of the most common ways are according to the (1) appearance and growth pattern, and (2) type of body tissue from which they arise.

Classification by appearance and growth pattern identifies neoplasms (tumors) as **benign** (beh-NINE) or **malignant** (mah-LIG-nant). Tumors that are confined to a local area and do not spread are called benign. If the tumor spreads into local tissue (**invasion**) or to distant sites or different organs (**metastasis**; meh-TAS-tah-sis), it is called a malignant (deadly) tumor or neoplasm. The general term for any malignant neoplasm or tumor is cancer.

Benign tumors are generally harmless while malignant neoplasms are considered deadly as they exhibit characteristics of invasion and metastasis. Invasion refers

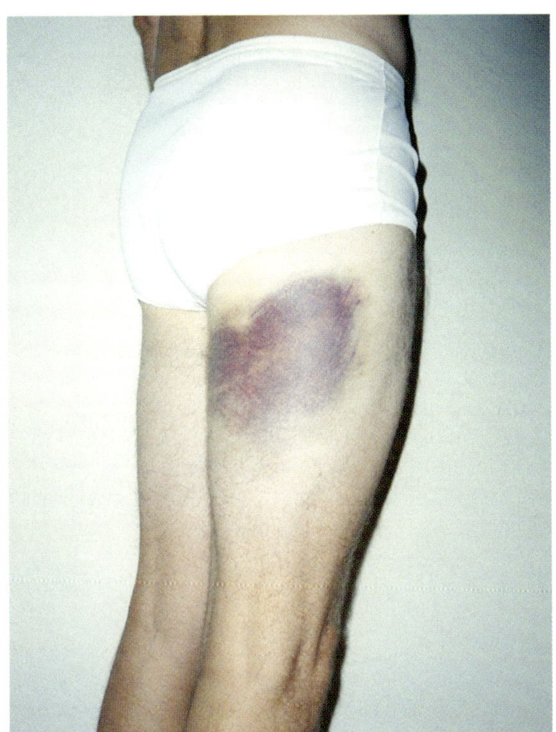

Figure 3–1 Hematoma.

to the spreading of the neoplasm into surrounding tissue. Metastasis is the spread of the neoplasm to distant sites.

Tumors are classified or named according to the tissue they resemble plus the suffix "oma" for tumor. A benign tumor will have the suffix "oma" added after the name of the tissue. An example would be lipoma, a benign tumor of fatty tissue. A malignant neoplasm will have the term **carcinoma** (KAR-sih-**NO**-mah) or **sarcoma** (sar-KOH-mah) added to the name of the tissue type.

Carcinoma is the largest group of malignant neoplasms and indicates a tumor of epithelial tissue found on external or internal body surfaces. A benign tumor of epithelial tissue such as a gland would be adenoma; if it is a malignant neoplasm the name becomes adenocarcinoma.

Sarcoma is used if the neoplasm is from connective tissue such as muscle, fat, and bone. Sarcomas are less common than carcinomas but spread more rapidly and are highly malignant. A benign tumor of connective tissue such as bone would be an osteoma; if it is a malignant neoplasm the name is osteosarcoma.

Leukemias and **lymphomas** (lim-FOH-maz) are malignant neoplasms of blood-forming organs and lymphatic tissues respectively. These malignant neoplasms do not have benign counterparts. All leukemias and lymphomas are malignant, although their prognoses may vary considerably (Figure 3–2).

There are, of course, some tumors that do not follow this pattern. For example, malignant melanoma, a malignant neoplasm of melanocytes, is not a benign tumor as its name would suggest. Glioma is used to refer to all tumors of the glial cells of the brain. Gliomas truly do not fit the terms of this classification system. They are benign in appearance and do not metastasize, but they are malignant (deadly) since most will kill the individual. Examples of benign and malignant neoplasms are listed in Table 3–1.

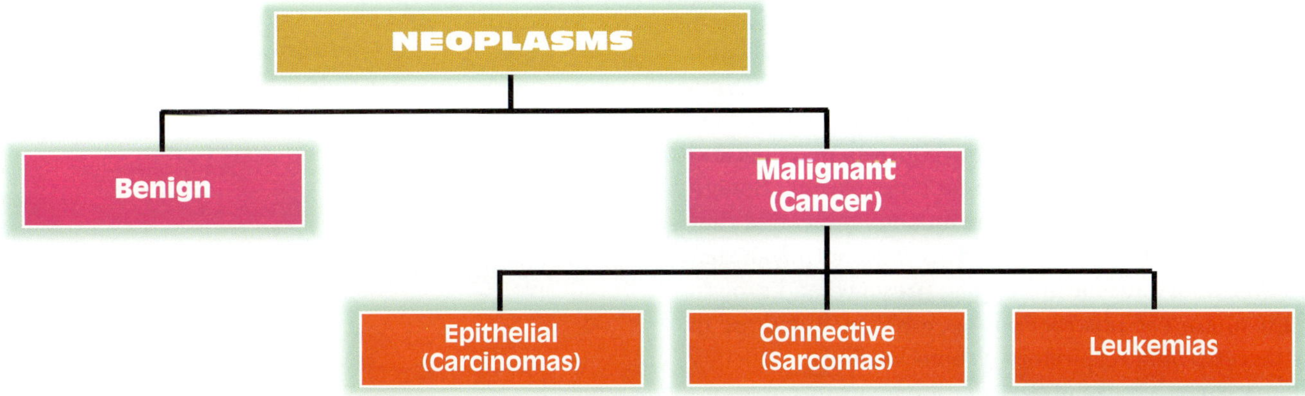

Figure 3–2 Classification of neoplasms.

TABLE 3-1 Origin and Names for Benign and Malignant Neoplasms

Cell or Tissue of Origin	Name of Benign Neoplasm	Name of Malignant Neoplasm
Glandular epithelium	Adenoma	Adenocarcinoma
Squamous epithelium	Epithelioma	Squamous cell carcinoma
Adipose (fat)	Lipoma	Liposarcoma
Cartilage	Chondroma	Chondrosarcoma
Bone	Osteoma	Osteosarcoma
Glial		Glioma
Blood		Leukemia

BENIGN AND MALIGNANT NEOPLASMS

Normal cells grow and function for a purpose. The growth of normal cells is regulated by several factors. First, the built-in genetic program of each cell regulates its growth pattern. Secondly, normal cellular growth is limited by contact with other cells. When two normal cells come in contact with one another they tend to stick together and transmit a signal to each other to stop growing (Figure 3–3). Lastly, normal cellular growth is regulated by growth-promoting or growth-inhibiting substances. Once the normal cells stop growing, they begin performing their specialized function. For example, epithelial cells begin functioning to cover and protect the organism while bone cells function to provide structure and support. This process of individual specialization is called **differentiation** (Figure 3–4).

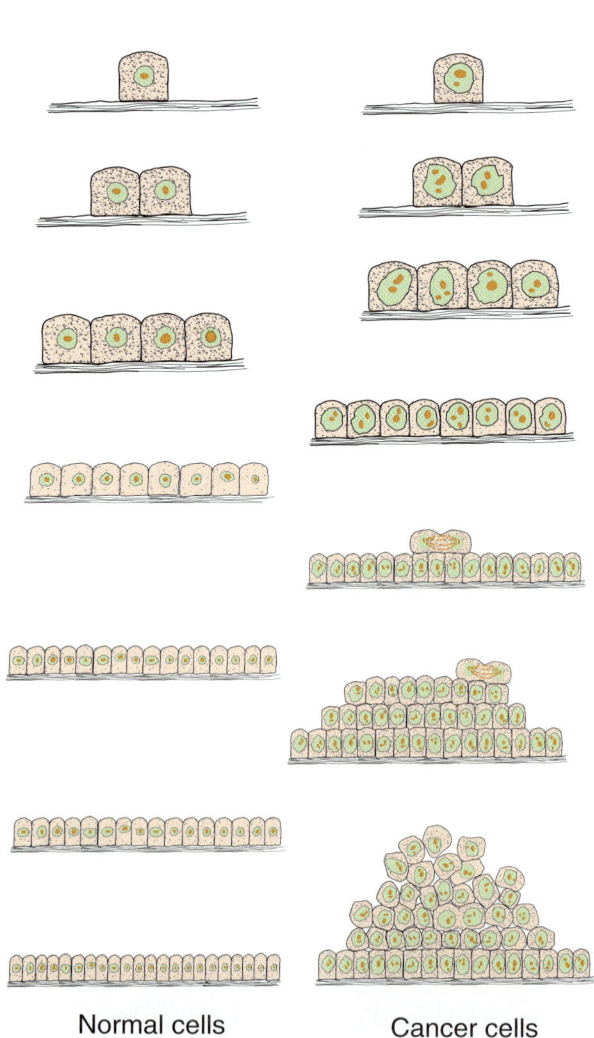

Figure 3–3 Cellular growth patterns.

Benign tumors may retain some normal structure and function. Cells of benign tumors often resemble cells of their origin and, even though they have an abnormal appearance, their appearance is uniform. These cells may also be able to function to some degree like normal cells. Benign tumors are encapsulated or covered with a capsule-like material that makes removal or excision easier. These tumor cells have a limited growth potential and are slower growing than metastatic neoplasms. Benign tumors are expansive (grow and enlarge in the area) but are not invasive or metastatic. This does not mean that benign tumors are harmless. The presence and growth of any tumor can obstruct passageways, such as those in the digestive and respiratory systems leading to difficulty with eating or breathing. Tumors also may exert pressure on nerves causing pain and loss of sensation or movement. Benign tumors affecting a gland may cause over- or undersecretion of hormones with resulting disorders. A benign tumor growing in an enclosed area such as the brain may

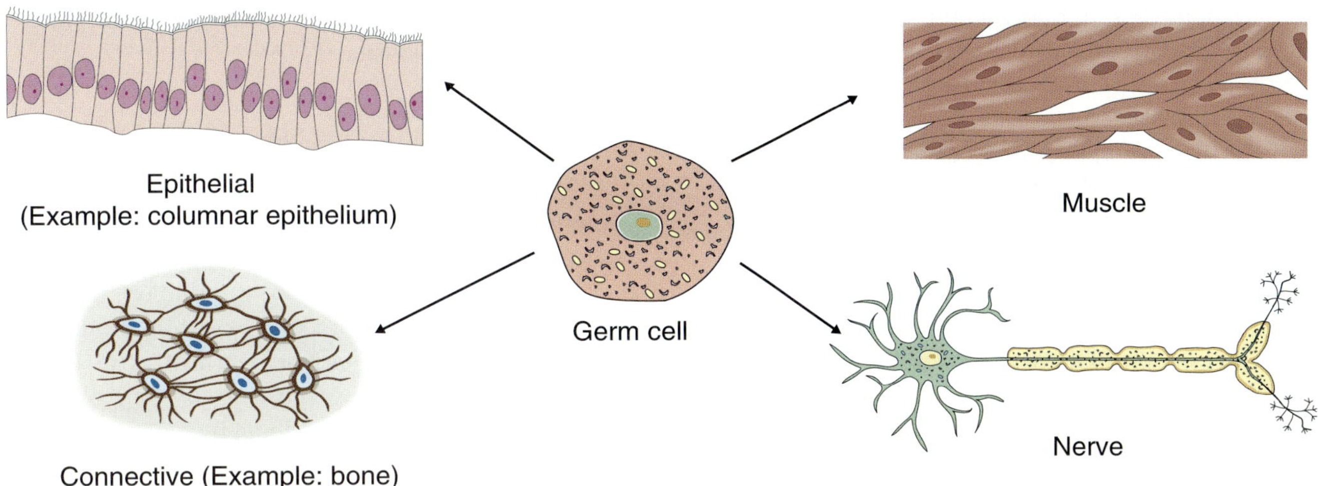

Figure 3–4 The process of cell differentiation.

place pressure on normal tissue leading to death of the tissue and, potentially, death of the individual.

Metastatic neoplasm describes cells whose growth pattern has no purpose and is uncontrollable. Neoplastic cells grow autonomously or independent of growth factors. These cells grow excessively without regard to normal regulatory factors such as contact inhibition. Neoplastic cells do not have the structure or function of cells of their origin. Unlike benign tumor cells, neoplastic cells do not look alike. Their structure is not uniform but haphazard and inconsistent. They are not differentiated and do not perform specialized functions. The surface area of the malignant neoplasm is not encapsulated, rather, it is more crab-like in appearance with multiple claw-like extensions that invade surrounding tissue. A malignant neoplasm (cancer) also metastasizes to distant areas or organs. A comparison of benign and malignant tumors is listed in Table 3–2.

Cancer cells are fast growing. The entire metabolism of the cancerous cell is aimed at rapid reproduction and growth far outpacing the growth of the normal cell. This increase in the metabolic needs of cancer cells leads to an increase in the need for nutrients and oxygen. To meet this need **angiogenesis** (AN-jee-oh-**JEN**-eh-sis; angio = vessel, genesis = growth or new growth of blood vessels) occurs. This increase in blood flow provides increased nutrients to the neoplasm allowing it to continue this rapid, uncontrolled growth. During this time normal cells are deprived of needed nutrients and the individual begins to lose weight and appear thin, frail, and weak. This condition is called **cachexia**.

HYPERPLASIAS AND NEOPLASMS

It is important to note that there is another type of cellular growth that closely resembles a neoplasm. **Hyperplasia** (HIGH-per-**PLAY**-zee-ah; hyper = too much, plasia = growth) and neoplasia (neo = new, plasia = growth) are both an overgrowth of cells that causes an increase

TABLE 3–2 Comparison of Benign and Malignant Tumors

Feature	Benign	Malignant
Growth	Slow, expansive	Fast, invasive, metastatic
Appearance	Symmetrical	Crab-like
Capsule	Yes	No
Tissue Type	Resembles tissue of origin	Does not resemble tissue of origin
Cells	Differentiated	Undifferentiated
Surface	Smooth	Irregular, may ulcerate and hemorrhage

in the size of the tissue. Both commonly produce masses that, once discovered, need to be identified as either hyperplasia or neoplasm, since the treatment of each is drastically different.

Hyperplasias and neoplasms differ in the cause and extent of their growth. Hyperplasia usually occurs in response to a stimulus and the growth stops when the stimulus stops. Neoplasm, as previously mentioned, grows independently, excessively, and usually, unceasingly.

Hyperplasias may be caused by a variety of different stimuli. An example of a hyperplasia caused by tissue irritation is a skin callus on the foot. The stimulus is the irritation or rubbing of a shoe on that particular area. When the shoe size is corrected and the stimulus has stopped, the hyperplasia stops and the callus eventually disappears. Hyperplasias may develop because of hormone excess or deficiency. An example of a hormone deficiency hyperplasia is the enlargement of the thyroid gland, called goiter. Chronic inflammation may lead to hyperplasia as in lymph node hyperplasia or adenoid hyperplasia. Lastly, the hyperplasia may be caused by an unknown stimulus as in the case of prostatic hyperplasia in elderly men.

Hyperplasias and neoplasms both represent an increase in cell number caused by an increase in mitosis (cellular division). Hyperplasias are an increase of cells that still look like cells of their origin. To simplify this concept, one might consider the cells as daughter cells that still look like their mother or the cell of their origin. Neoplasms are an increase in cell number, but the cells are new (neo = new) or different in their appearance from their cell of origin or their mother (Figure 3–5). This difference in appearance is important to the clinical pathologist who determines or diagnoses the mass as hyperplasia or neoplasm.

DEVELOPMENT OF MALIGNANT NEOPLASMS (CANCER)

Genetic alteration is the basis for the development of malignant neoplasm or cancer. Cells throughout the body may undergo genetic alteration or mutation, but amazingly few develop into cancer. A cell must undergo a change or series of changes in its DNA structure in order to acquire the altered growth pattern of cancer. Genetic mutation or change is brought about by some virus, chemical, **radiation** (the process of using light, short waves, ultraviolet or X-ray), or other biologic agent called a **carcinogen** (kar-SIN-oh-jen; carcino = cancer, gen = arising) or cancer-causing agent or substance.

Continued exposure to a carcinogen or to several carcinogens may increase or promote the abnormality of the cell. Abnormal cells may revert back to normal cells, appear as benign tumors, or digress to a malignant neoplasm. The body's immune system may prevent or reverse the development of cancer. Just removing or stopping the carcinogen may also reverse cancer development.

If development is not halted, abnormal cells begin to establish themselves in an effort to become cancerous. These cells must now grow rapidly enough to establish a site. They must fight for space and nutrition. The body and the abnormal cells are at odds with each other at this point. If the body wins, the abnormal cells may die out and disappear. If the abnormal cells get the upper hand, they may become established and thrive.

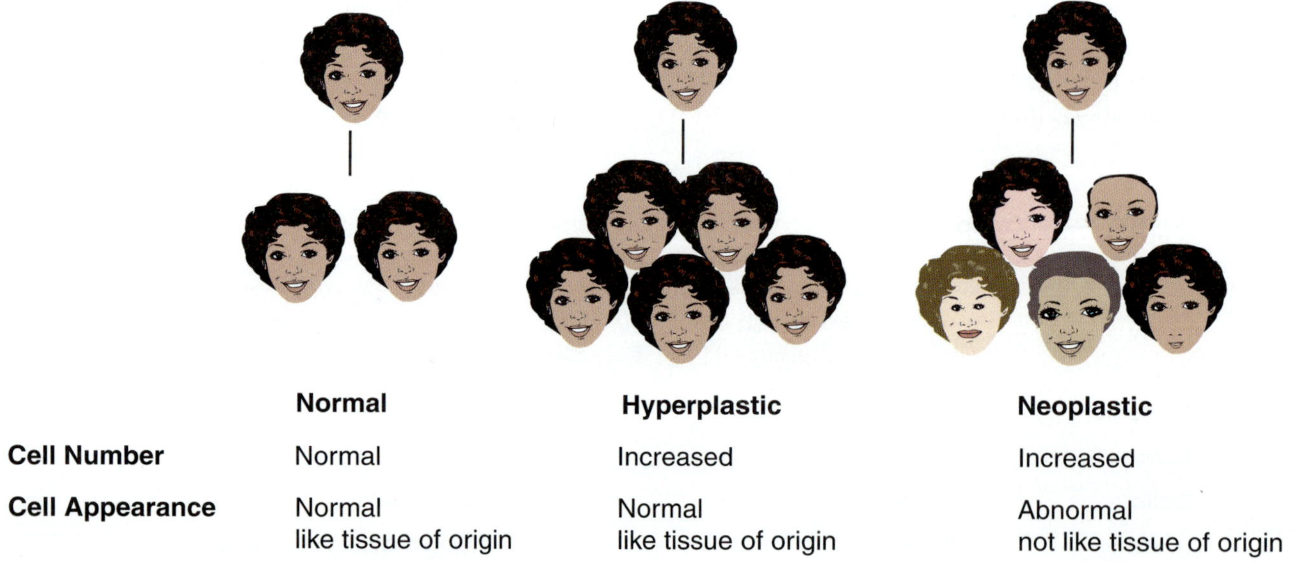

	Normal	Hyperplastic	Neoplastic
Cell Number	Normal	Increased	Increased
Cell Appearance	Normal like tissue of origin	Normal like tissue of origin	Abnormal not like tissue of origin

Figure 3–5 Comparison of hyperplasia and neoplasm.

As long as the abnormal cells are not firmly established they are considered preneoplastic or precancerous. If these cells are discovered at this point, surgical removal can be accomplished before cancer actually develops. Unfortunately, very few potential cancers are discovered at this stage. Squamous epithelial tissue often progresses through a slow series of changes including hyperplasia, abnormal hyperplasia called **dysplasia** (DIS-**PLAY**-zee-ah), and finally a stage called **carcinoma in situ**. In carcinoma in situ, the atypical cells are "just sitting" in the epithelial layer of the tissue and have not broken through the basement membrane and invaded the surrounding tissue. Carcinoma in situ commonly occurs in the uterine cervix, larynx, and mouth. Cancer can be avoided at this stage by surgical removal of the dysplasia or in situ tumor.

The final stage in cancer development is the invasion of the precancerous cells into the surrounding tissue. Local tissue invasion is the step that signifies a change from precancerous to malignant neoplasm. With epithelial tissue this is the point where neoplastic cells (carcinomas) break through the basement membrane that separates the epithelium from the connective tissue below (Figure 3–6). Once this break occurs the neoplastic cells can spread quickly, not only with local tissue invasion, but also via the lymphatic system (lymph fluid) and circulatory system (blood).

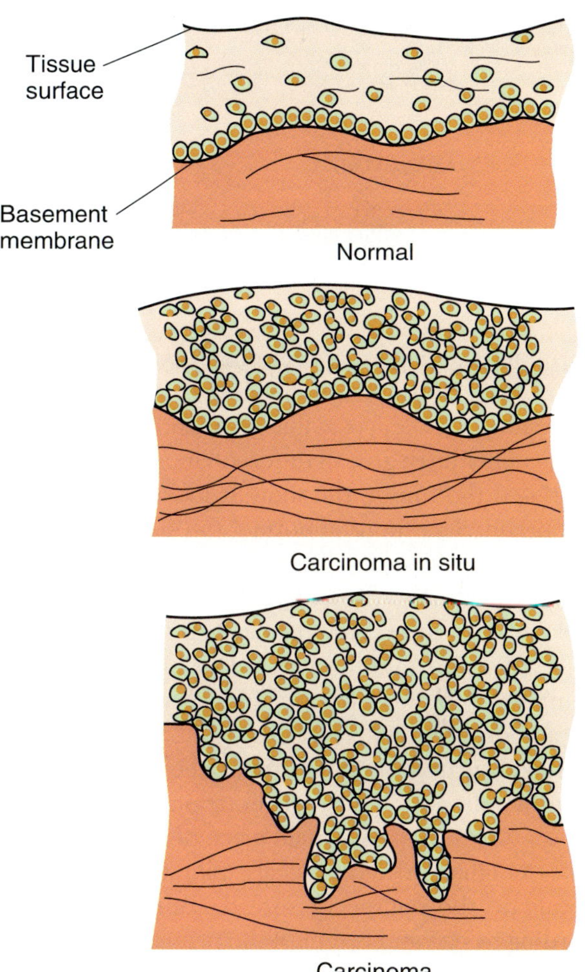

Figure 3–6 Carcinoma and carcinoma in situ.

INVASION AND METASTASIS OF CANCER

Local invasion of cancer is similar to the way plants sink their roots into the soil. The finger-like projections of the neoplasms force themselves along the lines of least resistance. Pressure from the growing tumor occludes blood supply, leading to local tissue necrosis, thus weakening the tissue, which eases further spread of the neoplasm. Spread of cancer from this primary location or site to other secondary sites in the body is called metastasis.

Carcinomas, epithelial tissue neoplasms, commonly spread through the lymphatics or lymphatic system. Lymph nodes can catch or filter cancer cells. For this reason lymph nodes are commonly removed surgically and examined for the presence of cancerous cells. Lymph nodes near the tumor are generally the first to filter cancerous cells. As more and more neoplastic cells spread into the lymphatic system the filters fill with neoplastic cells. Eventually the nodes become full and are unable to filter more cells. When this occurs the neoplastic cells may spill over into the bloodstream.

Absence of lymph node involvement with cancer is a favorable sign and may mean that surgical cure is possible. Usually, the higher the number of lymph nodes involved, the poorer the chance of survival.

Sarcomas do not utilize the lymphatic system as readily as carcinomas (Table 3–3). These tumors shed neoplastic cells directly into the blood. Once cancerous cells enter the bloodstream they may be widely distributed throughout the body. Common sites of bloodstream metastasis are the liver, lungs, and brain, all organs with a large blood flow. Frequently, it is the secondary cancer site that is discovered first.

Metastasis may also occur by invasion and implantation within a serous cavity. Once neoplastic cells reach a serous cavity, such as the pleural or peritoneal cavity, they may seed and implant freely within that cavity.

GRADING AND STAGING OF CANCER

Grading and **staging** of malignant tumors are utilized to plan treatment and predict possibility of a cure. Grading

TABLE 3–3 Comparison of Carcinomas and Sarcomas

Feature	Carcinoma	Sarcoma
Tissue	Epithelial	Connective
Occurrence	Very common	Less common
Growth	Slow	Rapid
Metastasis	Primarily through lymph	Primarily through blood

determines the degree of abnormality of the neoplasm while staging considers the degree of spread.

Grading is the microscopic examination of the tumor to determine the degree of differentiation. The more differentiated the tumor, the more it looks like the tissue of its origin. The more abnormal the tissue appears in comparison to its normal tissue the more undifferentiated or **anaplastic** (AN-ah-**PLAST**-ic) it is. The higher the degree of differentiation the better the prognosis. Tumors that are undifferentiated or anaplastic do not resemble the tissue of origin, are highly malignant, and have a poor prognosis.

Staging is utilized to determine the extent of spread of the neoplasm. Clinical examination, X-rays, **biopsy** (BYE-op-see; removing a small piece of tissue for microscopic examination) and surgical exploration may be used to evaluate the degree of spread. Tumors are staged according to size and extent of the primary tumor, number of lymph nodes involved, and metastasis to other sites. Of the two predictors, staging is the better indicator of the prognosis.

CAUSES OF CANCER

Unfortunately the actual cause of most cancer is unknown. Cancer appears to occur because of a variety of circumstances, which suggests that more than one factor is involved in its development. One thing remains constant in the development of cancer and that is the genetic alteration that allows the cell to grow independently and uncontrollably. It is thought that cellular mutations actually occur frequently in humans. It is further theorized that the human immune system catches and destroys these abnormal cells as soon as they occur. So, in some respects, cancer may represent some failure of the immune system in the involved individual.

Prevention and cure of cancer will depend on finding the initiating agents that cause the genetic alteration in the cell or the event that causes an altered cell to become malignant. Currently there are hundreds of carcinogenic compounds that have been identified. The process of **carcinogenesis** (KAR-sin-oh-**JEN**-eh-sis; cancer development) may take many years to develop, may stop and start, or may even be reversed, but usually there will be a continual progression of cellular changes from hyperplasia to dysplasia to **metaplasia** (MET-ah-**PLAY**-zee-ah) to neoplasia (Figure 3–7).

Chemical Carcinogens

Chemical carcinogenesis is quite complex. The frequency of exposure and the strength or potency of the chemical are important factors in the development of cancer. Chemicals that do not cause a problem by themselves

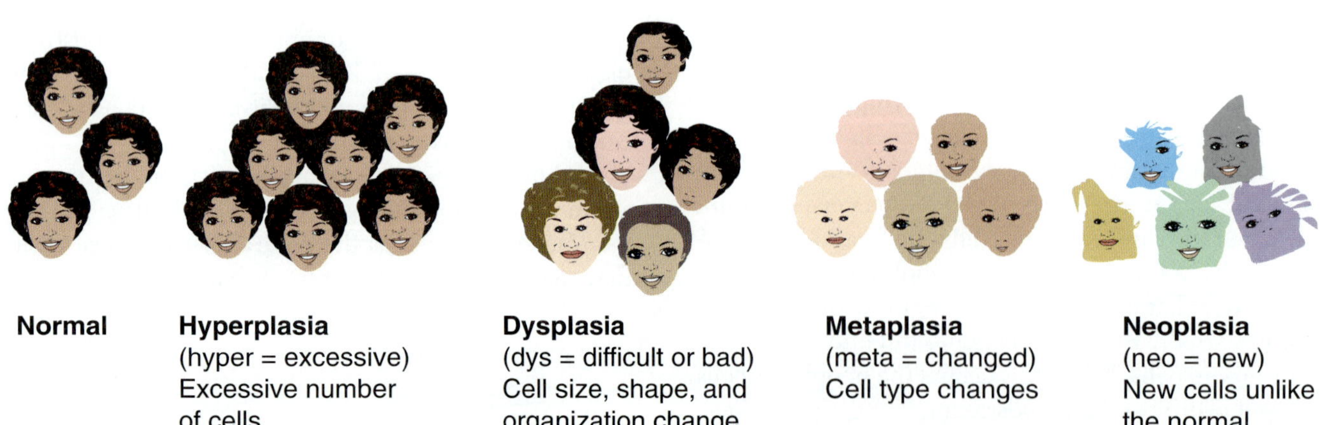

Figure 3–7 Cellular changes progressing to neoplasm.

may enhance cancer development when used in combination with other chemicals. Chemical carcinogens abound in our environment. Exposure to certain chemicals used in industry may lead to cancer in the workers. Naphthylamine, found in certain types of dye, has been found to cause bladder cancer. Asbestos, previously used in roofing and insulating materials, has been identified as a carcinogen leading to lung cancer. Miners of nickel ore have a high rate of nasal cancer. Farmers using arsenic as an insecticide often suffer with skin and lung cancers. Currently, chemicals used as food additives, cosmetics, and certain plastics are the focus of intensive research investigating the possible relationship with these chemicals and cancer.

Hormones

Hormones may increase the incidence of cancer, yet at times hormones may be used as a form of cancer treatment. The action of hormones as related to cancer is not clearly understood. For example, a benign mole never becomes malignant until sex hormones increase at puberty. Administration of diethylstil-bestrol, a synthetic estrogen compound, to pregnant women during the 1940s and 1950s led to an increase in a rare vaginal adenocarcinoma in their female children and to testicular abnormalities in their male children. Excessive production of estrogen in the female may lead to cancer of the breast and uterus. Estrogen medication used to treat menopausal symptoms in women has been shown to lead to an increase in endometrial cancer. The ovaries are sometimes removed after a female has breast cancer in an effort to decrease stimulation of other possible tumors. Although much research has been done to correlate cancer with birth control pills, the findings are inconclusive. The most widely used "combination" pill, combining estrogen and progesterone, may actually decrease the risk of cancer.

Cancer of the prostate is stimulated by the male hormone testosterone, but slowed or inhibited by estrogen treatment. Males who suffer with prostatic cancer may undergo treatment with estrogen medication to counteract the effects of testosterone. Treatment to decrease testosterone production may also include an orchiectomy, removal of the testes, in an effort to decrease or slow the growth of the prostatic tumor or decrease stimulation of other possible tumors.

Radiation

Ultraviolet (UV) radiation, x-radiation, and radioactive materials are all known carcinogens. About 1,000,000 cases of skin cancer are diagnosed each year (American Cancer Society, 1999). Sunbathers, farmers, fishermen, construction workers, mariners, and anyone else having an extended exposure to the UV rays of the sun or tanning lights have an increased risk of developing basal or squamous cell carcinomas. While basal and squamous cell carcinomas tend to occur because of cumulative exposure to the sun, melanoma occurs more frequently from extreme, blistering burns at a young age. Fair-skinned people are at greatest risk for skin cancer as they lack the protective effects of melanin. UV related skin cancer is uncommon among the black population.

X-rays have been used extensively as a diagnostic tool since discovery by Roentgen in 1895. Radiologists commonly developed cancers before the correlation of radiation and cancer. Roentgen himself developed skin cancer. In the late 1800s, radiation dosage was determined by taking repeated X-rays of the operator's hand. Soon after X-ray discovery the development of the first hand cancer was reported. Presently, radiation is considered a professional risk for radiologists and those working in the field of radiology, but with proper use of protective clothing and equipment the risk is minimal. High doses of radiation may be used as treatment for some cancers. This treatment does carry a risk of leading to the development of secondary tumors. These tumors usually develop after a lengthy period of time, twenty to twenty-five years, which makes the benefits of radiation therapy far outweigh the risk.

Radioactive materials that emit alpha, beta, and gamma rays are potential carcinogens. Most of these materials are used in medicine and research and are under strict regulation. With the use of protective clothing, the risk to workers in these areas is minimal. The most devastating and dramatic link between radiation and cancer was the increase shown in leukemia and thyroid cancers in the survivors of the atomic bomb dropped on Hiroshima and Nagasaki in 1945.

Viruses

Viruses have been proven to cause cancer in laboratory animals, but the proof is not as clear-cut in humans. Some examples that are worth noting include the Epstein-Barr virus, which causes infectious mononucleosis. The Epstein-Barr virus has been associated with Burkitt's lymphoma, a malignant neoplasm seen primarily in Africa. Hepatitis B virus has been closely connected to liver cancer. Individuals with cervical cancer tend to also have the herpes simplex virus.

Genetic Predisposition

There is some genetic predisposition for cancer as evidenced by the increased occurrence of certain types of cancers in the same family. This knowledge has led to intensive research. Discovery of certain cancer suppressor genes, and most recently a breast cancer gene, has aided research efforts, but complete understanding of the correlation of genetics and cancer has not yet been reached. It is known that colon and breast cancer have a higher incidence in certain families. A woman whose mother or sisters have or have had breast cancer runs a five-times greater chance of developing breast cancer than other women. Genetic testing is now available to test for the breast cancer gene.

Personal Risk Behaviors

There are several personal behaviors common in our society that put an individual at increased risk for developing cancer. These behaviors include smoking cigarettes and use of other tobacco products, some dietary practices, alcohol use, and certain sexual behaviors.

Smoking and Tobacco Products Use. Cigarette smoking is carcinogenic. Approximately 160,000–170,000 deaths occur yearly from tobacco use (American Cancer Society, 1999). It is the major cause of lung cancer. Cancer of the lung is fifteen times greater in smokers than non-smokers. Smoking also doubles the incidence of cancer of the bladder and pancreas. Chemicals in cigarette smoke affect all organs of the body because the chemicals are absorbed from the lungs into the blood and circulated to all organs. These chemicals are found in increased concentrations in the urine of smokers. Second-hand smoke has been proven to cause lung cancer in non-smokers.

The chemicals in smokeless tobacco are absorbed into the blood and again circulate to the entire body causing detrimental effects. Oral cancer occurs more frequently in smokeless tobacco users than in non-tobacco users.

Diet. Identifying the carcinogenic nature of dietary practices is difficult as many factors are involved. Diet seems to function over a period of time to place an individual at risk for cancer. There is a consistent relationship between increased weight in women and the risk of cancer, although there is not a relationship between the two for men. Obesity and a high consumption of dietary fat in women is a consistent risk factor for endometrial, breast, and colon cancer.

Much controversy exists concerning food additives, especially saccharin and nitrites. Saccharin has been shown to cause bladder cancer in rats, but this correlation has not been clear in humans. Nitrates are used as preservatives in meat and fish and have been shown to produce stomach cancer in animals. Countries with high nitrite consumption, Japan for example, have high rates of gastric cancer.

Colon cancer rates are lower in countries that have a lower consumption of dietary fat and a higher consumption of dietary fiber than the United States. The western plains area of the United States is high in selenium and has lower colon cancer rates, thus supporting the idea of some correlation between selenium levels and colon cancer.

Alcohol Use. Cancer of the mouth, throat, and esophagus occurs more often in people who smoke and consume large quantities of alcohol. Alcohol has not been proven as a carcinogen per se but recent studies have also shown a higher incidence of breast cancer in women who drink even moderate amounts (three drinks per week).

Sexual Behavior. The risk of developing cervical cancer is related to the age of first sexual intercourse and the number of sexual partners. The younger the female and the larger the number of sex partners the greater the risk. Females who have only one sexual partner are at risk if that partner has had multiple partners. True virgins do not experience cervical cancer (Coleman, 1992). The factor causing the increased risk may be the HPV (human papilloma virus) transmitted between the partners. The incidence of cervical cancer is two times greater in black women than in white and is found more commonly in women from lower socioeconomic groups. Women marrying men whose previous sexual partners had developed cervical cancer are at greater risk of also developing cervical cancer. Pregnancy and childbirth appear to be protective mechanisms for women from cancer of the ovary, endometrium, and breast. Females who start menstrual cycles at a later age, have early menopause, and/or bear the first child at an early age are at decreased risk for breast cancer.

CANCER PREVENTION

Cancers of the lung, breast, and colon are responsible for the majority of cancer deaths. Many of these cancers can be prevented by lifestyle changes. Smoking and tobacco use lead to approximately thirty percent of all cancers. Cigarette smoking is considered the single most preventable cause of not only lung cancer but of heart disease and other diseases of the lung, such as asthma or bronchitis.

Diet and nutrition play a significant role in the prevention of cancer. **Preventive** measures include reduction of fat intake and an increase in consumption of fruits, vegetables, and fiber.

Americans' passion for a suntan encourages people to lie in the sun and use tanning lights. The most widespread cancer, skin cancer, can be prevented by avoiding unnecessary exposure to the sun and tanning lights. If exposure to the sun is necessary, the use of a sun block agent with 15 or higher SPF is recommended.

The American Cancer Society recommends the following preventive measures:

- Do not smoke. The risk of developing lung cancer is fifteen times greater for smokers.
- Limit alcoholic intake. Heavy drinking increases the risk of cancer of the esophagus, mouth, throat, larynx, and liver.
- Protect skin from excessive sun exposure.
- Refuse needless X-rays. Special precautions must be taken to protect the unborn child if X-rays are necessary.
- Take hormone therapy to relieve menopausal symptoms only as long as necessary.
- Avoid heavily polluted air and long exposure to household solvent cleaners, paint thinners, and so forth.
- Follow label instructions carefully when using pesticides, fungicides and other home garden and lawn chemicals.
- Monitor caloric intake, and exercise properly. Eat fewer fatty foods and more high-fiber food such as bran, whole grains, and fibrous vegetables and fruits.
- Women should regularly perform breast examinations. Breast cancer has a peak incidence between forty-five and sixty-five years old, but can occur in women as young as the late teens.
- Men should regularly perform testicular examinations. Testicular cancer is most common in the twenty- to forty-year-old age group.
- Have regular checkups by physicians. For women over fifty, the doctor may recommend a mammogram as part of the routine examination. Also, the **Pap test** (a test to screen for cervical cancer) should be performed at regular intervals once the woman becomes sexually active. Men over forty should be regularly checked for prostate cancer. A rectal examination should be part of every medical checkup for men and women, and stool samples should be examined for blood, which may be an indication of colon cancer. Additionally, colonoscopies are recommended for men and women at age fifty and then every few years after to screen for polyps that can develop into colon cancer.

According to the American Cancer Society (1999) the relative survival rate for fifty percent of newly diagnosed cancer cases is about eighty percent, but this could increase to ninety-five percent if all individuals participated in regular screening programs.

FREQUENCY OF CANCER

Cancer is a focus of major concern for our society as it strikes over a million individuals per year. It is the second leading cause of death in the United States outranked only by heart disease. One in two men and one in three women will be diagnosed with cancer during their lifespan. Since 1990, eleven million cases of cancer have been diagnosed with five million deaths occurring. One out of four deaths (1,500 per day) is caused by cancer. It affects many lives causing extreme grief, suffering, and financial loss. However, almost seven and one-half million Americans who have or have had cancer are still alive. Today, four out of ten patients survive cancer five or more years (American Cancer Society, 1999).

The term cancer covers a large number of specific types of malignant neoplasms. Each of these types may vary considerably in behavior, treatment, and prognosis. The prognosis for these individual types will depend on the individual cancer's metastatic rate, the extent of spread when discovered and the effectiveness of current treatments. In general the overall survival rate of cancer is approximately fifty percent. Even though all malignant neoplasms may fit into a classification of carcinomas, sarcomas, leukemias, or lymphomas there is a great difference in the way they behave. Some types, such as pancreatic carcinoma, are usually deadly while skin carcinoma is seldom deadly.

Cancer affects people of all ages, young and old, both male and female. The most common types of cancer are basal and squamous cell skin cancers. These neoplasms are seldom fatal as they are very visible, slow growing, and can be completely excised. Because these tumors are generally treated in a physician's office, they are difficult to track statistically and are usually excluded in statistical data. Malignant melanoma, on the other hand, is a deadly form of skin cancer that only comprises approximately one percent of all skin malignancies, but is statistically recorded as skin cancer.

The most common types of cancer, excluding skin cancers, are cancers of the lung, colon, breast, uterus, and prostate. The common sites for cancer in the male and female are presented in Figure 3–8.

DIAGNOSIS OF CANCER

The prognosis for the individual with a malignant neoplasm is best if the cancer is located and treated early. Routine screening can be very effective in discovery and early diagnosis of cancer. Screening measures include monthly breast self-examinations, regular Pap tests, and mammograms for females. Screening for males includes routine testicular self-examinations. Occult stool examinations after age forty to screen for colon cancer and colonoscopies after age fifty are important for both sexes.

Discovery of tumors may occur through routine screening or accidentally during other diagnostic procedures. X-ray examinations of the chest prior to surgery may reveal a mass. Annual physical examinations may lead to the discovery. Recognition of cancer warning signals by an individual is important. The American Cancer Society lists several of these signs, with the initial letters forming the acronym **CAUTION**. They may be indicative of cancer development so the individual with one or more of these signs should be evaluated immediately by a physician.

- **C**hange in bowel or bladder habits
- **A** sore that does not heal
- **U**nusual bleeding or discharge
- **T**hickening or lump in breast or elsewhere
- **I**ndigestion or difficulty in swallowing
- **O**bvious change in a wart or mole
- **N**agging cough or hoarseness

Once discovered, the tumor must be diagnosed by microscopic examination of the cells and tissue. Examination of cells is called **cytology** (sigh-TOL-oh-jee; cyto = cell, ology = study) or a cytologic examination. Live tissue examination is a biopsy. A biopsy is the most definitive (clear-cut or without question) test used to diagnose a tumor.

To microscopically examine live tissue a biopsy must be done. A biopsy may be obtained by aspiration, needle biopsy, endoscopy, or surgery. Aspiration biopsy utilizes a needle attached to a suction device to remove a small piece of tissue from the tumor. Needle biopsy is obtained by punching a needle through the tumor and

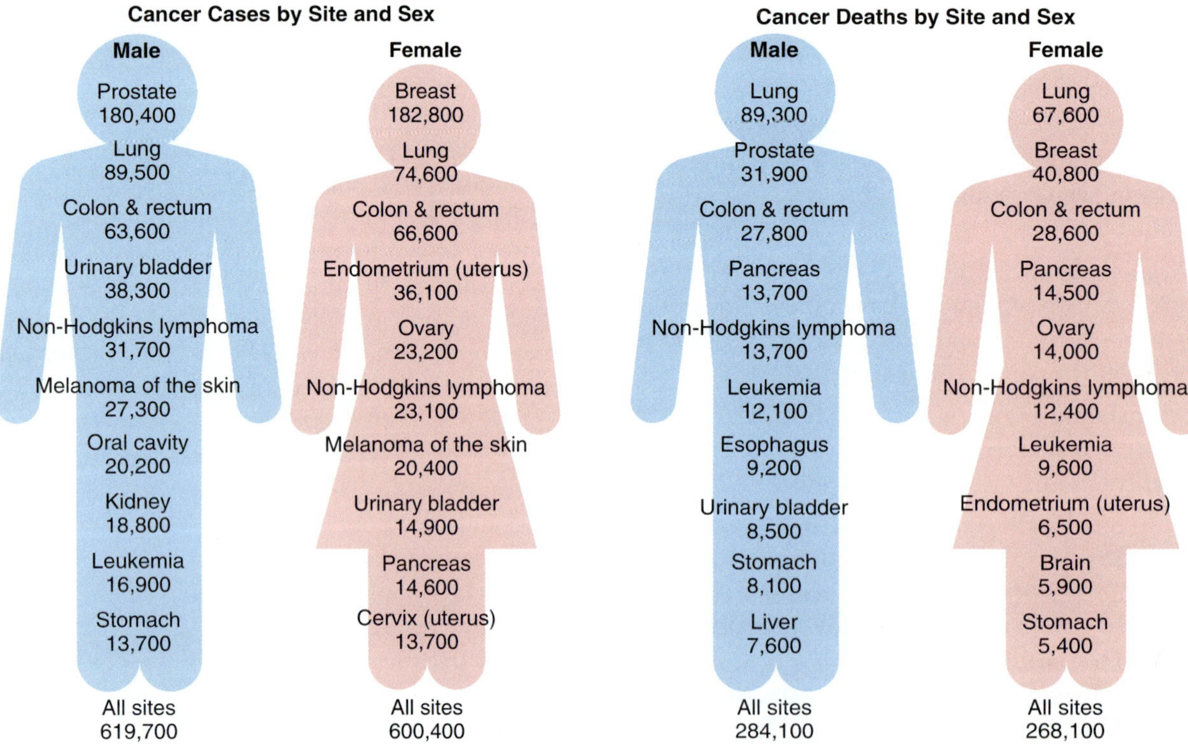

Figure 3–8 Leading sites of new cancer cases and deaths. (Cancer Facts and Figures—2000. Reprinted by the permission of the American Cancer Society, Inc.)

*Excludes basal and squamous cell skin cancers and in situ carcinomas, except urinary bladder.

using the tissue caught in the lumen of the needle for examination. If the size of the needle is quite small, the biopsy is called a fine needle biopsy. During endoscopy, the tissue is removed by use of the appropriate scope; for example bronchoscope, colonoscope, gastroscope. For surgical biopsy, the tissue is removed by cutting or incising the tissue (Figure 3–9).

Surgical biopsy may be performed with the patient's consent to surgically excise the tumor if it is found to be cancerous. Once the biopsy is obtained it is sent immediately to the pathologist for diagnosis. The patient often remains in the surgical suite under anesthesia while the surgeon awaits these results. Using a technique called a **frozen section** enables the pathologist to make a rapid determination of the tumor condition: benign or malignant.

SIGNS AND SYMPTOMS OF CANCER

Signs and symptoms of cancer are highly variable with the site and type of malignancy. Pain, obstruction, hemorrhage, anemia, fracture, infection, and cachexia may be manifestations of cancer. Any one of these symptoms may be present, or a combination may be present, but often cancer is asymptomatic until late in its developmental stage, including metastasis.

Pain from cancer is usually not an early sign. Cancer causes pain by growing to the point of causing destruction of normal tissue, obstruction of the lumen of hollow organs such as the intestine, placing pressure on nerve endings, and/or causing inflammation leading to discomfort.

Obstruction of a hollow organ may occur from a tumor growing inside the organ or from tumor growth outside the organ which compresses or pushes into the organ. Examples of obstruction could include the bronchus of the lung and any area of the intestine.

Hemorrhage may be caused by the cancerous tissue ulcerating and bleeding. This may lead to acute or chronic blood loss and often to anemia. Hidden blood in the feces may be detected by a Hemoccult stool test.

Anemia is very common in individuals with malignant neoplasm. The anemia may be the result of tumor hemorrhage as previously discussed. Anemia may also be caused by a decrease in red blood cell production as a result of cancer treatments.

Pathologic fractures may occur if a tumor has invaded the bone and caused weakness at that site. A fracture occurring with a minimal injury may be indicative of a cancer, but in the elderly it may also be caused by osteoporosis. The bone tumor may be primary or secondary with cancer of the lung, breast, and prostate readily metastasizing to the bone.

Infection is common and may lead to the final demise of the individual. Tumor ulceration may allow entry of microorganisms causing infection. The individual may have impaired immunity caused by **chemotherapy** (chemo = chemical, therapy = treatment) and radiation treatments, affecting the bone marrow and causing a decrease in production of white blood cells. Individuals with cancer often have a loss of appetite leading to a poor nutritional state increasing the chance of infection. Immune deficiency often leads to infection of

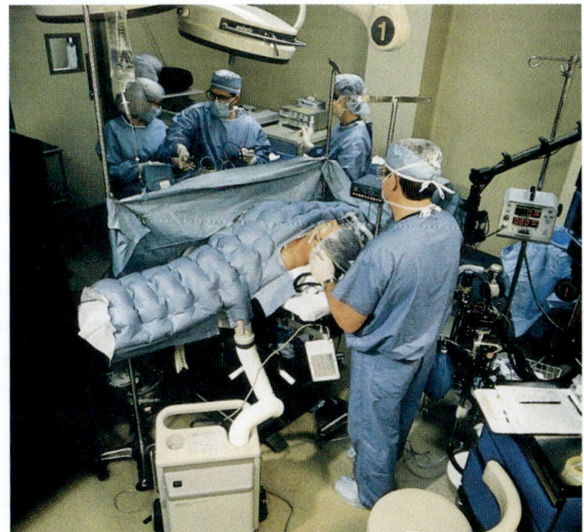

(A) A small piece of tissue is surgically removed. (Courtesy of Mallinckrodt Medical, Inc.)

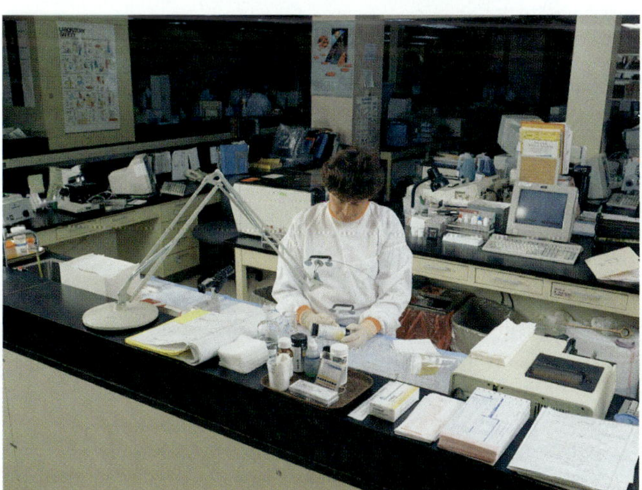

(B) A pathologist, looking for presence of disease, examines tissue in a laboratory .

Figure 3-9 Tissue biopsy.

the individual by a host of organisms such as fungi, viruses, protozoa and bacteria that are not usually pathogenic.

Cachexia is a condition of general ill health and malnutrition often seen in the terminally ill patient (refer to Chapter 2, Figure 2–3). This condition is evidence of the demands placed on the body by the rapidly growing tumor and treatment modalities, coupled with poor nutritional intake.

CANCER TREATMENT

New technological advances lead to ever changing treatment of malignant neoplasms. Treatment may be aimed at cure (**curative**) or at relief of symptoms (**palliative**; **PAL**-ee-AY-tiv) or at prevention (preventive). The three major types of treatment include surgery, chemotherapy, and radiation. Hormone treatment may be the treatment of choice in some instances. Immunotherapy and immunomodulation combat cancer cells by boosting specific immune cells or chemicals and are relatively new treatment modalities. The oncologist may recommend one of these treatments or a combination of them depending on the type of cancer and treatment plan.

Surgery for cancer may be curative, palliative, or preventive. Curative surgery is aimed at complete removal of the tumor. Cancer of the lung, stomach, skin, breast, intestine, and female reproductive organs respond well to this type of surgery. Palliative surgery is usually indicated when cure is not possible, but when surgery will alleviate pain and discomfort. The intestine is an area commonly undergoing this type of surgery for obstruction, bleeding, or perforation. Surgery may also be performed to sever nerves in an effort to reduce pain. Preventive surgery may be performed to prevent development of cancer. Polyps in the colon may be removed as they are thought to be precancerous. A woman may undergo prophylactic mastectomy if she has been identified as one at high risk for breast cancer.

Chemotherapy may be the treatment of choice or used in combination with surgery and radiation therapy. Generally chemotherapy is effective to treat rapidly growing metastatic neoplasms. Chemotherapy is aimed at rapidly growing neoplastic cells with the idea that it will kill or inhibit the growth of these cells while having minimal effect on normal cells. In some instances the growth rate of normal cells and neoplastic cells is not varied enough and normal body cells suffer from the effects of the treatment. Rapid growing normal cells such as those found in the epithelium, hair, and bone marrow suffer the most, leading to nausea, vomiting, loss of appetite, hair loss, anemia, and impaired immunity.

Radiation is generally used to treat tumors that are not surgically accessible nor operable and in treatment of residual neoplasm postoperatively. Palliative radiation treatments may shrink the tumor and thus relieve discomfort. Radiation treatment may be external with direct radiation or internal using radioisotope beads, seeds, or ribbons that are implanted inside the body. Both methods are aimed at disrupting DNA and interfering with cell growth and replication. The goal is to destroy as much of the tumor as possible without affecting the normal tissue surrounding it. Adverse effects generally occur in the skin, mucous membranes, and bone marrow, leading to nausea, vomiting, loss of appetite, hair loss, and impaired immunity.

Hormone therapy may cause regression in tumors of the breast and prostate. Administration of antagonistic hormones or excision of hormone producing organs such as the ovaries and testes may be effective in prolonging life. Hormone therapy is generally used as a palliative treatment for metastatic tumors.

Immunotherapy and immunomodulation involve altering the way the cells and chemicals of our immune system react towards cancerous cells. As mentioned earlier in this chapter, the immune system has the ability to detect and remove many of the genetic cell variations that occur before they turn into cancer. Altering the amount of these chemicals and cells can help the body's immune system more aggressively attack cancer. Malignant melanoma and renal cell carcinoma are two types of cancer that respond well to this form of treatment. Research into the development of vaccines against certain types of cancer, for example melanoma, is also underway. These vaccines theoretically enhance the immune system's ability to identify which cells are cancerous, much in the same way the chicken pox vaccine allows the body to identify the virus that causes chicken pox. Identifying the cancer cells may allow the body to attack and destroy these cells before they grow into a tumor.

SUMMARY

Neoplasms are new growths that can arise from cells almost anywhere in the body. They can be benign or malignant. Tumor is the term commonly used to describe a neoplasm but not all neoplasms form tumors. Hyperplasias are similar to neoplasms because they are an overgrowth of cells, but they are like their cell of origin and neoplasms are not. Neoplasms that are malignant are usually called cancers. They are usually named for the type of tissue from which they developed. Metastatic cancers are those that spread to other parts of the body.

The cause of most cancer is unknown but research has identified some carcinogens in the environment as well as high risk behaviors that may contribute to cancer development. The American Cancer Society has recommended preventive measures and lists seven warning signs of cancer. Although cancer is the second leading cause of death in our society, with early diagnosis and treatment there is a good prognosis for most types of cancer.

REVIEW QUESTIONS

Short Answer

1. What is the difference between a neoplasm and a tumor?

2. How are neoplasms classified?

3. What is the largest group of malignant neoplasms?

4. When a malignant neoplasm moves to various parts or organs of the body, it is said to be a ____________________ tumor.

5. What is the difference between hyperplasia and neoplasms?

True or False

6. T F Grading is the microscopic examination of the tumor to determine the degree of differentiation.
7. T F Tumors that are undifferentiated or anaplastic do not resemble the tissue of origin, are highly malignant, and have a poor prognosis.
8. T F Radioactive materials that emit alpha, beta, and gamma rays are not considered to be potential carcinogens.
9. T F There is no known genetic predisposition for cancer.
10. T F There are several personal risk behaviors common in our society that put an individual at increased risk for developing cancer.

Matching

11. Match the term in the left column with the phrase that best describes it from the column on the right.

_____ Metastatic neoplasm
_____ Cancer of the lung, breast, and colon
_____ CAUTION
_____ Basal and squamous cell skin cancer
_____ Biopsy
_____ Liver, lungs, and brain
_____ Ultraviolet (UV) radiation, x-radiation, and radioactive materials
_____ Routine screening
_____ Surgery, chemotherapy, and radiation
_____ Palliative

a. known carcinogens
b an acronym for the seven warning signs of cancer
c. microscopic examination of live tissue
d responsible for the majority of cancer deaths
e. cells whose growth pattern has no purpose and is uncontrollable
f. common sites of bloodstream metastasis
g. the most common type of cancer
h. major types of cancer treatment
i treatment aimed at relieving symptoms
j. very effective in discovery and early diagnosis of cancer

CASE STUDY

Mr. Holloway is a 65-year-old man who has made an appointment for a routine checkup. He has not complained of any unusual symptoms but feels he should have a yearly exam because of his age. What are some routine screening tests that should be done on Mr. Holloway because of his age and gender? What important cancer prevention strategies should you discuss with Mr. Holloway during his visit?

BIBLIOGRAPHY

Altman, L. K. (May 6, 1997). Surviving with AIDS is one problem; cancer is yet another. *New York Times*, C3.

American Cancer Society. (1999). Website: *http://www.cancer.org/frames.html*.

Coleman, R. L. (1992). Cervical cancer: Causes and prevention. *Online Journal*, 4(3). Website: *http://www.acsh.org/publications/priorities/0403/cancer.html*.

Fritz, A. G. (1996). Has there been a real drop in the number of expected cancer cases in the United States? *Topics in Health Information Management*, 17(3), 15–28.

Lecallois, P. (1995). Assessing exposure to carcinogens in drinking water. *American Journal of Public Health*, *85(9)*, 1298–1300.

Nabel, G. J., Chang, A.E., Felgner, P., Shu, S., & Cho, K. (1994). Immunotherapy for cancer by direct gene transfer into tumors. *Human Gene Therapy*, 5(1), 57–77.

Perera, F. P. (1996). Uncovering new clues to cancer risk. *Scientific American*, 274(5), 54-55.

Rabkin, C. S. & Yellin, F. (1994). Cancer incidence in a population with a high prevalence of infection with HIV type 1. *Journal of the National Cancer Institutes*, 86(22), 1711–1716.

Sorensen, G. (1996). Work site-based cancer prevention: Primary results from the working well trial. *American Journal of Public Health*, 86(7), 939–947.

Steen, R. G. (1997). Winning the war on cancer. *The Futurist*, 31(2), 24–28.

Trichopoulos, D. (1996). What causes cancer? *Scientific American*, 275(9), 80–87.

Willett, W. (1996). Strategies for minimizing cancer risk. *Scientific American*, 275(9), 88–91.

CHAPTER 4

Inflammation and Infection

CONTENT OUTLINE

- Defense Mechanisms
- Inflammation
- The Inflammatory Process
- Chronic Inflammation
- Inflammatory Exudates
- Inflammatory Lesions
    - Abscesses
    - Ulcer
    - Cellulitis
- Tissue Repair and Healing
    - Tissue Repair
    - Tissue Healing
    - Delayed Wound Healing
    - Complications of Wound Healing
- Infection
    - Frequency and Types of Infection
    - Testing for Infection

KEY TERMS

Abscess
Adhesion
Antibody
Antigen
Bacteria
Cellulitis
Chemotaxis
Culture and sensitivity
Débridement
Dehiscence
Diapedesis
Empyema
Exudate
Fistula
Fungi
Helminth
Histamine
Hyperemia
Induration
Infection
Inflammation
Keloid
Lesion
Leukocytosis
Macrophage
Malaise
Mast cells
Opportunistic infection
Primary union
Protozoa
Purulent
Pus
Pyogenic
Rickettsiae
Scar
Secondary union
Septicemia
Sinus
Tachycardia
Trauma
Ulcer
Virulent
Virus(es)

LEARNING OBJECTIVES

Upon completion of the chapter, the student should be able to:

1. Identify important terminology related to the defense mechanisms.
2. Describe the basic defense mechanisms in the body.
3. Explain the steps in the inflammatory process.
4. Describe the process of tissue repair and healing.
5. Identify complications of wound healing.
6. Describe the process of infection development.
7. Identify the common infectious microorganisms and the resulting diseases.
8. Identify the common laboratory test conducted to identify pathogenic organisms.

OVERVIEW

The human body is in a constant state of activity. The overall goal in the body's responses to foreign invaders or pathogens is to prevent trauma and maintain homeostasis. The defense mechanisms are responsible for this protection. Inflammation is a natural protective mechanism. When the protective mechanisms fail, the usual result is an infection. Infections are diagnosed and treated in a variety of ways.

DEFENSE MECHANISMS

The immune system has the difficult job of protecting the body against foreign invasion. Defense may be non-specific, protecting the body against any and all invaders, or it may be specific, identifying the invader prior to its demise. This system utilizes three basic lines of defense to accomplish this goal.

1. Physical or surface barriers (non-specific)—An intact skin is the body's first line of defense. The skin is not only a physical barrier, but the acidic surface is also anti-microbial. The normal bacterial flora of the skin acts as a placeholder preventing habitation by other **bacteria** (microscopic, one-celled organisms). Sebaceous (oil secreting) and odoriferous (perspiration secreting) glands secrete antibacterial acids and enzymes. Mucous membranes serve to trap invaders.
2. Inflammation (non-specific)—If physical barriers are broken and the foreign invader penetrates the cells and tissues, the inflammatory response occurs. This response begins within seconds of an unwanted invasion. It is a stereotypic vascular response. In other words, the process unfolds or follows the same pattern no matter the type of invader. The primary goals of the inflammatory response are to isolate or wall off the invader, destroy it, and clean up the debris, thereby promoting healing.
3. Immune response (specific)—The third and last line of defense reacts to invasion more slowly than inflammation, but with specific killing ability. All cells, even human body cells, have protein or saccharide markers on their surfaces that identify the cell. This marker is called an **antigen** (AN-tih-jen). During the immune response the body actually identifies the invader by the antigen. Once the antigen is identified, antibodies are produced by lymphocytes. Antibodies link with the cell antigen thus killing the cell or rendering it helpless. This immunologic defense has the unique ability to remember the invader and produce more antibodies if the invader returns (Figure 4–1).

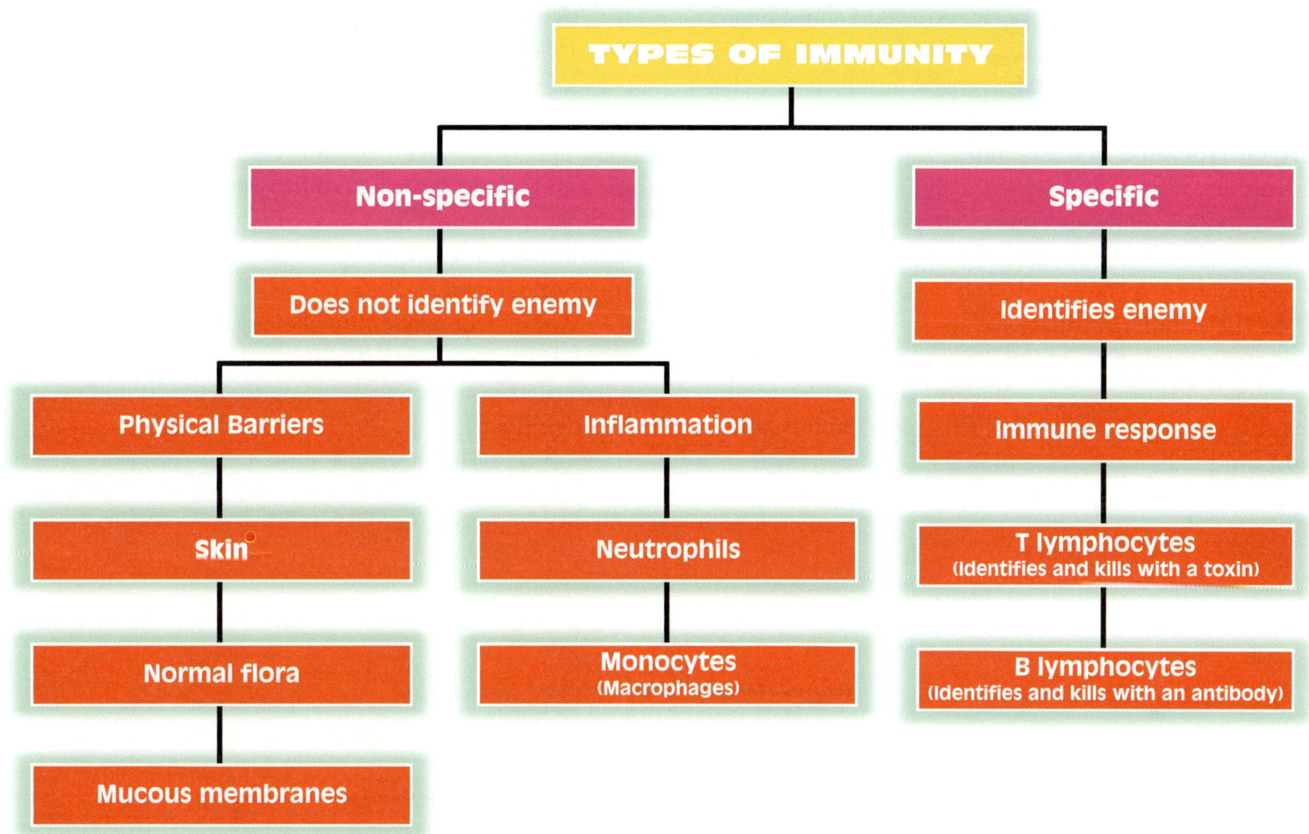

Figure 4–1 Immunity—lines of defense.

INFLAMMATION

Inflammation is a non-specific cellular and vascular reaction to any tissue **trauma** (TRAW-mah; injury). The primary goals of the inflammatory response are to isolate or wall off the invader, destroy it, and clean up the debris, thereby promoting healing. One limiting factor of inflammation is that it cannot occur in tissue that does not have a blood supply.

If tissue is destroyed by injury, the inflammatory process will only occur along borders of the injury where blood supply is maintained. Gangrene is an example of this process. In gangrenous tissue, inflammation cannot occur in the dead or necrotic tissue, but there is an observable reaction along the borders of the necrotic tissue.

The fact that inflammation will only occur in vascularized (supplied with blood) tissue is important in forensic medicine. Evidence of inflammation in tissue confirms that an injury occurred while the individual was alive. If no evidence of inflammation exists the pathologist can be assured that the person was dead when the injury was inflicted.

Inflammation is designed to be a beneficial, protective defense mechanism. In some instances the reaction may become so intense that it becomes harmful to tissues. An acute hypersensitivity reaction may lead not only to local tissue damage but also to anaphylactic shock and death of the individual. If the process goes awry, producing an autoimmune reaction, the body begins to destroy itself. Anti-inflammatory medications may be needed to stop the reaction if it becomes injurious.

THE INFLAMMATORY PROCESS

When any tissue undergoes trauma (injury), regardless of the cause, inflammation will occur. The trauma may be caused by physical injury, invasion of microorganisms, ischemia (decreased oxygen in cells), freezing, burning, electrocution, radiation, or chemical irritation, to name a few.

Mast cells, also called tissue histocytes, are found in all tissues of the body, and play a major role in the inflammatory process. When injured or irritated these cells release **histamine**. Histamine causes local arterioles, venules, and capillaries to dilate, resulting in an increase in blood flow to the area. This increase in blood flow, called **hyperemia** (HIGH-per-**EE**-me-ah; hyper = increased, emia = blood), causes the increased redness and heat in this area.

Hyperemia also brings increased numbers of leukocytes (white blood cells) to the area. The white cells that move into this area first and in the greatest numbers are neutrophils, also called polymorphonuclear leukocytes (PMNs)(poly = many, morphic = shaped nucleus). These white cells line the endothelium of the vessels awaiting the opportunity to move into the tissue.

As the capillaries dilate under the influence of histamine, vascular permeability increases. In other words, the capillary becomes permeable or leaky as the endothelial cells are stretched apart. This permeability allows blood fluid called **exudate** (ECKS-you-dayt) to leak into the tissue. This leakage of fluid is the cause of the swelling or edema observed with inflammation.

As edema increases, more pressure is exerted on nerve endings leading to increased pain. With increased pain and tenderness, the individual tends to guard this area and experiences loss of function. These vascular and cellular responses produce the five cardinal signs of inflammation: heat, redness, swelling, pain, and loss of function (Figure 4–2).

Vascular permeability also allows the awaiting neutrophils to escape into the tissue. The neutrophil extends a part of its body between the epithelial cells and squeezes through the capillary wall by a process called **diapedesis** (DYE-ah-pe-**DEE**-sis) (see Figure 4–2). The process of dia-

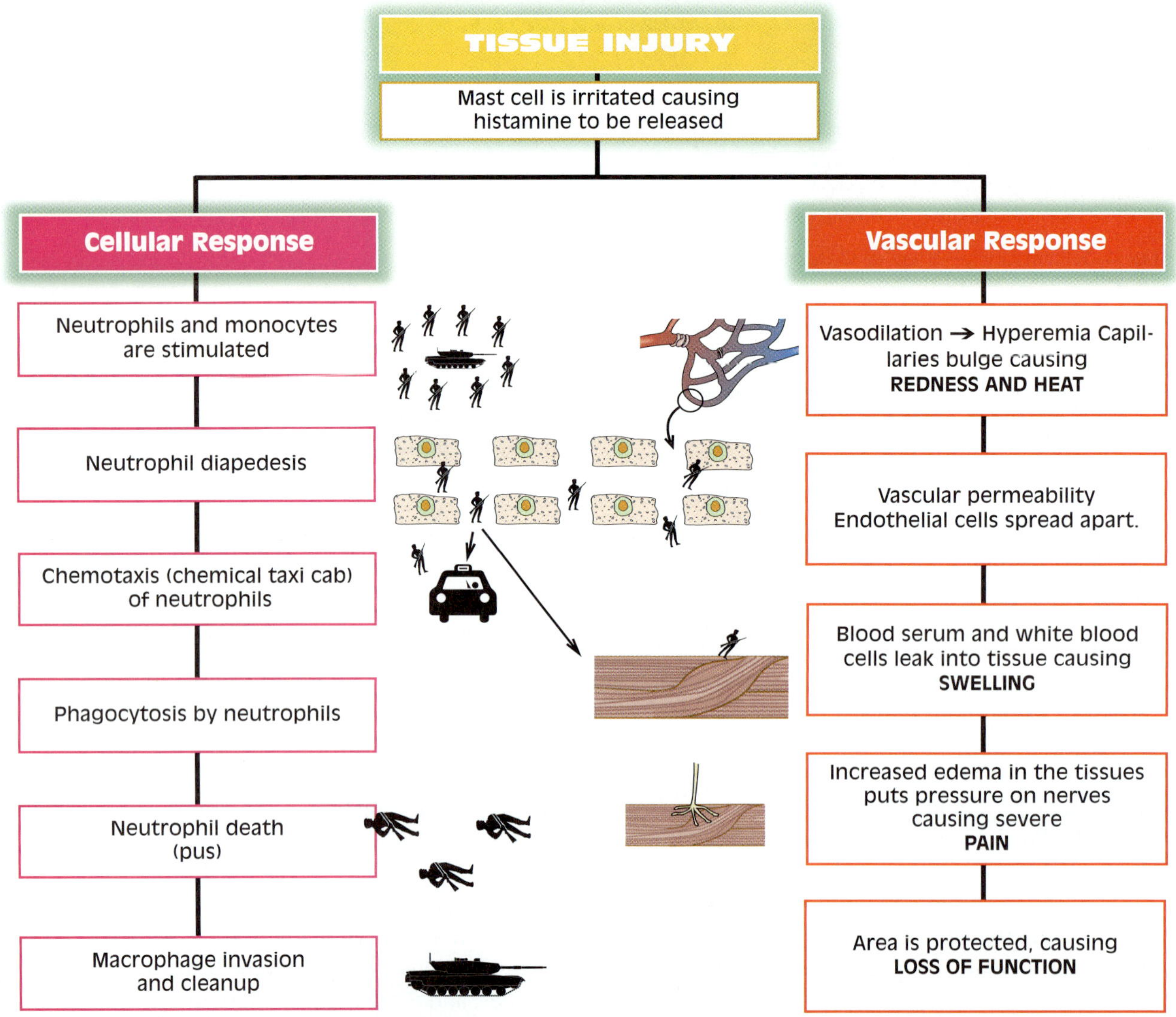

Figure 4–2 Acute inflammation—cellular and vascular response.

pedesis is very effective, delivering millions of neutrophils to the area within a few hours.

Neutrophils can be considered the "foot soldiers" of the inflammatory process. They arrive first, they arrive in great numbers, and they readily move into action in the tissue. Neutrophils are drawn or directed to the injured area by a process called **chemotaxis**. One might think of this process as a "chemical taxi cab." Chemicals are released by a variety of things including bacteria, injured tissue, sensory nerve fibers, and plasma proteins. Such chemicals are detected through chemoreceptors on the neutrophil's outer membrane which draw the neutrophil in the direction of the highest chemical concentration (see Figure 4–2).

Once the neutrophil arrives at the scene of the trauma it begins the job of phagocytosis or cell eating. The neutrophil eats and destroys microorganisms, foreign materials, and dead cells. The life of the neutrophil is short-lived, and like the foot soldier, it dies on the battlefield. Death of numerous neutrophils mixed with exudate or blood fluid make up, in part, the white fluid identified as **pus**.

Approximately three to four days after the inflammatory process begins, large numbers of another type of white cell begin to arrive at the scene. This large, slow-moving cell is the monocyte. As the monocyte leaves the bloodstream and moves into the tissue it becomes phagocytic and is called a **macrophage** (macro = large, phage = eat). As the name suggests, a macrophage is a large eater of microorganisms, foreign material, and dead cells. This cell might be considered the "tank" of the war as it is slower moving but more effective in killing power than the neutrophil. Another job of the macrophage is to act as the clean-up crew, cleaning up the dead neutrophils and tissue debris in the inflamed area.

Until this point the **inflammation** is considered to be an acute (short-lived) situation. If the inflammation persists for a longer period of time, it is considered to be a chronic problem. This time period is difficult to establish because some chronic inflammations will exhibit periods of exacerbation (flare-up), eliciting a new outpouring of neutrophils. Similarly, some acute inflammations will trigger the response of an unusually high number of macrophages.

After approximately seven to ten days, if the inflammatory process has not overcome the invader, the nuclear warheads of the defense system, the lymphocytes, are called to respond. Lymphocytes are slow but powerful killers. They are part of the body's third line of defense—the immune response. They are specific killers. They identify the enemy, make an **antibody** to kill it, then remember the enemy and the killing process (see Figure 4–1). Refer to Chapter 12 for more detailed information on the immune system.

CHRONIC INFLAMMATION

Generally speaking a chronic inflammation may be considered as one that lasts two weeks or longer. If the acute attack by neutrophils and macrophages is unsuccessful the battle may become chronic. Microscopic examination of chronic inflammation will reveal a large number of macrophages and fewer neutrophils.

If macrophages are unable to overcome the invader and protect the host, the body may try to wall off and isolate the area by forming a granuloma. A granuloma is formed by macrophages and fibrous deposits of collagen, and may be hardened by calcium deposits. This granuloma protects the surrounding tissue and allows healing to begin. A classic cause of granuloma formation is tuberculosis. Granulomas may become quite large, form a fibrous rim, and eventually calcify. Another cause of granuloma is foreign body involvement. If foreign materials, such as a wood splinter, gravel, suture, glass sliver, or metal fragments, are embedded in the tissue, the body walls off the material to protect the adjacent tissue. This granuloma may become hardened with fibrous tissue and remain for the life of the individual.

INFLAMMATORY EXUDATES

The duration and extent of an inflammatory **lesion** (LEE-zhun; any discontinuity of tissue) may be determined by direct visualization of the site. External inflammatory lesions are easily observed while internal inflammatory lesions in organs and cavities may require radiographic, surgical, or endoscopic examination. The appearance and amount of exudate or blood fluid may assist in identifying an acute or chronic condition.

Serous exudate is a clear serum-like fluid containing small amounts of protein. It implies a lesser degree of damage and occurs in the acute stage of inflammation. Examples of serous exudate include the fluid in skin blisters, cold sores, and injured joints to name a few. Serous exudate is easily reabsorbed once the inflammatory response is halted and healing begins.

Fibrinous exudate is composed of fluid and large amounts of fibrinogen. In comparison to serous exudate, the leakage of fibrinogen indicates a larger injury with more severe inflammation. Fibrinous exudate may be observed in strep throat or bacterial pneumonia forming a mesh-like lesion. A superficial skin wound may be covered with dried fibrinous exudate commonly called a scab.

Purulent (PURR-you-lent) exudate is loaded with dead and dying PMNs or neutrophils, tissue debris, and **pyogenic** (PYE-oh-JEN-ick; pyo = pus, genic = arising) or pus-forming bacteria. Purulent exudate is commonly called pus. A localized collection of pus is called an **abscess**. An accumulation of pus in a body cavity is called **empyema** (EM-pye-**EE**-mah). For example, pus accumulated in the chest or thoracic cavity would be called thoracic empyema.

INFLAMMATORY LESIONS

Any discontinuity or abnormality of tissue is called a lesion. Lesion is a broad term that includes wounds, ulcers, wheals, blisters, vesicles, pustules, or tumors to name a few. Lesions are caused by physical or pathologic injury. Inflammatory lesions include abscesses, ulcers, and **cellulitis** (SELL-you-**LYE**-tis; inflammation of connective tissue).

Abscesses

Abscesses are typically caused by streptococcal and staphylococcal (pyogenic) bacteria. During the inflammatory response, the body attempts to contain or stop the spread of the bacteria into adjacent tissue by forming a wall around the area. When this wall forms around a purulent exudate, an abscess is formed. Boils, furuncles, and pimples are examples of abscesses.

Typically, a small abscess shows signs of acute inflammation: redness, heat, swelling, and pain. When the central portion of the abscess softens or develops a "head," puncturing the head will cause an outpouring of pus, relief of pain, and onset of healing. Puncturing the abscess before the area is walled off and the head is soft may lead to a spread of the infecting organism.

A small abscess may also rupture and heal spontaneously, but a large abscess may need to be surgically incised and drained. Draining an abscess speeds healing. Without drainage the body must continue to battle the invading organisms. If the body is successful, it will eventually win the battle, reabsorb the exudate, and replace the area with fibrous tissue. A large abscess, if not contained, may spread and become fatal. An example of this process is the abscess formation occurring in appendicitis. If a large abscess ruptures it tends to form a tract or opening to the surface of the body called a **sinus**. If this tract connects two organs or cavities to each other or to the surface of the skin it is called a **fistula** (FIS-tyou-lah) (Figure 4–3).

Ulcer

An **ulcer** is a crater-like lesion in the skin or mucous membranes. It is the result of an injury and the subsequent inflammatory response. The tissue in this area becomes necrotic (dead) and sloughs off leaving a crater or excavated area. Ulcers are commonly seen in the stomach and duodenum as a result of injury by bacteria and stomach acid. Pressure ulcers, commonly called bedsores or decubitus ulcers, are caused by excessive pressure on tissue. Pressure ulcers primarily appear over bony prominences of the body, especially those affected in the lying position, such as the heel, sacrum, elbow, and scapula (Figure 4–4).

Cellulitis

Cellulitis is a diffuse or widespread acute inflammatory process. It is usually seen in the skin and subcutaneous tissues. Cellulitis is characterized by general edema, redness, and localized pain and heat. Cellulitis of the face

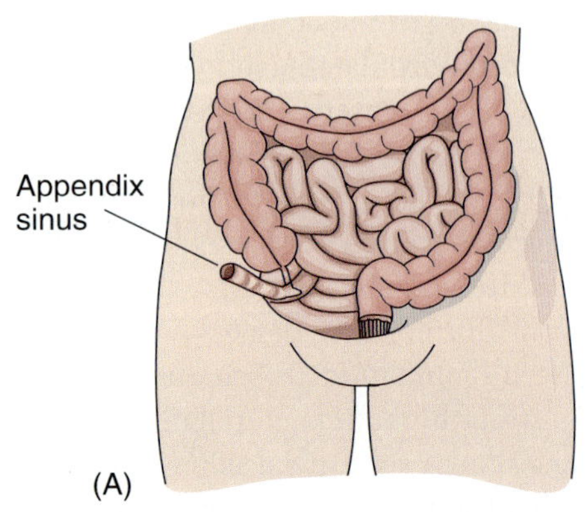

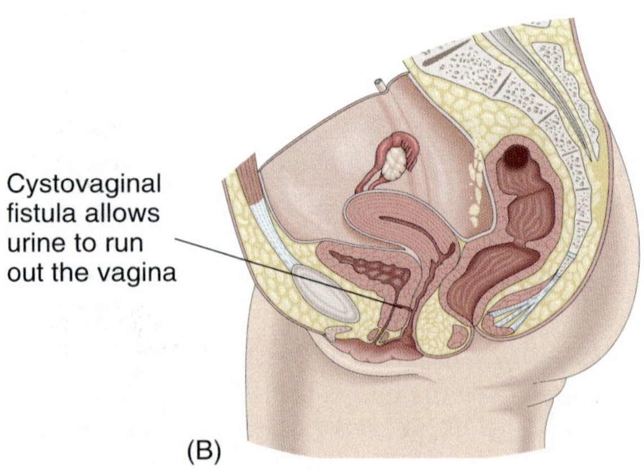

Figure 4–3 (A) Sinus, (B) Fistula.

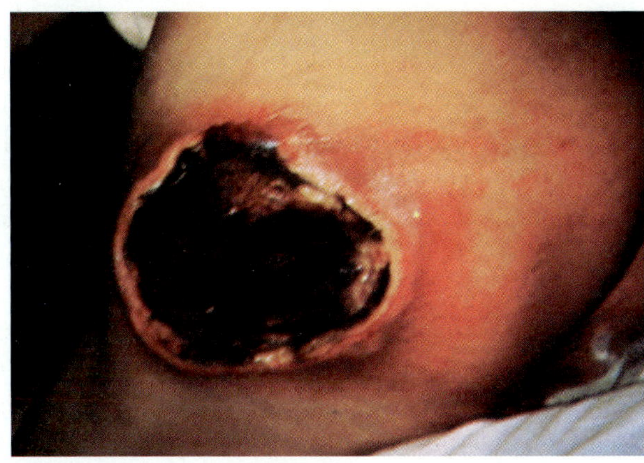

Figure 4–4 Pressure ulcer.

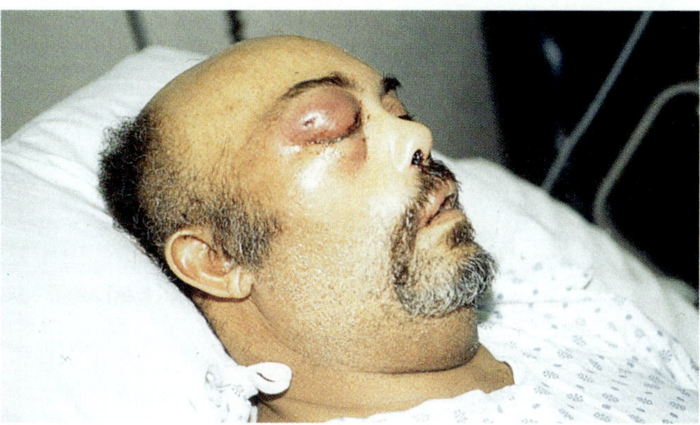

Figure 4–5 Cellulitis. (Courtesy of Dr. Mark Dougherty, Lexington, KY.)

primarily involves the cheeks and periorbital (peri = around, orbital = eye) areas. This type of cellulitis must receive special attention as it may spread to the brain. Cellulitis is often caused by streptococcus or staphylococcus bacteria and the body's inability to confine or wall off the causative organism. Cellulitis is potentially dangerous but usually can be treated effectively with antibiotics (Figure 4–5).

TISSUE REPAIR AND HEALING

Tissue repair and healing is an ongoing process much like any other body process. Proper repair and healing occurs in most instances but this process can be influenced by many other factors. Healing may be impaired or slowed when secondary diseases are present, the body is malnourished, or the immune system is compromised.

Tissue Repair

During the final phase of the inflammatory process, macrophages are responsible for cleaning up the area and producing growth factors that aid in the repair process. Repair of tissue also depends on cellular regeneration and the type of cells that make up the tissue. Some cells divide quite readily while others do not. Cellular proliferation or division can be grouped into three general categories.

1. Mitotic Cells—continuously divide throughout life. These cells are found in the skin and mucosa of internal organs. They readily replace damaged tissue.
2. Facultative Mitotic Cells—do not divide regularly, but can be stimulated to divide when necessary. These cells are found in such organs as the liver and kidney. Some part of these organs must remain intact for these cells to be available to divide and replace the lost tissue.
3. Non-dividing cells—are those that do not divide under any condition. Cells of this type include nerves, brain cells, and heart muscle cells. Repair of these tissues is by fibrous scarring.

The body's two basic methods of repair involve healing by regeneration, and fibrous connective tissue repair or **scar** formation. Regeneration is the better type of repair as it usually leads to restoration of normal function while fibrous connective tissue repair does not.

Regeneration. Regeneration involves mitotic cell division. During regeneration the damaged tissue is replaced by cellular division of healthy tissue (Figure 4–6A). For example, skin tissue is replaced by epithelial cell division, and bone tissue is replaced by osteocyte division. Regeneration can usually occur in internal organs if the major framework of the organ has not been destroyed. Complex structures such as lung tissue and glomeruli (in the kidney) do not regenerate. Regeneration is particularly important when there is damage to a large amount of tissue. Epithelial regeneration is very beneficial with massive burns. Bone cells have a remarkable ability to regenerate from a few remaining cells or may be transplanted from another individual by bone marrow transplant.

Fibrous Connective Tissue Repair (Scar Formation). Fibrous connective tissue repair or scar formation may occur in any tissue with the same result no matter the location, namely, a tough fibrous tissue called a scar. A scar provides a bridge between the normal tissue and the wound, but does not restore function. Wound repair of nerves, brain tissue, and heart muscle is by fibrous connective tissue repair (Figure 4–6B).

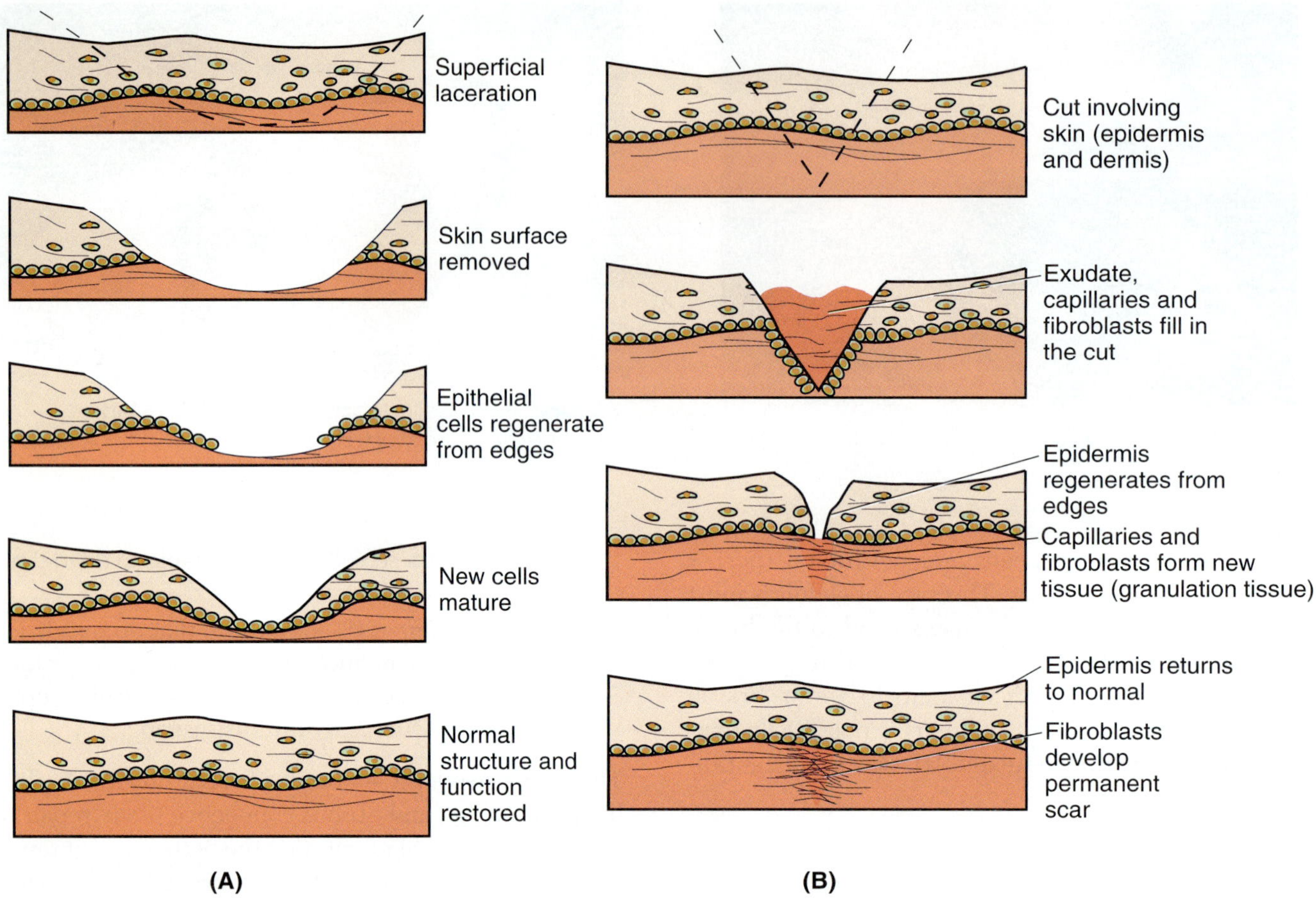

Figure 4–6 Tissue repair—(A) Complete regeneration. (B) Fibrous connective repair.

Tissue Healing

Tissue healing can be separated into categories of healing by primary union or secondary union. Categorization is determined by whether the wound edges are approximated (pulled together) or left separated during the healing process.

Primary Union (First Intention). **Primary union**, also called healing by first intention, involves approximating the edges of the wound. A classic example of healing by primary union is the healing process following a clean surgical incision. The wound edges are clean, there is minimal tissue damage, and the edges are approximated or brought together with sutures, staples, or tape.

Primary healing occurs in an orderly fashion and includes the following steps:

1. The incisional line quickly fills with serum forming a scab.
2. Within one to two days, new capillaries begin to bridge the gap between the wound edges.
3. In the next few days fibroblasts grow across the deeper wound layers and begin to deposit collagen in this fibrous network. This tissue is called granulation tissue.
4. The collagen begins to contract, pulling the wound edges together and forming a scar.

After a few weeks, the incision may appear healed, but the deeper layers of tissue may not be healed for a month or more. Usually an incisional scar will pale in color and shrink in size over a period of months or years (Figure 4–7A).

Secondary Union (Secondary Intention). Large wounds and those infected by dirt, debris, and bacteria cannot be pulled together to heal by primary intention. The process of healing by **secondary union** is the same process as primary union but involves a larger degree of tissue damage and more inflammation to resolve (Figure 4–7B). In order to fill the wound large numbers of capillaries, fibroblasts, and collagen must be produced. After a

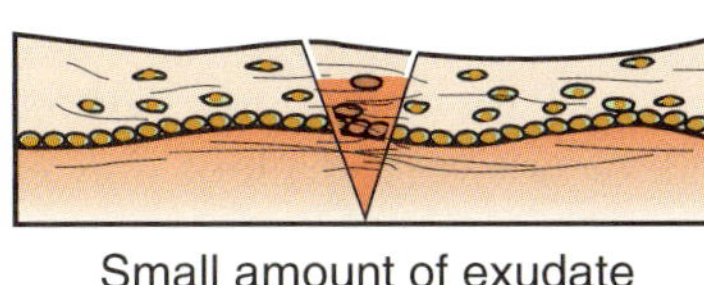
Small amount of exudate

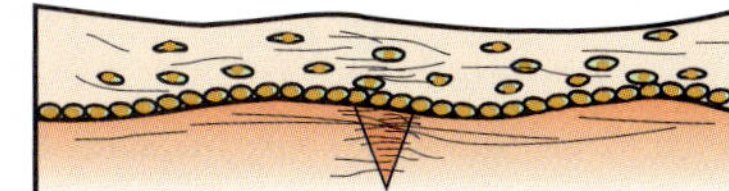
Small amount of granulation tissue

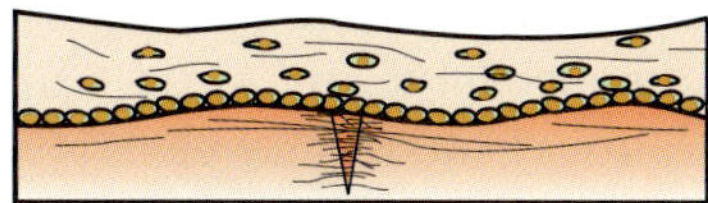
Small-sized scar

(A) Primary union

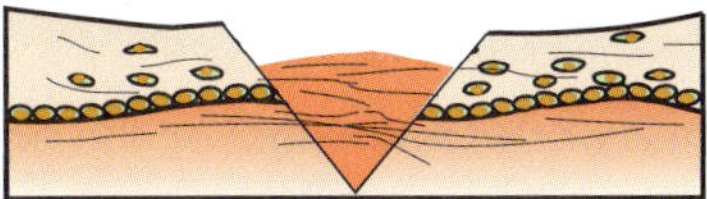
Large amount of exudate

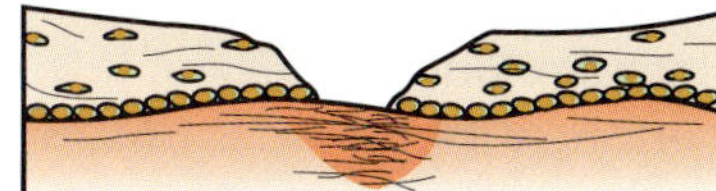
Large amount of granulation tissue

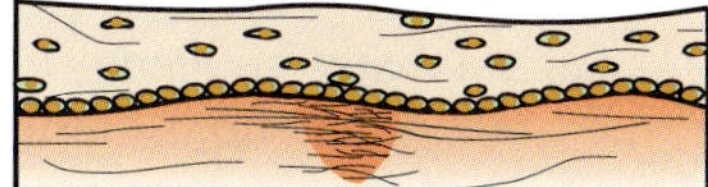
Large-sized scar

(B) Secondary union

Figure 4–7 Tissue healing—(A) Primary union. (B) Secondary union.

week or so the new soft red tissue is called granulation tissue. Granulation tissue is eventually replaced as more collagen is deposited in the area. The collagen contracts, pulling the wound edges together and beginning the formation of a scar. Healing time varies depending on the size of the wound. Large wounds may take a long time to heal by secondary union. Additional time may be needed for the scar to develop the strength of the surrounding tissue. If the wound is too large, the epithelium may not be able to bridge the gap and a skin graft may be needed.

Delayed Wound Healing

One of the greatest impediments to wound healing is the amount of dead tissue and debris in the wound. The debris may be dirt, bacteria, dead leukocytes, or a variety of other contaminates. It may take the body's leukocytes weeks or months to phagocytize (eat up) all the debris. In the meantime, bacteria may be producing dead cells and necrotic tissue as fast as the cleanup effort can advance. In order to speed healing, dirty wounds are cleaned and débrided. **Débridement** (day-breed-MON) is a process of washing or cutting away necrotic tissue and foreign material.

Other factors affecting healing time include:

1. Age—Younger people heal more rapidly than older people.
2. Size—Smaller wounds heal faster than larger ones.
3. Location—Epithelial tissue heals more rapidly compared to other tissue types.
4. Nutrition—Good nutritional status promotes wound healing. Protein and vitamin C are essential to healing.
5. Immobility—Wound tissue heals more rapidly if it is kept immobile.
6. Circulation—Tissue with good blood supply heals more rapidly. Epithelial tissue heals more readily than cartilage. Individuals with diabetes have small blood vessel disease (diabetic microangiopathy) leading to ischemia of the tissue and poor wound healing.
7. Organism virulence—Wounds infected with **virulent** (VIR-you-lent; poisonous) microorganisms are slower to heal than those that are not infected.
8. Steroids—Steroid therapy inhibits the inflammatory response prolonging healing time.

Complications of Wound Healing

Prolonged wound healing may occur as a result of any one or a combination of the factors previously discussed. Other complications of wound healing involve poor or excessive scar formation. A scar that does not have adequate strength may lead to wound **dehiscence** (dee-HISS-ens) or separation of tissue margins. Excessive collagen formation often results in a hard raised scar called a **keloid** (KEE-loid) (Figure 4–8). Keloid scars are often unsightly but harmless, and occur more often in the black population. Surgical removal may result in the formation of another keloid.

Adhesions from scar tissue may be a complication of surgery, especially abdominal surgery. As normal fibrous

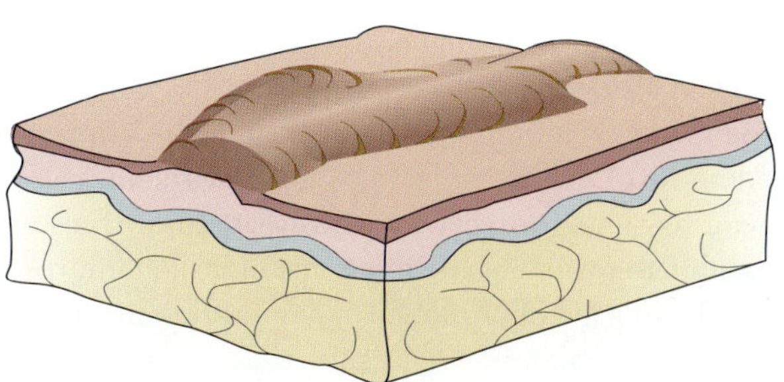
Figure 4–8 Keloid.

scar tissue develops in the operative organ, a part of this tissue may cling to the surface of the adjoining organs. The fibrous band that develops is called an **adhesion** (ad-HE-zhun). Adhesions are often asymptomatic and cause no difficulties, but in some cases they may become painful and lead to obstruction of the adjacent organ. The intestine is an organ that is frequently obstructed by adhesions following abdominal surgery. Further surgery may be needed to release painful or obstructive adhesions.

INFECTION

Chapter 2 briefly discusses the difference between inflammation and infection. Inflammation is a protective immune response and can occur without bacterial invasion. **Infection**, on the other hand, refers to the invasion of microorganisms into the tissue causing cell or tissue injury, thus leading to the inflammatory response.

Humans live with disease-causing microorganisms all around them. Some bacteria live on the skin surface, in the respiratory tract, and in the intestine without causing illness. Some bacteria are beneficial, for example, those in the gut that produce Vitamin D. These bacteria are called normal flora.

Microorganisms that produce disease are called pathogenic. Normal flora may become pathogenic when the host immune defense is compromised or when other normal flora are eliminated, allowing the remaining bacteria to grow unchecked. When this occurs, the normal flora bacteria cause an **opportunistic infection**.

Certain conditions must be present for a microorganism to cause an infection in the host. A pathogen must have an area to enter, be resistant enough to survive, enter in great enough number to survive, and overcome the defenses of the individual.

First the microorganism must successfully gain access into the body through a portal of entry. Any break in the skin allows entry of microorganisms. Common openings such as the nose, mouth, eyes, and ears are portals of entry. The most common port of entry is the respiratory system. Other portals include the digestive system, urinary tract, and reproductive tract.

The pathogen must also be resistant to the defenses of the host. The ability of a microorganism to overcome the defense of the host is its virulence. A virulent microorganism has an aggressive or invasive nature. It also has the ability to produce a toxin or poison, which injures tissues. The degree of virulence of a microorganism varies. Generally speaking, organisms that come from an infected host are more virulent than those grown in laboratory conditions.

The number of invading pathogens also plays a part in the conditions necessary for infection. Pathogenic organisms that are weak or not very virulent may cause infection if they invade in large enough numbers to overcome the body's defense system. Generally speaking the higher the number of invading pathogens the greater the risk of infection.

Finally the condition of the individual or the host is a determinant of infection risk. An individual who is in good physical and emotional health, has good nutrition, practices risk-reducing living habits, and is relatively young has a good chance of avoiding infection.

Frequency and Types of Infection

Infectious diseases are the leading cause of death in the world. A country's ability to track and identify infectious diseases is an important weapon in the control of disease. In the United States, the Centers for Disease Control and Prevention (CDC), based in Atlanta, provide these services.

Respiratory infections, including upper respiratory infections, influenza-like infections, pneumonia, and bronchitis, account for over eighty percent of all infections. Childhood infections, wound infections, viral infections, and other types of infection account for the remaining number of infections diagnosed.

Microorganisms that produce infection in humans include bacteria, **viruses**, **fungi**, **rickettsiae** (RIC-**KET**-see-ah), **protozoa**, and **helminths** (Table 4–1). These organisms can produce infections in the host that range from very mild to life threatening.

Bacteria. Bacterial infections may occur as a primary or secondary disease. Primary bacterial infections occur when one is exposed to a pathogen. Secondary infection occurs after the onset of another disease process or condition. Secondary infections are very common. The most common cause for secondary infection is obstruction of a body passageway. For example, nasal obstruction may lead to sinusitis, and obstruction of the eustachian tubes may lead to otitis media or middle ear infection.

Bacteria normally live on or in the skin, mouth, nose, genital tract, and intestines of humans. These normal flora bacteria often become pathogenic when they gain access into the body or when the body's resistance is less than normal. Staphylococcus is a bacterium of the skin that often enters the body and can infect any organ. *Staph aureus* is an important member of the staphylococcus family because it has the ability to develop strains that are resistant to penicillin and other antibiotics. Methicillin Resistant Staphylococcus Aureus (MRSA) is such a strain.

TABLE 4–1 Some Common Infections Caused by Microorganisms in Man

Bacteria	Virus	Fungus
Staphylococcus	Common Cold	Ringworm (Tinea)
Streptococcus	Herpes Simplex	Athlete's Foot
Escherichia Coli	Mononucleosis	Candidiasis
Klebsiella	HIV	Thrush
Pseudomonas	Measles	Vaginitis
Shigella	Mumps	Histoplasmosis
Salmonella	Rubella	Coccidioidomycosis
	Influenza (flu)	
Rickettsial	**Protozoan**	**Helminths**
Rocky Mountain Spotted Fever	Malaria	Roundworms
	Giardiasis	Flatworms
		Pinworms
		Tapeworms

These antibiotic-resistant strains are particularly dangerous as they are difficult to control and eliminate (Healthy Highlight 4–1).

Streptococcus bacteria normally live on the skin and in the throat. Common infections caused by streptococcus bacteria include strep throat, scarlet fever, pneumonia, and meningitis. Strep throat in a select group of individuals may lead to rheumatic fever and glomerulonephritis.

Enteric bacteria are those living in the intestinal tract. Common enteric bacteria include *Escherichia coli (E. coli), Klebsiella, Pseudomonas, Shigella*, and *Salmonella. E. coli* causes enteritis in infants and adults and may be the cause of travelers' diarrhea. *E. coli* and *Klebsiella* are common causes of urinary tract infections. *Pseudomonas* commonly infects wounds and is associated with a foul odor and green pus production. *Shigella* and *Salmonella* infections cause diarrhea. *Salmonella* is the causative organism of food poisoning.

Viruses. Viruses are the smallest infective organisms and must be visualized by an electron microscope. Viruses cannot reproduce or live outside the cell. They must invade the cell and use it to reproduce their genetic information. Lymphocytes of the immune system are the body's primary defense against viruses. Some viruses have the ability to mutate or change, so the body cannot develop just one antibody to kill that type of virus.

HEALTHY HIGHLIGHT 4–1

Medication Precautions

WARNING! Anyone taking a prescribed antibiotic medication should always take ALL the medication. Even if the symptoms stop, the medication should be taken until it is completed. Antibiotics should not be "saved" for the next illness. Failure to complete antibiotic therapy may lead to the development of antibiotic resistant strains of bacteria. In other words, the first doses of medication may kill weaker bacteria and stun the stronger ones. If therapy is halted, the stronger bacteria may survive and reproduce strains that can resist the antibiotic. When this occurs, stronger and usually more expensive medications must be used to treat the same infection at a later date. Mismanagement of antibiotic therapy has led to development of strains of bacteria that now must be treated with stronger oral antibiotics or IV antibiotics.

Viral infections cannot be treated easily. There are some antiviral agents that can be given to individuals with reduced resistance to infections to try to prevent the viral infection. Antibiotic therapy does not kill a virus. Handwashing and ensuring that all equipment and surfaces are cleaned between patient contacts is the best method of reducing the transmission of most viruses. Usually supportive care is given by treating the symptoms that the virus causes. Symptoms may include fever, sore throat, runny nose, headache, and chest congestion. Antibiotics may help in treatment of a secondary bacterial infection occurring with the viral infection.

Viral infections of the upper respiratory system, including the common cold, far outnumber other viral diseases. Cold sores, also known as herpes simplex, are very common and affect many individuals. Infectious mononucleosis frequently affects adolescents and young adults. Human immunodeficiency virus (HIV) is the cause of acquired immune deficiency syndrome (AIDS) and has become the most noted virus because of its usually fatal outcome.

Immunizations are effective in preventing many viral diseases, such as measles, mumps, rubella, and small pox. Influenza virus (flu) mutates and requires new vaccines with each mutation. Some viruses are latent, meaning they live inside the cell causing no harm until the body becomes stressed or impaired. Latent viruses, such as those in the herpes family, replicate and cause symptoms during stressful periods.

Fungi. Fungi are microscopic plant-like organisms that cause diseases referred to as mycoses. Fungi are larger than bacteria and only a few types are pathogenic. Single-celled forms of fungi are called yeast.

Fungal infections of the skin, such as those of the tinea family (ringworm and athlete's foot), are common. Candida, commonly called candidiasis or yeast infection, often occurs in individuals with suppressed immune systems, anyone on long-term antibiotic therapy, and diabetic patients. Candida is a superficial infection of the skin and mucous membranes appearing commonly in the moist folds of the skin, the mouth (thrush), vaginal cavity (vaginitis), and genital area.

Other fungal infections include histoplasmosis and coccidioidomycosis. These infections are common to certain geographical locations, but are not common in the general population. Fungal infections can be treated with anti-fungal and antibiotic medications but often are difficult to cure and may require long-term therapy.

Rickettsiae. Rickettsiae are microscopic organisms that are intermediate between bacteria and virus. They must live in the host cell like a virus. Rickettsiae are spread by fleas, ticks, mites, and lice and can cause fatal infections in humans. The most common rickettsial infection is Rocky Mountain spotted fever.

Protozoa. Protozoa are single-celled microscopic members of the animal kingdom. They are found in the soil and live on dead or decaying material. Infection is by ingestion of spores or by infected insect bites.

Malaria is the most prevalent protozoan infection worldwide, but is uncommon in the United States. The protozoan causing malaria lives in and destroys the red blood cell of the host. Malaria is spread by mosquitos. Giardiasis is an intestinal infection caused by the protozoan *Giardia lamblia*. It is caused by drinking infected water and is treated with antibiotic therapy.

Helminths. Helminths are any of the round or flatworms. Helminth infestation is common worldwide, but not as common in the United States. Pinworms and tapeworms are the most common helminths. Pinworms cause anal itching, but do not cause serious illness. Tapeworms may cause intestinal disease in humans. All tapeworms are acquired by eating uncooked or inadequately cooked meat.

Testing for Infection

Symptoms of infection in an individual may include fever, **tachycardia** (TACH-ee-**KAR**-dee-ah; tachy = rapid, cardia = heart rate), and **malaise** (general ill feeling). Often blood studies will reveal **leukocytosis** (leuko = white, cyto = cell, osis = condition) or an increase in white cell count. Blood from an individual with **septicemia** (SEP-tih-**SEE**-me-ah) will reveal the presence of the pathogen in the blood. Infection in the meninges or meningitis may show presence of pathogens in the individual's spinal fluid.

A culture is the process of growing pathogenic cells on or in a gelatin-like substance called media. Pathogenic organisms use this media for food (Figure 4–9). Media may be made of different nutrient agars. A common nutrient agar is sheep's blood agar. Laboratory studies of how the microorganism utilizes this food assist in the determination of the type of pathogen.

A culture is the most definitive test for organisms in a lesion or wound. Cultures are most commonly utilized for bacteria identification, but may also be utilized for identification of fungal or some viral infections. Most bacterial specimens are obtained from the throat, urine, sputum, purulent wound lesions, feces, blood, and spinal fluid.

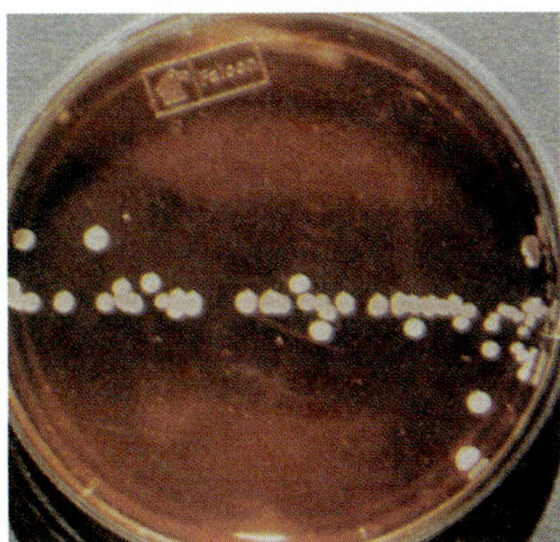

Figure 4–9 Bacterial culture.

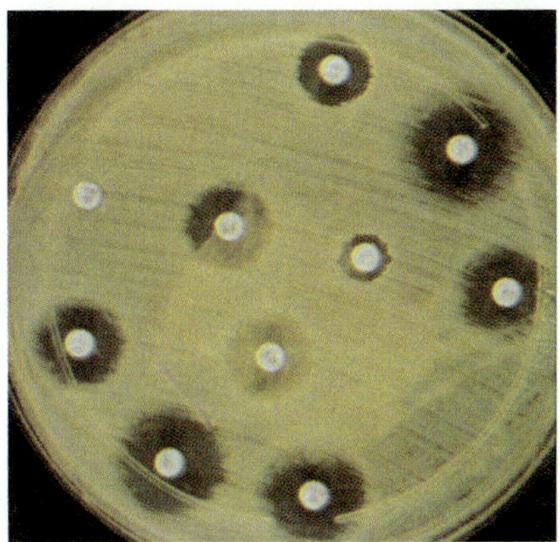

Figure 4–10 Bacterial sensitivity.

A culture helps identify the pathogen. After identification of the pathogen, a sensitivity test is utilized to identify the type of treatment needed. The combined test for these is called a **culture and sensitivity** test. During a sensitivity test, the microorganisms are smeared on the nutrient agar and small antibiotic permeated disks are placed on the agar (Figure 4–10). After incubation the agar plate is observed for killing zones around the disk. Disks that display a large killing zone are the most effective in treatment.

Specific antigen-antibody reactive tests may be utilized to determine the presence of pathogens. For example, a rapid diagnosis of strep throat may be made by testing for the presence of an antigen in a throat specimen. For example, the streptococcus antigen will clot or clump when mixed with laboratory streptococcus antibody.

Bacterial, rickettsial, viral, and some other pathogenic infections may be determined by serologic testing. Serologic testing uses the individual's blood serum to test for antibodies against the pathogen.

Skin testing also utilizes antibody presence to determine exposure to pathogens. Tuberculosis (TB) skin testing is one of the most common skin tests. This test (also called the Mantoux test) involves the intradermal (under the skin) injection of tuberculin bacteria particles (antigen) (Figure 4–11). If an individual has been exposed to TB and has developed the TB antibody, this antibody will attack the antigen and cause an **induration** (**IN**-dur-RAY-shun; hardened tissue). Presence of an induration at the injection site greater than a certain size is a positive skin test.

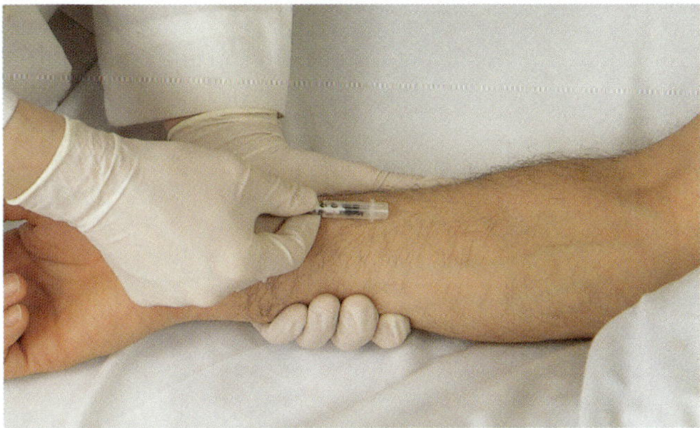

Figure 4–11 Tuberculosis (TB) skin test.

A positive skin test and serology testing may not indicate current infection or the degree of infection, but may only indicate that the individual has been exposed to the pathogen and has developed antibodies. These are only a few of the many laboratory tests used in diagnosing pathogenic infections.

SUMMARY

The body responds to the invasions of pathogens by utilizing its defense mechanisms. Inflammation is a natural protective mechanism that occurs when physical barriers are broken and the invader penetrates the tissues. The inflammatory process consists of a series of events that eventually, if functioning properly, destroy the invading pathogen. When this system of protection fails, infection may occur. Infections are caused by a variety of organisms, most commonly by bacteria and viruses. They are diagnosed and treated in a variety of ways. Several laboratory tests can be used to identify the organism and determine the appropriate therapy.

REVIEW QUESTIONS

Short Answer

1. Describe the three defense mechanisms of the body.
2. What are the steps in the inflammatory process?
3. How do inflammatory exudates and inflammatory lesions differ?
4. What are the five cardinal signs of inflammation?
5. What is the difference between a keloid and an adhesion?
6. Compare some microorganisms that produce infection in humans.
7. What type of testing is used to identify the organism causing an infection?

Fill in the Blank

8. Cellular proliferation can be grouped into the three categories of __________, __________, and __________.
9. The body's two main methods of repair involve __________ and __________.
10. Primary union is also called __________.
11. The process of secondary union involves a larger degree of __________ and more __________ to resolve than primary union.
12. The greatest impediments to wound healing are __________ and __________.

CASE STUDY

You are transporting Mr. Jordan to the nursing home for rehabilitation after a long hospital stay following complicated surgery and infection. As you are talking with Mr. Jordan, you recall learning about wound healing and wound infection. What steps are involved in primary union? What are common organisms that cause a wound infection? What is the best method to prevent spread of organisms?

BIBLIOGRAPHY

Beat the yeast. (1997). *Prevention, 49*, 143.

Boland, M. (1997). What's wrong with this kitchen? *American Health for Women, 16(6)*, 72–3.

Breiman, R. F. (1996). Impact of technology on the emergence of infectious diseases. *Epidemiology Review, 18(1)*, 4–9.

Cliver, D. O. (1997). Hepatitis A from strawberries: who's to blame? *Food Technology, 51(6),* 132.

Day, M. W. (1997). Using a personal ventilation mask: Your protection from infection. *Nursing 97, 27(4),* 56–57.

Desowitz, R. S. (1997). Viruses without frontiers. *Natural History, 106(6),* 10–11.

Hospital Infection Control Practice Advisory Committee. (1994). Guideline for prevention of nosocomial pneumonia: Part II. *American Journal of Infection Control, 22,* 266–292.

Hughes, J. M. (1996). Emerging pathogens: An epidemiologist's perspective on the problem and priorities for the future. *Western Journal of Medicine, 164(1),* 21–22.

Infection control update: 97. (1997). *Nursing 97, 27(6),* 60–61.

Jeffries, D. J. (1995). Viral hazards to and from health care workers. *Journal of Hospital Infections, 30(5),* 140–155.

Nightingale, S. L. (1997). Safety alert re risk of misdiagnosis of group B streptococcal infection. *Journal of the American Medical Association, 277,* 1343.

Ostfeld, R. S. (1997). The ecology of Lyme disease risk. *American Scientist, 85(3),* 338–346.

Rogues, A. M., Dupon, M., Morlat, P., Lacoste, D., Pelligrin, J. L., Ragnaud, J. M., & Gachie, J. P. (1996). Hospital-acquired infections in patients with HIV/AIDS. *Journal of Hospital Infection, 34(4),* 333–336.

Sissons, J. G. P., Borysiewicz, L. K., & Cohen, J. (1995). Immunology of infection. *Virus Research: An International Journal of Molecular and Cellular Virology, 39(2),* 386.

Taubes, G. (August 24, 1997). A mosquito bites back. *New York Times Magazine,* 40–46.

The new suburban health threat. (1997). *Good Housekeeping, 224(6),* 177–179.

Walter, T. (1997). Iron, anemia, and infection. *Nutrition Reviews, 55(4),* 11–124.

Woolery, W. A. (1997). Atypical infections in older adults. *Geriatrics, 52(3),* 51.

Zuger, A. (May 27, 1997). Rapid test for common infection is proving elusive. *New York Times,* C3.

CHAPTER

5

Fluid, Electrolyte, and Acid-Base Balance

CONTENT OUTLINE

- Physiology of Fluid and Acid-Base Balance
  - Fluid Compartments
  - Body Fluid Distribution
  - Electrolytes
  - Movement of Body Fluids
  - Regulators of Fluid Balance
  - Acid-Base Balance
  - Regulators of Acid-Base Balance
- Factors Affecting Fluid and Electrolyte Balance
- Disturbances in Fluid, Electrolyte, and Acid-Base Balance
  - Fluid Disturbances
  - Electrolyte Disturbances
  - Acid-Base Disturbances
- Assessment
  - Health History
  - Physical Examination
  - Diagnostic and Laboratory Data
- Management
  - Parenteral Fluids
  - Blood Transfusion

KEY TERMS

Acid
Acid-base balance
Acid-base buffer system
Acidosis
Alkalosis
Arterial blood gases (ABGs)
Base
Colloid
Crystalloid
Diffusion
Edema
Electrochemical gradient
Electrolyte
Filtration
Homeostasis
Hydrostatic pressure
Hypercalcemia
Hyperchloremia
Hyperkalemia
Hypermagnesemia
Hypernatremia
Hyperphosphatemia
Hypertonic
Hypocalcemia
Hypochloremia
Hypokalemia
Hypomagnesemia
Hyponatremia
Hypophosphatemia
Hypotonic
Hypoxemia
Isotonic
Osmolality
Osmolarity
Osmole
Osmosis
Osmotic pressure
Permeability
Semipermeable
Skin turgor
Solute
Solvent

LEARNING OBJECTIVES

1. Describe the physiological processes responsible for the maintenance of body fluid and acid-base balance.
2. Describe the common alterations in body fluid and acid-base balance.
3. Describe the common signs and symptoms that occur in patients with alterations in body fluid and acid-base balance.
4. Identify common interventions for patients with fluid and acid-base imbalances.

OVERVIEW

The human body is dependent upon the availability of the proper amount of electrolytes and regulation of the acid-base system. Electrolytes are important for nerve conduction, muscle contraction, and regulation of the cardiac conduction system. Alterations outside normal ranges may result in complaints as benign as muscle weakness or as severe as cardiac arrest. Just as the electrolyte balance must be maintained, the body needs to maintain the circulating blood and body fluids at a certain pH to allow important metabolic processes to occur at the cellular level. Some alterations in pH may be caused by long-term and chronic changes of certain disease processes, such as chronic obstructive pulmonary disease (COPD), while other alterations in pH are acute and life-threatening as in hypoxia. The EMS provider needs to be able to understand the consequences of alterations in electrolytes and the acid-base balance and understand how some of these alterations may change management of certain patients.

The physiological functions and alterations of body fluid and acid-base balance are presented in this chapter. The term *body fluid* is used to denote both water and electrolytes, whereas the term *body water* refers to water alone. **Homeostasis**, or equilibrium of the internal environment, refers to the state of balance of body fluid.

PHYSIOLOGY OF FLUID AND ACID-BASE BALANCE

The body normally maintains a balance between the amount of fluid taken in and the amount excreted. Alterations in this balance can be caused by many disease processes.

Fluid Compartments

The body's fluid is contained within three compartments: cells, blood vessels, and the tissue space (space between the cells and blood vessels). To understand this concept, visualize cars on a freeway. The cars represent cells; the lanes represent the blood vessels, and the space between the cars in the lanes represents the tissue space. The freeway itself is the body with defined structure.

Just as traffic is ongoing and continuous, fluids move constantly from one compartment to another to accommodate the cell's metabolic needs (Figure 5–1). Specific terms are used in describing compartmentalized body fluid:

- *Intra*cellular fluid: *within* the cell
- *Intra*vascular fluid: *within* blood vessels

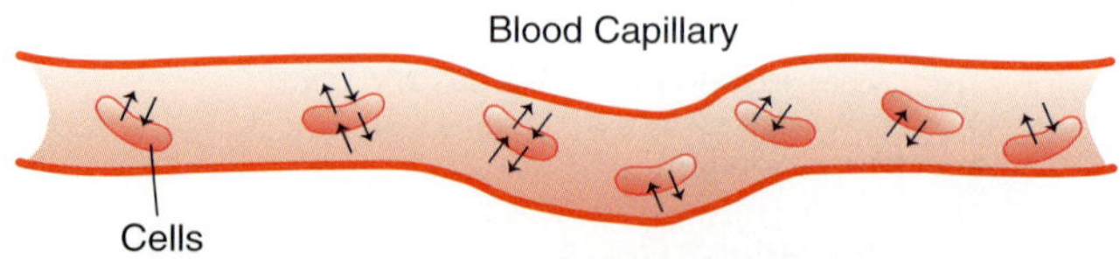

Figure 5–1 The movement of fluid between the intracellular and extracellular compartments.

- *Inter*stitial fluid: *between* cells; fluid that surrounds cells

There are two types of body fluid: intracellular (ICF) and extracellular (ECF). Because intravascular and interstitial fluid are outside the cells, these fluids are extracellular. Key terms used in explaining the movement of molecules in body fluids are:

- **Solute:** Substance dissolved in a solution
- **Solvent:** Liquid that contains a substance in solution
- **Permeability:** Capability of a substance, molecule, or ion to diffuse through a membrane (covering of tissue over a surface, organ, or separating spaces)
- **Semipermeable:** Selectively permeable (All membranes in the body allow some solutes to pass through the membrane without restriction but will prevent the passage of other solutes.)

Cells have permeable membranes that allow fluid and solutes to pass into and out of the cell. Permeability allows the cell to acquire the nutrients it needs from extracellular fluid to carry on metabolism and to eliminate metabolic waste products.

Blood vessels have permeable membranes that bathe and feed the cells. The intravascular fluid of arterioles carries oxygen and nutrients to the cells. The venules take in the waste products from the cells' metabolic activity.

Cells and capillaries form a meshlike structure that creates a tissue space between cells and the vascular system to allow cellular access to the vascular system. Interstitial space promotes access of the cells to the arterioles and venules.

Body Fluid Distribution

Water is the largest single constituent of the body, representing 45% to 75% of the body's total weight. About two-thirds of the body fluid is intracellular. The remaining one-third is extracellular, with one-fourth of this fluid being intravascular and three-fourths being interstitial fluid. Body fat is essentially free of water; therefore, the ratio of water to body weight is greater in leaner people than in obese people.

Body fluid is replenished by the ingestion of liquids and food products such as meats and vegetables, which contain 65% to 97% water. The third source of body fluid is the metabolism of foods, which yields water of oxidation. The kidneys excrete the largest quantity of fluid; other avenues for water loss are the lungs, skin, and gastrointestinal tract.

Electrolytes

An **electrolyte** is a compound that, when dissolved in water or another solvent, forms or dissociates into ions (electrically charged particles) (Figure 5–2). The electrolytes provide inorganic chemicals for cellular reactions and control mechanisms. Electrolytes have special physiological functions in the body that promote neuromuscular irritability, maintain body fluid osmolarity, regulate acid-base balance, and distribute body fluids between the fluid compartments.

Electrolytes are measured in terms of their electrical combining power, the quantities of cations and anions in a solution, expressed as milliequivalents per liter (mEq/l). Because electrolytes produce either positively charged ions (cations) or negatively charged ions (anions), they are critical regulators in the distribution of body fluid. The main electrolytes in body fluid are: sodium (Na^+), potassium (K^+), calcium (Ca^{2+}), and magnesium (Mg^{2+}).

Table 5–1 discusses the distribution of electrolytes in body fluid, their regulatory functions, and dietary sources. As shown in Table 5–1, the extracellular fluid contains the largest quantities of sodium, chloride, and bicarbonate ions, but only small quantities of potassium, calcium, magnesium, phosphate, sulfate, and organic acid ions. The intracellular fluid contains only small quantities of sodium and chloride ions and almost no calcium ions. Large quantities of potassium and phosphate ions with moderate quantities of magnesium and sulfate ions are contained within intracellular fluid (see the accompanying display).

Movement of Body Fluids

The physiological forces that affect the movement of body fluids through cell walls and capillaries can be perceived as a mass-transportation system that carries traffic between

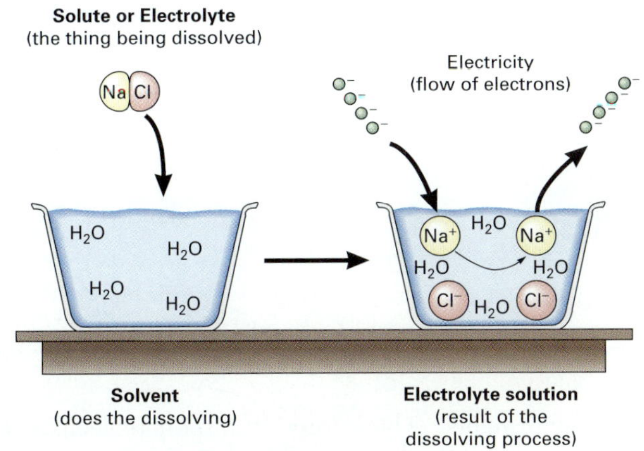

Figure 5–2 Dissolution of electrolytes.

TABLE 5-1 Common Electrolytes

Electrolyte Ion	Distribution in Body Fluid		Basic Functions	Dietary Sources
	Extracellular (mEq/l)	Intracellular (mEq/l)		
Sodium (Na^+)	135–154	15–20	Regulates fluid volume within extracellular fluid (ECF) compartment. Increases cell membrane permeability. Regulates vascular osmotic pressure. Controls water distribution between ECF and intracellular fluid (ICF) compartments. Stimulates conduction of nerve impulses. Maintains neuromuscular irritability.	Table salt (NaCl), 40% of which is sodium; cheese, milk, processed meat, poultry, shellfish, fish, eggs, and foods preserved with salt (e.g., ham and bacon)
Potassium (K^+)	3.5–5	150–155	Regulates osmolality of ICF. Promotes transmission of nerve impulses. Promotes contraction of skeletal and smooth muscles. Promotes enzymatic action for cellular energy production by transforming carbohydrates into energy and restructuring amino acids into proteins. Regulates acid-base balance by cellular exchange of hydrogen ions.	Fruits, especially bananas, oranges, and dried fruits; vegetables, meats, and nuts
Calcium (Ca^{2+})	4.5–5.5	1–2	Provides strength and durability to bones and teeth. Establishes thickness and strength of cell membranes. Promotes transmission of nerve impulses. Decreases neuromuscular excitability. Is essential for blood coagulation. Promotes absorption and utilization of vitamin B_{12}. Activates enzyme reactions and hormone secretions.	Dairy products (milk, cheese, and yogurt), sardines, whole grains, and green leafy vegetables
Magnesium (Mg^{2+})	4.5–5.5	27–29	Activates enzyme systems, mainly those associated with vitamin B metabolism and the utilization of potassium, calcium, and protein. Promotes regulation of serum calcium, phosphorus, and potassium levels. Promotes neuromuscular activity.	Green leafy vegetables, whole grains, fish, and nuts

the compartments. These forces transport molecules of water, foods, gases, wastes, and ions to maintain a physiological balance between extracellular and intracellular fluid volumes. These transport processes account for fluid shifts between the compartments (see Table 5–2).

TABLE 5-2 Movement of Body Fluid

Physiological Force	Process	Related Factors
Diffusion The rate of **diffusion** (continual movement of molecules in a solution or a gas is influenced by: • The size of the molecule (smaller molecules diffuse faster than larger molecules) • The concentration of the molecules (molecules move from an area of greater concentration to an area of lesser concentration) • The temperature of the solution (higher temperatures increase the rate of diffusion)	Particles move across a permeable membrane and disperse in all directions through a solution or a gas (Figure 5–3).	The particle's electrical charge can also affect the process of diffusion because ions with opposite charges are pulled toward other ions.
Osmosis The process of **osmosis** (passage of a solvent from an area of lesser concentration to an area of greater concentration) is influenced by: • The net movement of water • The semipermeability of the membrane	Solvent molecules move across a membrane to an area where there is a higher concentration of solute that cannot pass through the membrane (Figure 5–4).	**Osmotic pressure** is force created when two solutions of different concentrations are separated by a selectively permeable membrane. An **osmole** is the unit of measure of osmotic pressure.
Active Transport An **electrochemical gradient** (sum of all the diffusion forces acting on the membrane, from either a concentration gradient or an electrical or pressure gradient) exists when there is active transport.	Occurs when a cell membrane moves molecules or ions against an electrochemical gradient from an area of lesser concentration to an area of greater concentration.	In order for active transport to occur, there must be a carrier and adenosine triphosphate (ATP) molecules inside the cell membrane (Figure 5–5).
Hydrostatic Pressure **Hydrostatic pressure** (force a liquid exerts on the sides of the container that holds it) is governed by: • The force by which the heart pumps • The rate of blood flow • The arterial blood pressure • The venous blood pressure	The force of fluid presses outward against the blood vessel wall.	The hydrostatic pressure is twice as great at the arterial end than at the venous end, causing fluid and solutes to go from the arterial end of the capillary into the interstitial space.
Filtration **Filtration** is governed by the presence of a greater hydrostatic pressure in the arterial end capillaries than in the interstitial spaces.	The movement of fluid through a semipermeable membrane from an area with higher hydrostatic pressure to an area with lower hydrostatic pressure creates an outward gain of fluid in the interstitial spaces.	The body achieves total fluid balance when the excess fluid and solutes remaining in the interstitial spaces are returned to the intravascular compartment by the lymphatic system.

(continues)

TABLE 5-2 Movement of Body Fluid (continued)

Physiological Force	Process	Related Factors
Colloid Osmotic Pressure		
Created by solutes or **colloids** (proteins or nondiffusible substances) in the plasma	There is a movement of fluid between the intravascular and interstitial compartments, based on the number of solute particles on the concentrated side and the presence of a semipermeable membrane.	Because the protein content of intravascular fluid is 16 times as great as that of interstitial fluid, the fluids move into the capillary or intravascular compartment when the heart pumps effectively.

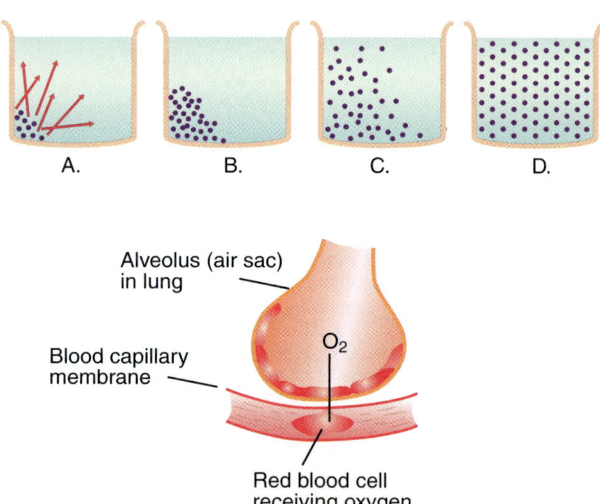

Figure 5-3 The process of diffusion. A. A small lump of sugar is placed in a beaker of water, its molecules dissolve and begin to diffuse outward. B. C. The sugar molecules continue to diffuse through the water from an area of greater concentration to an area of lesser concentration. D. Over a long period of time, the sugar molecules are evenly distributed throughout the water, reaching a state of equilibrium. Examples of diffusion in the human body: Oxygen diffuses from lung alveoli, where it is in greater concentration, across the capillary membrane into a red blood cell, where it is in lesser concentration.

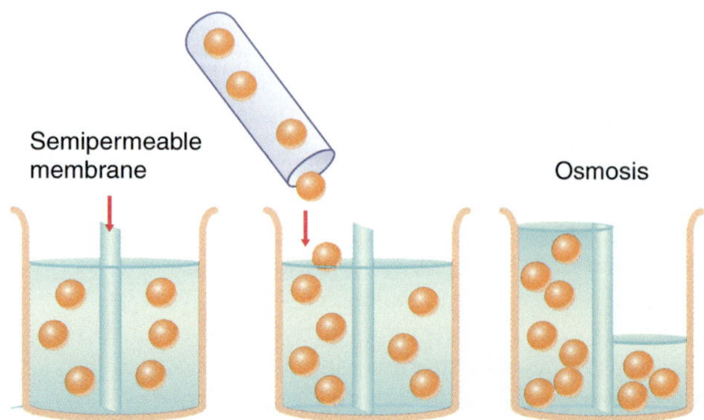

Figure 5-4 The process of osmosis.

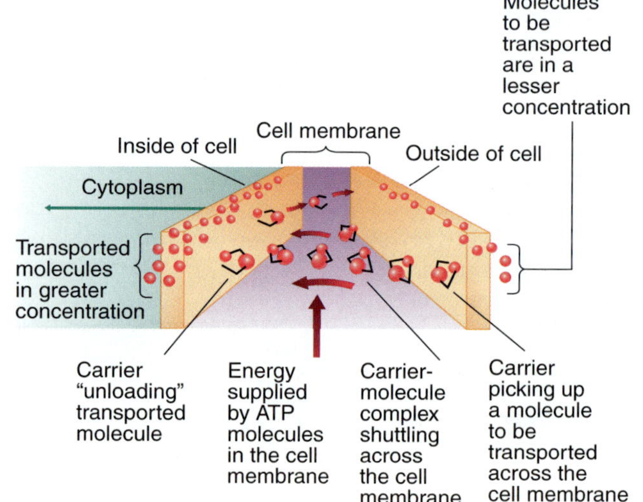

Figure 5-5 The active transport of molecules from an area of lesser concentration to an area of greater concentration.

Regulators of Fluid Balance

The body has many regulators that maintain fluid balance, including fluid and food intake, skin, lungs, gastrointestinal tract, and kidneys. When all organs are functioning normally, the body is able to maintain homeostasis.

Fluid and Food Intake. There are three natural sources by which water enters the body: oral liquids; water in foods; and water formed by metabolism of foods. A normal diet provides the electrolytes required by the body. Ingested liquids account for approximately 1,500 ml of fluid intake daily. Approximately 700 ml of water comes from foods and approximately 200 ml is produced by processing of food within the body.

Skin. An estimated water loss of 300 to 400 ml per day occurs by diffusion through the skin of an adult. Because the person is not aware of this water loss, it is called *insen-*

sible loss. Water is also lost through the skin by perspiration; however, the total amount of water lost by perspiration can vary from 1.5 to 3.5 l per hour, depending on environmental factors and body temperature.

Lungs. An estimated insensible water loss of 300 to 400 ml per day occurs in an adult through expired air, which is saturated with water vapor. This amount may vary with the rate and depth of respirations.

Gastrointestinal Tract. Although a large amount of fluid—about 8,000 ml per day in the adult—is secreted into the gastrointestinal tract, almost all this fluid is reabsorbed by the body. In adults, about 200 ml of water is lost per day in feces. Severe diarrhea can cause a fluid and electrolyte deficit because the gastrointestinal fluids contain a large amount of electrolytes.

Kidneys. The kidneys play a major role in maintaining fluid balance by excreting 1,200 to 1,500 ml per day in the adult. The excretion of water by healthy kidneys is proportional to the fluid ingested and the amount of waste or solutes excreted.

When an extracellular fluid volume deficit occurs, hormones play a key role in restoring the extracellular fluid volume. The release of the following hormones into circulation causes the kidneys to conserve water:

- Antidiuretic hormone (ADH) from the posterior pituitary gland acts on the distal tubules of the kidneys to reabsorb water.
- Aldosterone (produced in the adrenal cortex) causes the reabsorption of sodium from the renal tubules (see Chapter 14). The increased reabsorption of sodium causes water retention in the extracellular fluid, increasing its volume.
- Renin, which is released from the juxtaglomerular cells of the kidneys, promotes vasoconstriction and the release of aldosterone.

The interaction of these hormones with regard to renal functions serves as the body's compensatory mechanism to maintain homeostasis.

Sodium is the main electrolyte that promotes the retention of water. An intravascular water deficit causes the renal tubules to reabsorb more sodium into circulation. Because water molecules go with the sodium ions, the intravascular water deficit is corrected by this action of the renal tubules.

Acid-Base Balance

Acid-base balance refers to the homeostasis of the hydrogen ion concentration in body fluids. The slightest variation in the hydrogen ion concentration causes marked alterations in the rate of cellular chemical reactions. The pH symbol is used to indicate the hydrogen ion concentration of body fluids; 7.35 to 7.45 is the normal pH range of extracellular fluid. Hydrogen ions (H^+), which carry a positive charge, are protons. Depending on the number of hydrogen ions present, a solution can be either acidic, neutral, or alkaline.

As the number of hydrogen ions increases, the fluid becomes acidic. *Acidity of a solution increases as the pH value decreases.* An **acid** is a substance that donates hydrogen ions. For example, hydrochloric acid (HCl) ionizes in water (a solution) to form hydrogen ions and chloride ions. HCl, which is found in gastric juices, has a strong tendency to form ions, discharging hydrogen ions into the solution.

As the number of hydrogen ions decreases, the fluid becomes alkaline. *Alkalinity of a solution increases as the pH value increases.* A **base** is a substance that accepts hydrogen ions (proton acceptor).

A neutral solution has a pH of 7. In such a solution there are equal numbers of hydrogen ions (H^+) and hydroxyl ions (OH^-), which can combine to form water (H_2O). When the number of hydrogen ions is increased, the solution becomes acidic (pH value below 7); a decrease in the number of hydrogen ions causes the solution to become alkaline (pH value above 7). When the number of free hydrogen ions in a solution increases to the point that the pH value becomes less than 7.35, the body is in a state of **acidosis**. The opposite occurs with **alkalosis**, in which a pH value higher than 7.45 results from a low hydrogen ion concentration.

Regulators of Acid-Base Balance

The body has three main control systems that regulate acid-base balance to counter acidosis or alkalosis: the buffer systems; respiration; and renal control of hydrogen ion concentration. These systems vary in their reaction time in regulating and restoring balance to the hydrogen ion concentration of a solution.

Buffer Systems. All body fluids are supplied with an **acid-base buffer system** (a solution containing two or more chemical compounds that prevents marked changes in hydrogen ion concentration when either an acid or a base is added to a solution). The buffer system reacts within a fraction of a second to prevent excessive changes in the hydrogen ion concentration.

There are several *chemical* buffer systems of body fluids, which are activated under different conditions; however, the bicarbonate-carbonic acid system (carbonate system) is the body's primary buffer system. The carbonate system consists of a mixture of carbonic acid (H_2CO_3) and sodium bicarbonate ($NaHCO_3$). The pH of the extracellular fluid can be returned to normal limits by this system because carbonic acid is a weak acid and bicarbonate is a weak base.

Bicarbonate helps to stabilize pH by combining reversibly with hydrogen ions. Most of the body's bicarbonate is produced in red blood cells, where the enzyme carbonic anhydrase accelerates the conversion of carbon dioxide to carbonic acid.

Respiratory Regulation of Acid-Base Balance. The respiratory buffering system helps to maintain acid-base balance by controlling the content of carbon dioxide in extracellular fluid. The *rate of metabolism* determines the formation of carbon dioxide. Carbon dioxide is continually being formed in the body by different intracellular metabolic processes. The carbon in foods is oxidized by oxygen to form carbon dioxide.

It takes the respiratory regulatory mechanism several minutes to respond to changes in the carbon dioxide concentration of extracellular fluid. With the increase of carbon dioxide in extracellular fluids, respirations are increased in rate and depth so that more carbon dioxide is exhaled. As the respiratory system removes carbon dioxide, there is less carbon dioxide in the blood to combine with water to form carbonic acid. Similarly, if the blood level of carbon dioxide is low, respirations are depressed to maintain a normal ratio between carbonic acid and basic bicarbonate.

Renal Control of Hydrogen Ion Concentration. The kidneys control extracellular fluid pH by eliminating either hydrogen ions or bicarbonate ions from body fluids. If the bicarbonate concentration in the extracellular fluid is greater than normal, the kidneys excrete more bicarbonate ions, making the urine more alkaline. Conversely, if more hydrogen ions are excreted in the urine, the urine becomes more acidic. The renal mechanism for regulating acid-base balance cannot readjust the pH within seconds, as can the extracellular fluid buffer system, nor within minutes as can the respiratory compensatory mechanism, but it can function over a period of several hours or days to correct an acid-base imbalance.

FACTORS AFFECTING FLUID AND ELECTROLYTE BALANCE

The balance of fluids and electrolytes in the body is dependent on many factors and will vary depending on such elements as age and lifestyle.

Age

Body water distribution is relative to body size. The smaller the body, the larger the fluid content:

- Adult, 60% water
- Child, 60% to 77% water
- Infant, 77% water
- Embryo, 97% water

In the elderly, body water diminishes because of tissue loss; the percentage of total body weight that is fluid may be reduced to 45% to 50% in persons over age 65.

Lifestyle

Loss of body fluids can result from stress, exercise, or a warm or humid environment. Stress leads to increased blood volume and decreased urine production, with a subsequent intensification of antidiuretic hormone levels. Sweating and exercise cause the body to lose water and sodium, thus necessitating electrolyte replacement and intensifying the thirst response. Warm climates can exert a similar effect.

An individual's diet will also determine fluid and electrolyte levels. Adequate intake of fluids, carbohydrates, potassium, calcium, sodium, fats, and protein is essential in helping the body maintain homeostatis and function properly. Dehydration is one of the most common yet most serious fluid imbalances that can occur from poor monitoring of diet. It is important to ensure that all patients understand the role water plays in health and to see that patients understand how to maintain adequate hydration status.

DISTURBANCES IN FLUID, ELECTROLYTE, AND ACID-BASE BALANCE

Disturbances in fluid balance can be divided into fluid volume excess and fluid volume deficit. Similarly, electrolyte disturbances involve either too little electrolyte or too much electrolyte. Acid-base imbalances caused by a disturbance in the level of either carbonic acid or bicarbonate are also discussed.

Fluid Disturbances

The fluid balance in the body is important, not only to provide enough water for the body to perform the needed chemical processes, but because many of the body's systems depend upon having a normal amount of fluid available to function properly.

Fluid Volume Excess. Fluid volume excess (FVE) exists when the patient has increased interstitial and intravascular fluid retention and edema. FVE is related to the excess fluid either in tissues of the extremities (peripheral edema) or in lung tissues (pulmonary edema). Factors that put the patient at risk for FVE are:

- Excessive intake of fluids (e.g., intravenous therapy, sodium)
- Increased loss or decreased intake of protein (chronic diarrhea, burns, kidney disease, malnutrition)
- Compromised regulatory mechanisms (kidney failure)
- Decreased intravascular movement (impaired myocardial contractility)
- Lymphatic obstruction (cancer, surgical removal of lymph nodes, obesity)
- Medications (steroid excess)
- Allergic reaction

Assessment findings in the patient with FVE include acute weight gain; decreased serum osmolality, protein and albumin, BUN, Hgb, Hct; increased central venous pressure (greater than 12–15 cm H_2O); and signs and symptoms of edema. The clinical manifestations of edema are relative to the area of involvement, either pulmonary or peripheral (see Table 5–3).

Fluid Volume Deficit. Fluid volume deficit (FVD) exists when the patient experiences vascular, interstitial, or intracellular dehydration. The degree of dehydration is classified as mild, marked, severe, or fatal on the basis of the percentage of body weight lost. There are multiple causes of FVD (see Table 5–4).

TABLE 5–3 Clinical Manifestations of Edema

Pulmonary Edema	Peripheral Edema
Constant cough	Pitting edema in extremities
Dyspnea	Edematous area: tight, smooth, shiny, pale, cool skin
Engorged neck and hand veins	Puffy eyelids
Moist rales in lungs	Weight gain
Bounding pulse	

TABLE 5–4 Causes of Fluid Volume Deficits

- Excessive fluid loss from diaphoresis, vomiting, diarrhea, hemorrhage, burns, ascites, wound drainage, indwelling tubes, or suction
- Diabetes insipidus
- Diabetes mellitus
- Addison's disease (adrenal insufficiency)
- Gastrointestinal fistula or draining abscess
- Intestinal obstruction

Assessment findings in the patient with FVD include thirst and weight loss, with the amount varying with the degree of dehydration. With marked dehydration, the mucous membranes and skin are dry. There is poor skin turgor; low-grade temperature elevation; tachycardia; respirations 28 or greater; a decrease (10–15 mm Hg) in systolic blood pressure; slowing in venous filling; a decrease in urine; concentrated urine; and an acid blood pH (less than 7.4).

Severe dehydration is characterized by the symptoms of marked dehydration. Also, the skin becomes flushed. The systolic blood pressure continues to drop (60 mm Hg or below). There are behavioral changes (restlessness, irritability, disorientation, and delirium). The signs of fatal dehydration are anuria and coma that leads to death.

Electrolyte Disturbances

In health, normal homeostatic mechanisms function to maintain electrolyte and acid-base balance. In illness, one or more of the regulating mechanisms may be affected, or the imbalance may become too great for the body to correct without treatment. Table 5–5 describes common causes and clinical manifestations for electrolyte disturbances.

Sodium. Sodium is the primary determinant of extracellular fluid concentration because of its high concentration and inability to cross the cell membrane easily. As presented in Table 5–5, alterations in sodium concentration can produce profound central nervous system effects on cognition and sensory perception and on the circulating blood volume. When the kidneys reabsorb sodium ions, chloride and water are reabsorbed with the sodium to maintain the body's fluid volume.

TABLE 5-5 Manifestations of Common Electrolyte Disturbances

Disturbance/Causes	Clinical Manifestations
Hyponatremia	
Nutrition and metabolism • Low sodium intake • High water intake • Anorexia nervosa • Loss of GI secretions (vomiting, diarrhea, bulimia, suctioning or drainage, tap-water enemas) • Loss of ECF sodium (peritonitis, burns) • Excessive ingestion of water or administration of IV solutions (D_5W) • ECF sodium dilution (congestive heart failure [CHF], cirrhosis, nephrosis) Elimination • Advanced renal disorders • Diuretics • Antidiuretic hormone (ADH) • Syndrome of inappropriate antidiuretic hormone (SIADH)	Cognitive and sensory • Headaches • Apprehension • Lethargy • Confusion • Depression • Convulsion Activity/mobility • Muscular weakness Skin and mucous membranes • Dry, pale skin • Dry mucous membranes Oxygenation and ECG • Tachycardia • Hypotension Nutrition and metabolism • Nausea • Vomiting • Diarrhea • Abdominal cramps Biochemical • Serum sodium ↓ 135 mEq/l • Specific gravity ↓ 1.008 • Serum osmolality ↓ 280 mOsm/kg
Hypernatremia	
Nutrition and metabolism • High sodium intake • Low water intake • Severe GI loss (diarrhea and vomiting) • Excessive insensible loss (perspiration) • Salt-water drowning • Administration of IV solutions (hypertonic or isotonic saline, sodium bicarbonate) • Hypertonic saline abortions Elimination • Renal dysfunction (nephritis) • Peritoneal dialysis with glucose solution • Uncompensated diabetes insipidus Hemostatic dysfunction • CHF (↓ cardiac output, ↓ renal flow, ↑ sodium retention) • Nephrotic syndrome and cirrhosis (↑ aldosterone leading to ↑ sodium retention)	Cognitive and sensory • Restlessness • Agitation • Delirium • Twitching • Convulsions • Coma Activity/mobility • ↑ Muscle tone • Hyperreflexia Skin and mucous membranes • Flushed, dry skin • Red, dry tongue • Sticky mucous membranes Oxygenation and ECG • Tachycardia

(continues)

TABLE 5-5 Manifestations of Common Electrolyte Disturbances (continued)

Disturbance/Causes	Clinical Manifestations
Hypernatremia (continued)	Nutrition and metabolism • Nausea • Vomiting • Anorexia Elimination • Polyuria (nephritis and uncompensated diabetes insipidus) Biochemical • Serum sodium ↑ 146 mEq/l • Urine sodium ↓ 40 mEq/l • Specific gravity ↑ 1.025 • Serum osmolality ↑ 295 mOsm/kg
Hypokalemia Nutrition and metabolism • Malnutrition • Starvation • Crash diets • Alcoholism • Anorexia nervosa • Stress • Licorice abuse • GI loss (vomiting, diarrhea, gastric or intestinal suctioning, intestinal fistula) • NPO and potassium-free IV fluids • Diabetes mellitus • Hyperaldosteronism • Adrenal tumor, cirrhosis, CHF Elimination • Laxative abuse • Bulimia • Enemas • Potassium-depleting diuretics (thiazide and furosemide) • Diuretic phase of acute renal failure • Dialysis • Steroids • Cushing's syndrome Skin and cellular integrity: • Trauma • Tissue injury • Surgery Redistribution of potassium • Insulin • Alkalotic state • Healing phase of burns • Recovery from diabetic acidosis	Nutrition and metabolism • ↓ Motility (hypoactive → absent bowel sounds) • Abdominal distention • Paralytic ileus • Nausea • Vomiting Cognitive and sensory • Malaise • Disorientation • Coma • Loss of tactile discrimination Activity/mobility • Muscle weakness • Hyporeflexia Elimination • Constipation • Polyuria Oxygenation and ECG • Diminished breath sounds • Shallow, rapid, ineffective respirations • Tachycardia • ↓ Peripheral pulses • Postural hypotension • ↑ Sensitivity to digitalis • ST depression • T wave inverted • U wave prominent • Heart block • Cardiac arrest (severe hypokalemia) Biochemical • Serum potassium ↓ 3.5 mEq/l • Serum osmolality ↓ 280 mOsm/l

(continues)

TABLE 5-5 Manifestations of Common Electrolyte Disturbances (continued)

Disturbance/Causes	Clinical Manifestations
Hyperkalemia Nutrition and metabolism • Oral potassium supplement • IV potassium Elimination • Acute and chronic renal failure • Potassium-sparing diuretics • Addison's disease Skin and cellular integrity • Massive trauma and crushing injuries • Hemolysis • Tourniquet application • Phlebotomy • Burns	Nutrition and metabolism • Abdominal cramps (intermittent GI pain) • Nausea • Diarrhea Activity/mobility • Muscular weakness • Paresthesia • Muscle cramps and pain Elimination • Oliguria or anuria Oxygenation and ECG • Bradycardia → arrest • T wave tented • P wave small → nonvisible • QRS complex widened • Life-threatening dysrhythmias (supraventricular and/or ventricular tachycardia, premature ventricular beats, and ventricular fibrillation → arrest) Biochemical • Serum potassium ↑ 5.3 mEq/l • Serum osmolality ↑ 295 mOsm/l
Hypocalcemia Nutrition and metabolism • Inadequate dietary intake of calcium-rich foods (e.g., during pregnancy and lactation, when calcium requirements are high) • Poor vitamin D intake and absorption • Associated disorders: hypoparathyroidism, pancreatitis, acute metabolic acidosis, and accidental surgical removal of parathyroid glands during a thyroidectomy Elimination • Diarrhea • Wound drainage	Cognitive and sensory • Anxiety, irritability • Tingling and numbness of fingers • Tetany • Convulsions Activity/mobility • Abdominal and muscle cramps • Positive Trousseau's sign (carpopedal spasm with hypoxia) • Positive Chvostek's sign (contraction of facial muscles when facial nerve is tapped) • Pathologic fractures (persistent deficit) Oxygenation and ECG • ↓ Stroke volume • ECG changes: ST segment lengthened and prolonged PR interval Biochemical • ↓ Prothrombin • Serum calcium ↓ 4.5 mEq/l (total) • Elevated serum phosphorus

(continues)

TABLE 5-5 Manifestations of Common Electrolyte Disturbances (continued)

Disturbance/Causes	Clinical Manifestations
Hypercalcemia Activity/mobility • Excessive movement of calcium out of bones: multiple fractures, bone tumors, immobility Nutrition and metabolism • Overconsumption of milk or dietary salts • Overactivity of parathyroid glands Elimination • Renal impairment • Thiazide diuretics • Steroid therapy	Cognitive and sensory • Depression and lethargy Activity/mobility • ↓ Muscle tone and deep tendon reflexes • Osteoporosis • Osteomalacia • Pathologic fractures • Deep bone pain Oxygenation and ECG • Heart block • Arrest (hypercalcemia crisis) Nutrition and metabolism • Nausea, vomiting, anorexia • Constipation Elimination • Flank pain from calculi • Polyuria Biochemical • Serum calcium >5.5 mEq/l (total)
Hypomagnesemia Nutrition and metabolism • Prolonged inadequate dietary intake of magnesium (e.g., malnutrition and alcoholism) • Excessive losses of magnesium (e.g., vomiting, gastric suction) • Prolonged administration of IV solutions without magnesium additives Elimination • Severe renal disease • Thiazide diuretics • Aldosterone excess • Polyuria	Cognitive and sensory • Disorientation, confusion • Vertigo • Irritability, tremors Activity/mobility • ↑ Tendon reflexes • Positive Chvostek's & Trousseau's signs Oxygenation and ECG • ↑ BP • Tachycardia • Dysrhythmias • T wave flat or inverted • ST segment depressed Biochemical • Serum magnesium ↓ 1.5 mEq/l
Hypermagnesemia Nutrition and metabolism • Excessive treatment of magnesium deficit Elimination • Renal failure	Cognitive and sensory • Lethargy, drowsiness • Coma Activity/mobility • Muscle weakness, paralysis • ↓ Deep-tendon reflexes

(continues)

TABLE 5-5 Manifestations of Common Electrolyte Disturbances (continued)

Disturbance/Causes	Clinical Manifestations
Hypermagnesemia (continued)	Oxygenation and ECG • ↓ respirations, 10 to 12 per minute • ↓ BP • Bradycardia • AV block • Respiratory and cardiac arrest (severe hypermagnesemia) • QRS complex widening • QT interval prolonged Biochemical • Serum magnesium ↑ 2.5 mEq/l
Hypophosphatemia Nutrition and metabolism • Inadequate intake: malnutrition, chronic alcoholism • Prolonged administration of IV solutions that are phosphorus-poor or phosphorus-free • Acid-base imbalances (e.g., diabetic ketoacidosis and respiratory alkalosis) • Increased secretion of parathyroid hormone • Overuse of aluminum-containing antacids	Cognitive and sensory • Confusion, seizures, coma • Fatigue, memory loss Activity/mobility • Muscle pain, weakness • Paresthesia • Hyporeflexia • Bone pain • Joint stiffness Oxygenation and ECG • Tissue hypoxia • Hyperventilation • Possible bleeding • Weak pulse Safety • Possible infection Nutrition and metabolism • Anorexia • Dysphagia Biochemical • Serum phosphate ↓ 1.7 mEq/l • ↓ Platelet count • ↓ Leukocyte • ↓ Oxygen saturation • ↑ Cardiac enzymes
Hyperphosphatemia Nutrition and metabolism • Excessive administration of oral and IV solutions containing phosphate substances • Hypoparathyroidism • Laxatives containing phosphate Elimination • Renal insufficiency	Activity/mobility • Tetany • Muscle weakness • Flaccid paralysis • Circumoral paraesthesia • Hyperreflexia Oxygenation and ECG • Tachycardiac • ST segment shortened • QT interval shortened

(continues)

TABLE 5-5 Manifestations of Common Electrolyte Disturbances (continued)

Disturbance/Causes	Clinical Manifestations
Hyperphosphatemia (continued)	Nutrition and metabolism • Nausea, anorexia, vomiting, diarrhea Biochemical • Serum level ↑ 2.6 mEq/l • ↓ Serum calcium

Hyponatremia. **Hyponatremia** is a deficit in the extracellular level of sodium. With hyponatremia, there is either a sodium deficit or a water excess; a hypo-osmolar state exists because the ratio of water to sodium is too high. The water moves out of the vascular space into the interstitial space and then into the intracellular space, causing edema.

Hypernatremia. **Hypernatremia** is an excess in the extracellular level of sodium. With an excess of sodium or a loss of water, a hyperosmolar state exists because the ratio of sodium to water is too high. This ratio causes an increase in the extracellular osmotic pressure, which pulls fluid out of the cells into the extracellular space. The symptoms of this increase depend on the cause and the location of the edema (see Table 5–5).

Potassium. The normal range of extracellular potassium is narrow (3.5–5.0 mEq/l). The slightest decrease or increase can cause serious or life-threatening effects on physiological functions. A reciprocal relationship exists between sodium and potassium; large sodium intake results in an increased loss of potassium, and vice versa. When potassium is lost from the cells, sodium enters the cells. Intracellular potassium deficit may coexist with an excess of extracellular potassium. There are two main categories of diuretics that can cause hypokalemia:

1. *Potassium-wasting diuretics* excrete potassium and other electrolytes, such as sodium and chloride. Furosemide is an example of a potassium-wasting diuretic.
2. *Potassium-sparing diuretics* retain potassium but excrete sodium and chloride. Spirmolactine is an ecample of a potassium-sparing diuretic.

Hypokalemia. **Hypokalemia** is a decrease in the extracellular level of potassium. Gastrointestinal-tract disturbances and the use of diuretics can place the client at risk for hypokalemia and an acid-base imbalance (metabolic alkalosis). Potassium-wasting diuretics can cause hypokalemia. Besides diuretics, other major drug groups that can cause hypokalemia are laxatives, corticosteroids, and antibiotics. Hypokalemia can cause cardiac arrest when the potassium level is very low. Hypokalemia also enhances the action of digitalis, placing the patient taking digitalis at risk for toxicity (see Chapter 8, Cardiovascular System, and Chapter 15, Toxicology, for more information).

Hyperkalemia. **Hyperkalemia** is an increase in the extracellular level of potassium. There are major drug groups that may cause hyperkalemia:

- Potassium-sparing diuretics
- Central nervous system agents
- Oral and intravenous replacement potassium salts

Hyperkalemia can also inhibit the action of digitalis.

Calcium. Most of the body's calcium (99%) is deposited in bone as phosphate and carbonate. The remaining 1% is in the blood plasma (serum). Normally, 50% of the serum calcium is ionized (physiologically active), with the remaining 50% bound to protein. Free, ionized calcium is needed for cell membrane permeability. The calcium that is bound to plasma protein cannot pass through the capillary wall and therefore cannot leave the intravascular compartment.

A stable blood level of calcium is maintained by a negative-feedback system controlled by vitamin D, parathyroid hormone, calcitonin (thyrocalcitonin), and the serum concentrations of calcium and phosphate ions (see Chapter 11). A decreased blood level stimulates the parathyroid gland to secrete parathyroid hormone, which in turn mobilizes the release of calcium from the bone, increases the renal reabsorption, and increases intestinal absorption in the presence of vitamin D. Similarly, calcitonin, secreted by the thyroid gland, reduces the blood calcium concentration.

Calcium ions are never completely absorbed from the gastrointestinal tract. Dietary calcium absorption and utilization require an adequate amount of protein and vitamin D. Besides being needed by the body for bone and tooth formation, calcium is an important ion in the blood-clotting mechanism, maintaining the integrity of the neuromuscular system, and driving muscle contraction.

Hypocalcemia. **Hypocalcemia** is a decrease in the extracellular level of calcium. The rapid administration of citrated blood, alkalosis, and elevated levels of serum albumin increase the activity of calcium binders, thereby decreasing the amount of free calcium.

Hypercalcemia. Hypercalcemia is an increase in the extracellular level of calcium. The clinical symptoms result from a decrease in neuromuscular activity, reabsorption of calcium from bone, and the kidney's response to a high serum calcium concentration.

Magnesium. Magnesium plays an important role as a coenzyme in the metabolism of carbohydrates and proteins and as a mediator in neuromuscular activity. Magnesium has the unique characteristic of being the only cation that has a higher concentration in cerebrospinal fluid than in extracellular fluid.

Hypomagnesemia. **Hypomagnesemia** is a decrease in the extracellular level of magnesium and usually occurs with hypokalemia and hypocalcemia. It is probably the most undiagnosed electrolyte deficit because it is asymptomatic until the serum level is very low.

Drugs that may cause hypomagnesemia include: digitalis, potassium-wasting diuretics, cortisone, aminoglycosides, and amphotericin B; the chronic use of laxatives may also cause the condition. Clinical manifestations are related to the neuromuscular, neurologic, or cardiovascular system (see Table 5–5).

Hypermagnesemia. **Hypermagnesemia** refers to an increase in the extracellular level of magnesium. It rarely occurs from excessive dietary ingestion; however, overuse of magnesium-containing drugs (antacids, laxatives, and intravenous magnesium sulfate) can cause hypermagnesemia. The clinical manifestations of hypermagnesemia are nonspecific (refer to Table 5–5).

Phosphate. Phosphate is the main intracellular anion; it appears as phosphorus in the serum. Phosphorus is similar to calcium in that vitamin D is needed for its reabsorption from the renal tubules.

Hypophosphatemia. **Hypophosphatemia** is a decreased extracellular level of phosphorus. An increase in parathyroid hormone causes decreased renal reabsorption and increased excretion of phosphates. The aim of nursing care is to protect the client from injury and to correct the deficit (see Table 5–5).

Hyperphosphatemia. **Hyperphosphatemia** is an increased extracellular level of phosphorus. Excessive administration (oral or intravenous) of phosphate-containing substances can cause hyperphosphatemia. Other causes of hyperphosphatemia are hypoparathyroidism, renal insufficiency, and laxatives containing phosphate.

Chloride. As previously stated, chloride and water move in the same direction as sodium ions, influencing the osmolality of extracellular fluid. Although chloride losses usually follow sodium losses, the proportion will differ because a loss of chloride can be compensated for by an increase in bicarbonate. Therefore, signs and symptoms of a chloride imbalance will be similar to those of a metabolic acid-base imbalance, discussed later in this chapter. A deficit of either chloride or potassium will lead to a deficiency of the other electrolyte.

Hypochloremia. **Hypochloremia** is a decrease in the extracellular level of chloride. Gastrointestinal tract losses may cause a decrease in chloride because of the acid content of gastric juices, mainly hydrogen chloride. Because the bicarbonate ion compensates for the loss of chloride, the client is at risk for developing metabolic alkalosis. The signs and symptoms of hypochloremia are muscle twitching and slow, shallow breathing. With a severe loss of chloride and extracellular fluid volume, there may be a drop in blood pressure.

Hyperchloremia. **Hyperchloremia** is an increase in the extracellular level of chloride. It usually occurs with dehydration, hypernatremia, and metabolic acidosis. The signs and symptoms of hyperchloremia are muscle weakness, deep, rapid breathing, and lethargy progressing to unconsciousness if untreated.

Acid-Base Disturbances

The common types of acid-base imbalances are respiratory acidosis and alkalosis and metabolic acidosis and alkalosis.

Laboratory Data. The biochemical indicators of acid-base imbalance are assessed by measurement of arterial blood gases (ABGs). **Arterial blood gases** measure the levels of oxygen and carbon dioxide in arterial blood. The levels of blood pH, bicarbonate ion, sodium, potassium, and chloride are also important in the assessment of acid-base imbalance.

In the determination of whether the acid-base imbalance is caused by a respiratory or a metabolic alteration, the key indicators are bicarbonate and carbonic acid levels (Figure 5–6). With respiratory acidosis and alkalosis, the bicarbonate level is normal and carbonic acid is either increased (acidosis) or decreased (alkalosis). With metabolic acidosis and alkalosis, the carbonic acid is normal and the bicarbonate level is either decreased (acidosis) or increased (alkalosis).

Respiratory Acidosis (Carbonic Acid Excess). Respiratory acidosis is characterized by an increased hydrogen ion concentration (a blood pH below 7.35), an increased arterial carbon dioxide pressure (greater than 45 mm Hg), and an excess of carbonic acid. Respiratory acidosis is caused by hypoventilation or any condition that depresses ventilation (see Table 5–6).

Hypoventilation can begin in the respiratory system, as occurs with respiratory failure, or outside the respiratory system, as occurs with drug overdose. Common drugs that can cause central nervous system depression and place the client at risk for respiratory acidosis are narcotics, barbiturates, and anesthetic agents.

Patients with respiratory acidosis experience neurologic changes resulting from the acidity of the cerebrospinal fluid and brain cells. Hypoventilation causes **hypoxemia** (decreased oxygen levels), which causes further neurologic impairments. Hyperkalemia may accompany acidosis. See Table 5–7 for the clinical manifestations of respiratory acidosis.

Respiratory Alkalosis (Carbonic Acid Deficit). Respiratory acidosis is characterized by a decreased hydrogen ion concentration (a blood pH above 7.45) and a decreased arterial carbon dioxide pressure (less than 35 mm Hg). Respiratory alkalosis is caused by hyperventilation (excessive exhalation of carbon dioxide) resulting in hypocapnia (decreased arterial carbon dioxide concentration). Hyperventilation can be triggered by hypoxia at high altitudes, anxiety, fear, pain, fever, and rapid mechanical ventilation. Other causes of hyperventilation, which involve overstimulation of the respiratory center, include salicylate poisoning, hyperthyroidism, pneumonia, atelectasis, asthma, adult respiratory distress syndrome, congestive heart failure, pulmonary edema and embolus, brain tumors, meningitis, and encephalitis; refer to Table 5–7 for the clinical manifestations of respiratory alkalosis.

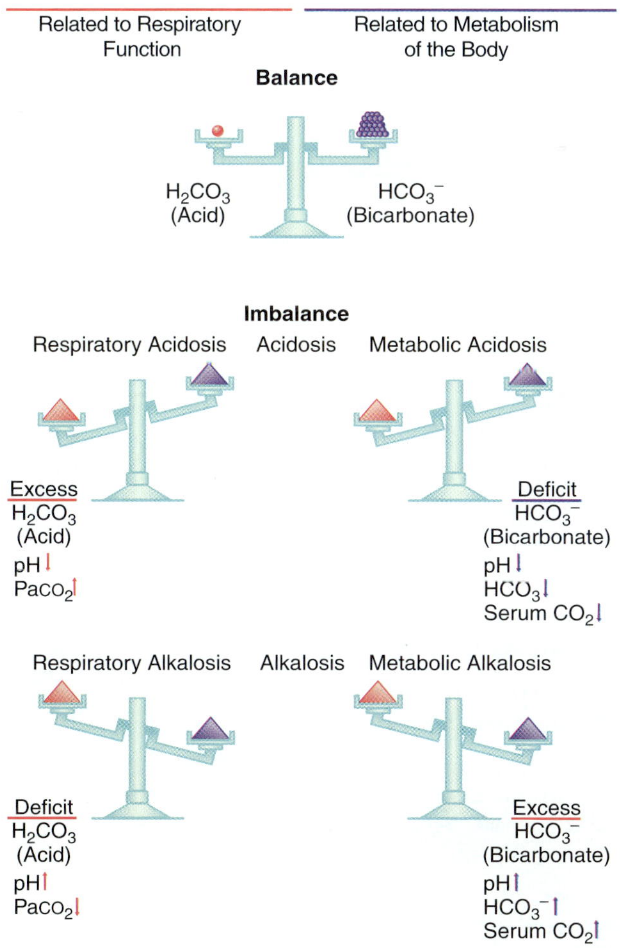

Figure 5–6 Acid-base balance and imbalance.

TABLE 5–6 Common Causes of Acute and Chronic Respiratory Acidosis

Acute	Chronic
Drug-induced CNS depression	Asthma
Pneumonia and atelectasis	Cystic fibrosis
Pulmonary edema	Emphysema
Respiratory distress syndrome	
Pneumothorax	
Hypoventilation	
Poliomyelitis	
Chest trauma	
Brain and spinal cord injury	

TABLE 5-7 Respiratory and Metabolic Acidosis and Alkalosis

Imbalance/Causes	Clinical Manifestations
Respiratory Acidosis (Retention of Carbon Dioxide)	
• CNS disorders • Drug overdose • Pneumonia • Pulmonary edema • Pneumothorax • Restrictive lung disease	Cognitive and sensory • Disorientation • Depression • Weakness → stupor Skin and mucous membranes • Flushed and warm Oxygenation and ECG • Dyspnea • Tachycardia • Dysrhythmia Biochemical • ↓ pH (<7.35) • ↑ $Paco_2$ (>45 mm Hg) • ↑ HCO_3 (>28 mEq/l, indicating metabolic renal compensation)
Respiratory Alkalosis (Hyperventilation)	
• Anxiety, fear • CNS disorders • Pain • Fever • Pneumonia, atelectasis • Asthma • Adult respiratory distress syndrome (ARDS) • Congestive heart failure, pulmonary edema • Pulmonary embolus	Cognitive and sensory • Hyperactive reflexes • Tetany • Positive Chvostek's sign • Positive Trousseau's sign • Vertigo • Unconsciousness Skin and mucous membranes • Sweating (may occur) Oxygenation and ECG • Rapid, shallow breathing • Palpitations Biochemical (uncompensated respiratory alkalosis) • ↑ pH (>7.45) • ↓ $Paco_2$ (<35 mm Hg)
Metabolic Acidosis (Gain of Metabolic Acids or Loss of Base)	
Increased acids: • Renal failure • Diabetic ketoacidosis • Anaerobic metabolism • Drug overdose (salicylates, methanol) Loss of base: • Diarrhea	Cognitive and sensory • Restlessness, disorientation • Stupor, coma Activity/mobility • Weakness, lethargy Skin and mucous membranes • Warm, flushed skin Oxygenation and ECG • Kussmaul breathing (deep, rapid respirations) • Bradycardia, decreased cardiac output • Dysrhythmias Nutrition and metabolism • Nausea, vomiting • Abdominal pain

(continues)

TABLE 5-7 Respiratory and Metabolic Acidosis and Alkalosis (continued)

Imbalance/Causes	Clinical Manifestations
Metabolic Acidosis (Gain of Metabolic Acids or Loss of Base) (continued)	
	Biochemical • ↓ pH (<7.35) • ↓ HCO_3^- (<24 mEq/l) • ↓ BE (base excess <2 mEq/l) • ↓ Serum CO_2 (<22 mEq/l)
Metabolic Alkalosis (Gain of Base of Loss of Metabolic Acids)	
Gain of base: • Excess ingestion of antacids • Excess administration of sodium bicarbonate Loss of metabolic acids: • Vomiting • Nasogastric suctioning or lavage • Low potassium or chloride • Increased aldosterone • Administration of steroids or diuretics	Cognitive and sensory • Irritability, confusion Activity/mobility • Tetany • Hypertonic muscles • Hypertonic reflexes Oxygenation and ECG • Depressed rate and depth of respirations Nutrition and metabolism • Vomiting Biochemical • ↑ pH (>7.45) • ↑ HCO_3^- (>28 mEq/l) • ↑ BE (base excess >2 mEq/l) • ↓ Serum levels of potassium and chloride

(From Hartshorn, J., Lamborn, M., & Noll, M. [1993]. *Introduction to critical care nursing.* Philadelphia: Saunders; Kee, J. L., & Paulanka, B. J. [1994]. *Fluids and electrolytes with clinical applications* [5th ed.]. Albany, NY: Delmar Publishers.)

Metabolic Acidosis (Bicarbonate Deficit). Metabolic acidosis is characterized by an increase in hydrogen ion concentration (blood pH below 7.35) or a decrease in bicarbonate concentration. Causes of metabolic acidosis can be divided into two categories: loss of base and gain in metabolic acids. Chronic diarrhea causes an excessive loss of bicarbonate and sodium ions from the small intestines. With the loss of sodium ions, chloride ions are in excess and combine with hydrogen to produce a strong acid (hydrochloric acid).

Clients with certain medical diagnoses are at risk for metabolic acidosis. Such conditions include:

1. Diabetic ketoacidosis: The cells are deprived of glucose (decrease or absence of insulin) for metabolism; the liver, in response to the needs of the cells, increases the metabolism of fatty acids, which causes an increase in ketone bodies, making the extracellular fluid more acidic (see Chapter 11).
2. Renal failure: The normal mechanism of the kidneys to conserve sodium and water and excrete hydrogen is compromised (see Chapter 14).
3. Anaerobic metabolism: Cellular catabolism and acid accumulation occur with starvation, severe malnutrition, infection, fever, trauma, shock, and excessive exercise.
4. Drug overdose: Acid accumulation results from excessive ingestion of salicylate, paraldehyde, and methanol (see Chapter 15).

In response to metabolic acidosis, the respiratory center is stimulated, causing an increase in the rate and depth of respirations (Kussmaul's respirations); to lower the acid concentration in extracellular fluid by increasing the exhalation of carbon dioxide. The respiratory compensatory mechanism is usually ineffective in decreasing acids, especially if the client has chronic obstructive pulmonary disease or is in ketoacidosis. The renal compensatory mechanism tries to increase the pH by exchanging sodium ions with hydrogen ions to increase the excretion of hydrogen; refer to Table 5–7 for the clinical manifestations and treatment of metabolic acidosis.

Metabolic Alkalosis (Bicarbonate Excess). Metabolic alkalosis is characterized by an increased loss of acid from the body or a gain in base (increased levels of bicarbonate). The blood pH is above 7.45. A gain in base may result from excessive ingestion of antacids and milk, often used in the treatment of gastric ulcers. These substances neutralize acids, producing alkalosis and hypercalcemia. The excessive oral or parenteral administration of sodium bicarbonate or other alkaline salts (e.g., sodium or potassium acetate, lactate, or citrate) increases the amount of base in extracellular fluids.

The following clinical conditions can place clients at risk for metabolic alkalosis:

1. Vomiting and nasogastric suctioning or lavage cause a loss in hydrochloric acid and chloride; with the loss of the hydrogen and chloride ions, bicarbonate ions are absorbed, unneutralized, into the bloodstream and the pH of the extracellular fluid rises (alkalosis).
2. Diarrhea, and steroid or diuretic therapy can cause the excessive loss of potassium, chloride, and other electrolytes; the potassium deficit causes the kidneys to exchange hydrogen ions (instead of potassium ions) for sodium ions, which promotes the loss of hydrogen, thereby increasing bicarbonate level.

The respiratory and renal compensatory mechanisms respond to an increased bicarbonate-carbonic acid ratio. The rate and depth of respirations are decreased in an effort to retain carbon dioxide. The arterial carbon dioxide concentration rises, creating respiratory acidosis, to counter the pH imbalance of metabolic alkalosis.

A normal serum potassium level is a prerequisite to renal compensation. In alkalosis, potassium ions enter the cells in exchange for hydrogen ions, causing hypokalemia. Hypokalemia further potentiates metabolic alkalosis because the kidneys conserve hydrogen ions by excreting potassium ions in exchange for sodium ions. When hypokalemia is present, the kidneys cannot function as a compensatory mechanism; therefore, they continue to excrete hydrogen, and bicarbonate excess continues. Refer to Table 5–7 for the clinical manifestations and treatment of metabolic alkalosis.

ASSESSMENT

Assessment data are used to identify patients who have potential or actual alterations in fluid volume. Patients receiving certain treatments, such as medications and IV therapy, are at risk for developing imbalances. The key assessment indicators that identify imbalances are changes in weight, vital signs, changes in intake and output, and the physical findings of the skin, oral cavity, eyes, venous filling, and neuromuscular system.

Health History

Some of the key history items relevant to fluid and electrolyte disturbances are listed in Table 5–8.

Physical Examination

The EMS provider performs a complete physical examination and identifies all abnormalities because fluid alterations may affect any body system. The physical assessment of patients with altered fluid status is discussed in this section.

Vital Signs. Measurement of vital signs provides the EMS provider with information regarding the patient's fluid, electrolyte, and acid-base status and the body's compensatory response for maintaining balance. An elevated temperature places the patient at risk for dehydration caused by an increased loss of body fluid.

Changes in the pulse rate, strength, and rhythm are indicative of fluid alterations. Fluid volume alterations may cause the following pulse changes:

- Fluid volume deficit (FVD): increased pulse rate and weak pulse volume
- Fluid volume excess (FVE): increased pulse volume and third heart sound

TABLE 5-8 Health History

• Lifestyle (sociocultural and economic factors, stress, exercise)
• Dietary intake (recent changes in the amount and types of fluid and food, increased thirst)
• Religion (whether illness has had an effect on beliefs or religion; query whether the client would like a visit from his or her religious counselor)
• Weight (sudden gain or loss)
• Fluid output (recent changes in the frequency or amount of urine output)
• Gastrointestinal disturbances (prolonged vomiting, diarrhea, anorexia, ulcers, hemorrhage)
• Fever and diaphoresis
• Draining wounds, burns, trauma
• Disease conditions that could upset homeostasis (renal disease, endocrine disorders, neural malfunction, pulmonary disease)
• Therapeutic programs that can produce imbalances (special diets, medications, chemotherapy, administration of interavenous fluid or total parenteral nutrition, gastric or intestinal suction)

Respiratory changes are assessed by inspecting the movement of the chest wall, counting the rate, and auscultating the lungs. Changes in the rate and depth may cause respiratory acid-base imbalances or may be indicative of a compensatory response in metabolic acidosis or alkalosis, as previously described in Table 5–7.

Blood pressure measurements can be used to assess the degree of FVD. FVD can lower the blood pressure with or without orthostatic hypotension. A narrow pulse pressure (less than 20 mm Hg) may indicate FVD that occurs with severe hypovolemia.

Edema. **Edema** (the detectable accumulation of increased interstitial fluid) is the main symptom of FVE. Edema may be localized (confined to a specific area) or generalized (occurring throughout the body's tissue). Localized edema is characterized by taut, smooth, shiny, pale skin. The body may retain 5 to 10 pounds of fluid before edema is noticeable. Inspect the dependent body parts—sacrum, back, and legs—to assess peripheral edema. Pitting edema can be described as trace, mild, moderate, or severe depending upon the amount of fluid in the affected area.

Skin Turgor. **Skin turgor** is the normal resiliency of the skin. When the skin is pinched and released, it springs back to a normal position because of the outward pressure exerted by the cells and interstitial fluid. With dehydration there is a decreased skin turgor, as manifested by lax skin that returns slowly to the normal position. Increased skin turgor, which occurs with edema, is manifested by smooth, taut, shiny skin that cannot be grasped and raised.

Buccal (Oral) Cavity. Inspect the buccal cavity. With FVD, there is a decrease in saliva, which causes sticky, dry mucous membranes and dry cracked lips. The tongue has longitudinal furrows.

Eyes. Inspect the eyes. FVD causes sunken eyes, dry conjunctiva, and decreased or absent tearing. Puffy eyelids (periorbital edema, or papilledema) are characteristic of FVE; the patient may also have a history of blurred vision.

Jugular and Hand Veins. Circulatory volume is assessed by measuring venous filling of the jugular and hand veins. Place the patient in a low Fowler's position. Then:

1. Palpate the jugular (neck) veins: FVE causes a distention in the jugular veins (Figure 5–7).

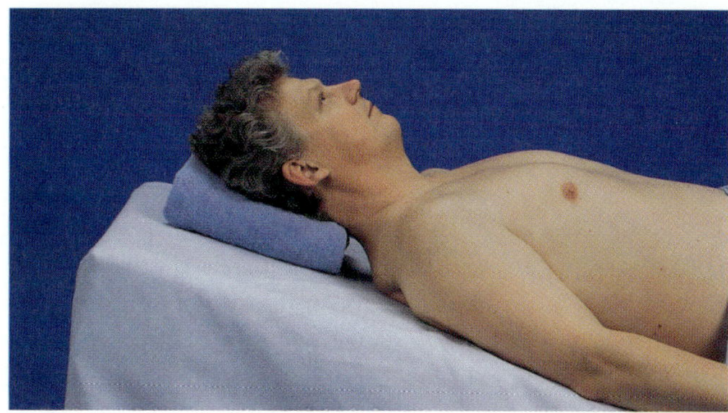

Figure 5–7 Positioning the patient to assess jugular vein distention.

2. Place the client's hand below the heart level, and palpate the jugular veins; with FVD there is decreased venous filling (flat neck veins).

Neuromuscular System. Fluid and electrolyte imbalances may cause neuromuscular alterations: The muscles lose their tone and become soft and underdeveloped, and reflexes are diminished. Calcium and magnesium imbalances cause an increase in neuromuscular irritability.

Other neurologic signs include inability to concentrate, confusion, and emotional lability, as previously described in Tables 5–5 and 5–7.

Diagnostic and Laboratory Data

Biochemical assessment in the emergency department is another essential source of objective data. Laboratory results can be used to detect imbalances before clinical symptoms are assessed in the physical examination. Laboratory tests used in assessing patients with common alterations in extracellular fluid volume are discussed in the following paragraphs.

Hemoglobin and Hematocrit Indices. The hematocrit is affected by changes in plasma volume. For instance, with severe dehydration and hypovolemic shock, the hematocrit is increased, whereas overhydration decreases the hematocrit. Hemoglobin levels are decreased with severe hemorrhage.

Osmolality. **Osmolality** is a measurement of the total concentration of dissolved particles (solutes) per kilogram of water. Osmolality measurements are performed on both serum and urine samples to determine alterations in fluid and electrolyte balance. Osmolality can also be explained in relation to the specific gravity of body fluids.

Specific gravity expresses the weight of the solution when compared with an equal volume of distilled water; the osmolality of a solution can be estimated by the specific gravity.

Serum Osmolality. Serum osmolality is a measurement of the total concentration of dissolved particles per kilogram of water in serum, recorded in milliosmols per kilogram (mOsm/kg). The particles measured in serum osmolality include electrolyte ions, such as sodium and potassium, and electrically inactive substances dissolved in serum, such as glucose and urea. Water and sodium are the main entities that control the osmolality of body fluids. Serum sodium is responsible for 85% to 90% of the serum osmolality.

The normal serum osmolality is 280 to 295 mOsm/kg. It can increase with dehydration and loss of body water and decrease with water excess.

In clinical practice, the terms *osmolality* and **osmolarity** (the concentration of solutes per liter of cellular fluid) are often used interchangeably to refer to the concentration of body fluid. However, these terms are actually different, in that osmolality refers to the concentration of solutes in the total body water (solutes per kilogram of body weight) rather than in cellular fluid. Figure 5–8 relates osmosis to the osmolality of a solution. The appropriate term to use in intravenous fluid therapy is *osmolarity*. An osmolaritic solution is described as:

- **Hypotonic** (hypo-osmolar) when there are fewer solutes in proportion to the volume of water than is the case in the body
- **Isotonic** (iso-osmolar) when body water and solutes (sodium) are in amounts equal to those in the body
- **Hypertonic** (hyperosmolar) when there are more solutes in proportion to the volume of water than is the case in the body

Urine Osmolality. Urine osmolality is a measurement of the total concentration of dissolved particles per kilogram of water in urine, recorded in milliosmols per kilogram (mOsm/kg). The particles measured in urine osmolality come from nitrogenous waste (creatinine, urea, and uric acid), with urea contributing most. Urine osmolality varies greatly with diet and fluid intake and reflects the ability of the kidney to adjust the concentration of urine in order to maintain fluid balance. With normal kidney function, a dehydrated patient will have an elevated urine osmolality, whereas patients with shock, hyperglycemia, hemoconcentration, and acidosis will have elevations in both urine and serum osmolality.

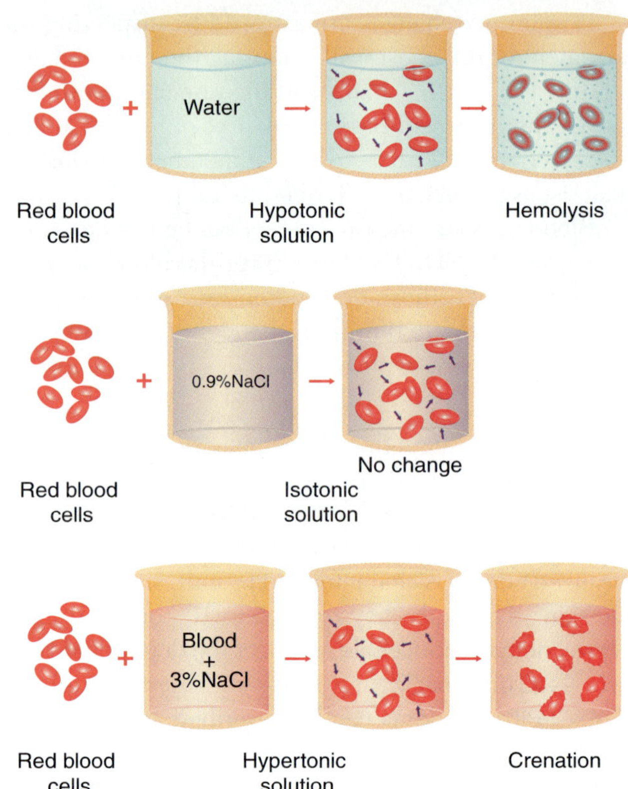

Figure 5–8 Osmosis as it relates to the osmolarity of a solution. The movement of water through a membrane from a lower concentration to a higher concentration is called osmosis. In a hypotonic solution, the water moves into the cells, causing them to swell and burst. The cells in the isotonic solution are normal in size and shape because the same amount of water is entering and leaving the cells. Cells in the hypertonic solution are losing water because water moves from a weaker concentration inside the cell to a greater concentration outside the cell membrane.

Urine pH. The measurement of the pH of urine reveals the hydrogen ion concentration of the urine to determine its acid or alkaline status. When the kidney buffering system is compensating for either metabolic acidosis or alkalosis, the pH of the urine should be within normal range. This is considered a sign of normal function. However, when the renal compensatory function fails to respond to the pH of the blood, the urine pH will increase with acidosis and decrease in alkalosis.

Serum Albumin. Albumin is synthesized in the liver from amino acids. Serum albumin plays an important role in fluid and electrolyte balance by maintaining the colloid osmotic pressure of blood, which prevents the accumulation of fluid (edema) in the tissues. Clinically, this blood test is used to measure prolonged protein depletion, which occurs in chronic malnutrition.

Arterial Blood Gas. Arterial blood gas samples are taken in the emergency department, typically from the radial artery, to assess the patient's acid-base status and oxygenation level. As with many numerical tests, trends may indicate a potential problem before the patient decompensates, allowing intervention earlier. Refer to Figure 5–6 and Table 5–7 for a description of acid-base imbalances.

MANAGEMENT

Intravenous (IV) access is obtained by EMS providers for a variety of reasons, from trauma resuscitation to medication access lines. While the actual equipment and procedure is outside the scope of this text, certain aspects of parenteral fluid and blood product administration are pertinent to the EMS provider.

Parenteral Fluids

Table 5–9 describes the common types of intravenous solutions the EMS provider is likely to encounter in either EMS practice or during interfacility transports. The fluids are divided into three groups by their tonicity and some of the clinical implications of the use of each fluid are presented.

Crystalloids (electrolyte solutions with the potential to form crystals) are used to replace concurrent losses of water, carbohydrates, and electrolytes. Sodium chloride and Ringer's lactate are commonly used crystalloids in EMS practice. Crystalloid solutions can be isotonic (equal to the sodium concentration of the blood, 0.9%); hypotonic (lower than the sodium concentration of the blood); or hypertonic (greater than the sodium concentration of the blood).

Colloids (non-diffusible substances) function like the plasma proteins in the blood by exerting a colloidal pressure to replace intravascular volume only. Examples of colloidal solutions are albumin, dextran, Plasmanate, and hetastarch (artificial blood substitute). During the administration of these solutions, the EMS provider needs to continually monitor the patient for hypotension and allergic reactions.

Blood Transfusion

The EMS provider may have the occasion to transport a patient undergoing a blood transfusion. The purpose of a blood transfusion is to replace blood loss (deficit) with whole blood or blood components. On the basis of the patient's unique needs, the physician determines the type of transfusion to administer, either whole blood or a component of whole blood.

Whole Blood and Blood Products. Patients with a demonstrated deficiency in either whole blood or a specific component of blood are given a blood transfusion. Whole blood contains red blood cells (RBCs) and plasma components of blood. It is used when the patient needs all the components of blood to restore blood volume after severe hemorrhage and to restore the capacity of the blood to carry oxygen. Various types of blood components are used in the clinical setting (see Table 5–10).

Plasma or fresh frozen plasma is separated and frozen within 8 hours after blood collection. Albumin (protein colloid) is a volume expander that maintains the colloid osmotic pressure of the blood. Albumin, hetstarch, and dextran (non-protein colloids) are agents that increase intravascular volume in order to maintain hemodynamic stability and to provide adequate tissue perfusion. Cryoprecipitate is the most expensive of all blood components because it is constituted from many units of whole blood.

When the physician prescribes the administration of whole blood or a blood product, the patient's blood is typed and crossmatched (refer to Chapter 16 for a complete discussion of blood groups and Rhesus [Rh] factor). The blood is stored in the blood bank after typing and crossmatching until it is ready to be administered.

Although whole blood has a refrigerated shelf life of 35 days, platelets must be administered within 3 days after they have been extracted from whole blood. If the RBCs and plasma are frozen, their shelf life can be extended up to 3 years.

Initial Assessment and Preparation. The EMS provider must perform an initial assessment before administering blood. The viscosity of whole blood usually requires the use of an 18- or 19-gauge or larger catheter to prevent damage to the red cells.

Prior to administering any blood products or assuming care for a patient receiving blood products, the EMS provider should confirm that the label on the blood product matches the identity of the patient. The patient should be assessed or re-assessed when assuming care, during the transfusion, and, if multiple bags of blood product are being administered, after each change in bag.

Administering Whole Blood or a Blood Component. The agency's blood protocol may require that a licensed

TABLE 5-9 Common Intravenous Solutions

Tonicity	Solution	Contents (mEq/l)	Clinical Implications
Hypotonic	Sodium chloride 0.45%	77 Na^+, 77 Cl^-	Daily maintenance of body fluid and establishment of renal function.
Isotonic	Dextrose 2.5% in 0.45% saline	77 Na^+, 77 Cl^-	Promotes renal function and urine output.
	Dextrose 5% in 0.2% saline	38 Na^+, 38 Cl^-	Daily maintenance of body fluids when less Na^+ and Cl^- are required.
	Dextrose 5% in water (D_5W)		Promotes rehydration and elimination; may cause urinary Na^+ loss; good vehicle for K^+.
	Ringer's lactate	130 Na^+, 4 K^+, Ca^{2+}, 109 Cl^-, 28 lactate	Resembles the normal composition of blood serum and plasma; K^+ level below body's daily requirement.
	Normal saline (NS), 0.9%	154 Na^+, 154 Cl^-	Restores sodium chloride deficit and extracellular fluid volume.
	Dextran 40 10% in NS (0.9%) or D_5W		A colloidal solution used to increase plasma volume of clients in early shock; *it should not be given to severely* dehydrated clients and clients with renal disease, thrombocytopenia, or active hemorrhaging.
	Dextran 70% in NS		A long-lived (20 hours) plasma volume expander; used to treat shock or impending shock due to hemorrhage, surgery, or burns. *It can prolong bleeding and coats the RBCs (draw type and crossmatch prior to administering).*
Hypertonic	Dextrose 5% in 0.45% saline	77 Na^+, 77 Cl^-	Daily maintenance of body fluid and nutrition; treatment of FVD.
	Dextrose 5% in saline 0.9%	154 Na^+, 154 Cl^-	Fluid replacement of sodium, chloride, and calories (170).
	Dextrose 10% in saline 0.9%	154 Na^+, 154 Cl^-	Fluid replacement of sodium, chloride, and calories (340).
	Dextrose 5% in lactated Ringer's	130 Na^+, 4 K^+, 3 Ca^{2+}, 109 Cl^-, 28 lactate	Resembles the normal composition of blood serum and plasma; K^+ level below body's daily requirement; caloric value 180.
	Hyperosmolar saline 3% and 5% NaCl	856 Na^+, 865 Cl^-	Treatment of hyponatremia; raises the Na osmolarity of the blood, and reduces intracellular fluid excess.
	Ionosol B with dextrose 5%	57 Na^+, 25 K^+, 49 Cl^-, 25 lact., 5 Mg^{2+}, 7 PO^{4-}	Treatment of polyionic parenteral replacement caused by vomiting-induced alkalosis, diabetic acidosis, fluid loss from burns, and postoperative FVD.

person sign a form to release the blood from the blood bank and that a blood product be checked by two licensed personnel prior to infusion. The following information must be on the blood bag label and verified for accuracy: the patient's name and identification number, ABO group and Rh factor, donor number, type of product ordered by the practitioner, and the expiration date.

Observe the blood bag for any signs of puncture, gas bubbles, color, and consistency (RBCs clumping). When the information has been verified, both licensed personnel sign the appropriate form. If any of the information does not match exactly or if the product has expired, do not accept the product and notify the nurse caring for the patient.

TABLE 5-10 Blood-Component Therapy

Type	Use	Special Considerations
Fresh or frozen plasma	Replaces deficient coagulation factors. Increases intravascular compartment.	Use within six hours with any straight-line administration set. Client is at risk for hepatitis.
Platelet	Corrects bleeding disorders (e.g., thrombocytopenia). Replaces platelets.	Infuse at rate of 10 minutes a unit with special platelet administration set.
Albumin	Restores intravascular volume. Treats shock and hypoproteinemia.	Available in 5% and 25% solution. Infuse slowly with special tubing that accompanies solution.
Granulocyte (white blood cell)	Restores the leukocyte count, usually depressed in clients receiving radiation or chemotherapy.	Infuse slowly, over 2- to 4-hour interval with Y-type blood filters, and prime with normal saline.
Cryoprecipitate	Restores factor VIII and fibrinogen in treating hemophilia A.	Infuse with a straight-line administration set. Observe for febrile reactions.

Blood should be administered within 30 minutes after it has been received from the bank, to maintain RBC integrity and to decrease the chance of infection. Whole blood should not go unrefrigerated for more than 4 hours. Room temperature will cause RBC lysis, releasing potassium and causing hyperkalemia.

Safety Measures. The patient should be observed for the initial 15 minutes for a transfusion reaction. Vital signs are usually taken every 15 minutes for the first hour, then every hour while the blood is transfusing.

To prevent blood contamination, change the blood tubing and filter every 4 hours or after each unit of blood. Transfuse each unit of blood over a 2- to 4-hour interval. Use only normal saline with a blood product. Blood transfusions are incompatible with dextrose and with Ringer's solution. Together, they cause hemolysis, clumping of RBCs.

As a precaution against a blood transfusion reaction, prepare a bag of normal saline, as directed by protocol. The normal saline is prepared as a secondary infusion system; it should not be connected to the Y-set tubing that is transfusing blood. If the patient has a reaction, and the blood is discontinued, the secondary bag of normal saline should be connected and infused. This action prevents the patient from receiving all the blood that is in the Y-set tubing, approximately 20 to 30 ml. Even though the procedure for infusing packed cells, and sometimes whole blood, requires a Y-set for coadministering normal saline, the secondary bag of normal saline is a precautionary measure for transfusion reactions.

There are three basic types of transfusion reactions: allergic, febrile, and hemolytic. Other complications include sepsis, hypervolemia, and hypothermia. An allergic reaction may be mild or severe, depending on the cause. Hemolytic reactions may be immediate or delayed up to 96 hours, depending on the cause of the reaction. The classic symptoms of a reaction and sepsis are fever and chills.

The immediate actions for all types of reactions and complications are: stop the transfusion, keep the vein open with normal saline, and notify the physician. Other measures include holding the IV tubing and bag of blood to send back to the blood bank; obtaining a blood specimen; labeling the specimen "Blood Transfusion Reaction"; documenting the transfusion reaction on the run report; and monitoring vital signs every 15 minutes until stable.

A delayed hemolytic reaction results when the donor and patient's anti-A or anti-B agglutinins are mismatched or when there has been improper storage of the blood unit. This reaction causes the cells to clump and form plugs in small blood vessels. Within a few hours or days, the phagocytic WBCs and the reticuloendothelial system destroy agglutinated cells, releasing hemoglobin into the plasma. (See Chapters 4 and 16.)

An immediate hemolytic reaction is a rare occurrence. It results from a mismatch of donor and client's blood, causing immediate hemolysis of RBCs. The antibodies cause lysis of RBCs, which release proteolytic enzymes that rupture the cell membranes. The clinical manifestation are headache, dyspnea, cyanosis, chest pain, and tachycardia.

Febrile reactions are common and result from the patient's sensitivity to WBCs, platelets, or plasma proteins. Warm, flushed skin, headache, muscle pain, and anxiety are the symptoms of a febrile reaction. It is treated with antipyretic medication. To help prevent a febrile reaction, keep the patient warm during the transfusion.

Mild allergic reactions are common, resulting from a sensitivity to infusing plasma proteins. Allergic reactions cause a rash, itching, hives (urticaria), and wheezing. Patients with these symptoms should be monitored for anaphylactic shock. Antihistamines may be prescribed to counter the allergic response (see Chapter 17).

Severe allergic reaction results from an antibody-antigen response as demonstrated by shortness of breath and chest pain; if untreated, it may cause circulatory collapse and cardiac arrest. If this occurs, initiate CPR after the blood has been discontinued.

Sepsis results from the administration of contaminated blood (containing gram-negative bacteria). It is a serious complication. Clinical manifestations include chills and fever, vomiting, abdominal cramping, diarrhea, shock, and renal failure. It is treated with broad-spectrum antibiotics and steroids. EMS measures are directed toward maintaining hydration.

Hypervolemia from fluid overload is a preventable complication. Patients at risk for FVE are placed in a sitting position. The blood is transfused at a reduced flow rate; request the blood laboratory to divide the unit into 2 containers of blood so that none of it is unrefrigerated for more than 2 hours during transfusion. Clinical manifestations of hypervolemia are similar to those of FVE (dyspnea, cough and rales, distended neck veins, hypertension, tachycardia, and pulmonary edema). Administer oxygen and IV diuretics per protocol to treat circulatory overload.

Patients needing rapid transfusions are at risk for transfusion-induced hypothermia. Such patients may include neonates needing exchange-transfusions and trauma victims who require large volumes of whole blood. A blood-warming device may be used to prevent transfusion-induced hypothermia. The symptoms of transfusion-induced hypothermia result from the rapid transfusion of large amounts of cold blood. If the infusing blood temperature is below 30°C (86°F), the myocardial temperature decreases, causing hypotension and myocardial irritability that may progress to ventricular fibrillation and cardiac arrest. EMS interventions are directed toward warming the client with temperature-regulating blankets after the transfusion has been stopped. Obtain an ECG to assess for cardiac arrhythmias.

SUMMARY

Fluid, electrolyte, and acid-base balance plays an important role in allowing the human body to perform the functions necessary for life. Fluid imbalances include fluid volume deficit, resulting in dehyrdration, and fluid volume excess that can result in edema, both pulmonary and peripheral. Electrolyte balance is essential for proper functioning of the nervous, musculoskeletal, cardiovascular, and renal systems. Electrolyte imbalances can affect these systems or any of the other body systems, ranging in severity from muscle weakness to cardiac arrest. The body must maintain the proper acid-base balance to allow the cells to perform their functions, as all of the chemical reactions that take place are dependent on the proper level of hydrogen ion (pH) to allow the reactions to occur. Alterations in acid-base balance can have a respiratory or metabolic origin and result in an acidosis or alkalosis. The EMS provider should be aware of the manifestations of fluid, electrolyte, and acid-base disturbances during the management of all patients.

REVIEW QUESTIONS

Short Answer

1. What are the three sources of body water replacement?

2. Which electrolyte regulates the osmotic pressure of extracellular fluid?

3. What is the most common indication of a fluid volume deficit?

4. What effect does an acid-base imbalance have on the body's cells?

5. Jennifer has been vomiting for 3 days and is unable to keep any food or water in her stomach. Besides having a fluid volume deficit, what other alterations would you expect from the excessive loss of gastric juices?

6. All of the following are clinical manifestations of FVE, except:
   a. Edema
   b. Weight gain
   c. Increased serum osmolality
   d. Decreased serum osmolality

7. Besides potassium-wasting diuretics, what other drugs can cause hypokalemia?

8. What effect does potassium have on digitalis?

9. Which type of intravenous solution is sodium chloride (0.45%)?
   a. Hypotonic
   b. Isotonic
   c. Hypertonic

10. Which type of intravenous solution is dextrose 5% in water (D_5W)?
   a. Hypotonic
   b. Isotonic
   c. Hypertonic

CASE STUDY

You are transporting Gloria Small, a teenager who is being transferred to a tertiary care center for inpatient cancer treatment. Gloria began receiving a blood transfusion just prior to transport. You are about to take the second set of vital signs fifteen minutes into the transport when Gloria states, "I am cold. I think I'm having chills, and my chest hurts." What do you think is causing her chills? Her chest pain? What should you do?

BIBLIOGRAPHY

Asbaghi, Z. (1995). Questions and answers about blood transfusions. *Nursing 95*, 25(2), 32C–32G.

Bulechek, G. M., & McCloskey, J. C. (1992). *Nursing interventions: Essential nursing treatments* (2nd ed.). Philadelphia: Saunders.

Carpenito, L. J. (1992). *Nursing diagnosis: Application to clinical practice* (4th ed.). Philadelphia: Lippincott.

Cochran, L. (1995). What you need to know about potassium imbalances. *Nursing 95*, 25(2), 32H–32N.

Gettrust, K. V., & Brabec, P. D. (1992). *Nursing diagnosis in clinical practice: Guides for care planning*. Albany, NY: Delmar Publishers.

Guyton, A. C., & Hall, J. (1995). *Textbook of medical physiology* (9th ed.). Philadelphia: Saunders.

Hartshorn, J., Lamborn, M., & Noll, M. L. (1993). *Introduction to critical care nursing*. Philadelphia: Saunders.

Hogstel, M. O. (1994). *Nursing care of the older adult* (3rd ed.). Albany, NY: Delmar Publishers.

Kee, J. L., & Paulanka, B. J. (1994). *Fluids and electrolytes with clinical applications* (5th ed.). Albany, NY: Delmar Publishers.

Kim, M. J., McFarland, G. K., & McLane, A. M. (1993). *Pocket guide to nursing diagnoses* (5th ed.). St. Louis, MO: Mosby Yearbook.

Masoorli, S. (1995). Know the pitfalls of I.V. therapy. *NSO Risk Advisor*, 20(2), 1, 4.

McCloskey, J. C., & Bulechek, G. M. (Eds.) (1996). *Iowa Intervention Project: Nursing interventions classification* (NIC) (2nd ed.). St. Louis, MO: Mosby.

McFarland, G. K., & McFarland, E. A. (1993). *Nursing diagnosis and interventions: Planning for patient care* (2nd ed.). St. Louis, MO: Mosby.

McFarland, M., & Grant, M. (1994). *Nursing implications of laboratory tests* (3rd ed.). Albany, NY: Delmar Publishers.

Noe, D., & Rock, R. (1994). *Laboratory medicine*. Baltimore: Williams & Wilkins.

Skretkowicz, V. (Ed.). (1992). *Florence Nightingale's notes on nursing*. London: Scutari Press.

Wolfrum, J. (1994). A follow-up evaluation to a needle-free IV system. *Nursing Management*. 25(12), 33–35.

CHAPTER

6

Pathophysiology of Shock

CONTENT OUTLINE

- Classification of Shock
  - Hypovolemic Shock
  - Cardiogenic Shock
  - Neurogenic Shock
  - Vasogenic Shock
- Assessment of Shock
- Age-Related Differences in Shock

KEY TERMS

Anaphylaxis
Cardiogenic shock
Compensated shock
Decompensated shock
Endotoxin
Hypoadrenal shock
Hypovolemic shock
Insensible fluid loss
Multiple organ dysfunction syndrome (MODS)
Neurogenic shock
Pulse pressure
Sepsis
Septic shock
Systemic inflammatory response syndrome (SIRS)
Traumatic shock
Vasogenic shock

Learning Objectives

Upon completion of the chapter, the student should be able to:

1. Define the term shock.
2. Describe the three components of the cardiovascular system affected in the pathophysiology of shock.
3. List the four main classifications of shock and the component(s) of the cardiovascular system affected.
4. Describe the pathophysiology for each specific classification of shock.
5. Describe the important assessment findings for a patient in shock.

Overview

Shock is a general term used to describe a state of poor perfusion of the tissues with oxygen-rich blood. There are many causes for this state, but they all involve one or more of the components of the circulatory system, the blood (the fluid), the vessels (the piping), or the heart (pump). This chapter explores the different classifications of shock and describes the pathophysiology of the different forms of shock. EMS providers will undoubtedly encounter many patients each year in various states of shock and knowledge of the underlying pathophysiology will aid the EMS provider in effective and efficient treatment.

CLASSIFICATION OF SHOCK

The common denominator of shock is inadequate perfusion of the tissues with oxygen-rich blood. This poor perfusion can occur if any one of the three main components of the circulatory system is compromised: the volume of blood in the system, the integrity of the vascular system, and the ability of the heart to pump blood into the circulation. A cascade of events will begin that, if not treated aggressively, may end in death.

These three components of the cardiovascular system, the volume of blood in the system, the blood vessels, and the heart can be affected resulting in a decrease in blood pressure and impaired delivery of oxygen-rich blood to the tissues:

- Blood. If the volume of blood in the system drops, the blood pressure will also fall because there is less blood to pump through the system (Figure 6–1A).
- Vessels. If the size of the blood vessels changes so the diameter is larger, the blood pressure will decrease. This drop in blood pressure occurs because the "container" becomes significantly larger than the volume of blood, less blood returns to the heart, the blood pressure drops, and the tissues do not get sufficient oxygen (Figure 6–1B).
- Heart. If the heart is unable to pump efficiently, the amount of blood flow will decrease, the blood pressure will drop, and the tissues will not get enough oxygen (Figure 6–1C).

The brain and heart are important tissues, but even the "nonessential" tissues, for example, the gastrointestinal system, play an important role in the development of shock. The body will initially attempt to maintain perfusion to the heart and brain, shunting blood away from other organs (Figure 6–2). For short periods of time in a relatively healthy person, this diversion of blood can be life-saving, allowing the EMS provider time to intervene. However, this shunting of blood will become detrimental if it continues for a longer period of time.

There are four main classifications of shock: hypovolemic shock, cardiogenic shock, neurogenic shock, and vasogenic shock. These four classifications all have a dysfunction in one of the three components of the circulatory system with a different pathophysiology. Table 6–1 lists the common causes for each of these classifications.

Hypovolemic Shock

The component of the circulatory system affected in **hypovolemic shock** is the volume of blood in the sys-

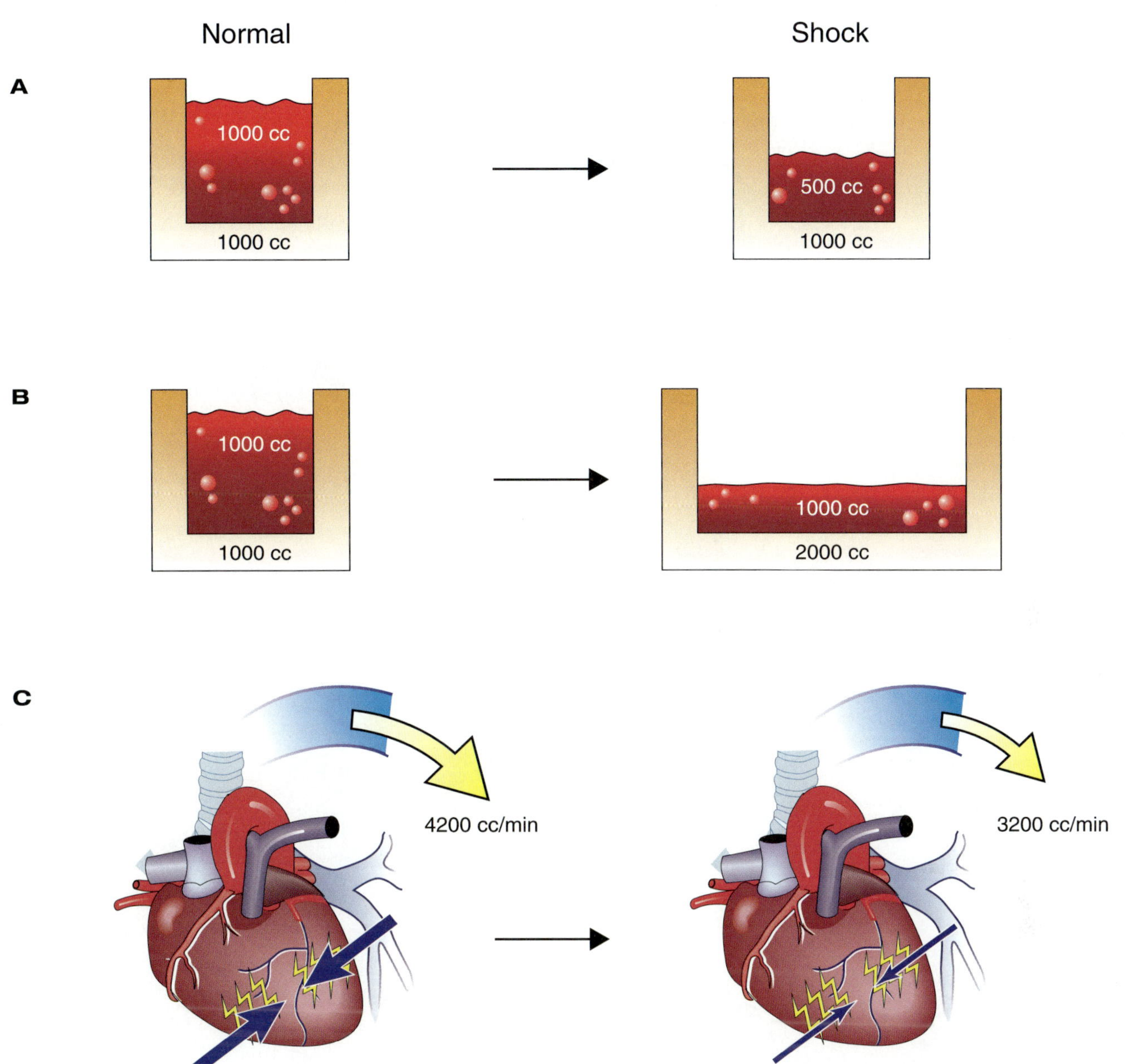

Figure 6–1 Circulatory system components and their relation to shock. (A) Blood volume. (B) Blood vessels. (C) The heart.

tem. As depicted in Figure 6–1A, the fluid volume in the system decreases, directly causing the pressure within the system to decrease. A second reason for the drop in blood pressure is that less blood is available to be pumped through the system. The volume of blood can decrease for two reasons: blood loss or loss of plasma, the fluid component of blood.

Loss of blood is a common cause of shock in the pre-hospital setting. According to 1997 statistics, traumatic injury is the overall fifth leading cause of death and the most common cause of death for people under forty-five years old. Blood loss in trauma is generally acute in nature; however, some abdominal injuries can cause slower blood loss that may not declare itself for a period of time after the initial injury. Blood loss can occur acutely in medical conditions, for example, a ruptured aneurysm or ruptured esophageal varices. Blood loss can also occur chronically as in the case of a colon tumor that bleeds as stool passes. The amount of blood volume lost relative to the total body blood volume can be used to gauge the severity of shock (Table 6–2).

Plasma is the liquid component of blood and is essentially water with some dissolved compounds. As discussed in Chapter 5, fluid can cross between compartments. This

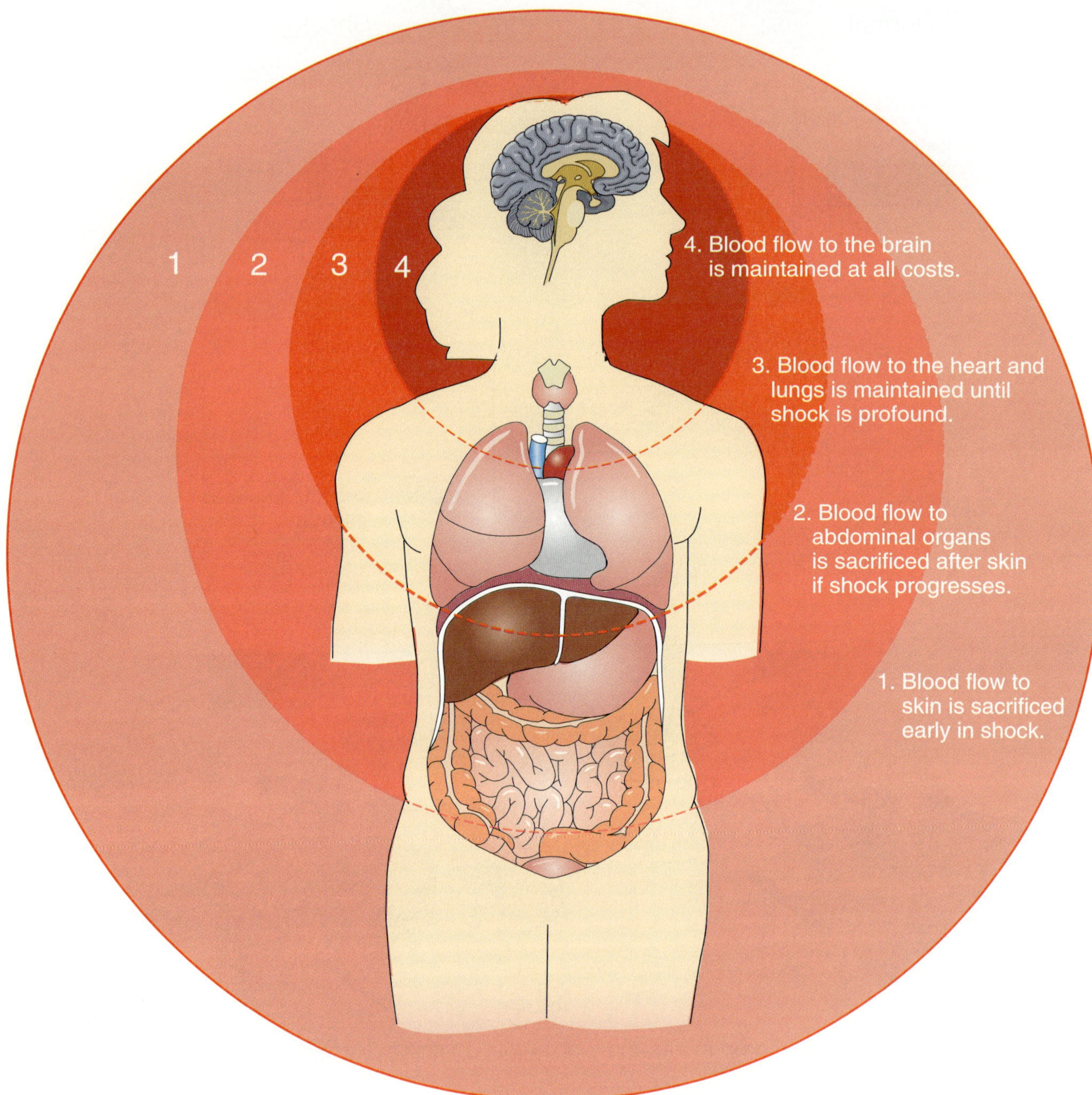

Figure 6-2 If faced with hypoperfusion, the body will sacrifice the perfusion of particular organs to maintain the blood supply to others.

shift of fluid from the vascular compartment to the extravascular compartment can cause a hypovolemia because less fluid is available to pump through the circulation as blood. One example of this fluid shift is in patients who have been severely burned.

Plasma volume can be lost via the gastrointestinal system, renal system, or through insensible fluid loss. The cause of prolonged diarrhea or vomiting, whether infectious or toxic, results in a fluid shift from the circulation to the GI system. This drain on the circulatory system can easily cause a patient to become dehydrated and progress to a state of mild shock within 24 to 36 hours. In the case of a bowel obstruction, fluid is drawn into the bowel in an attempt to soften and expel the obstruction.

Plasma volume loss can occur because of changes in renal system function. Excessive urination, which can occur in a patient who is hyperglycemic, can also drain plasma volume from the circulation as the body is trying

TABLE 6–1 Classifications and Causes of Shock

Classification	Common Etiologies
Hypovolemic	Hemorrhage
	Loss of plasma (e.g., burn, GI loss)
Cardiogenic	Pump failure (MI, valve problem, arrhythmia)
	Tension pneumothorax
	Pericardial tamponade
	Pulmonary embolism
Neurogenic	Spinal cord injury
	Traumatic brain injury
Vasogenic	Systemic inflammatory response
	Anaphylaxis
	Hypoadrenal
	Traumatic

to dilute and filter and dispose of the excess glucose. The hormones that regulate the fluid balance in the body can also function improperly, resulting in excessive urination and fluid loss.

Insensible fluid loss is fluid that is lost from evaporation and cannot be measured. In average healthy people, a certain amount of fluid is lost via the lungs during respiration. In certain patients, for example, burn patients, the protective barrier of the skin is damaged and a significant amount of fluid can be lost to evaporation.

As the patient becomes hypovolemic, she can initially compensate by increasing her heart rate, constricting the blood vessels, and selectively shunting blood from nonessential tissues to the heart and brain. The patient's heart rate will increase as additional blood is lost until the heart does not have enough time to adequately fill between contractions. While the heart rate is increasing, the **pulse pressure**, or difference between the systolic and diastolic blood pressure, will decrease or narrow. This narrowing pulse pressure indicates in this case that the heart is not adequately filling, even though it is maintaining a sufficient cardiac output. Once the heart does not fill completely between beats, the blood pressure will begin to fall not only because of loss of blood but also from inability to pump blood through the system. In a young, otherwise healthy patient, the initial sign of shock may be a slight tachycardia that persists once the situation has calmed. This is especially true in children who have an amazing ability to compensate for hypovolemia for a long period of time before suddenly crashing. Other signs and symptoms of hypovolemic shock include restlessness, thirst, anxiety, decreased mental status, and cool, clammy skin. The difference between **compensated shock** and **decompensated shock** is the drop in systolic blood pressure below 90 mmHg in decompensated shock. A patient in compensated shock can maintain an adequate systolic blood pressure (> 90 mmHg). The dividing line between compensated and decompensated shock for adults according to the American College of Surgeons classification described in Table 6–2 is usually between Class II and Class III, or somewhere around 30% blood loss.

TABLE 6–2 Class of Shock Related to Percent of Total Blood Volume Lost (as described by the American College of Surgeons). The volumes in ml are based on an average size person with a total blood volume of approximately 5 liters (5000 ml).

Class	% Blood Loss
I	< 15% (< 750 ml)
II	15–30% (750–1500 ml)
III	30-40% (1500–2000 ml)
IV	> 40% (> 2000 ml)

Treatment of hypovolemic shock involves replacing the fluid volume lost. In the field, this is performed with either lactated Ringer's or normal saline. Once at the hospital, blood can be added to the resuscitation to provide needed erythrocytes to carry oxygen. Vasopressors, for example, dopamine and dobutamine, are not used in the treatment of hypovolemic shock because the problem is not with the piping but with the lack of fluid. The body has used some of its natural vasopressors to maximally vasoconstrict the vascular system and adding additional vasopressors will not provide additional constriction of the blood vessels. The use of the pneumatic anti-shock garment (PASG) has generally fallen out of favor, especially for the use of penetrating thoracic injuries; however, it may be beneficial for localized bleeding control under the garment.

Cardiogenic Shock

In **cardiogenic shock**, the heart is not able to pump out enough blood to maintain the patient's blood pressure. This pump problem can be caused by either intrinsic or extrinsic factors. Intrinsic factors include damage to the heart muscle or structures that cause the heart to function abnormally. Extrinsic factors impair the ability of the reasonably healthy heart to function. In some cases, both intrinsic and extrinsic factors are at work, and it can be difficult to identify the cause.

Intrinsic Factors. Intrinsic causes for cardiogenic shock include problems with the myocardium, the valves, or the conduction system, or a combination of the three. If the heart muscle is damaged from a significant myocardial infarction (MI), a heart attack, the muscle fibers will not contract efficiently. The heart may be damaged to the point where certain sections do not contract at all. A heart that has to work harder, for example, in a patient who has hypertension or high blood pressure, will be stretched over time and also not pump efficiently. Once another event occurs, for example, another MI, the heart may not be able to pump enough blood to maintain an adequate blood pressure. The myocardium can also be damaged as a result of direct or indirect trauma that disrupts the ability for the muscle fibers to contract.

The valves in the heart (Figure 6–2) are designed to permit flow in the forward direction. When these valves are damaged by chronic disease, a portion of the blood in the chamber can leak around the valve and flow in the reverse direction. In an MI, the muscles that attach to the valves can rupture and cause a significant leak. As with chronically damaged myocardium, all the patient needs is another event, such as an MI, to place him into pump failure and cardiogenic shock.

Conduction system dysrythmias can occur for a variety of reasons, such as the result of damage to the conduction system from trauma or an MI. They can also be caused by electrolyte imbalances or congenital differences in the conduction system. Whatever the cause, certain dysrhythmias impair the coordinated effort that occurs with each heartbeat to pump blood away from the heart. When this coordinated effort is disrupted, the cardiac output is decreased. Dysrhythmias such as ventricular tachycardia impair the ability of the heart to pump blood to the point where the patient is in danger of losing a pulse and rapidly progressing into ventricular fibrillation and subsequently cardiac arrest. Even if the patient does not lose a pulse, she may become unconscious from the lack of sufficient oxygen supply to the brain.

Extrinsic Factors. Extrinsic factors are external to the heart and disrupt its ability to mechanically pump blood through the circulatory system. The heart may be healthy and require significant outside influence to fail, or may be damaged from chronic cardiovascular disease so that a small insult can disrupt what little adequate function remained. Two common examples of extrinsic factors that affect the heart's ability to pump are tension pneumothorax (see Chapter 7) and pericardial tamponade (see Chapter 8). Both of these conditions result in decreased blood return to the heart and a drop in cardiac output.

In a pneumothorax, the buildup of pressure in the affected side can grow to the point where blood return to the heart is diminished. This can occur from compression of the vena cava or compression of the atria (see Figure 6–3). The heart will not be able to fill properly, and as a result, will pump a smaller volume of blood. This decrease in the cardiac output will cause a drop in blood pressure.

A pericardial tamponade operates on the same principle but with a different mechanism. In tamponade, fluid or blood fills the pericardium, the tough "bag" that surrounds the heart. As this is a very small space, it takes relatively little fluid to put pressure on the chambers. This outside pressure decreases the ability of the chambers to fill properly and, as in the case of a pneumothorax, decreases cardiac output. The source of the fluid in tamponade can occur traumatically, as in the case of a ruptured blood vessel that leaks into the pericardial sac, or from a fluid shift as occurs in some renal diseases.

Neurogenic Shock

In **neurogenic shock**, the capacity of the circulatory system is significantly greater than the blood volume available to fill the system (see Figure 6–1B). In effect, the container size has increased while the volume of blood in that container stayed the same, with a drop in blood pressure as the end result. The cause of neurogenic shock involves the central nervous system control of the blood vessel diameter.

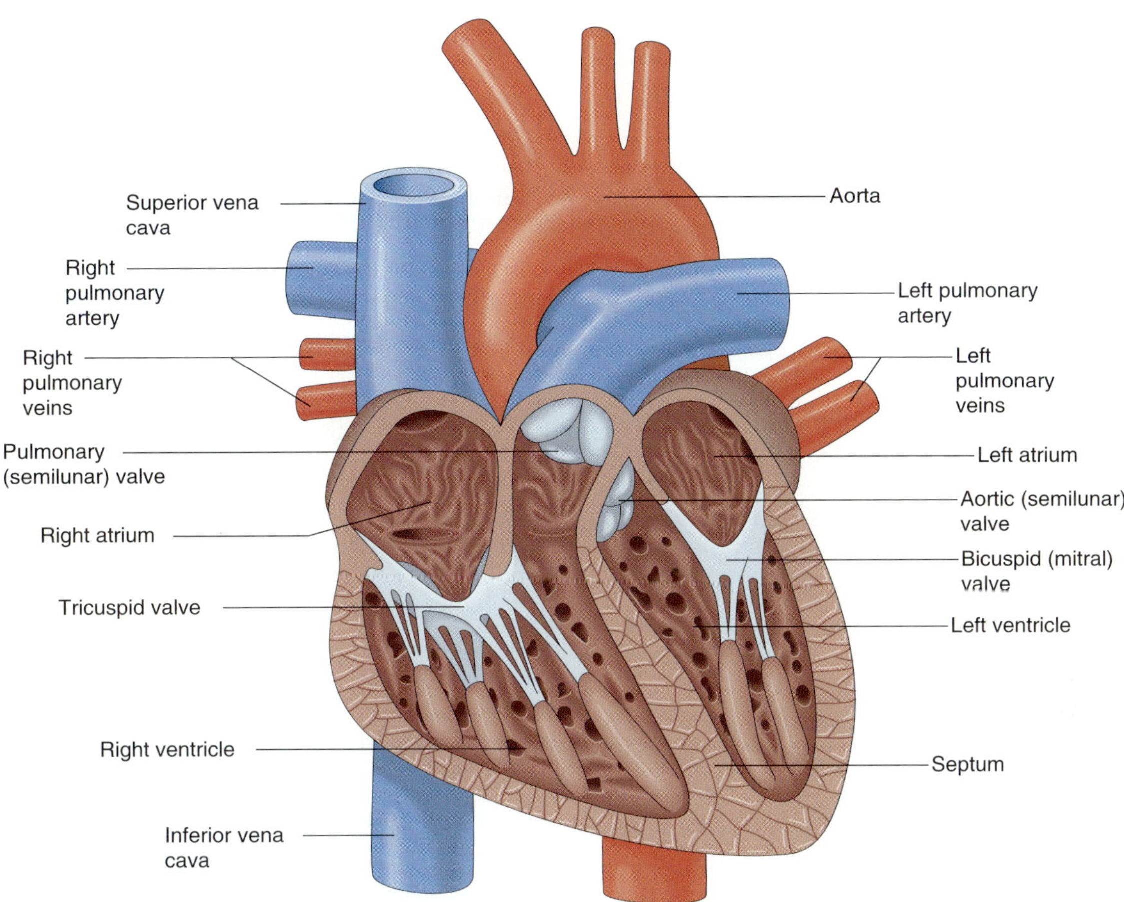

Figure 6-3 The heart.

Blood vessel size and heart rate are controlled automatically by the body in an effort to maintain the blood pressure within a certain range for each individual. The range will change automatically based upon the body's activity, stresses on the body, and the need for additional oxygen. For example, an individual's blood pressure and pulse are expected to increase during a basketball game to provide additional oxygen to the player's muscles and brain. Once the game is over and the basketball player sits down to read the newspaper, the heart rate and blood pressure should return to a normal resting level. The part of the nervous system responsible for this control is the autonomic nervous system, and it is mediated at both the brain and spinal cord level (see Chapter 9).

Injury to the spinal cord is a classic example used to describe neurogenic shock. In a complete spinal cord injury, the nerve cells that make up the autonomic nervous system are damaged. The autonomic nervous system acts to decrease the diameter of the blood vessels, so if that control is lost, the blood vessels in the body that are controlled by the damaged nerve cells will relax or dilate. When this occurs over a significant portion of the body, as in a spinal cord injury, the size of the circulatory system quickly increases. The drop in blood pressure occurs for two reasons. The amount of blood in the system is not adequate to fill the system and maintain the blood pressure. The blood also tends to pool within the circulatory system below the injury, with the decreased blood return to the heart decreasing the cardiac output and blood pressure.

Neurogenic shock can also occur as a result of traumatic brain injury. The centers of the brain or the pathways that transmit the information from the brain centers down to the spinal cord can be damaged by traumatic injury.

Vasogenic Shock

Vasogenic shock, like neurogenic shock, involves a problem with blood vessel size. However, vasogenic shock involves chemical mediators of inflammation (described in Chapter 4) rather than loss of autonomic nervous system control in the pathogenesis of the condition. These chemical mediators cause a loss of vasomotor control, and cause the container (the vascular system) to become very large in size (Figure 6–1B).

There are four major subcategories of vasogenic shock: anaphylaxis, hypoadrenal shock, systemic inflammatory response syndrome, and traumatic shock.

Anaphylaxis. **Anaphylaxis** is an extreme allergic reaction to a substance. The main player in anaphylaxis is the mast cell. The mast cell, as described in Chapter 4, plays a significant role in the inflammatory process. When the allergen, or substance the patient has an allergy to, comes in contact with the patient, the patient's antibodies react. These antibodies bind to the surface of the mast cell and cause the cell to release histamine into the surrounding tissue. Histamine causes capillaries to dilate and become leaky, drawing fluid from the vascular space. This fluid shift causes the edema and hyperemia seen in hives, a skin manifestation of an allergy.

In anaphylaxis, the patient has an extreme reaction to allergens. For those patients, a significant amount of fluid can shift from the vascular space and the blood vessels in the entire body can dilate, resulting in shock, generalized edema, edema of the airway, and spasm of the smaller airways. For these patients, the allergic reaction is life threatening and rapid treatment with epinephrine, intravenous fluids, and diphenhydramine is essential for stopping the progression of and reversing this process.

Hypoadrenal Shock. A second form of vasogenic shock, **hypoadrenal shock**, is a relatively uncommon form of shock. As described in Chapter 11, the adrenal glands are responsible for production of a variety of hormones. The glucocorticosteroids in particular are produced to assist the body in dealing with stressors, both internal and external. They assist the autonomic nervous system with some of the "fight or flight" events that occur when a person is stressed. Some patients do not have the ability to produce enough glucocorticosteroids to mount an appropriate stress response in traumatic situations. Hypoadrenal shock should be considered in patients who either have been on long-term glucocorticosteroid therapy, for example prednisone, or who remain in shock despite an aggressive fluid resuscitation and use of vasopressors. Intravenous steroids are administered to augment the production of glucocorticosteroids. The patient should also be evaluated for adrenal insufficiency in either the emergency department or intensive care unit.

SIRS, Sepsis, MODS. **Systemic inflammatory response syndrome** (SIRS) is a condition where the body's normal inflammatory response to infection or other stress is out of control. SIRS occurs either with infection, as in the case of sepsis, or without infection. The criteria used to define SIRS are described in Table 6–3. **Sepsis** may be suspected in the field by the patient's history and is confirmed in the hospital by blood cultures that demonstrate the presence of bacteria in the blood. **Septic shock** is sepsis that causes hypotension and evidence of poor tissue perfusion. This can progress to **multiple organ dysfunction syndrome** (MODS), where there is damage or dysfunction to more than one organ in an acutely ill patient. Patients who progress to MODS can be very difficult to treat, with a mortality of between twenty and one hundred percent depending upon the number of organs that have failed.

In sepsis, it may not be the bacteria itself that causes the inflammatory response, but the **endotoxin** that is released by the bacteria. The endotoxin is a component of the cell wall that is antigenic in humans, causing an inflammatory response against the bacteria. Certain bacteria invoke a significant inflammatory response that includes vasodilation, fluid shifts, and shock. It is important to note that while antibiotics will kill bacteria, they do nothing against the endotoxins released by the bacteria. A patient can be well treated with antibiotics but still exhibit signs of SIRS or septic shock because the endotoxin remains in the blood for a period of time after the death of the bacteria. Some newer treatments aimed at attacking specific endotoxins or modulating the systemic inflammatory response have had mixed results. A significant amount of research is underway as sepsis and

TABLE 6-3 Systemic Inflammatory Response Syndrome (SIRS) Criteria. The patient meets the criteria for SIRS if he has at least two of these four criteria.

Criteria	
Temperature	Greater than 38°C (100.4°F)
	Less than 36°C (96.8°F)
Heart	Rate greater than 90
Respiratory	Rate greater than 20
	Or
$PaCO_2$	Less than 32 mmHg
WBC Count	Greater than 12,000
	Lower than 4,000

SIRS remain difficult to treat and have a high mortality and morbidity associated with these conditions.

The GI system can also play a significant role in the development of vasogenic shock. As mentioned earlier in the chapter, early in shock the body attempts to divert blood away from "nonessential organs" to the heart and brain to reduce damage to these organs. The GI tract, specifically the stomach and intestines, is a large organ that becomes poorly perfused early in shock. Ischemia in the gut lining develops, causing damage or death to the protective lining. Bacteria that normally live in the gut but do not cause any harm may be able to cross this protective barrier into the blood stream, causing a bacteremia and ultimately SIRS. When the gut finally becomes reperfused with oxygen-rich blood, the acids and toxins that built up during the period of ischemia are returned to the normal blood stream and can cause damage to cells throughout the body or instigate an inflammatory response. Aggressive and early treatment of shock to maintain adequate perfusion can prevent these significant consequences of gut ischemia.

Traumatic Shock. The fourth form of vasogenic shock, **traumatic shock**, is one that is probably not seen in the field but may be observed by EMS providers involved in critical care transportation. Traumatic shock begins as hypovolemic shock which involves more significant blood loss and fluid shifts. This sets up an environment for significant tissue ischemia and the release of inflammatory mediators. In contrast to hypovolemic shock, traumatic shock may persist even with significant fluid resuscitation and may require treatment with vasopressors. Traumatic shock may progress to MODS even with aggressive treatment.

ASSESSMENT OF SHOCK

Almost every patient encountered in the field should be assessed for the signs of shock during the physical exam. Even for a non-acute interfacility transport, most of the signs of shock are contained within a set of vital signs. As discussed above, shock can have several different etiologies with similar signs and symptoms.

In hypovolemic shock, a decrease in circulating blood volume is the problem. The baroreceptors in the aortic arch and the carotid arteries sense the drop in blood pressure and signal an increase in heart rate, an increase in the strength of myocardial contraction force, and a constriction of the systemic blood vessels to maintain an adequate blood pressure. The vasoconstriction that occurs is selective and the skin becomes pale and cool as blood is diverted away from the skin and other organs to the heart and brain. As additional volume is lost, these changes continue to occur. The respiratory rate will also increase in an attempt to increase the amount of oxygen in the blood. A significant drop in blood pressure is a late sign of shock and signals the transition from ACS Class II to ACS Class III hypovolemic shock, corresponding to approximately a thirty percent or one-and-one-half-liter loss of blood for the average 70 kg person. Finally, as the blood pressure falls, the patient's mental status diminishes. Table 6–4 describes the transition in vital signs corresponding to the different ACS classes of shock.

In cardiogenic shock where pump failure is the problem, some additional signs and symptoms may occur. If the failure is caused by an MI, dysrhythmia, pneumothorax, or pericardial tamponade, then chest pain is typically present. Bradycardia, diminished heart sounds, and pulmonary edema may also be present as the heart is not able to pump efficiently or filling is impaired by an extrinsic factor.

In both neurogenic and vasogenic shock, systemic vasodilation is a key problem. In neurogenic shock caused by spinal cord injury, this vasodilation occurs below the level of the injury, with the skin below the injury becoming warm and flushed and the skin above the injury pale and cool. Neurologic deficiencies will also be present in the areas affected by the injury. In vasogenic shock, the skin over the entire body is typically warm and flushed. The patient may have a fever from infection or the inflammatory mediators.

It is important for the EMS provider to recognize shock early and treat it aggressively before the patient decompensates. A young and otherwise healthy individual

TABLE 6–4 Assessment Findings Related to American College of Surgeons Class of Shock (HR = heart rate; BP = blood pressure; CR = capillary refill; RR = respiratory rate).

Class	Assessment Findings
I	Normal vitals, few symptoms
II	HR > 100; narrow pulse pressure; CR > 2 seconds; RR 20–30
III	HR > 120; BP falls; CR > 2 seconds; RR 30–40
IV	HR > 120; Low BP; confused/lethargic; CR > 3–4 seconds

may present with a significant blood loss and only a mild tachycardia because their body is able to effectively compensate for the loss. Awareness of the mechanism of injury in trauma and knowledge of pathophysiology will assist the EMS provider in detecting and managing the patient in shock.

AGE-RELATED DIFFERENCES IN SHOCK

Patients at both of the age extremes compensate differently for shock. Infants have a very small total blood volume and even a blood loss of 50–100 cc can place the infant in shock. Children have a very resilient circulatory system and can compensate very well for blood loss. Their bodies tend to overreact to stimulus and adjust very quickly. The disadvantage is that children tend to compensate well for a long period of time and then suddenly decompensate. Signs of shock can be very subtle in children. As humans age, their circulatory system adjusts slower to changes in blood pressure. This is caused in part by aging but cardiovascular disease plays a significant role in the slow adjustment. Certain medications, for example, beta-blockers, can blunt the body's natural response to increase heart rate in the face of hypovolemia. Patients who are taking beta-blockers and sustain a traumatic injury should be carefully assessed for other signs of shock, as tachycardia may never develop. These age-related differences in the signs of shock can present a challenge and underscore the need for the EMS provider to evaluate thoroughly patients in these age groups.

SUMMARY

The term shock is used to describe the general state of inadequate perfusion of the tissues with oxygen-rich blood. The four major classifications of shock, hypovolemic shock, cardiogenic shock, neurogenic shock, and vasogenic shock, each involve problems with one of the three components to the circulatory system: the blood volume, the blood vessels, or the heart. The patient is said to be in compensated shock while she can still maintain an adequate blood pressure and decompensated shock once the systolic blood pressure begins to fall below 90 mmHg. Young children and older adults respond differently in shock states, with younger children maintaining an adequate blood pressure for a longer period of time before quickly decompensating. Older adults often do not have the ability to mount an adequate physiologic response because of a combination of chronic disease, normal aging, or pharmacological interference.

REVIEW QUESTIONS

Matching

1. Match the forms of shock on the left with the descriptions on the right.

_____ Cardiogenic shock	a. mast cell histamine release
_____ Hypovolemic shock	b. systemic inflammatory response syndrome
_____ Neurogenic shock	c. pump failure
_____ Anaphylactic shock	d. associated with spinal cord injury
_____ Septic shock	e. plasma volume loss from diarrhea

Multiple Choice

Choose the letter that *best* answers the question.

2. Your average size patient has lost an estimated 1700 cc of blood in a chain saw accident. What classification of shock is he in according to the American College of Surgeons?
   a. Class I
   b. Class II
   c. Class III
   d. Class IV

3. An extrinsic cause for cardiogenic shock is:
   a. Ruptured mitral valve
   b. Massive anterior wall MI
   c. Tension pneumothorax
   d. Ventricular tachycardia refractory to treatment

4. The etiology of vasogenic shock involves:
   a. Blood loss.
   b. Loss of autonomic system control of the blood vessel diameter
   c. Spinal cord or traumatic brain injury
   d. Inflammatory mediators that produce vasodilation

5. In neurogenic shock caused by a spinal cord injury:
   a. The skin is cool and clammy above the level of the injury.
   b. The skin is cool and clammy below the level of the injury.
   c. The skin is warm and flushed above the level of the injury.
   d. Tachycardia may never develop because of to nerve injury.

6. Which of the below can generally interfere with an elderly individual's body's ability to mount a proper response to blood loss?
   a. Certain commonly prescribed medications (e.g. beta-blockers).
   b. Slow response to changes in blood pressure.
   c. Stiffer vascular system.
   d. All of the above.

CASE STUDY

You are called to the scene of a motor vehicle crash and are assigned to a conscious 75-year-old male who was an unrestrained front seat passenger. His vehicle was hit at 45 mph with the impact on his side just to the rear of his seat. What signs of shock are you specifically looking for when you assess him? How do his age, medications, and mechanism of injury factor into your assessment? What is your treatment plan for this patient?

BIBLIOGRAPHY

Centers for Disease Control. (June 30, 1999). *National Vital Statistics Reports* (Vol. 47, No. 19.) Atlanta.

Sabitson, D.C., (Ed.). *Textbook of surgery: the biological basis of modern surgical practice* (15th ed.). (1997). Philadelphia: W. B. Saunders.

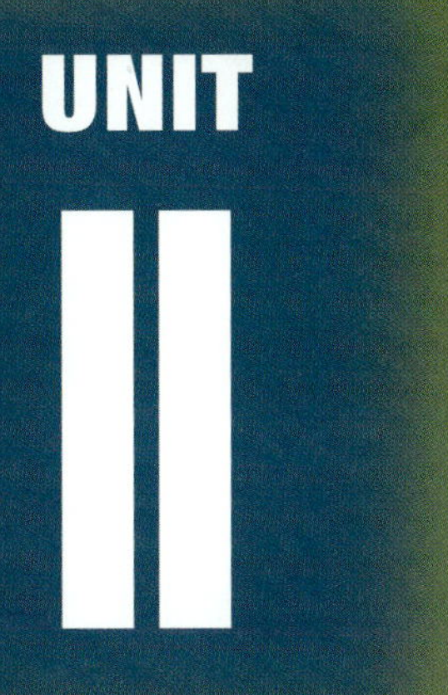

Common Diseases and Disorders

CHAPTER

7

Respiratory Diseases and Disorders

CONTENT OUTLINE

- Anatomy and Physiology
- Common Signs and Symptoms
- Diagnostic Tests
- Common Diseases of the Respiratory System
  - Diseases of the Upper Respiratory Tract
  - Diseases of the Bronchi and Lungs
  - Diseases of the Pleura and Chest
  - Diseases of the Cardiovascular and Respiratory Systems
- Trauma
  - Rib Fracture
  - Flail Chest
  - Sternal Fracture
  - Pneumothorax and Hemothorax
  - Pulmonary Contusion
  - Traumatic Asphyxia
  - Diaphragmatic Injury
- Developmental and Genetic Disorders
  - Cystic Fibrosis
- Effects of Aging on the System

KEY TERMS

Agonal respirations
Analgesics
Antipyretics
Apnea
Arterial blood gases
Biot's respiration
Bradypnea
Bronchiectasis
Bronchoscopy
Central neurogenic hyperventilation
Cheyne-Stokes respiration
Clubbing
Cyanosis
Dead space
Dyspnea
Exocrine glands
Epistaxis
Expiratory reserve
FiO_2
Forced expiratory volume in one second (FEV_1)
Functional reserve capacity
Hemoptysis
Hyperventilation
Hypoventilation
Hypoxemia
Hypoxia
Inspiratory capacity
Inspiratory reserve
Kussmaul's respirations
Minute volume
Obstructive disease
Orthopnea
Paradoxical respiration
Percussion note
Productive cough
Pulsus paradoxus
Rales
Residual volume
Restrictive disease
Rhinorrhea
Rhonchi
Sputum
Subcutaneous emphysema
Tachypnea
Tidal volume
Total lung capacity
Viscous
Vital capacity
Wheezing

LEARNING OBJECTIVES

Upon completion of the chapter, the student should be able to:

1. Define the terminology common to the respiratory system and the disorders of the system.
2. Identify the common disorders of the respiratory system.
3. Discuss the basic anatomy and physiology of the respiratory system.
4. Identify the important signs and symptoms associated with common respiratory system disorders.
5. Describe the common diagnostic tests used to determine type and/or cause of the respiratory system disorders.
6. Describe the typical course and management of the common respiratory system disorders.
7. Describe the effects of aging upon the respiratory system and the common disorders of the system.

OVERVIEW

The respiratory system includes the chest, lungs, and internal airway structures. In order to continue life, the individual must breathe and have a continuous exchange of oxygen for carbon dioxide. Breathing and the exchange of gases that takes place within the system are complex processes involving the respiratory system as well as the neurological and circulatory systems. Diseases of the respiratory system include some of the most well-known disorders, such as the common cold and pneumonia. Trauma to the respiratory system can range from minor, as in the case of an uncomplicated rib fracture, to life-threatening, as in the case of a tension pneumothorax. The respiratory and cardiovascular systems are interdependent upon each other, with some conditions shared between the two systems. Respiratory diseases affect all ages, but the elderly are the most susceptible to both chronic and acute disorders of the system.

ANATOMY AND PHYSIOLOGY

The respiratory system consists of the chest (thorax), lungs, and conducting airways. The chest or thorax is the structure that houses the lungs and the mediastinum (includes heart and vessels). The respiratory system structures in the thorax include the lungs, twelve pairs of ribs, part of the vertebral column, and the sternum. The diaphragm, a large muscle of respiration, separates the thorax from the abdomen (Figure 7–1). The lungs are two spongy organs divided into three lobes in the right lung and two lobes in the left lung. The lungs lie in the pleural cavity in the thorax. This cavity is lined with a membrane called the pleura. The lungs are also covered with a second membrane or pleura. Between the two pleural membranes is a lubricating liquid that prevents friction as the process of breathing and lung expansion occurs.

Usually the airways of the respiratory system are divided into two parts. The upper respiratory system includes the nose (nasal cavities), mouth, sinuses, pharynx, and larynx. The lower respiratory system includes the trachea, bronchi, and bronchioles (Figure 7–2). The alveoli are found at the distal end of the terminal bronchioles. They are grape-like clusters of air sacs that are surrounded by capillaries (Figure 7–2). This is where the oxygen-carbon dioxide gas exchange in the lungs occurs.

The mechanism of ventilation and gas exchange is a complex process. Ventilation is the movement of air into and out of the respiratory system. This requires both inhalation and exhalation to occur. Ventilation is controlled by chemosensory receptors in spinal fluid and in the carotid and aortic arteries, arterial carbon dioxide tension, and oxygen deficiency. As the receptors detect increases or decreases in carbon dioxide and/or oxygen, ventilation is increased or decreased as needed to meet body requirements. This process can be altered by respiratory or neurologic disease, as the respiratory control center is located in the medulla of the brain.

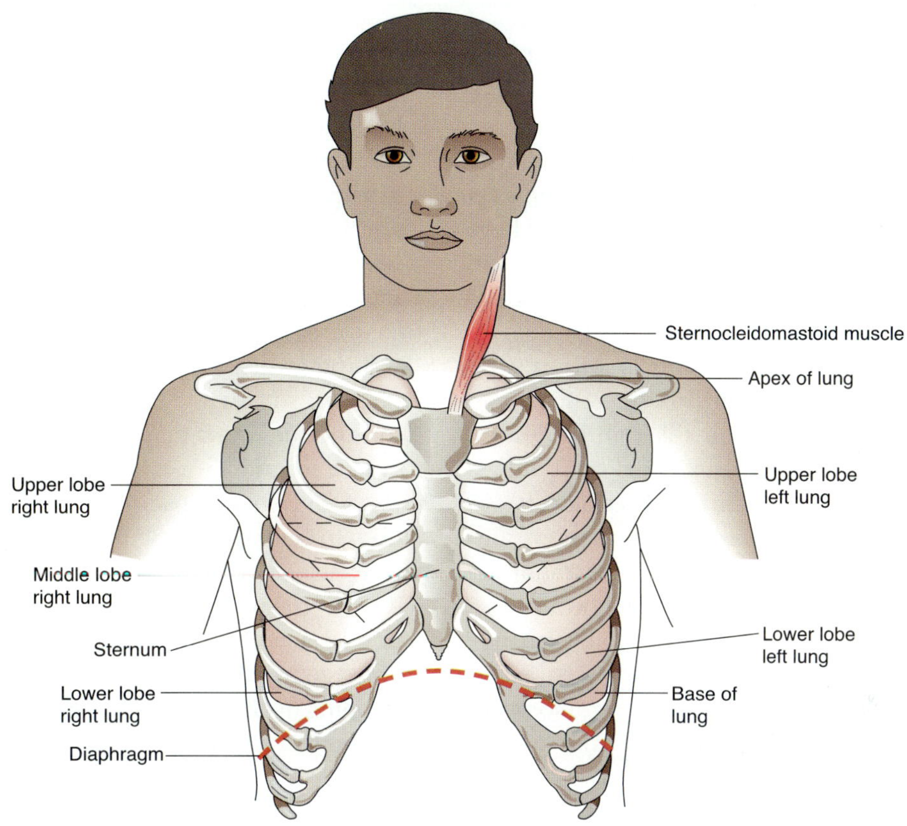

Figure 7–1 The respiratory system.

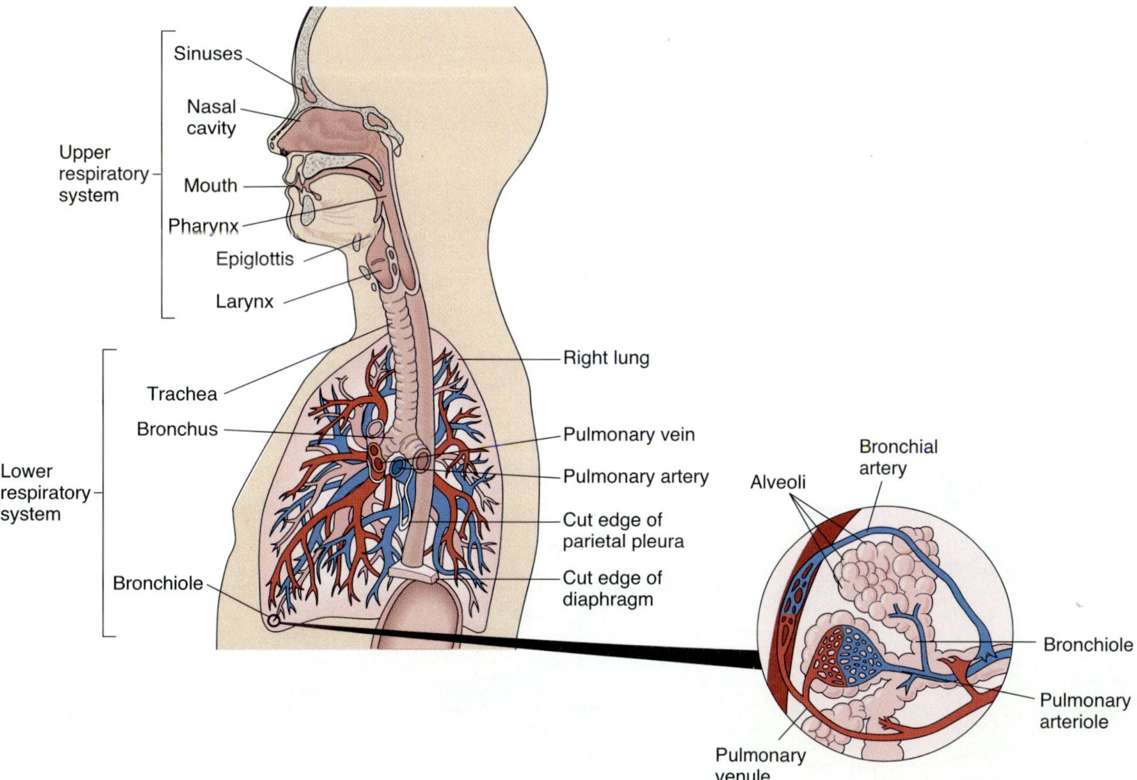

Figure 7–2 Airway divisions and terminal bronchiole/alveoli.

The exchange of gases occurs both in the lungs and throughout the body at the tissue level (Figure 7–3). In the lungs, carbon dioxide is released from the capillary beds into the alveolar spaces by the process of diffusion. In the same way, oxygen moves from the air spaces into the capillaries for transport to the tissues. This process is reversed at the tissue level throughout the body where oxygen moves from the bloodstream into the tissues, and carbon dioxide moves from the tissues into the blood for transport to the lungs and removal from the body.

The EMS provider should be familiar with several respiratory measurements (Figure 7–4). **Total lung capacity** is the total amount of air that can be held in the lung. The **tidal volume** is the volume of air that is inhaled and exhaled in one breath and is equal to 10–15 cc/kg for both adults and children. The **functional reserve capacity** is the amount of air remaining in the lungs after a normal exhalation. **Dead space** comprises the sections of the respiratory system where gas exchange does not occur, for example, in the nasopharynx and mainstem bronchi, and the **residual volume** or amount of air left in the lungs after exhalation. The **inspiratory capacity** is the volume of air inhaled during maximal inhalation. The **vital capacity** is the maximum volume of air that can be exhaled from the lungs after a maximal inspiration. The **expiratory reserve** is the volume of air that can be exhaled during forced exhalation. The **inspiratory reserve** is the additional volume of air over normal tidal volume that can be inhaled during maximal inhalation. The **minute volume** is the volume of air that travels through the respiratory system during one minute of ventilation, and is calculated by multiplying the tidal volume by the respiratory rate. The **forced expiratory volume in one second**, abbreviated **FEV_1**, measures the volume of air that is forcibly exhaled over a period of one second after a full inhalation.

FEV_1, vital capacity, and total lung volume can be used to classify respiratory conditions as either **obstructive disease** or **restrictive disease**. In an obstructive disease, the pathological process that occurs obstructs the flow of air out of the lung. This decreases the amount of oxygen-rich air that can fill the lungs because of the trapping of air. A restrictive disease process is one where the flow of air into the lungs is decreased. Disease pro-

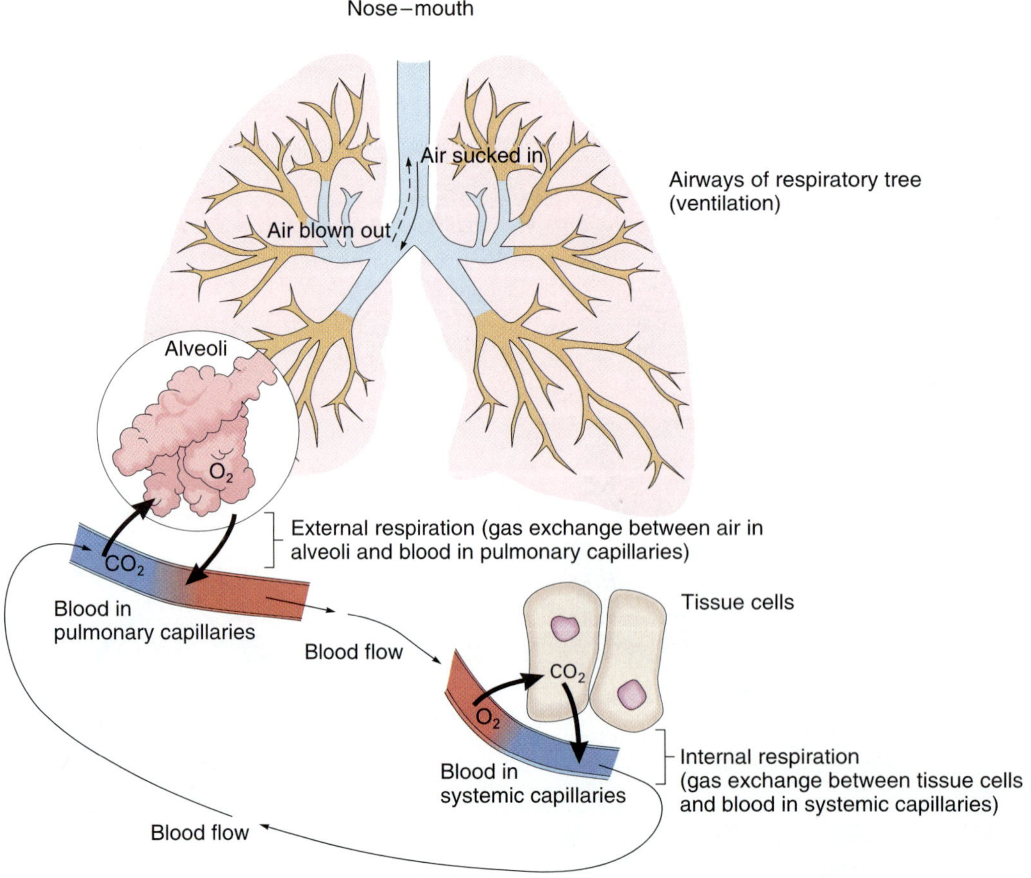

Figure 7–3 Gas exchange in the lungs and tissues.

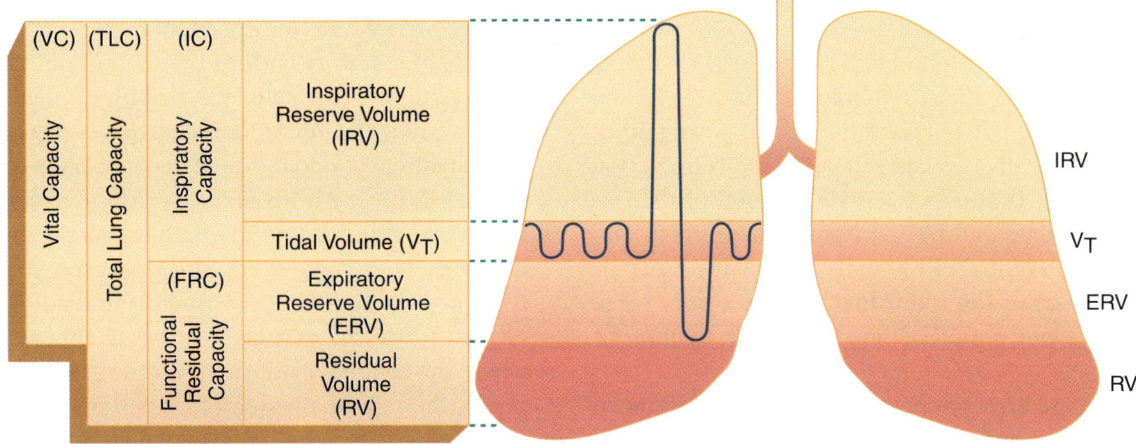

Figure 7–4 Normal lung volumes and capacities.

cesses may also be a combination of the two or may begin as one type and then develop characteristics of both types.

The level of oxygen in the blood is affected by several factors. **FiO_2** is the fraction of inspired air that consists of oxygen. FiO_2 is typically reported as a decimal form of the percentage. Average atmospheric air contains approximately 21 percent oxygen, so the FiO_2 of room air is 0.21. Supplemental oxygen received through a non-rebreather mask is close to 100 percent oxygen, or an FiO_2 of 1.00. The higher the FiO_2, the higher the oxygen content of the blood. The blood oxygen content is also dependent upon the ability of the oxygen molecules to diffuse across the cell wall from the alveoli to the blood. Disease processes that impede this diffusion, for example, increased mucus production in the lower airways seen in bronchitis and pneumonia or fluid in the alveoli as seen in pulmonary edema, will lower the oxygen content of the blood. Other factors that can decrease oxygen carrying content of the blood are a decrease in the number of red blood cells (Chapter 16), a decrease in the amount of iron and other nutrients ingested by the patient, the presence of carbon monoxide or lead in the blood, and the patient's respiratory rate and tidal volume.

COMMON SIGNS AND SYMPTOMS

There are many common signs and symptoms of respiratory disease. These symptoms can range from mild, as seen in the common cold, to severe, as seen in pneumonia. Dyspnea, orthopnea, apnea, wheezing, coughing, and nasal discharge are some of the most common symptoms. Changes in the rate and pattern of respirations can also occur.

Dyspnea (DISP-nee-ah; dys = difficulty, pnea = breathing) is a common sign of respiratory disease. Dyspnea may be in the form of **orthopnea** (or-THOP-nee-ah; ortho = straight, pnea = breathing) where an individual has difficulty breathing in a lying down position or is able to breathe with less difficulty when standing or sitting "straight" up. **Apnea** (ap-NEE-ah; a = without, pnea = breathing) for an extended amount of time is a life-threatening emergency. Dyspnea caused by a partial obstruction of the airways will produce **wheezing**. Severe dyspnea may lead to **hypoxemia** (high-POX-**SEE**-me-ah; hypo = not enough, ox = oxygen, emia = blood) or low blood-oxygen level. A common sign of hypoxemia is **cyanosis** (SIGH-ah-**NO**-sis; cyano = blue, osis = condition) or a blue color often observed in the nail beds and lips.

Coughing is another common symptom caused by irritation of the airways or a build-up of fluid in the lung tissue. **Sputum** (SPYOU-tum) is fluid or secretions coughed up from the lungs, not to be confused with saliva or spit from the digestive system. A **productive cough** is one in which there is a bringing up of sputum or excessive mucus. Coughing up blood, **hemoptysis** (he-MOP-tih-sis; hemo = blood, ptysis = saliva) may be a sign of serious respiratory disease.

Nasal discharge is frequently present in infections, inflammation, and in allergic respiratory reactions. It is the most frequent symptom of the common cold, but is also present in other respiratory disorders and may be a serious symptom of a chronic problem.

Hiccoughs, commonly called "hiccups," are the result of a sudden spasm of the diaphragm. They commonly occur after eating or drinking and can be stopped by a variety of techniques, including holding the breath and drinking water through a straw. Hiccoughs may accompany disease and in this instance are more difficult to eliminate.

Chronic respiratory conditions often lead to abnormal, permanent signs, such as clubbing and barrel-chested appearance. **Clubbing** is a condition of unknown pathogenesis, but it usually is related to poor distal circulation and oxygenation. It affects the distal portion of the finger and is characterized by soft tissue enlargement and an abnormal curvature of the nail (Figure 7–5). A barrel chest appears as the individual uses accessory chest muscles over a long period of time in an effort to improve breathing.

Wheezes are high-pitched sounds that are produced by air flowing through constricted respiratory passages. Wheezes that are auscultated during inspiration are called inspiratory wheezes, while wheezes auscultated during exhalation are called expiratory wheezes. Inspiratory wheezes are more common with small airway obstruction while expiratory wheezes are more common in asthma and chronic obstructive pulmonary disease.

The respiratory rate and volume are valuable signs that should be assessed by the EMS provider in every patient. **Tachypnea** (TACK-ihp-**NEE**-ah; tachy = rapid, pnea = referring to breathing) is a respiratory rate that is faster than normal and **bradypnea** is a respiratory rate slower than normal. Conditions such as infection, fever, fear, and neurological insults to the brain are among the vast list of conditions that can cause tachypnea. Bradypnea can be the result of drug overdose, hypothermia, or other neurological problems. **Hyperventilation** is an increased tidal volume above the normal range and **hypoventilation** is a decreased tidal volume below the normal range. Hyperventilation can occur from infection, fever, or fear, and hypoventilation can occur from overdoses or head injury. As the level of carbon dioxide in the blood is affected by the quantity of ventilation, hyperventilation will cause a decrease in blood carbon dioxide level and hypoventilation will result in an increased blood carbon dioxide level. Normal ranges for respiratory rate are indicated in Table 7–1.

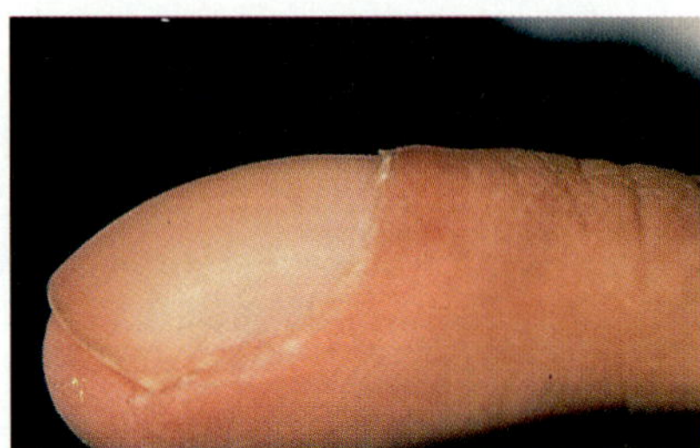

Figure 7–5 Clubbing. (Courtesy of Robert A. Silverman, M.D., Clinical Associate Professor, Department of Pediatrics, Georgetown University.)

The respiratory pattern is also important to assess in every patient. Normally, the respiratory pattern is regular, meaning the inhalation/exhalation cycle occurs within the same time period between one inhalation and the next (Figure 7–6A). An irregular pattern may not necessarily reflect pathology, although there are several patterns that have been named because they accompany certain types of conditions, both respiratory and non-respiratory. **Cheyne-Stokes respiration** is an abnormal pattern where the ventilation rate and volume gradually increases, peaks, then gradually decreases with interspersed periods of apnea (Figure 7–6B). Cheyne-Stokes respiration can occur with injury to the brain stem (see Chapter 9). **Kussmaul's respirations** can occur in conditions such as diabetic coma (see Chapter 11) and consists of deep, gasping respirations (Figure 7–6C). **Biot's respiration** (Figure 7–6D) consists of an irregular pattern, rate, and volume, with intermittent periods of apnea, and can occur in situations of increased intracranial pressure (see Chapter 9). **Central neurogenic hyperventilation** (CNH) is similar to Kussmaul's in that the volume is increased accompanied by an increased ventilation rate. CNH is also associated with increased intracranial pressure. **Agonal respirations** are known to the lay public as the "dying breath" and consist of slow, shallow, irregular, and sometimes gasping respirations (Figure 7–6E). Agonal respirations generally result from brain anoxia and are a terminal respiratory pattern unless aggressive intervention is performed.

One sign that highlights the interdependence of the respiratory and cardiovascular systems is **pulsus para-**

TABLE 7-1 Normal Respiratory Rates by Age.

Age	Normal Respiratory Rate
Premature	40–60
Term	30–60
3 months	30–50
6 months	25–35
9 months	23–33
1 year	20–30
2–4 years	20–28
5–6 years	20–25
8–12 years	16–24
14 years–Adult	12–20

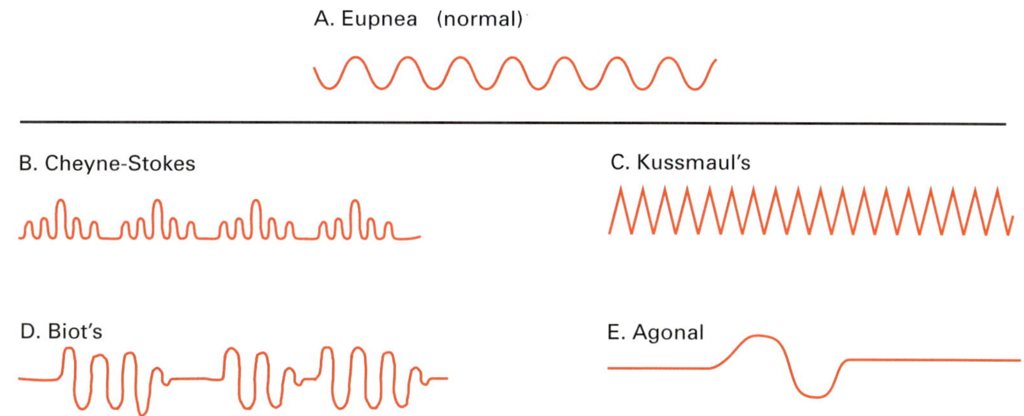

Figure 7-6 Respiratory patterns (A) Normal (B) Cheyne-Stokes (C) Kussmaul's (D) Biot's (E) Agonal.

doxus. Pulsus paradoxus is present when there is a greater than 10 mmHg drop in systolic blood pressure during inspiration; it can occur in respiratory diseases, such as chronic obstructive pulmonary diseases (COPD), and cardiovascular diseases, such as pericardial tamponade (see Chapter 8). This drop in systolic blood pressure is caused by an increase in intrathoracic pressure which decreases the ability for the heart to properly fill with blood. The less blood that returns to the heart, the lower the systemic blood pressure. Chapter 8 discusses the relationship between heart filling and blood pressure.

DIAGNOSTIC TESTS

A physical examination, including auscultation (listening to the chest with a stethoscope) should be completed to assess for normal as well as abnormal breathing quality. Abnormal breath sounds including wheezes, rales, and rhonchi are common with respiratory diseases. **Rales** are abnormal musical sounds heard on inspiration and are often called crackles. **Rhonchi** are dry rattling sounds in the bronchi caused by obstruction of the airways.

In addition to using the stethoscope, the EMS provider can gain useful information from percussing the chest. It is often best to percuss the chest prior to transporting the patient, as the noise of the ambulance makes the percussion note difficult to hear. To percuss the chest, the EMS provider places one finger on the tissue between the ribs and then taps that finger with a finger on the other hand. This produces a **percussion note** that can identify the presence of certain lung abnormalities. When percussing a normal chest, a mid-range tone is heard that is neither too high-pitched nor too low-pitched. As the EMS provider percusses from an area of normal lung to an area that is filled with fluid or pus, as in the case of pneumonia, the note changes to a dull sound. As the EMS provider percusses from an area of normal lung to an area that is filled with a greater amount of air than normal, as in the case of pneumothorax, the percussion note will change to a higher pitched or hyperresonant sound. Percussion can be used to localize and correlate findings with the auscultated breath sounds.

Two instruments assist the EMS provider in assessing the amount of respiration that is occurring during ventilation. Pulse oximetry is used to detect the percentage of arterial hemoglobin that has taken in oxygen. The higher the percentage, the better the uptake. To take the reading, a clip is placed either on the finger or earlobe. The pulse oximetry reading can be inaccurate in situations where the hemoglobin is altered; in carbon monoxide poisoning; if the patient is wearing fingernail polish; and in cold weather where blood flow to the skin is reduced. Capnometry is generally used after a patient is intubated to assess for endotracheal tube placement and to monitor gas exchange. In the situation of an intubated patient, the percentage of carbon dioxide, a normal byproduct of cellular metabolism present in inspired air, is extremely low. If the endotracheal tube is in place, the air will reach the alveoli, oxygen and carbon dioxide will be exchanged, and the expired air will have a much greater amount of carbon dioxide present. Capnometry can be continuously monitored, either with a colormetric device or an electronic device, to allow continual assessment of endotracheal tube placement or can be used just to confirm initial endotracheal tube placement.

A peak flow meter can be used to assess the ability of a patient to exhale air. Patients with chronic obstructive disease and asthma typically have peak flow meters at home, and regularly assess their peak flow. The normal peak flow is adjusted for sex, age, and height. Peak flows can be assessed before and after treatment with bronchodilators to objectively assess patient response to the medication.

A chest roentgenogram (X-ray) is a major diagnostic tool utilized in the emergency department to diagnose lung diseases such as tumors, tuberculosis, abscesses, and pneumonia. Sputum cultures are effective in determination of infectious disease. A tissue biopsy may be obtained as a definitive test for lung disease. Tissue biopsy is often obtained during a **bronchoscopy** (brong-KOS-koh-pee; broncho = bronchus or lung passageways, oscopy = procedure to look into the bronchus). Lung tissue may be biopsied utilizing a fine needle technique through the body wall.

The best indicator of lung function is measurement of the amounts of carbon dioxide (waste) and oxygen in the blood. This measurement is done on arterial blood and is called **arterial blood gases** (ABGs). Normal arterial blood gases should be high in oxygen and low in carbon dioxide. The reverse of these readings is indicative of poor pulmonary function.

Pulmonary function tests (PFT) are a group of tests that measure volume and flow of air as discussed earlier. PFTs are valuable in assisting in the diagnosis of a respiratory problem. PFTs may also be performed before and after brochodilation treatment to measure treatment effectiveness. PFTs are measured against a norm for the individual's age, height, and sex.

COMMON DISEASES OF THE RESPIRATORY SYSTEM

Chronic lung diseases affect over thirty million Americans. Approximately 350,000 Americans die annually from lung diseases, making it the number three killer responsible for an estimated four out of every seven deaths.

Diseases of the respiratory system range from simple, like the common cold, to very serious, like cancer of the lung. The symptoms of the various disorders are often similar in the early stages with most conditions manifesting in shortness of breath, coughing, and/or wheezing. However, some disorders may not present symptoms until late in the disease development. Smoking is the number one risk behavior for developing chronic respiratory disease.

Diseases of the Upper Respiratory System

Respiratory illnesses, which are mostly viral infections, account for approximately fifty percent of all acute illnesses. Respiratory infections account for over eighty percent of all infections. Most disorders of the upper respiratory system are not life-threatening.

Upper Respiratory Infection (URI). Upper respiratory infection is a broad term referring to several infectious diseases of the upper respiratory system. These infections are the most common cause for lost days of work for adults. Most URIs (not to be confused with UTI—urinary tract infection) are caused by viruses. The most common is a group called *Rhinovirus*. General treatment for viral diseases includes rest, drinking increased amounts of fluids, taking **antipyretics** (anti = against, pyretic = fever) and **analgesics** (an = without, algesic = pain). Antibiotics are not effective against viral infections, but may be needed for secondary bacterial infection. The common cold is the most frequent URI and often leads to secondary infectious diseases.

Common Cold (Acute Rhinitis). The common cold is an acute inflammation of the mucous membranes of the upper respiratory system. Most individuals are very familiar with the symptoms of runny nose (**rhinorrhea**—rhino = nose, orrhea = run through), watery eyes, stuffy head, sore throat, sneezing, and fever. There are several hundred different virus strains that cause a cold. Developing immunity to one strain does not provide immunity to others.

A cold is very contagious and is usually passed from one individual to another through touch and air droplets. Good hand washing is the best preventive for a cold. Many individuals believe that getting chilled and/or wet is the cause of a cold. In actuality these actions do not directly cause a cold, however they lower an individual's resistance to invasion by a cold-causing virus. Children, the elderly, and individuals in generally poor health are at increased risk of contracting a cold.

Hay Fever (Allergic Rhinitis). Allergic rhinitis is an inflammation of the mucous membranes caused by allergies. This sensitivity to an allergen tends to run in families. Ragweed and grasses are two common allergens. Hay fever is discussed in detail in Chapter 12.

Sinusitis. Sinusitis is an inflammation of the mucous membrane lining the sinuses. The sinuses are air-filled cavities in the bony tissue of the head. The membranes that line the nose extend into the sinuses. For this reason acute rhinitis often leads to sinusitis. It is also believed that blowing the nose too hard may spread infection into the sinuses. Other causes of sinusitis include tooth infections, air pollution, and nasal deformities. As mucous membranes become swollen, the drainage system becomes blocked. Mucus accumulates in the sinuses causing increased pressure and often leads to sinus headaches, dizziness, and difficulty breathing. Treatment often includes decongestants to promote better drainage. Antibiotics are sometimes required if an infection is suspected.

Pharyngitis. Pharyngitis is an inflammation of the throat (pharynx = throat, itis = inflammation) commonly called a "sore throat." The most common cause is viral infection. Bacterial infection by streptococcus may also occur and is common in children. Irritation to the mucous membranes may also lead to pharyngitis. Irritants may include breathing extremely hot or cold air, chemical fumes, or smoke. Treatment may include throat lozenges, antiseptic or salt-water gargles, and analgesics. Additionally, bacterial infections require antibiotic treatment.

Laryngitis. Laryngitis is an inflammation of the larynx (lar-INKS) and vocal cords. Most individuals are familiar with the hoarse voice quality caused by laryngitis. Other symptoms include difficulty swallowing (dysphagia), throat pain, and fever. Laryngitis may be caused by viral or bacterial infections, or by breathing irritants such as extremely hot or cold air, chemical fumes, and smoke. Laryngitis frequently follows other URIs such as the common cold, pharyngitis, and sinusitis. Another cause may be overuse of the voice for an extended time. Treatment may include voice rest, increased fluid intake, analgesics, throat lozenges, and removal of causative factors.

Epistaxis. **Epistaxis**, or nosebleed, is a very common condition. Almost every person can remember a situation when he had a nosebleed. Most of the time, the nosebleed is a minor inconvenience and will stop without significant intervention; however, there are cases where the bleeding can be serious and life-threatening.

There are two types of epistaxis, *anterior* and *posterior*. Anterior epistaxis is a bleed located anterior on the nasal septum (see Figure 7–2). A posterior epistaxis is located posteriorly deep in the nasopharynx. Anterior bleeds usually stop within a reasonable amount of time with direct pressure to the nostrils. Posterior bleeds can be more difficult to stop because the blood vessels are not as accessible to apply direct pressure. A posterior bleed is suspected if bleeding occurs from both nostrils or continues without visualizing a source in the anterior portion of the nasal septum.

Treatment in the field consists of direct pressure to the nostrils and leaning the patient forward to both minimize drainage into the throat and encourage pooling and clotting. The airway should be maintained and all patients should be assessed for signs of shock. In the case of a significant bleed, an IV should be started and fluid treatment provided based upon vital signs. In the emergency department, the bleed may be chemically cauterized by applying silver nitrate to the source, or the nostril may be packed with gauze or a commercial packing.

Epiglottitis. Epiglottitis can be a life-threatening condition where the epiglottis (see Figure 7–2) becomes inflamed to the point where it occludes the trachea. In children, epiglottitis is caused by a bacterium *Haemophilus influenzae B* (HiB) and is prevalent among children age 1–5 years old. As an HiB vaccine has been available in this country now for several years, the occurrence of epiglottitis in children has markedly decreased. Currently epiglottitis has an occurrence that begins around 7 years of age and involves a bacterial infection by other organisms. In children, the onset of high fever, sore throat, stridor, and drooling is abrupt over a period of 1–2 days. The child will look very sick and may have an ashen gray skin color. Additionally, the child may have retractions between the ribs when inhaling, excessive drooling, and no cough. A decrease in activity and lack of eye contact for a toddler are signs of significant illness.

Emergency treatment involves supplemental oxygen and transport in a position of comfort. This is a serious emergency; however, the patient should be kept calm. Oxygen may be administered by allowing the parent to hold a mask several inches away from the face to reduce anxiety in the child. Endotracheal intubation will be very difficult in this child because of the extensive swelling of and around the epiglottis and generally should not be attempted in the field. At the emergency department, the child will likely receive intravenous antibiotics to combat the bacteria and steroids to reduce inflammation.

In adults, the situation can be just as serious as with children, but typically develops over a period of hours to days in contrast to the abrupt onset in children. The adult will complain of throat pain and dysphagia. Drooling may be present, but generally not to the same extent as in children. Treatment is the same as with children, consisting of oxygen and aggressive airway management if indicated. Again, endotracheal intubation is generally not recommended in the field, and should only be attempted if local protocols allow it in this situation and the EMS provider is experienced with difficult airway management.

Croup. Croup is a viral condition that produces inflammation in the larynx, trachea, and bronchi, and is known medically as laryngotracheolbronchitis. This condition is common among toddler age children and is discussed in Chapter 23, Childhood Diseases and Disorders.

Diseases of the Bronchi and Lungs

Diseases of the bronchi and lungs are usually more severe than diseases of the upper respiratory system. Many of these can be life-threatening, such as influenza, especially in the elderly population.

Asthma. Asthma is a hypersensitivity reaction that causes constriction of the bronchi leading to difficulty in breathing. Asthma, also called bronchial asthma, is discussed in detail as a hypersensitivity disorder in Chapter 12. Asthma is characterized by episodes of wheezing and dyspnea.

Field management of an acute asthma attack primarily concerns ensuring a patent airway and adequate ventilation. Continuous nebulization of albuterol, a beta–2 receptor agonist, or providing three treatments in an hour is generally the first line treatment. Atropine can also be nebulized and administered in conjunction with albuterol (Combivent), augmenting bronchodilation by blocking parasympathetic tone in the respiratory tree. Epinephrine can be administered subcutaneously to assist with bronchodilation and methylprednisolone can be administered intravenously or intramuscularly to treat the swelling that is associated with asthma. The use of magnesium has not played out to be as beneficial as once thought; however, it may be used in difficult cases. Some patients may require intubation and ventilation if respiratory failure is imminent.

Acute Bronchitis. Acute bronchitis is inflammation of the mucous membrane lining of the bronchus. It often involves the trachea (tracheobronchitis). Acute bronchitis is a short-term disorder commonly following an upper respiratory infection. Inhaling fumes, smoke, dust, cold air, and other irritants may also cause acute bronchitis. Symptoms include fever, a tight feeling behind the sternum, and a dry cough that later progresses to a productive cough (coughing up or expectorating mucus sputum). Treatment consists of rest, drinking increased amounts of fluids to help liquefy secretions, cough syrup, analgesics, and antipyretics. Antibiotics are helpful only if secondary bacterial infections occur. Prognosis is generally good for most individuals. Infants and small children may become seriously ill because the bronchioles are very small and may become obstructed by swollen tissue or mucus plugs. The elderly and chronically ill may have a poor prognosis because they have an increased risk for developing secondary bacterial infections such as pneumonia.

Influenza (Flu). Influenza is an acute, highly contagious respiratory infection. Influenza is characterized by sudden onset of fever, chills, headache, back and muscle pain. Other symptoms may include cough, runny nose, sore throat, sneezing, hoarseness, nausea, vomiting, and diarrhea. Influenza is a viral infection commonly spread by coughing of respiratory secretions.

There are many strains of influenza (flu) virus. The flu virus also has great genetic variation. The number of strains and variations help to explain how this virus causes epidemics year after year. Unfortunately, like the common cold, immunity to one viral strain does not provide immunity to another, and for this reason an individual may have the flu multiple times. Flu epidemics commonly occur in the winter and early spring.

Treatment of influenza is symptomatic and may include bedrest, analgesics (an = without, algesia = pain), and antipyretics (anti = against, pyretic = fever). Antibiotics are not indicated unless secondary bacterial infections occur. Pneumonia in the very young, old, and chronically ill may be fatal. For this reason, influenza vaccination should be given to the elderly and those individuals with chronic disease. Generally the prognosis is good if complications do not occur.

Health care workers, including EMS providers, are also encouraged to get an annual flu shot to help prevent contracting and to help reduce the spread of flu.

Chronic Obstructive Pulmonary Disease (COPD). Chronic obstructive pulmonary disease is a name for a group of pulmonary diseases characterized by the inability to get air into or out of the lungs. Ninety percent of the time these problems are caused by cigarette smoking. The two most common diseases classified as COPD are chronic bronchitis and emphysema. Since the etiology is the same, namely, cigarette smoking, these two diseases usually coexist. There can be pure forms of either but they usually occur together. For this reason the diagnosis of COPD may describe the condition more adequately.

Individuals with COPD often become debilitated in the final stages of the disease. Loss of normal respiratory response is not unusual. Normally, individuals are stimulated to breathe by an increase of carbon dioxide in the blood. A secondary or backup stimulus is a decrease of oxygen in the blood. Individuals with COPD commonly have high levels of carbon dioxide in the blood. Initially the body attempts to correct this by increasing breathing in an effort to blow out excessive CO_2. When this effort fails the respiratory system adapts to the high CO_2 levels and begins responding to the secondary system, low blood oxygen levels; this is called the hypoxic drive. Giving oxygen to these individuals may be fatal as high oxygenation removes the stimulus to breathe. However, the EMS provider should *never* withhold oxygen from a COPD patient who is complaining of increased dyspnea. In general, overriding this hypoxic drive to breathe is rare, requiring a longer period of oxygen administration than occurs during a typical EMS encounter. The pulse oximetry reading may be useful in guiding oxygen administration in these patients.

Diagnosis of COPD is made by history and physical examination and by ruling out other pulmonary diseases. Chest X-rays, pulmonary function tests (PFT), and arterial blood gases (ABGs) help confirm the diagnosis. There is no cure for end stage COPD. Cessation of smoking may slow or reverse the disease in the early stages and ease symptoms in the later stages. Symptomatic treatment includes use of bronchodilator medications, inhalers, mucolytics, and cough medications. Avoiding exposure to individuals with respiratory tract infections is important because these diseases aggravate COPD. Influenza vaccination is recommended. Prognosis is poor caused by progressive deterioration of pulmonary function which often leads to respiratory failure and death. Emergency treatment consists of oxygen, bronchodilators, and possible steroids for the same resaons they are used in asthma.

Chronic Bronchitis. Chronic bronchitis is a long-term inflammation of the mucous membranes of the bronchus. It is characterized by increased mucus production with a productive cough. Chronic inflammation leads to hypertrophy of the mucus-secreting glands, thickening of the mucous membrane, and **bronchiectasis** (BRONG-kee-**ECK**-tah-sis) or a chronic dilatation of the bronchus. Bronchiectasis allows mucus to pool in the bronchus, producing a foul smelling cough. Chronic bronchitis may be mild in nature for many years. This form is commonly called a "smoker's cough" and occurs primarily in the morning hours. As the disease progresses, obstruction of the bronchi and bronchioles becomes more pronounced, leading to difficulty getting air into the lungs. Coughing, dyspnea, and **hypoxia** (HIGH-**POCK**-see-ah; hypo = low, oxia = oxygen) occur. During bouts of hypoxia, the individual often becomes cyanotic. In the final or end stage, the symptoms are more continuous, causing lung damage, debilitation of the individual, and eventual death.

Emphysema. Emphysema comes from the Greek word emphysan, meaning to inflate. This chronic disease is characterized by an increased production of mucus, causing trapping of air in the tiny alveoli or air sacks of the lung. As air becomes trapped in the alveoli, they become overinflated, leading to destruction of the alveoli wall. Destruction of the alveoli wall allows the alveoli to fuse with other alveoli, forming a larger air sack and trapping more air (Figure 7–7). The individual with emphysema is able to get air in, but the air becomes trapped and must be forced out before more air can be taken in. These enlarged alveoli have a decreased surface area thus decreasing the ability to oxygenate the blood. Air trapping and decreased oxygen exchange lead to dyspnea, tachypnea, wheezing, and coughing.

Individuals with emphysema often lean over a table or chair to more adequately use accessory respiratory muscles in an effort to blow out the trapped air. Pursing of the lips also helps hold the alveoli open while pushing the air out (Figure 7–8). This extra pressure often causes the face and skin to become reddened. Extra pressure on the chest muscles also produces a characteristic "barrel chest" appearance (see Figure 7–8). Individuals with emphysema use large amounts of energy in their rerspiratory eddorts and can quickly develop respiratory failure if not treated aggressively.

Atelectasis. Atelectasis is the collapse or airless state of part or all of a lung. More commonly it affects only a

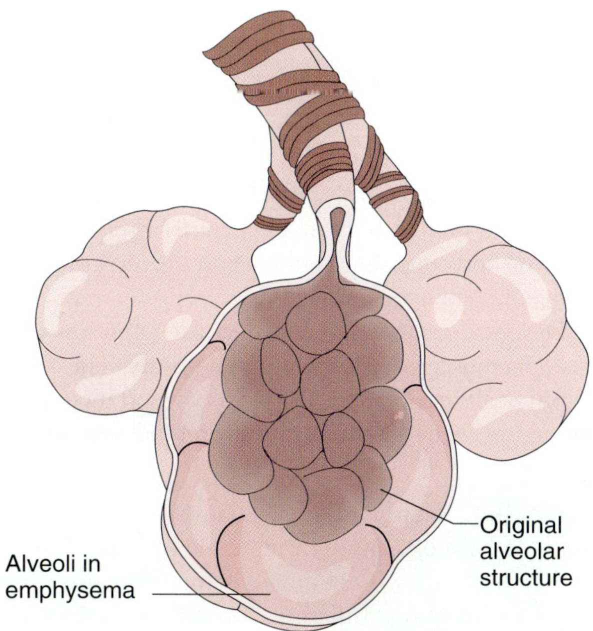

Figure 7–7 Normal vs. emphasematous alveoli.

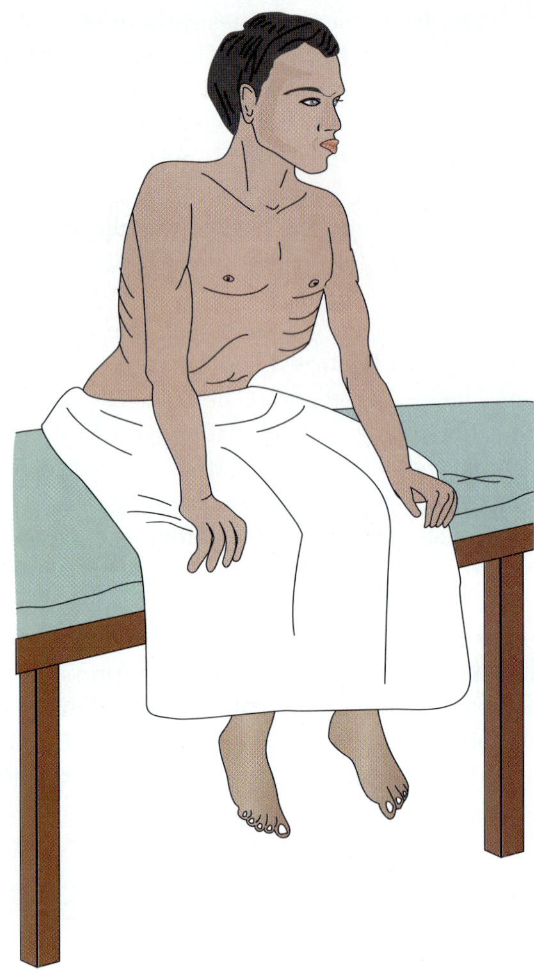

Figure 7–8 Pursed lips and barrel chest of emphysema.

Pneumonia may be identified in several ways. The cause may be included in the name, as pneumococcal, aspiration, and tuberculous pneumonia. The location may be identified in the name, as in a lobar, bilateral, and double pneumonia. Secondary pneumonia indicates a connection to another cause. Often the location and cause may be combined to describe the pneumonia, as in bilateral pneumococcal pneumonia. No matter the cause and location, pneumonia affects approximately four million individuals each year. It is the most common cause of infectious death in the United States.

Pneumonia may range from mild to life-threatening. Actions that inhibit the normal protective mechanisms of the respiratory system may lead to pneumonia. Such actions include smoking, immobility, general anesthesia, and endotracheal intubation. Pneumonia occurs more often in the elderly, chronically ill, and immunosuppressed and is a significant cause of death in these individuals.

Pathogens may reach the lung tissue through the respiratory system or through the blood as a result of septicemia. Invasion of pathogens into the alveoli leads to inflammation of the alveolar tissue. Inflammation causes the classic outpouring of blood fluid and white cells from the capillaries into the tissues, filling the alveoli. This filling of the alveoli causes a decrease in gas exchange leading to hypoxia (Figure 7–9).

Symptoms of pneumonia are related to the area and the amount of tissue involved. Symptoms include dyspnea, weakness, fever, chills, chest pain, and cough. Diagnosis is made after completion of a chest X-ray, history, and physical examination. Treatment depends on cause.

small section of the lung. Atelectasis is often related to inadequate breathing patterns related to pain. Surgical pain and fractured ribs often cause inadequate breathing leading to atelectasis. Blockage of the airway by a mucus plug may also cause atelectasis. Frequent deep breathing and coughing help to open the airway, expand the alveoli, and avoid atelectasis.

Dyspnea, cyanosis, and anxiety are common symptoms. Diagnosis is confirmed after a positive chest X-ray and physical examination. Prognosis is good if complications do not occur. Pneumonia is a common complication.

Pneumonia. Pneumonia is an inflammation of the bronchioles and alveoli caused by infection by bacteria, virus, or other pathogens. Pneumonia is the term specifically related to infection. Inflammation without infection is termed pneumonitis. Pneumonitis is inflammation generally caused by a hypersensitivity to dusts and chemicals.

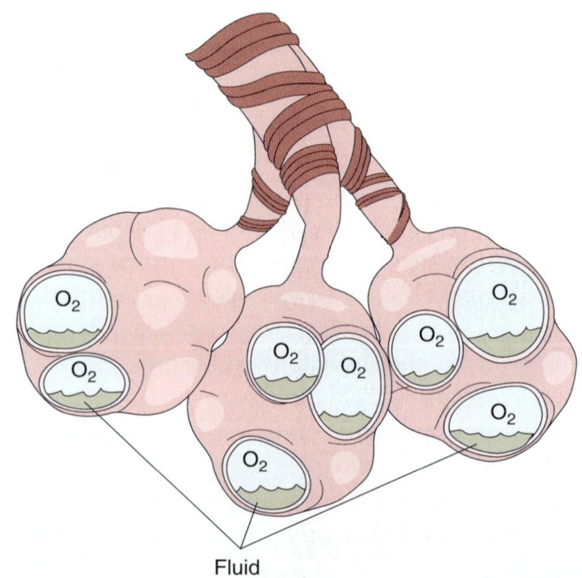

Figure 7–9 Pneumonia: alveolar filling with fluid.

Bacterial infection is treated with antibiotics. Viral infection is treated symptomatically. Rest, analgesics, oxygen therapy, and increased fluid intake are common for all types of pneumonia. Bronchodilators may also assist in opening the airways and improving oxygenation.

Pulmonary Abscess. Pulmonary abscess, also called lung abscess, is a collection of infectious material contained within a capsule (Figure 7–10). Abscess formation was discussed in detail in Chapter 4. Abscess formation may be a complication of bacterial pneumonia or aspiration of food or foreign objects. Symptoms include chills, fever, chest pain, and cough. Coughing of bloody or foul smelling sputum and foul smelling breath may also be indicative of a pulmonary abscess. Diagnosis is made by completion of a history and physical examination, chest X-ray, and sputum cultures. Pulmonary abscesses are commonly treated with long-term antibiotic therapy. Surgical resection may be indicated if the abscess are quite large or if antibiotic therapy is unsuccessful.

Pulmonary Tuberculosis (TB). Tuberculosis is a bacterial infection caused by *Mycobacterium tuberculosis*. It is acquired by breathing air that is infected with the bacteria and is spread by coughing and sneezing. The lungs are most often affected although the disease may spread to the kidneys, bones, and brain. Tuberculosis in an otherwise healthy individual often is asymptomatic. For this reason testing is needed to determine the presence of the disease. If symptoms appear they are often vague and include loss of weight, energy, and appetite. As the disease progresses, the individual may become symptomatic with a chronic productive cough, dyspnea, fever, and night sweats.

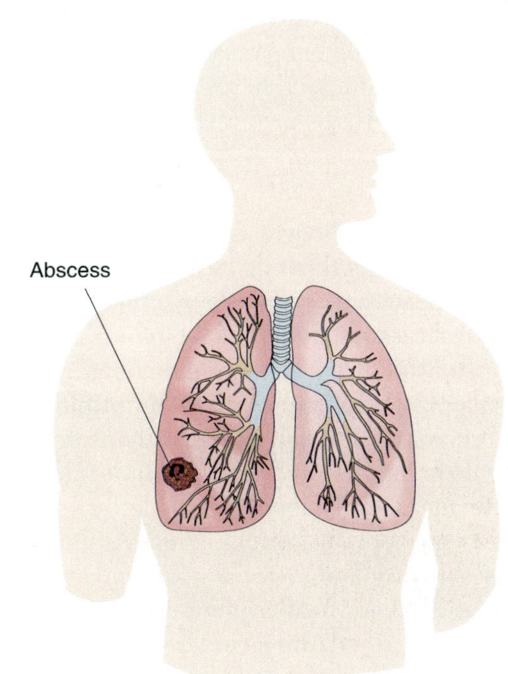

Figure 7–10 Pulmonary abscess.

Mycobacterium tuberculosis is protected in a strong coating that enables it to live outside the body for a lengthy amount of time. Infected droplets that are coughed or sneezed may dry up and remain on inanimate objects as dust. The tuberculosis bacteria can be killed by bactericidal solutions or by direct sunlight. TB is often prevalent in areas of overcrowding and poor sanitation. The incidence of tuberculosis was greatly reduced decades ago with the introduction of effective antibiotics. More recently, the number of TB cases in the United States has seriously risen because of the influx of high numbers of infected immigrants, the homeless, individuals with AIDS who have a poor resistance to infection, and the development of drug-resistant bacteria.

The infection begins with a primary lesion in the lungs. *Mycobacterium tuberculosis* does not attract PMNs and thus does not cause an acute inflammation. Lymphocytes and macrophages are attracted to these encapsulated bacteria. These immune cells begin producing antibodies and walling off the infection by forming a type of granuloma called a tubercule, hence the name tuberculosis. The inside of the tubercule contains dead bacteria, lung tissue, and immune cells that together exhibit a cheesy appearance called caseous necrosis.

After necrosis the tubercules change by fibrosing and calcifying. If the immune system is effective in walling off the bacteria, the disease may be arrested or rendered inactive for a long period of time (months to years). During this time the individual is often asymptomatic and not aware that he/she has tuberculosis. If the disease is not arrested the individual will become symptomatic with progressive primary tuberculosis. The antibodies that are produced during this time will circulate in the blood for the remainder of the infected individual's life in readiness to attack future tuberculosis bacteria. These circulating antibodies are the basis for the positive reaction of a TB skin test.

Secondary tuberculosis occurs when an individual is re-infected with *Mycobacterium tuberculosis* or the primary disease is reactivated because of a decline in the individual's resistance. Antibodies formed during the primary stage of the disease activate quickly and lead to larger areas of necrosis in the lung tissue. During secondary tuberculosis the individual becomes symptomatic. The tubercule mass becomes liquified and is coughed up leaving a cavity in the lung tissue (Figure 7–11). Frequent coughing often ruptures capillaries in

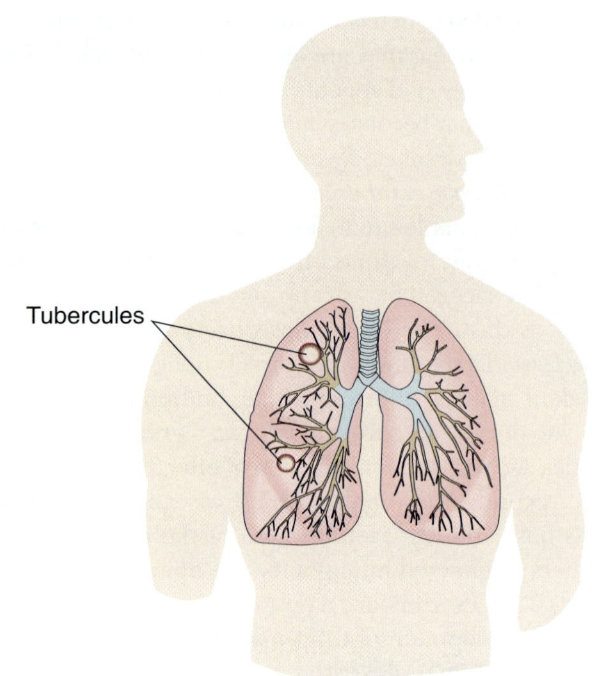

Figure 7–11 Tuberculosis.

the lung tissue, leading to hemoptysis or coughing and/or spitting of blood. Coughing by the infected individual fills the surrounding air with contagious bacteria thus increasing the spread of the disease.

As large cavities are formed in the lung tissue, the ability of the tissue to oxygenate the blood is decreased. The individual becomes dyspneic and cachectic with a general appearance of being "consumed" by the disease. For this reason, historically this disease was called consumption. During that time individuals were placed in sanitariums to prevent the spread of TB and to provide much needed rest. Without effective treatment, many infected individuals died from tuberculosis. Currently, tuberculosis is diagnosed by skin testing, chest X-ray, and sputum culture. Extended antibiotic therapy is needed to rid the individual of the infection.

Adult Respiratory Distress Syndrome (ARDS). Adult respiratory distress syndrome (ARDS) is a syndrome that occurs in response to a significant trauma to the body. In ARDS, there is diffuse damage to the alveoli. The capillaries surrounding the alveoli become leaky, and protein-rich fluid leaks into the alveoli. This protein-rich fluid also contains inflammatory products that damage the endothelium, or lining, of the alveoli. This damage decreases the ability for oxygen to diffuse into the blood. The protein-rich fluid is also very thick, and decreases the ability for oxygen to gain access into the blood.

Conditions that cause ARDS include multiple or major trauma, prolonged shock, aspiration, sepsis, major burns, near drowning, inhalation of chemical irritants, or through treatment with certain medications or street drugs. As oxygen transport into the blood is significantly impaired, patients who develop ARDS require prolonged ventilatory support. ARDS has a high mortality rate, and for those who do recover, permanent lung damage often remains.

Lung Cancer. Lung cancer is the leading cause of cancer deaths in the United States. It is often asymptomatic until metastasis has occurred. Metastasis to the brain, bone, and liver are common. Often the first symptoms are those related to other organs affected by metastasis. Discovery by metastasis makes for a very poor prognosis. Approximately ten percent of lung cancer victims survive five years. Symptoms related to the lung tumor are dyspnea, coughing, and hemoptysis. Ninety percent of lung cancer victims are smokers (Healthy Highlight 7–1). Men are affected more commonly than women, although the increase in female smokers after World War II has increased the number of female lung cancer victims. Diagnosis is made by X-ray, CT scan, and tissue biopsy. Treatment includes chemotherapy, surgery, and radiation. If the tumor is discovered early, surgical removal may mean cure, but this is rarely the case.

Diseases of the Pleura and Chest

Diseases of the pleura and chest may be caused by infection, trauma, or other diseases. Pain and shortness of breath are the common symptoms. The severity of the disorders can range from mild to severe, depending on the cause, the individual's age, medical history, and other complicating factors.

Pleurisy (Pleuritis). Pleurisy is the inflammation of the membranes covering the lung (visceral pleura) and lining the chest cavity (parietal pleura). Pleurisy may be caused by bacterial infection of the pleura. Secondary pleurisy often follows trauma, pneumonia, tuberculosis, and neoplasm. The main symptom of pleurisy is a sharp chest area pain that increases with inspiration and coughing. Pain may be so severe that it limits movement in the affected area. Diagnosis is made by completion of a history and physical examination. Auscultation of the lungs may produce a squeaky, rubbing sound during inspiration, known as a pleuralrub. Treatment is aimed at the cause and also includes symptomatic treatment with analgesics. This pain must be differentiated from cardiac pain.

HEALTHY HIGHLIGHT 7–1

The Harmful Effects of Smoking

Smoking tobacco products is the main cause of preventable death in the United States. Some of the other harmful effects of smoking include:

- its link to cancer, particularly cancer of the lung, larynx, esophagus, pancreas, bladder, kidney, and mouth; thirty percent of cancer deaths are linked to smoking
- heart and cardiovascular disease, especially stroke
- increased heart rate
- chronic bronchitis and emphysema
- associated with more frequent attacks of asthma and otitis media in children exposed to secondhand smoke
- decreased rate of lung tissue growth
- impaired level of lung function
- shortness of breath, especially with exercise, and increased phlegm production
- heartburn and peptic ulcers
- premature birth and low birth weight if used during pregnancy
- higher incidence of sudden infant death syndrome (SIDS) in infants whose parent(s) smokes, even outside the home
- shortened life span with increased risk of morbidity
- it is addictive

Pneumothorax. Pneumothorax is a collection of air in the pleural cavity often resulting in partial or complete collapse of the lung on the affected side (Figure 7–12). Spontaneous pneumothorax occurs when air is leaked into the pleural space from within or from the lung. Common causes include pulmonary disease, tumor, or pulmonary tissue tear.

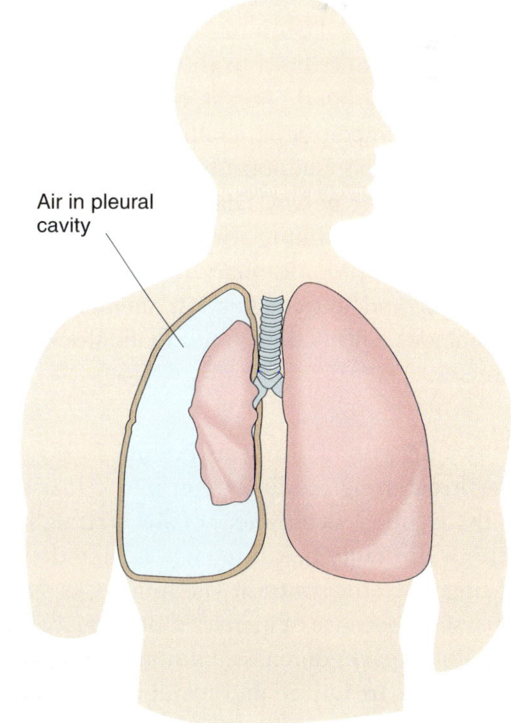

Figure 7–12 Pneumothorax.

Pleural Effusion (Hydrothorax). Pleural effusion or hydrothorax is a collection of fluid in the chest cavity. Causes of hydrothorax may include congestive heart failure, tuberculosis, cancer, pulmonary thromboembolism, or pneumonia. The affected individual may be asymptomatic or may exhibit signs of dyspnea and chest or pleuritic pain. Diagnosis may be confirmed by X-ray. Treatment in the hospital may include thoracentesis to remove the excess fluid. Correction of the condition causing hydrothorax is needed to prevent re-occurrence.

Empyema. Empyema is the collection of pus (py = pus) in the chest cavity. It may be the result of a ruptured lung abscess or an ulcerated tumor. Empyema is not as common as it was prior to the development of antibiotics. Symptoms include coughing, dyspnea, and chest pain on the affected side. Diagnosis is by X-ray and thoracentesis. Microbiologic cultures may be performed on the fluid to identify the infective organism. Surgical débridement of the empyema is sometimes necessary to allow healing.

Diseases of the Cardiovascular and Respiratory Systems

The cardiovascular and respiratory systems are so closely related that many diseases affect both systems, making it difficult to classify the disease by one system from the other. For this reason these diseases need further consideration.

Pulmonary Thromboembolism (PTE). Pulmonary thromboembolism is a sudden blockage of an artery in the pulmonary system by an embolism (Figure 7–13). Chapter 8 discusses the pathology of an embolism. The floating material may be a blood clot, fat globule, or piece of tissue. Commonly a blood clot or thrombus develops in the veins of the lower legs, thighs, and pelvis. This clot then breaks loose, floats in the vascular system and sticks in a pulmonary artery, resulting in a pulmonary thromboembolism. Symptoms of a PTE vary greatly depending on the size of the clot and the area affected. Dyspnea, cough, chest pain, and apprehension are common symptoms. If the PTE is severe, sudden symptoms of cyanosis and shock may occur. Death may also result.

Factors that contribute to the development of an embolism are prolonged bedrest, obesity, birth control pills, smoking, cancer, genetic alterations in the coagulation cascade (see Chapter 16), and trauma or fractures of the legs or pelvis. Diagnosis is confirmed by X-ray examination and lung scans. Treatment is aimed at maintaining cardiopulmonary function by administering oxygen and anticoagulation medications. Prevention includes ambulation, antiembolic stockings, and leg exercises.

Pulmonary Edema. Pulmonary edema, if severe, may be a life-threatening medical emergency. It is characterized by dyspnea, orthopnea (ortho = straight, pnea = breath) or difficulty breathing when lying down, and a blood-tinged, frothy sputum. The fluid leaks out of the vascular system because of increased pulmonary vascular pressure. Pulmonary edema is commonly seen as a result of congestive heart failure and resulting fluid buildup. Any disease that affects blood pressure, heart function, and blood fluid levels may lead to pulmonary edema.

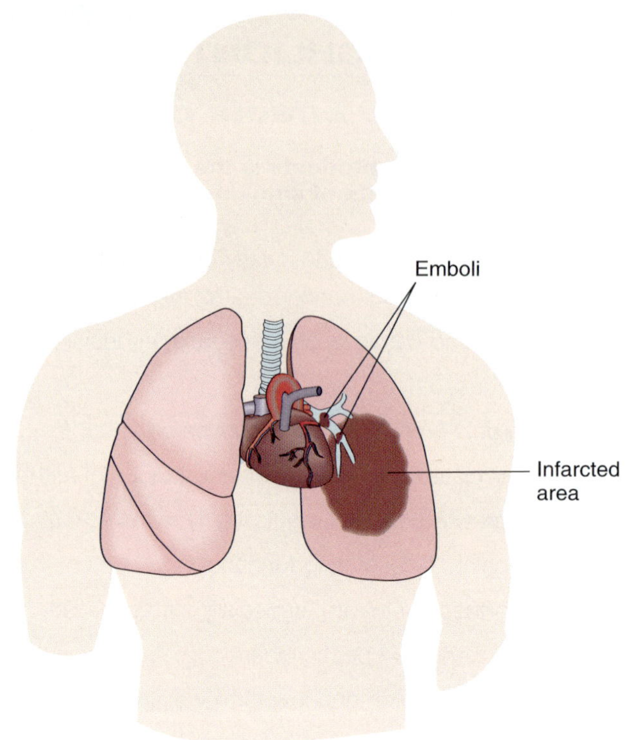

Figure 7–13 Pulmonary emboli.

These diseases include hypertension, pulmonary thromboembolism, and renal failure. Pulmonary edema is diagnosed by utilizing arterial blood gases (ABGs) and chest X-ray. ABGs will show an increased carbon dioxide level and chest X-rays will exhibit increased opacity or whiteness. Treatment is aimed at reducing pressure and blood volume and generally follows the LMNOP mnemonic (Lasix, morphine, nitrates, oxygen, and position), CPAP devices, and vasopressors. Diuretics to increase urine output, cardiogenics to increase the contraction of the heart and morphine to bring about venous dilatation may be prescribed. Mechanical respiratory ventilation may also be needed by either intubating the patient and placing on a ventilator or by using a Continuous Positive Airway Pressure (CPAP) or Bi-level Positive Airway Pressure (BiPAP) device to assist the patient's respiratory efforts. CPAP and BiPAP both utilize a fitted mask placed over the patient's nose or mouth and nose to produce a constant pressure in the patient's respiratory tree to allow the lower airways and alveoli to stay open during exhalation. In pulmonary edema, the increase in blood pressure in the lungs causes the alveoli and lower airways to collapse so the patient must expend additional energy to open these collapsed airways to allow gas exchange to occur. CPAP provides a continuous pressure throughout the entire respiratory cycle. BiPAP allows the operator to set different airway pressures for the inhalation and exhalation phases. The use of CPAP and BiPAP is a temporary measure that may allow time for medications to work in reducing systemic blood pressure and volume and avoid intubation.

Cor Pulmonale. Cor pulmonale, discussed further in Chapter 8, is a right-sided heart failure related to acute or chronic pulmonary disease. Increased pulmonary blood pressure causes enlargement of the right ventricle and decreased pumping ability. Polycythemia (poly = many, cyt = cell, red cell, emia = blood) develops as the body tries to compensate for hypoxemia (hypo = not enough, ox = oxygen, emia = blood) leading to a thickening of the blood and increased workload on the heart.

TRAUMA

Trauma to the respiratory system can have a devastating effect on the patient. Even a rib fracture can cause severe enough pain to produce hypoventilation and hypoxia, especially in a supine and immobilized patient. Tension pneumothoracies can be life-threatening if not rapidly treated. The EMS provider must use the information gained by observing the mechanism of injury and have a high index of suspicion when assessing the trauma patient for traumatic injuries to the respiratory system.

Rib Fracture

Rib fractures are caused by direct trauma to the thorax. This can occur by various mechanisms, including penetrating trauma and blunt trauma from a variety of sources. Rib fractures are painful, and many patients are reluctant to take a deep breath because of the pain. The patient may become tachypnic, breathing at an increased rate to compensate for the decreased tidal volume in order to maintain a normal minute volume. As tachypnea is an early sign for a tension pneumothorax, the EMS provider must carefully assess for other signs of a pneumothorax.

Complications of a rib fracture include significant bleeding, nerve damage, pheumothorax, or punctured abdominal organs. The intercostal blood vessels (artery and vein) and nerve run along the underside of each rib, and can be damaged by a rib fracture. The bleeding may be difficult to find and control, and in rare cases enough bleeding may occur to become dangerous. The patient who has a fracture of one of the lower ribs on either side is more at risk for hemorrhage by puncturing either the liver on the right side or the spleen on the left. Both organs are solid organs with a significant amount of blood flowing through them. Both organs also normally sit in the lower thoracic cavity. A tension pneumothorax can occur if a fractured rib punctures a lung. Air may leak out into the subcutaneous fat and create a bubbly, crinkly feel that can extend up into the face and down to the abdomen. This condition, called **subcutaneous emphysema**, is common in rib fractures and pneumothoracies.

Treatment can include taping a bulky dressing over the fractured rib to help stabilize it during breathing. Constricting bands around the chest may limit the ability for the patient to breathe, and are generally not used. In the field, administering high flow oxygen can allow each breath to be more efficient and may allow the patient to decrease their respiratory rate to a more normal level.

Flail Chest

A flail chest (see Figure 7–14) is defined as two or more adjacent ribs that are fractured in two or more places. This creates a segment of the chest wall that is isolated from the rest of the chest. This segment of chest wall is sucked in when the chest expands during inhalation, and pushed out during exhalation. This movement of the flail segment opposite the rest of the chest during normal respiration is called **paradoxical respiration**. Complications of a flail chest are the same as for a rib fracture, although the chance of bleeding and pneumothorax is increased because more ribs are involved. Treatment includes padding the area with a bulky dressing that is taped securely to the chest. The dressing should be large enough to splint the segment and encourage it to move with the rest of the chest. High flow oxygen is needed as the patient will likely hypoventilate because of impaired respiratory mechanics.

Sternal Fracture

A fracture of the sternum can occur through either a direct blow to the chest, as occurs when the chest strikes the steering wheel during an automobile accident, or can occur from the body's force against the seatbelt. It has been estimated that sternal fractures occur in approximately three percent of automobile collisions. Patients who have a sternal fracture will have significant pain in the anterior chest and tenderness along the fracture site. These patients are at risk for injury to the great vessels and blunt cardiac injury. Both conditions are covered in detail in Chapter 8.

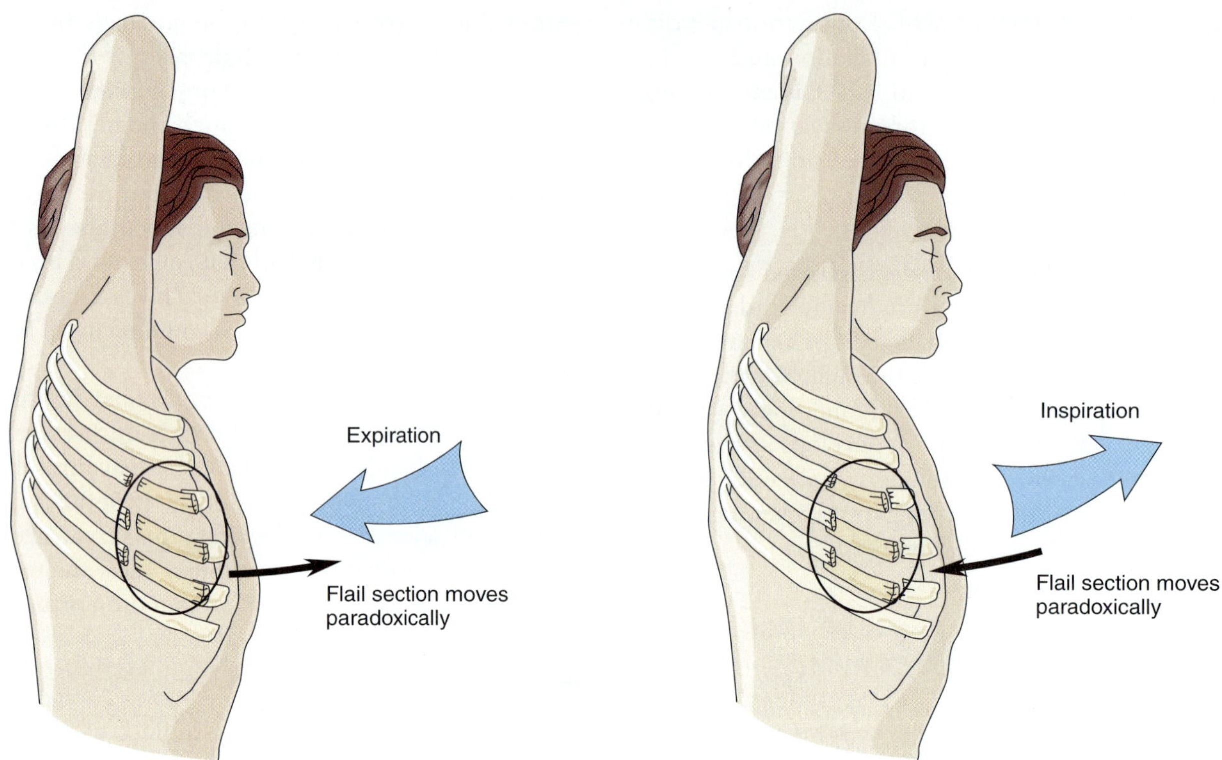

Figure 7–14 Flail segment and paradoxical respiration.

Pneumothorax and Hemothorax

Pneumothorax and hemothorax often occur from some type of trauma. Traumatic pneumothorax occurs when air enters the pleural cavity from outside the chest. Causes include gunshot wound, stabbing, or crushing of the chest. A rib fracture often causes a traumatic pneumothorax. Complete lung collapse causes a sudden severe chest pain followed by severe dyspnea and symptoms of shock. Respirations are weak and shallow. Sucking breath sounds may be heard at the site of a traumatic wound. Increased air pressure on the affected side may cause a shift of the mediastinum and trachea toward the unaffected side. The condition of mediastinal shift is a medical emergency. Emergency treatment of an open chest wound includes placing an occlusive dressing, clean hand, or plastic material over the sucking chest wound to prevent additional air from entering the chest.

Emergent treatment of a tension pneumothorax involves performing a needle decompression. The second intercostal space at the mid-clavicular line on the affected side is identified and the skin prepared with an antiseptic solution. The EMS provider then places a long (at least 2 inch) large bore (10 to 14 gauge) needle into the chest passing over the third rib to allow the increased pressure of the tension pneumothorax to escape. The needle is passed over the third rib to avoid damaging the neurovascular bundle that runs along the underside of each rib. The patient is at risk for continued development of a tension pneumothorax until more definitive treatment is performed in the emergency department. All patients who receive a needle thoracic decompression in the field must receive a chest tube in the emergency department.

Identification in the field is performed by assessing the patient's history and physical exam. Findings that suggest a tension pneumothorax include an extreme sudden onset of dyspnea, a hyperresonant percussion note on the affected side, decreased chest motion on the affected side, decreased or absent breath sounds on the affected side, shock, and, in later stages, tracheal deviation away from the affected side. Additional signs that may be present suggesting a tension pneuomothorax include an increase in jugular venous pressure, muffled heart sounds, and a sudden drop in oxygen saturation. In an intubated and ventilated patient, a pneumothorax should be suspected if there is a loss of compliance to positive pressure ventilation. A pneumothorax can be confirmed in the emergency department by a chest X-ray. Depending upon the amount of air in the chest, the physician may choose to place a chest tube in the affected side to relieve the pressure. This tube is placed on suction until the leak closes. A minor pneumothorax may just require careful observation and may resolve over time. Analgesics are often administered for pain control once the emergent stage is over.

Hemothorax is the collection of blood in the chest cavity. Cause, symptoms, diagnosis, and treatments are the same as pneumothorax. Blood pressure and blood loss are monitored and treated as necessary.

As in the case of a tension pneumothorax, the hemothorax can be treated emergently by needle decompression. Clotting of the catheter quickly occurs, making this intervention temporary at best. A chest tube is placed in the patient in the emergency department, surgical suite, or intensive care unit to allow blood drainage and healing.

Pulmonary Contusion

A pulmonary contusion is a bruising of the lung that predominantly occurs as a result of blunt trauma. The bleeding represents leakage from damaged pulmonary capillaries. This blood can cause inflammatory reaction in the lung tissue, which decreases the ability for oxygen to get from the alveoli into the blood, and the lung tissue becomes stiff. High flow oxygen is administered to help make the transport of oxygen more efficient. If the contusion is large, the patient may require ventilatory support. Generally, the patient will improve within a few days of the injury provided no additional complications occur.

Traumatic Asphyxia

Traumatic asphyxia occurs after a sudden, forceful, crushing blow to the chest that often occurs as the patient is inhaling. There is a sudden increase in thoracic pressure and blood that normally returns to the heart via the vena cava (see Chapter 8) is dispersed and typically engorges the vessels and tissues in the neck and head. These patients tend to look near death; however, the recovery course is closely tied to the severity of any underlying injury that may be present (see Figure 7–15). Signs and symptoms include distended neck veins, blue or gray appearing head, neck, and shoulders, bulging eyes, swollen lips and tongue, and a large chest deformity. Treatment includes high flow oxygen, and ventilatory support and circulatory support as needed. A tension pneumothorax may occur, but can be treated through needle chest decompression by an advanced EMS provider.

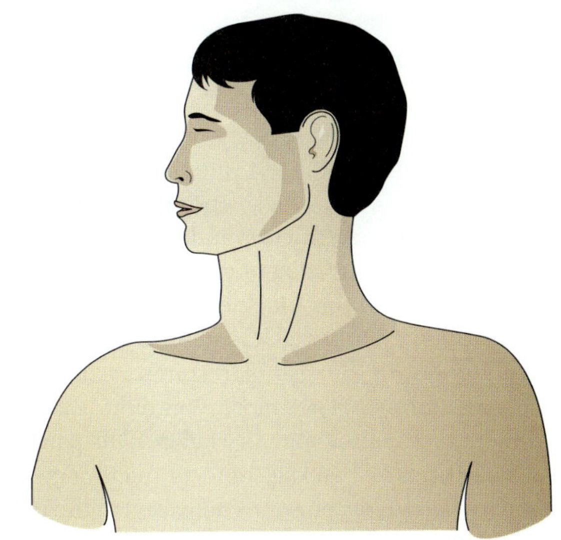

Figure 7–15 Traumatic asphyxia.

Diaphragmatic Injury

Diaphragmatic injuries normally result from penetrating injury, for example, a knife or bullet that passes through the diaphragm, but can occur during significant blunt injury to the abdomen. The diaphragm is the primary muscle of respiration and the amount of negative pressure developed in the thorax is dependent more on the action of the diaphragm than on the movement of the ribs. If the diaphragm is injured, the patient will not be able to produce an adequate negative pressure in the chest to support sufficient ventilation. Diaphragmatic injury is often missed during initial assessment and treatment because of other injuries that may be present. The EMS provider should have a high index of suspicion of a diaphragmatic injury on all patients with penetrating thoracic or abdominal injury. High flow oxygen should be administered and ventilatory support is often required. If the diaphragm tears, abdominal contents may extrude through the tear and become trapped, producing signs similar to a bowel obstruction (see Chapter 13). Abdominal contents in the thorax can also impair the ability for the lungs to expand, reducing ventilation. The majority of diaphragmatic tears caused by blunt injury occur in the left diaphragm because the liver, located on the right on the abdominal side of the diaphragm, protects the right diaphragm and distributes the force applied to it.

DEVELOPMENTAL AND GENETIC DISORDERS

There are many developmental abnormalities that can occur in the respiratory system, many of which are discovered before the baby is discharged from the newborn nursery. One genetic disorder that significantly impacts the health of the patient and which the EMS provider will surely encounter during his career is cystic fibrosis.

Cystic Fibrosis

Cystic fibrosis is a hereditary recessive disorder affecting young children. It is passed to the child by a recessive gene from each parent. Cystic fibrosis affects all the **exocrine glands** (glands that excrete through a duct) of the body causing **viscous** (thick) secretions. These viscous secretions cause obstruction in body passageways. The most serious complication of cystic fibrosis is in the lungs. The thick secretions block bronchi causing difficulty with breathing. These thick secretions also trap bacteria, thus increasing the risk of respiratory infections including pneumonia. The most common cause of death with this disease is respiratory failure. The pancreas is also affected because blockage of these ducts decreases the amount of pancreatic enzymes delivered to the intestine, resulting in poor digestion and weight loss. The sweat glands are also affected. Affected children perspire excessively and lose large amounts of salt or sodium. This loss of sodium causes an increase in the risk for heat exhaustion and electrolyte imbalances. This abnormal excretion of salt is usually the first sign that parents recognize as abnormal. Parents may bring the child in to the physician and complain that the child, when kissed, tastes salty or has "sweaty baby kisses." This excessive salt excretion is the basis for the "sweat test" that confirms the diagnosis of cystic fibrosis. Major improvements in treatment of cystic fibrosis have been made in the past few decades, but it is still considered a fatal disease. Life expectancy may reach into the late twenties or early thirties.

Treatment is directed toward reducing complications and improving quality of life. Aggressive respiratory treatments include postural drainage, chest-clapping, antibiotics, bronchodilators, expectorants, and oxygen therapy. A high-calorie, high-sodium diet is provided with pancreatic enzyme supplementation. Emotional support and extensive education are needed for the affected individual and family members.

EFFECTS OF AGING ON THE SYSTEM

The effects of aging on the respiratory system increase the risk for the older adult to develop respiratory disease. Over time the respiratory system loses some of its elasticity, becomes less efficient, and has less reserve. Weakened respiratory muscles contribute to the ineffectiveness of the system. It can also be adversely affected by changes in posture occurring with aging, by the long-term effects of chronic diseases such as COPD, and by the changes occurring in other systems. The older adult usually has a lower tolerance for exercise because of the increased need for oxygen during exercise and the inability of the body to meet that demand.

Changes in the immune responses that occur with aging put the older adult at increased risk for acute respiratory infections. Influenza and pneumonia are common but very serious diseases affecting older adults. Pneumonia is the leading cause of death from infections in the elderly population. Another respiratory disease that the elderly are at increased risk for developing is tuberculosis. Their reduced immunity contributes to the high incidence of TB among older adults.

Chronic respiratory diseases are particularly difficult for the elderly. The nature of the disease, symptoms, effects, and treatments may all contribute to the increased respiratory dysfunction, and thus, the debilitation of the individual. Many elderly individuals have been heavy smokers for years. The effects of smoking may have already severely damaged respiratory function and may continue to inhibit effective breathing if the individual continues to smoke. Smoking is the major cause of the high incidence of cancer of the lung in the elderly. Cancer of the lung is the second leading cause of death in the older adult.

SUMMARY

The respiratory system is responsible for the intake of oxygen for the body and the removal of carbon dioxide. Decreased respiratory function greatly limits the ability of other systems as oxygen is necessary at the cellular level for all activities to occur. Diagnostic tests for respiratory diseases include physical examination, chest X-rays, arterial blood gases, and pulmonary function tests. Respiratory diseases are a major cause of disability and death in the United States. Acute respiratory diseases such as the common cold and pneumonia occur in all age groups. Most chronic respiratory diseases are found in the older adult. Smoking is the greatest contributor to chronic respiratory disease, especially cancer of the lung.

REVIEW QUESTIONS

Short Answer

1. What are the functions of the respiratory system?

2. Which signs and symptoms are associated with common respiratory system disorders?

3. Which diagnostic tests are most commonly used to determine the type and/or cause of respiratory system disorders?

4. What is the significance of the percussion note when examining a patient?

5. What behavior puts an individual at highest risk for pulmonary disease?

Matching

6. Match the term on the left with the correct descriptive clause on the right.

_____ Asthma	a. inflammation of the mucous membranes of the sinuses
_____ Pneumothorax	b. high risk behavior for developing respiratory disease
_____ COPD	c. best preventive behavior for preventing respiratory infections
_____ Hemothorax	d. hypersensitivity reaction causing constriction of the bronchi
_____ Tuberculosis	e. bacterial infection causing a primary lesion in the lung
_____ Sinusitis	f. collapse of a part of the lung with blood in the space
_____ Cor pulmonale	g. group of chronic pulmonary diseases
_____ Hand washing	h. right-sided heart failure
_____ Smoking	i. collection of air in the pleural cavity

CASE STUDY

You respond to the residence of Mr. George Loftin, who is a 78-year-old male patient who was recently diagnosed with emphysema. He used to be a shipyard welder, and smoked two to three packs of cigarettes per day for the past sixty years. After his diagnosis, he cut back to one pack per day. He is complaining of dyspnea and states that he has had fevers and chills the past couple of days. What do you suspect as the likely causes of Mr. Loftin's COPD exacerbation? You auscultate his lungs and find an area of consolidation in his right lower lobe that corresponds to an area with a very dull percussion note. What do you suspect as Mr. Loftin's most likely diagnosis? How would you treat Mr. Loftin? What advice can you offer Mr. Loftin on decreasing the number of times he will call for ambulance assistance?

BIBLIOGRAPHY

Abzug, M. J. (March 15, 1997). Assault against respiratory syncytial virus. *Lancet, 349*, 743–744.

American Lung Association. http://www.lungusa.org/data/

Cancer facts and figures—1997. (1997). Atlanta, GA: American Cancer Society. Pamphlet 97-300M-No. 5008.97, 23–26.

Chisolm, S. (1997). Common questions about hantavirus pulmonary syndrome. *American Journal of Nursing, 97*(4), 68–70.

Cohen, M. R. (1995). Inhalation medications: The choice isn't clear. *Nursing 95, 25*(8), 15.

Conolly, M. J. (1996). Obstructive airways disease: A hidden disability in the aged. *Age and Ageing, 25*(7), 265–267.

Everard, M. L. (August 3, 1996). Acute bronchiolitis—A perennial problem. *Lancet, 348*, 279–280.

Harrison, T. R. & Isselbacher, K. J. (1994). *Harrison's principles of internal medicine* (Vol. 2). NY: McGraw-Hill.

Herbert, B. (February 10, 1997). Bad air day. *New York Times*, p. A15.

La Montagne, J. R. (January 18, 1997). RSV pneumonia, a community infection in adults. *Lancet, 349*, 149–150.

Leynaert, B. (April 13, 1996). Gas cooking and respiratory health in women. *Lancet, 347*, 1052–1053.

Lopez-Alarcon, M. (1997). Breast-feeding lowers the frequency and duration of acute respiratory infection and diarrhea in infants under six months of age. *The Journal of Nutrition, 127*(3), 436–443.

Lung protection for babies. (1996). *FDA Consumer, 30*(4), 2–3.

Metered-dose inhalers: Older patients need extra instructions. (1996). *Geriatrics, 51*(7), 20.

Moeller, J. L. (1996). Contraindications to athletic participation. *The Physician and Sportsmedicine, 24*(8), 47–49+.

Nearly all children become infected with this virus. (1996). *RN, 59*(3), 61.

Norman, D. C. (1997). Treating respiratory infections in the elderly: Current strategies and considerations. *Geriatrics, 52*(1), S1–S28.

Pneumonia is on the rise. (1997). *Current Health, 23*(2), 28–29.

Pneumonia: Tool helps identify low-risk patients. (1997). *American Journal of Nursing, 97*(7), 9.

Porterfield, L. M. (1997). Respiratory symptoms in an obese patient. *RN, 60*(4), 79.

Shils, M. E., Olson, J. A., & Shike, M. (1994). *Modern nutrition in health and disease* (Vol. 2). Philadelphia: Lea & Febiger.

Stoddard, J. J. (1997). Maternal smoking and medical expenditures for childhood respiratory illness. *American Journal of Public Health, 87*(2), 205–209.

Update: New CDC recommendations for pneumonia booster. (1997). *Geriatrics, 52*(7), 17.

Walling, A. D. (February 15, 1997). Effect of maternal smoking on neonatal respiratory function. *American Family Physician, 55*, 929.

Zimmer, J. G. (1997). Nursing home-acquired pneumonia: Avoiding the hospital. *Journal of the American Geriatrics Society, 45*(3), 380–381.

Zuckerman, M. (September 28, 1996). HIV-associated respiratory disease. *Lancet, 348*, 892–893.

CHAPTER

8

Cardiovascular Diseases and Disorders

CONTENT OUTLINE

- Anatomy and Physiology
- Common Signs and Symptoms
- Diagnostic Tests
- Common Diseases of the System
  - Diseases of Arteries
  - Diseases of the Heart
  - Diseases of Veins
- Trauma
  - Hemorrhage
  - Pericardial Tamponade
  - Blunt Cardiac Injury
  - Great Vessel Injury
- Developmental Diseases and Disorders
  - Atrial Septal Defect
  - Ventricular Septal Defect
  - Patent Ductus Arteriosus
  - Coarctation of the Aorta
  - Tetralogy of Fallot
- Effects of Aging on the System

KEY TERMS

Afterload
Angioplasty
Auscultation
Cardiac catheterization
Cardiac output
Cardiac palpitations
Chronotropism
Cyanosis
Diastolic
Doppler
Dromotropism
Dyspnea
Electrocardiogram
Embolus
Endarterectomy
Exsanguination
Hemothorax
Inotropism
Intermittent claudication
Ischemia
Lumen
Murmur
Patency
Plaque
Preload
Pulse deficit
Pulsus alternans
Pulsus paradoxus
Starling's law
Systolic
Tachycardia
Thrombus

LEARNING OBJECTIVES

Upon completion of the chapter, the student should be able to:

1. Define the terminology common to the cardiovascular system and the disorders of the system.
2. Identify the common disorders of the cardiovascular system.
3. Discuss the basic anatomy and physiology of the cardiovascular system.
4. Identify the important signs and symptoms associated with common cardiovascular system disorders.
5. Describe the common diagnostic tests used to determine type and/or cause of the cardiovascular system disorders.
6. Describe the typical course and management of the common cardiovascular system disorders.
7. Describe the effects of aging upon the cardiovascular system and the common disorders of the system.

OVERVIEW

The cardiovascular system is often regarded as the major body system because the individual cannot live without a functioning heart and circulatory system. A significant percentage of calls to EMS are for cardiovascular related complaints. The heart is responsible only for pumping blood while the vascular system transports the blood throughout the body. Disorders of the system often share common symptoms and problems. Other systems are affected when the cardiovascular system is malfunctioning as it is responsible for delivering necessary nutrients and oxygen to the body. Diseases of the cardiovascular system are a major cause of morbidity and mortality in all ages, but especially in older adults.

ANATOMY AND PHYSIOLOGY

The heart, arteries, and veins, along with the blood, make up the cardiovascular system. The heart is a four chambered muscular structure. It is about the size of a man's fist and weighs about 300 grams. The heart is situated approximately in the middle of the chest, slightly to the left, behind the sternum (breastbone). The heart is composed of the pericardium, the chambers, and the valves. The pericardium is a two-layer sac with fluid between the layers. The wall of the heart is divided into three layers. The epicardium is the outermost layer, the myocardium is the middle layer, and the endocardium is the innermost layer.

There are four chambers in the heart, the right atrium, right ventricle, left atrium, and left ventricle. The tricuspid valve is between the right atrium and ventricle; the mitral valve is between the left atrium and ventricle; the pulmonary valve is between the right ventricle and pulmonary artery; and the aortic valve is between the left ventricle and aorta.

Blood enters the heart from the superior vena cava, passes through the right atrium and the tricuspid valve into the right ventricle. It then passes through the pulmonary valve into the pulmonary artery and travels to the lungs where carbon dioxide is exchanged for oxygen. The oxygenated blood returns to the heart through the pulmonary vein to the left atrium through the mitral valve and into the left ventricle. It then passes through the aortic valve into the aorta and to the body (Figure 8–1). The heart itself is supplied with blood by the coronary arteries.

Cardiac muscle normally contracts continually throughout one's lifetime. Designated areas of the heart produce electrical stimulation causing the heart muscle to contract and pump the blood to the body. This

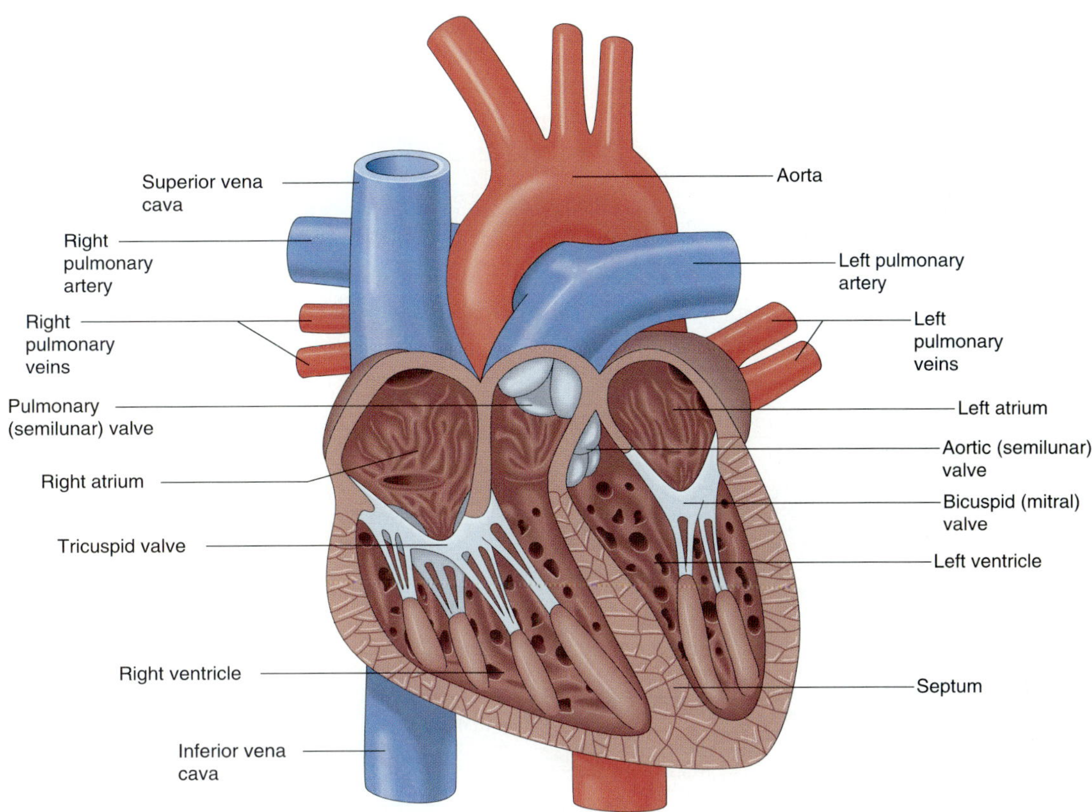

Figure 8–1 The heart: four chambers and great vessels.

sequence of events is termed the cardiac cycle. It begins in the sinoatrial (SA) node, passes to the atrioventricular (AV) node to the bundle of HIS and the Purkinje fibers (Figure 8–2).

One sequence of the conduction pathway is one cardiac cycle. This is represented on the electrocardiogram as the PQRST segment. The P wave represents the electrical stimulation beginning and passing over the atria (depolarization). The QRS wave is caused by the stimulation passing over the ventricles. The T wave represents the recovery of the ventricles (repolarization). The cardiac cycle repeats itself approximately 60–100 times per minute in the average adult. One cycle is one heartbeat. The pulsation (heartbeat) felt with the hand over the chest or the fingertips placed over an artery (such as at the wrist or neck) is called the pulse. The pulse rate is the number of pulsations felt in a minute. The closing of the heart valves produces the sounds heard when listening with a stethoscope over the heart.

Three terms that refer to different myocardial cell properties are inotropism, chronotropism, and dromotropism. These terms are commonly used when discussing the effects of medications or the nervous system on the heart. **Inotropism** refers to the strength of myocardial muscle cell contraction. An increase in the strength of contraction is called a positive inotropic effect and a decrease in strength of contraction is called a negative inotropic effect. **Chronotropism** refers to the rate of myocardial contraction. An increase in contraction rate, or heart rate, is a positive chronotropic event and a decrease in heart rate is a negative chronotropic event. **Dromotropism** refers to the speed of conduction of the electric impulse along the myocardial conduction system. A positive dromotropic effect increases the speed of impulse conduction and a negative dromotropic effect decreases the speed of impulse conduction. Many agents or medications will affect all three of these properties equally, while some will affect one property more than the other two. In general, agents that produce a positive effect will also increase myocardial oxygen demand.

The circulatory component of the cardiovascular system includes the arteries and veins (Figure 8–3). The three major subsystems include the portal unit, the pulmonary unit, and the systemic unit. Each of these circulatory subsystems has special functions in addition to delivering blood to the body. The portal unit or subsystem includes the circulation to the stomach, spleen, intestine, and pancreas. Blood from these organs goes through

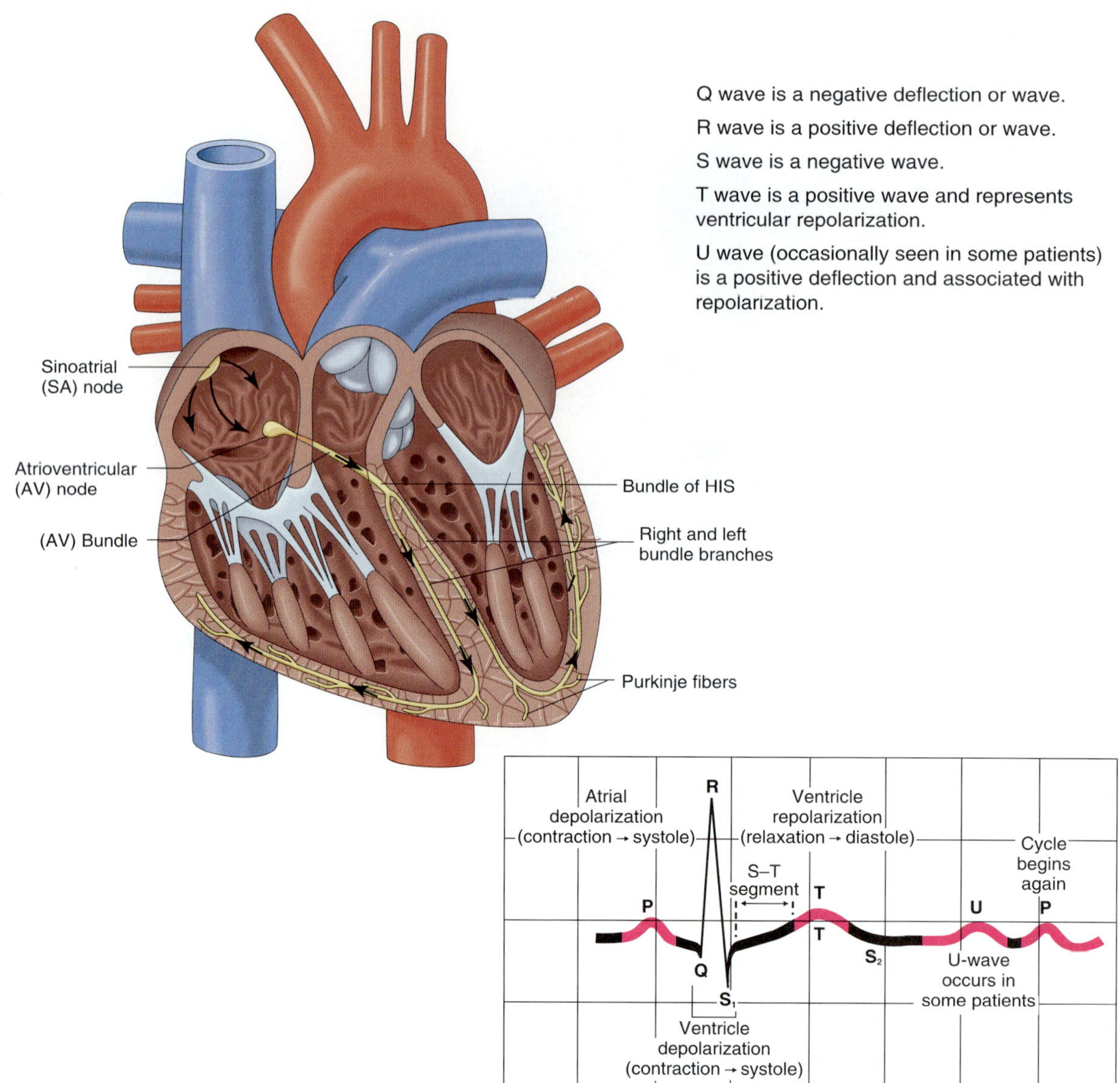

Figure 8-2 The conduction system.

the liver before returning to the heart (see Chapter 13). The pulmonary subsystem includes the pulmonary artery and its divisions, leading from the heart to the lungs, the circulation through the lungs, and the pulmonary vein leading from the lungs back to the heart. In this subsystem non-oxygenated blood from the systemic circulation passes through the lungs where an exchange of carbon dioxide for oxygen occurs. The oxygenated blood returns to the heart to be pumped throughout the body. The systemic subsystem includes all the arteries and veins and their capillaries not already included in the previous subsystems. This subsystem carries the oxygen and nutrients to the body cells, and removes waste products.

Several physiological concepts help the EMS provider in understanding many of the cardiovascular system disorders. These concepts, Starling's law, preload, afterload, and cardiac output, describe the relationship between blood volume and the heart's mechanical pumping ability. Many cardiovascular disorders as well as treatments affect one or more of these factors.

Starling's law describes the relationship between contractibility of cardiac muscle and the amount of stretch placed in that muscle. When cardiac muscle is stretched by additional blood volume, the muscle exerts an additional force on the next contraction in order to pump the additional blood out of the chamber. This property allows

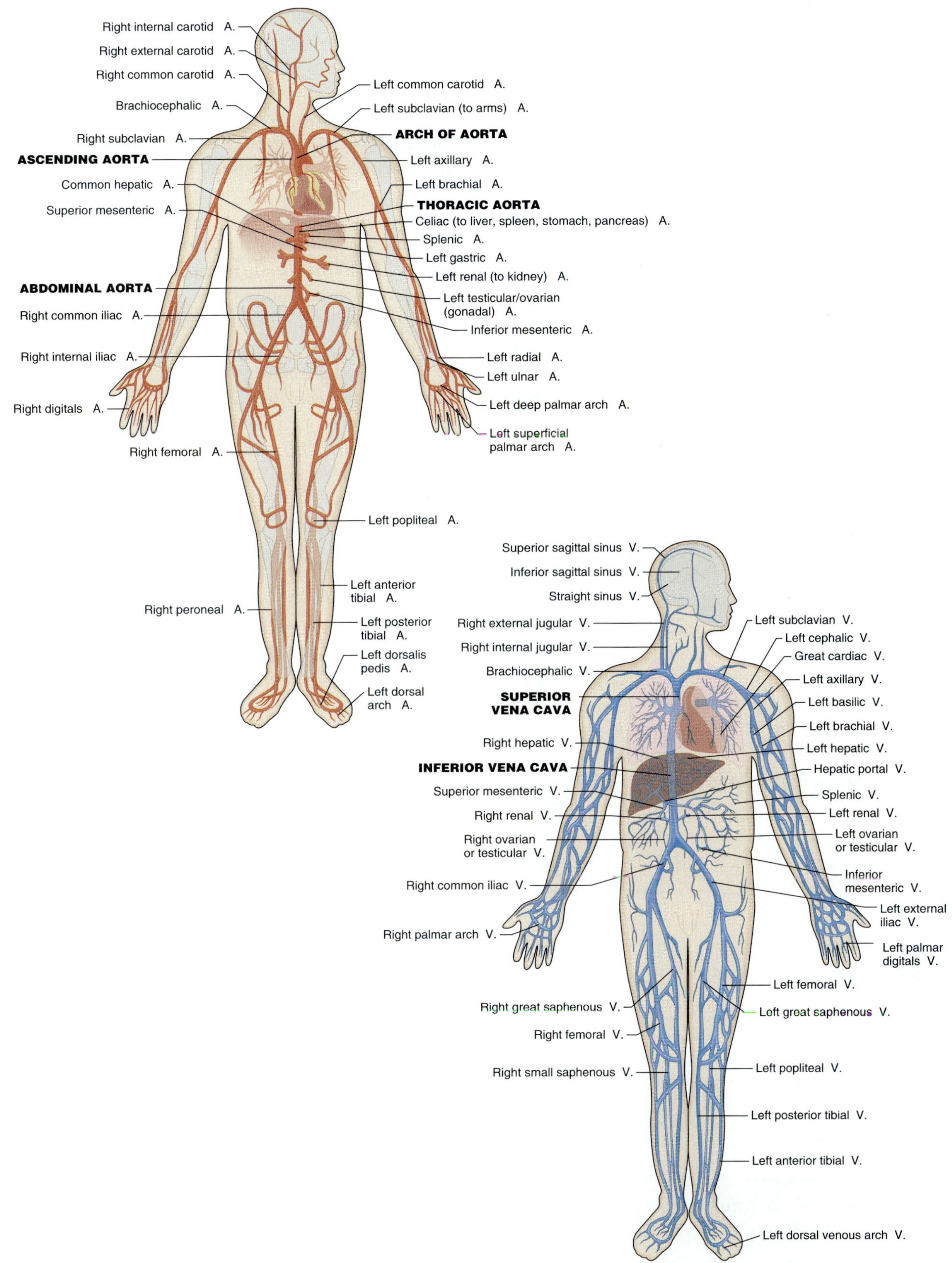

Figure 8–3 The circulatory system.

the heart to automatically compensate for additional volume of blood that enters the right side of the heart. As shown in Figure 8–4, the amount of force exerted by cardiac muscle will increase up to a point above which the muscle will contract inefficiently and the amount of force will actually decrease. This, in turn, will decrease the cardiac output because less blood will flow out of the heart.

Preload is defined as the pressure on the heart chamber exerted by the volume of blood returning to the heart. The volume of blood returning to the heart depends on circulating blood volume, the respiratory cycle, gravity, ventilator mode, and the action of the thoracoabdominal (diaphragm) and skeletal pumping mechanism to aid in blood return. Preload is increased by providing more volume to the heart, as in the case of fluid overload. As described above and in Figure 8–4, the greater the preload the greater the ventricular contraction, up to a point. After the peak of the curve, any additional volume will only dilate the ventricle and weaken the ability to contract.

Afterload is the amount of force the ventricle must overcome in order to provide blood flow through the circulatory system. The afterload can be equated to the resistance and capacitance in an electrical or hydraulic circuit. The afterload is dependent upon the circulating blood volume and vascular resistance. If the patient is in a fluid overload situation, the afterload will increase and the heart will have to pump harder to overcome the increased amount of fluid. If the patient is vasoconstricted, as in the case of the fight or flight response of the sympathetic nervous system (see Chapter 9), the peripheral resistance will increase, increasing the afterload. Vasodilation, and a decrease in blood volume will both decrease the afterload. The blood vessel can be thought of as a pipe. The larger the **lumen**, or hole in the center of the pipe, the less resistance to blood flow, resulting in a decreased systemic vascular resistance. The smaller the lumen (vasoconstriction), the resistance to blood flow increases, and the systemic vascular resistance increases.

The **cardiac output** describes the amount of blood the heart pumps out of the left ventricle every minute. It can be computed by multiplying the heart rate by the volume the left ventricle pumps with every contraction. Maintaining cardiac output by maintaining circulating volume and cardiac pumping is the goal in treating many disorders.

The blood pressure is the amount of pressure placed on the walls of the blood vessels by the circulatory system. Arterial blood pressure is commonly measured by health care providers. The **systolic** (sis-TALL-ick) pressure is the pressure against the vessel walls when the heart is contracting and the **diastolic** (dye-as-TOL-ick) pressure is the pressure exerted against the vessel walls when the heart is at rest. The blood pressure is dependent upon two factors, the cardiac output and systemic vascular resistance. If either the cardiac output or systemic vascular resistance increases, the blood pressure will increase. If either the cardiac output or systemic vascular resistance decreases, for example with significant blood loss or vasodilatation, the blood pressure will fall. The body works to maintain a certain blood pressure that can provide enough oxygen-rich blood to the brain to maintain normal brain function.

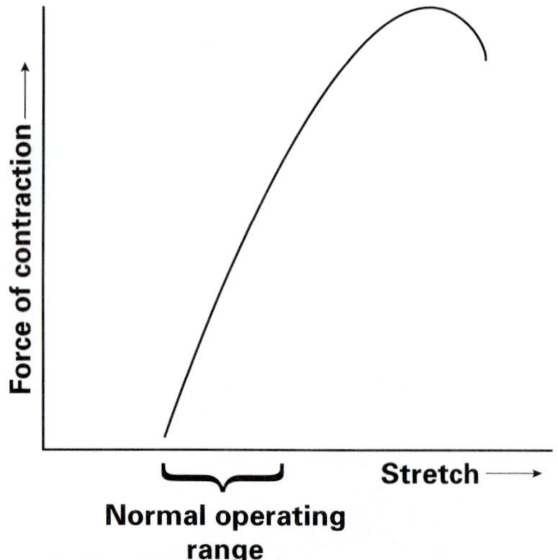

Figure 8–4 Starling's Law. The greater the cardiac muscle is stretched, the greater the force of contraction.

COMMON SIGNS AND SYMPTOMS

Common symptoms of heart disease include chest pain, **dyspnea** (DISP-nee-ah; dys = difficult, pnea = breathing), fatigue, and **tachycardia** (TACH-ee-**KAR**-dee-ah; tachy = rapid, cardia = heart). Chest pain may be described as a severe, crushing pressure as though someone is crushing the chest or the pain may be more mild and described as a constant feeling of indigestion. Pain may also radiate down the left arm or into the jaw. Dyspnea is also a common symptom as a lack of oxygen to the tissues stimulates the respiratory system. Individuals with heart disease often feel fatigued and experience episodes of tachycardia. Other symptoms include **cardiac palpitations** (an unusually strong, rapid or irregular heart rate that is so abnormal that the individual is aware or "can feel" it), sweating, edema in the extremities, and nausea and vomiting.

Pain, edema, and cyanosis are symptoms of diseases of the vascular system. Pain is often in association with poor blood perfusion to the tissues leading to **ischemia** (iss-KEE-me-ah; lack of oxygen) of the organ. Edema of the extremities is commonly caused by poor venous return leading to congestion of blood and fluids in the tissues. Tissues that lack oxygen often exhibit a characteristic blue color called **cyanosis** (SIGH-ah-**NO**-sis; cyano = blue, osis = condition).

Additional clues to cardiovascular system disease may be obtained from the physical exam. A **pulse deficit** is a difference between the apical pulse (as auscultated over the heart) and the peripheral pulse (often the radial or carotid pulse) that is found with dysrhythmias that do not allow the ventricles to fill prior to contraction. The EMS provider will hear a heart beat that does not correspond to a peripheral pulse on every beat. This can occur with dysrhythmias such as atrial fibrillation or with any rhythm that includes premature complexes. **Pulsus paradoxus** is a condition seen with pericardial tamponade and is defined as a decrease of greater than 10 mmHg in systolic blood pressure with inspiration. When fluid or blood builds up in the pericardial sac surrounding the heart, ventricular filling is impaired. As the patient takes a deep breath, blood pressure will normally fall slightly because of the pooling of blood in the pulmonary vasculature and drop in left ventricular filling. When tamponade occurs, left ventricular filling is significantly reduced, thus causing a more significant drop in systolic blood pressure. To assess for pulsus paradoxus, the EMS provider performs the usual procedure for obtaining a blood pressure. Once the systolic sound is auscultated, the sphygnometer pressure is held at that level and the patient is instructed to take and hold a deep breath. The EMS provider then continues to allow the sphygnometer pressure to slowly drop until the systolic sound is again heard. If the difference between these two sounds is greater than 10 mmHg, then the patient has a pericardial effusion and should be assessed for additional signs of tamponade as discussed later in this chapter. **Pulsus alternans** is the term used to describe a regular alternation in amplitude of the pulse. The cycle length does not change, but the power behind each pulse changes, producing a difference in palpated strength. This sign is common in patients who have heart failure with significant left ventricular dysfunction and is often accompanied by a loud S3 heart sound.

DIAGNOSTIC TESTS

Non-invasive procedures of the cardiovascular system involve listening to the heart and movement of blood in the vessels. This is accomplished by the use of a stethoscope in a procedure called **auscultation** (AUS-kul-**TAY**-shun). During auscultation the stethoscope may be placed on the chest to listen to the heart and over various arteries to listen for blood flow. Murmurs may be auscultated in the heart area and indicate abnormal flow through the heart valves. A **Doppler** device may also be placed over arteries to magnify the sound of blood flow. Decreased blood flow may be caused by heart and/or vessel disease.

Arterial blood pressure is simply referred to as blood pressure and is measured by a sphygmomanometer. A sphygmomanometer is a cuff and pressure gauge used to measure systolic and diastolic blood pressure. Venous blood pressure is an important measure of the heart's pumping ability and may be determined by examining the individual for edema. Edema in the extremities and distention of the jugular veins in the neck are common indicators of increased venous pressure.

The electrical component of the heart may be drawn or graphed by an electrocardiograph, a machine that receives electrical information and draws heart action. The picture produced is an **electrocardiogram** (ECG) (ee-LECK-troh-**KAR**-dee-oh-GRAM; electro = electrical, cardio = heart, gram = picture). ECG is helpful in evaluating most cardiac diseases.

Use of ultrasound for diagnostic purposes is valuable in the emergency department for both heart and vessel diseases. Echocardiography (ECK-oh-KAR-dee-**OG**-rah-fee) and ultrasound arteriography (AR-tee-ree-**OG**-rah-fee) both utilize sound waves to produce pictures of the heart and arteries, respectively. These procedures are non-invasive.

Cardiac catheterization (KATH-eh-ter-eye-**ZAY**-shun) is an invasive procedure used to sample the blood in the chambers of the heart to determine the oxygen content and blood pressure in the chambers. Cardiac output may also be checked. This procedure involves passing a small plastic catheter into the heart through a vein or artery. A vein is utilized for right-sided catheterization while an artery is used for a left-sided approach. Vessels of the arms and legs are commonly used (Figure 8–5).

X-rays of the heart and vessels may be beneficial in determining normal structure, size and **patency** (openness). These procedures involve injecting dye into the system and taking pictures of the heart and vessels. Common X-ray procedures include angiocardiography (AN-jee-oh-KAR-dee-**OG**-rah-fee; angio = vessel, cardio = heart, graphy = procedure), arteriography (arterio = artery, graphy = procedure), and venography (veno = vein, graphy = procedure). X-ray pictures produced are called angiocardiogram, arteriogram, and venogram, respectively.

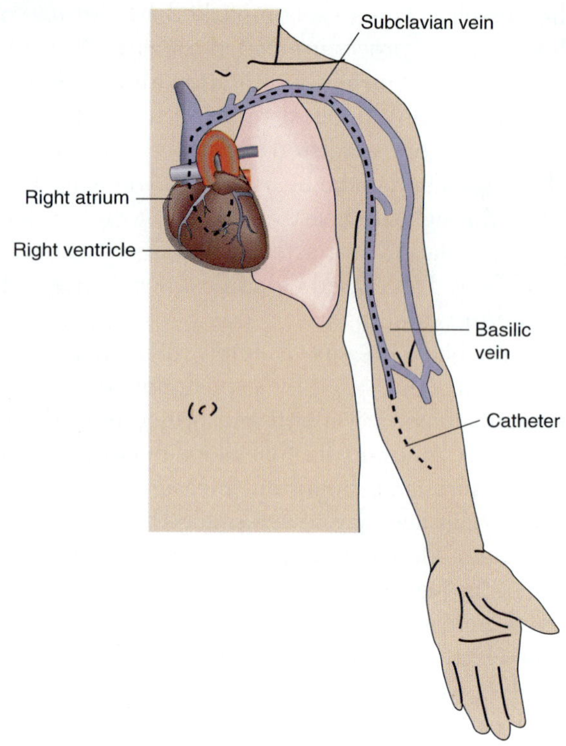

Figure 8–5 Cardiac catheterization.

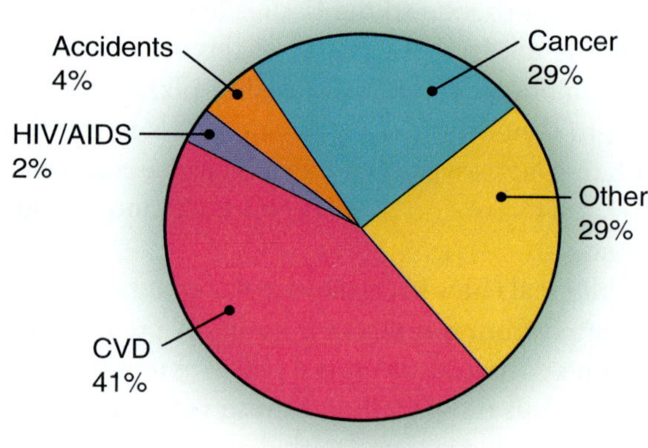

Figure 8–6 Mortality statistics comparing cardiovascular diseases with other diseases.

Blood tests of this system in the emergency department include enzyme studies that assist in determining if the individual has had a myocardial infarction (heart attack). As the heart muscle dies enzymes are released. The enzyme levels help determine the time and degree of the infarction. Common enzymes are creatinine phosphokinase (CPK), lactic dehydrogenase (LDH), and the troparins.

COMMON DISEASES OF THE CARDIOVASCULAR SYSTEM

Cardiovascular disease is the leading cause of death in the United States today (Figure 8–6). More than 2,600 Americans die each day from cardiovascular diseases. Over 57,000,000 individuals have some form of cardiovascular disease. High blood pressure accounts for most of these cases, but coronary heart disease, rheumatic heart disease, and other forms of cardiovascular disease also contribute to these staggering numbers (American Heart Association, 1999). Education about lifestyle behavioral changes has helped decrease some individuals' risk for cardiovascular disease.

Diseases of Arteries

Arterial disorders are the most common among all the cardiovascular diseases. High blood pressure (hypertension) accounts for the largest incidence of arterial disorders, but coronary artery disease (coronary heart disease) is the single leading cause of death overall.

Hypertension. Most people are familiar with the basic concept that hypertension is high arterial blood pressure. Other concepts include the fact that hypertension is not only a disease process, but also serves as an indicator of the development of cerebrovascular, cardiovascular, and kidney disease. Hypertension is a chronic disease and is the leading cause of stroke and heart failure. Life expectancy in all individuals regardless of age and sex is reduced when diastolic hypertension of greater than 90 mmHg is present.

Blood pressure varies from individual to individual but average adult blood pressure is considered to be approximately 120/80 mmHg. Medical parameters for diagnosing high blood pressure are a systolic blood pressure of 140 mmHg or greater and diastolic pressure of 90 mmHg or greater.

Specialized nerve receptors in the body help control pressure by bringing about vasoconstriction and vasodilatation at appropriate times. For example, when an individual stands up suddenly, the blood pressure to the head drops, often causing momentary dizziness. To correct this situation, nerves react and constrict blood vessels, raising blood pressure and restoring normal pressure in the head. If blood pressure is too high these nerve receptors dilate vessels leading to the kidneys. This increased blood flow leads to greater urine formation and output. Increased urine production decreases blood volume and thus lowers blood pressure. In this way the kidneys play a vital role in blood pressure. If pressure is too low, as often occurs in shock, blood flow to the kidneys is diminished, urine output is minimal, blood fluid is maintained and thus blood pressure is maintained or restored.

Because blood pressure and the kidneys have such a close relationship, one can see that any disease of the kidneys may cause an alteration in blood pressure. On the other hand, any change in blood pressure may have an adverse effect on the kidneys. The kidneys play a vital role in elimination of salt and water, two substances that also have a great effect on blood pressure. Retention of salt and water increases blood pressure, while elimination of these substances reduces blood pressure. Hypertension caused by kidney disease or some other type of disease process is called secondary hypertension. Only ten percent of all hypertensive cases are caused by secondary problems.

Primary or essential hypertension accounts for approximately ninety percent of all hypertensive cases. This type of hypertension is from an unknown cause and usually has a gradual onset over a number of years. Symptoms usually do not occur until significant heart and vessel damage has already occurred. For this reason, blood pressure screening is very important in diagnosing hypertension before the cardiovascular system is damaged. A random blood pressure of greater than 140/90 may be physiologic, thus screening with frequent blood pressure readings under varied conditions is needed to confirm the diagnosis.

Primary hypertension is idiopathic, but there are some identified genetic and environmental risk factors. These include:

- Heredity—hypertension affects black individuals twice as often as whites
- Diet—high salt and fat intake increases the risk of hypertension
- Age—blood pressure tends to rise with age
- Obesity—causes an increased workload on the heart
- Smoking—because of vasoconstriction by nicotine
- Stress—causes a rise in blood pressure from vasoconstriction
- Type A personality—such individuals tend to experience more stress

The effects of hypertension may take years to develop, but ultimately if untreated high blood pressure overworks the heart. Because the left ventricle works harder to pump blood, it is the area most often affected, leading to left ventricle hypertrophy or muscle enlargement. The vascular system or blood supply to the left ventricle does not increase with this enlargement of muscle. As a result, this extra tissue does not have adequate blood supply often leading to bouts of angina or chest pain from ischemia. This condition often leads to myocardial infarction or heart failure and death.

Hypertension not only affects the heart, but it also adversely affects the vessels. Over a period of years, the vessels become hardened (sclerotic) and lose elasticity, a contributing factor in arteriosclerosis (arterio = artery, scler = hardened, osis = condition of). Sclerotic (hardened) vessels are also more likely to form thrombi and to rupture. The results of thrombus or rupture may cause damage or death to the involved organs.

Treatment of chronic hypertension depends on the degree of hypertension and the number of risk factors involved. If blood pressure is extremely high, anti-hypertensive medications may be begun immediately. If hypertension is discovered in a milder form, lifestyle changes or reduction of risk factors may be the initial treatment. A low-salt, low-fat diet, stress reducing exercise and smoking cessation may solve the problem. If this treatment is ineffective or inadequate, the individual may be placed on diuretic medications. Diuretics increase urine output and thus lower blood pressure. If further control is needed, other anti-hypertensive medications may be prescribed. Patient compliance with hypertension is often a factor in the treatment of this chronic disease. Difficulty with lifestyle changes and following the medication regimen for the "rest of life" is often difficult for the individual to manage.

Hypertensive emergencies may be subdivided into four classifications depending upon the characteristics and patient history. A hypertensive emergency is defined as an elevated blood pressure in conjunction with neurological dysfunction or renal dysfunction. This category is sometimes termed hypertensive crisis or malignant hypertension. A hypertensive urgency involves a diastolic blood pressure (DBP) greater than 115 mmHg without any signs and symptoms of organ damage. An acute hypertensive episode is a pressure greater than 180/110, also without signs and symptoms of organ damage. Transient hypertension includes patients who are hypertensive but return to normal after whatever caused the hypertension has resolved. Examples of transient hypertension include pregnancy and severe anxiety.

In general, hypertensive emergency is severe and treatment of the patient's blood pressure is required. This may or may not occur in the field depending upon area protocols or medical control direction. Blood pressure can be controlled in a variety of ways, including nitrates, calcium channel blockers, or diuretics. Again, EMS providers should follow local protocol or medical control for pharmacological treatment of these patients.

Non-pharmacological treatment includes keeping the patient calm, administering supplemental oxygen if required and treating any other conditions that are present as required. The other classifications of hypertension often do not require immediate treatment and are treated in the emergency department, unless there is a long transport time to the ED.

Arteriosclerosis and Atherosclerosis. Arteriosclerosis is a group of diseases that are characterized by a loss of elasticity and a thickening of the artery wall. Atherosclerosis is the most common form of arteriosclerosis. For this reason these terms are often used interchangeably. Hardening of the arteries is a lay term describing this condition. The common result of arteriosclerosis is the gradual narrowing of the vessel lumen (Figure 8–7). This narrowing leads to a slowing or complete stoppage of blood flow to the organs supplied by those vessels. Without proper blood supply these organs become ischemic and eventually may die if blood supply is not restored.

An artery has a very smooth endothelium (inner lining). The lining may be thought of as Teflon-coated. As with Teflon-coated cookware, food particles normally do not stick to the surface. If the endothelium is damaged, then blood material begins sticking to the inner lining of the artery just as food particles begin sticking to scratched cookware. The artery wall surrounds this endothelium. Atherosclerosis is a condition characterized by deposits of fatty or lipid material in the wall of the artery (see Figure 8–7). These fatty, cholesterol containing deposits called **plaque** damage the artery and interrupt blood flow by:

- Pushing into the endothelium thus damaging the inner lining. Damage to this lining allows blood

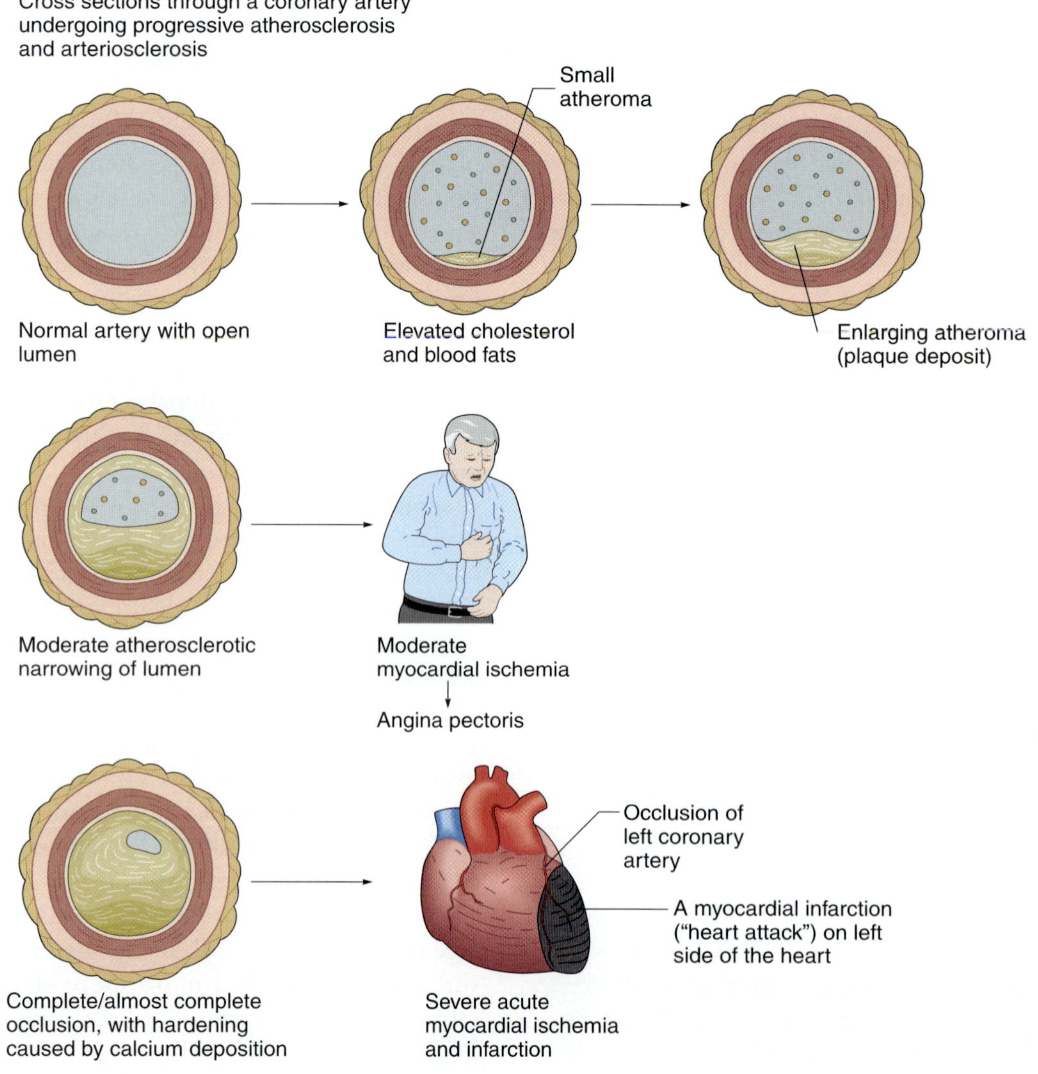

Figure 8–7 Atherosclerosis: narrowing of arterial lumen.

material to stick to the inner lining and occlude the lumen.

- Causing the artery wall to harden or lose elasticity. This loss of elasticity increases blood pressure and increases workload on the heart. A hardened vessel is not able to expand and accommodate the surge of blood caused by the beat of the heart.
- Thickening the artery wall to the point that the lumen is partially or completely occluded.
- Leading to formation of plaque that often ulcerates or breaks loose forming an **embolus** (EM-boh-lus; material floating in the blood) that may stick in a vessel and occlude or stop blood flow, leading to ischemia or death of the organs supplied by that vessel).

Narrowing of the lumen of the artery in these ways increases blood pressure, increases workload on the heart and decreases blood supply to the organs. Increased blood pressure stretches the hardened arteries causing further artery damage and further increasing workload on the heart.

Atherosclerosis may affect all arteries in the body. There are four major areas that are often affected by atherosclerosis often leading to disability or mortality (Figure 8–8).

The areas affected are the:

1. Coronary arteries—These arteries feed the muscle tissue of the heart. Atherosclerosis of these arteries leads to coronary artery disease, also called coronary heart disease. Consequences of coronary artery disease may include myocardial infarction or heart attack.
2. Cerebral arteries—These arteries feed brain tissue. Atherosclerosis of these arteries may lead to cerebrovascular accidents (CVA), commonly called stroke.

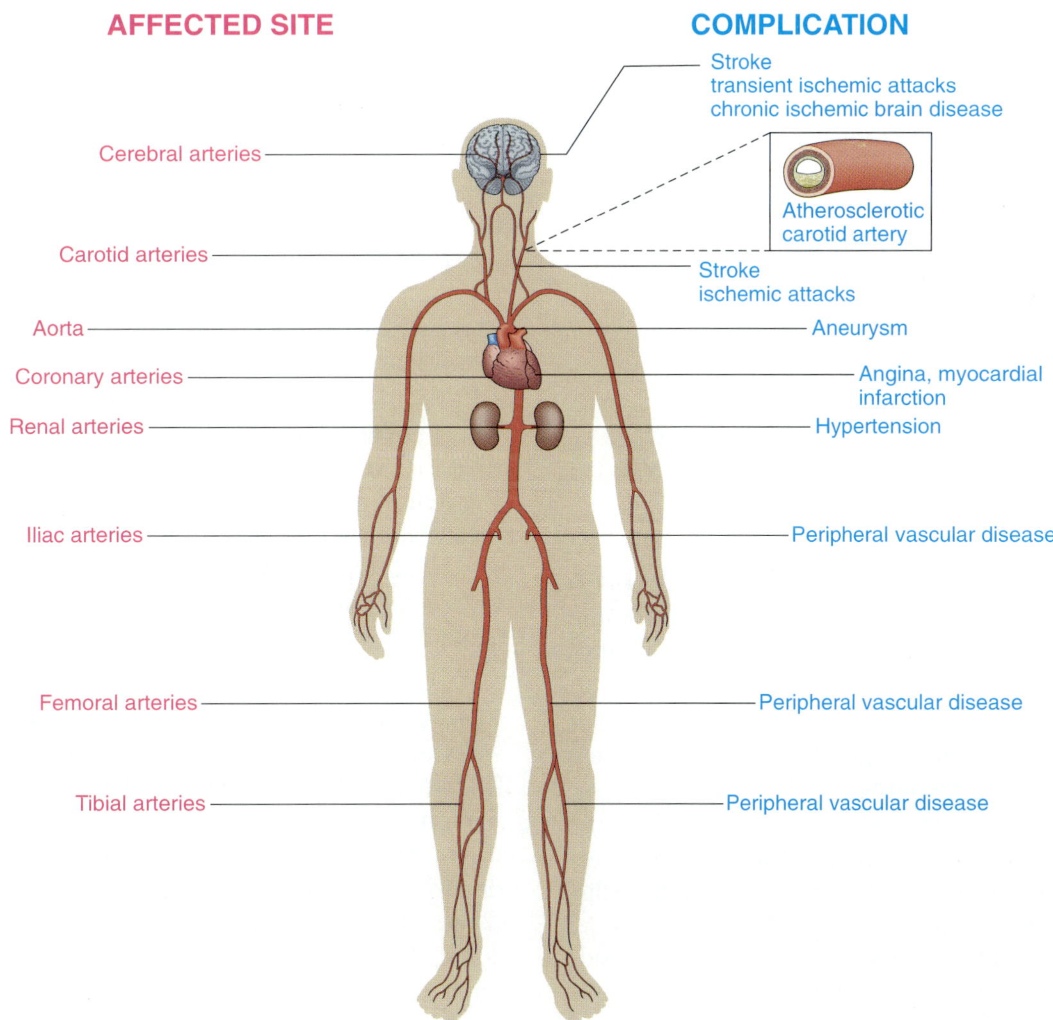

Figure 8–8 Atherosclerosis: major areas affected.

3. Aorta—This artery is the largest artery in the body and is responsible for carrying blood to the general circulatory system. Atherosclerosis of this artery in any area may lead to aneurysms.
4. Peripheral arteries—Peripheral arteries primarily feed the extremities (arms and legs). Atherosclerosis of these arteries may lead to peripheral vascular disease.

The cause of atherosclerosis is unknown, but it is thought to be the result of a combination of factors. Some of the factors are not controllable, but many are and may be altered by a change in lifestyle. Important risk factors include:

Non-Controllable Factors

- Heredity—Atherosclerosis appears to run in families. This may be related to common diet or, in some instances, a clear genetic tendency to develop hypercholesterolemia (hyper = increased, cholesterol, emia = blood) exists.
- Age—Atherosclerosis is considered a degenerative disease as all adults over the age of 30 have some degree of plaque formation. In general, the older the person, the more atherosclerosis present.
- Sex—Men have more atherosclerosis than women until after female menopause, at which time the incidence becomes more equal.
- Diabetes—Diabetic patients have more atherosclerosis than non-diabetic patients.

Controllable Factors

- Diet—Obese individuals have more atherosclerosis than individuals in normal weight range. The higher the diet in carbohydrates and fats, the higher the incidence of atherosclerosis.
- Sedentary lifestyle—Lack of exercise increases the risk of development of atherosclerosis.
- Cigarette smoking—This is one of the most important risk factors. To stop smoking is 10 times more effective in reducing risk than a combination of exercise and diet control.
- Stress—Stress increases blood pressure, but research does not support the idea that stress increases atherosclerosis.
- Hypertension—The higher the blood pressure, the greater the risk for development of atherosclerosis. It is difficult to determine which of these diseases occurs first. Atherosclerosis causes an increase in blood pressure, and hypertension leads to an increase in atherosclerosis. Often hypertension and atherosclerosis occur simultaneously with each complicating the treatment of the other.

Diagnosis of atherosclerosis is by blood pressure measurement, arteriograms, X-ray, and Doppler studies to determine blood flow through the affected area. Treatment aims to treat symptoms as they arise. Surgery to bypass occluded arteries and to remove plaque is commonly utilized. Prevention of atherosclerosis includes exercise, estrogen medication after menopause, and changing lifestyle to reduce risk factors.

Peripheral Vascular Disease (PVD) Peripheral vascular disease is caused by atherosclerotic plaque primarily in the arteries supplying blood to the legs. The occlusion by the plaque may be chronic or acute. Chronic occlusion is generally related to a progressive narrowing of the femoral and popliteal arteries. As these arteries become occluded, the blood supply to the leg muscles is decreased. Individuals with PVD have adequate blood supply to leg muscles during minimal activity like sitting or slow walking. If activity is increased to brisk walking or running blood supply becomes inadequate, causing leg muscle cramps. Resting the legs will relieve the muscle cramps. Rest allows the muscles to once again receive the needed amount of blood flow. This condition of developing muscle cramps that are relieved with rest and increase with activity is called **intermittent claudication** (KLAW-dih-**KAY**-shun). Treatment of chronic PVD often involves opening the artery and cleaning out the plaque. This surgical treatment is called **endarterectomy** (END-ar-ter-**ECK**-toh-me; endo = inside, arter = artery, ectomy = excision). If the artery is damaged, it may be bypassed with a graft. A femoral popliteal graft may be utilized to treat the symptoms of chronic occlusion.

Acute occlusion of the peripheral arteries often involves smaller arteries supplying blood to the feet and toes. This type of PVD often leads to necrosis and gangrene. Amputation or resection may be needed to treat acute occlusion.

Aneurysm. Aneurysm (AN-you-rizm) is a weakening in the wall of an artery that allows the vessel to bulge or rupture (Figure 8–9). This weakening is often caused by atherosclerosis, but may also be caused by a congenital defect or injury. Aneurysms are usually asymptomatic and are often discovered accidentally during physical examinations or X-rays. The most common area affected is the abdominal aorta. Rupture of an aneurysm is a medical emergency often causing death from massive hemorrhage and shock.

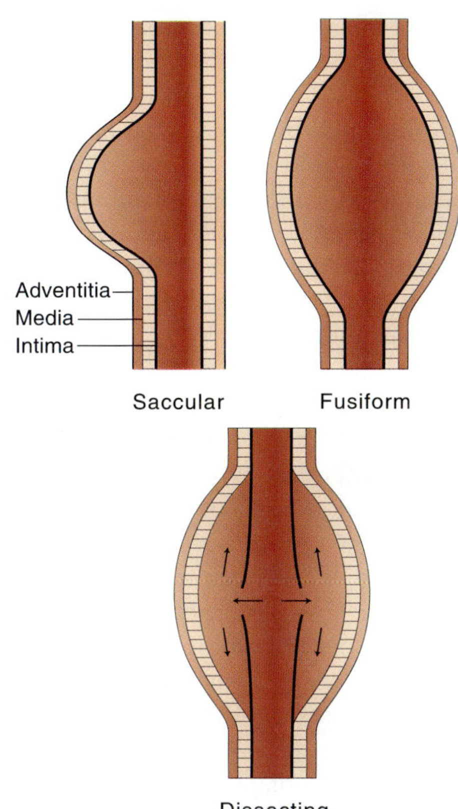

Figure 8–9 Three types of aneurysm.

Treatment aims to repair the aneurysm before rupture. Surgical resection and grafting are commonly performed.

Coronary Artery Disease. Coronary artery disease, often called coronary heart disease, is the narrowing of arteries that supply blood to the myocardium or heart muscle. It is the single leading cause of death in the United States today. This disease is commonly caused by atherosclerosis. Progressive or slow narrowing of the arteries leads to ischemia of the heart muscle and symptoms of angina. Some muscle cells may actually die and become replaced with scar tissue. This scar tissue cannot function like muscle tissue, causing an increase in the workload of the remaining heart muscle. Congestive heart failure often results.

If a coronary artery becomes blocked to the point that oxygen demands by the heart muscle cannot be met, the heart muscle dies. Occlusion may progress slowly as plaque builds up in the vessel or it may develop suddenly as a result of a **thrombus** (THROM-bus; a blood clot attached to a vein or artery) or embolus (traveling blood clot, free in the circulatory system, more dangerous than a thrombus). This dead muscle is called an infarct or myocardial infarct. The process of the myocardium dying is called myocardial infarction.

Slow, progressive occlusion of the arteries often leads to development of collateral arteries that extend into ischemic tissue. Collateral circulation provides some protection against ischemia and infarction. For this reason infarction caused by slow occlusion often has a better outcome than infarction caused by sudden occlusion of a vessel.

Diagnosis of coronary artery disease is made by a history of symptoms, ECG, and angiograms. Symptoms usually do not develop until the vessels are at least seventy percent occluded. Treatment of coronary artery disease is aimed at increasing blood flow or decreasing oxygen needs. Angina is often treated with rest and vasodilators. A coronary artery **angioplasty** (AN-jee-oh-**PLAS**-tee; angio = vessel, plasty = surgical repair) may be attempted to open the vessel. Angioplasty involves passing a catheter into the artery, inflating a balloon on the catheter to push the plaque against the vessel wall thus widening the lumen of the vessel (Figure 8–10). Another common surgical treatment for coronary artery disease is a coronary artery bypass graft, commonly called a CABG (pronounced cabbage). This procedure bypasses the occlusion (Figure 8–11). Mammary vessels and saphenous vessels from the legs are often used for the bypass.

It is very important that individuals with coronary artery disease reduce atherosclerotic risk factors. Diet, exercise, and a no-smoking regimen are prescribed to slow the progression of the disease.

Diseases of the Heart

Diseases of the heart are frequently caused by the atherosclerotic narrowing of the coronary arteries. The result of this is usually angina and/or a heart attack (myocardial infarction). Decreasing lifestyle behaviors that contribute to the development of atherosclerosis decreases one's risk for heart disease.

Angina Pectoris. Angina pectoris (an-JIGH-nah PECK-toh-riss) is is transient chest pain, caused by lack of oxygen to the myocardium or heart muscle. Angina is commonly a symptom of impending myocardial infarction. During an attack the individual may complain of a suffocating tightness in the chest that radiates to the left arm, neck, and jaw (Figure 8–12). Angina usually occurs during periods of increased workload on the heart, like those experienced with physical exercise, emotional stress, or digestion of a large meal.

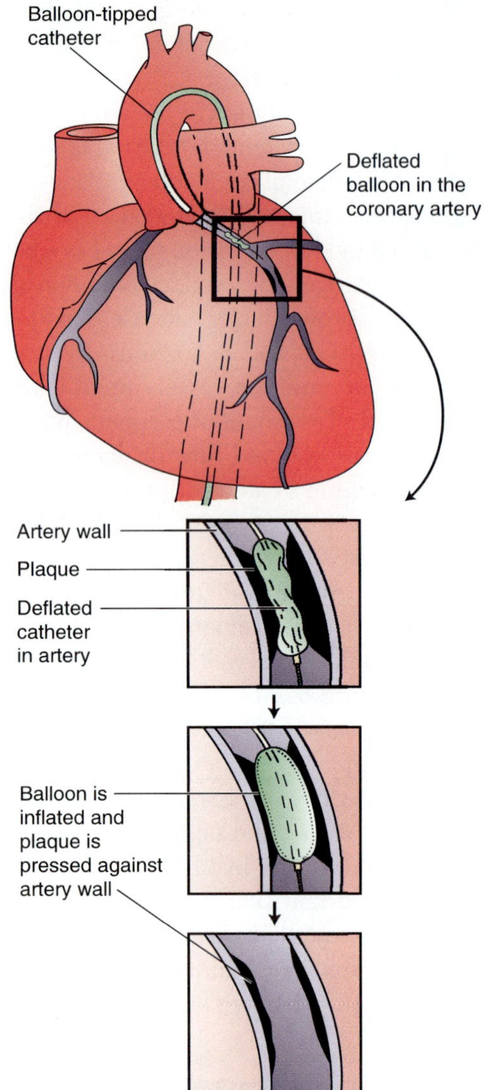

Figure 8–10 Coronary artery angioplasty.

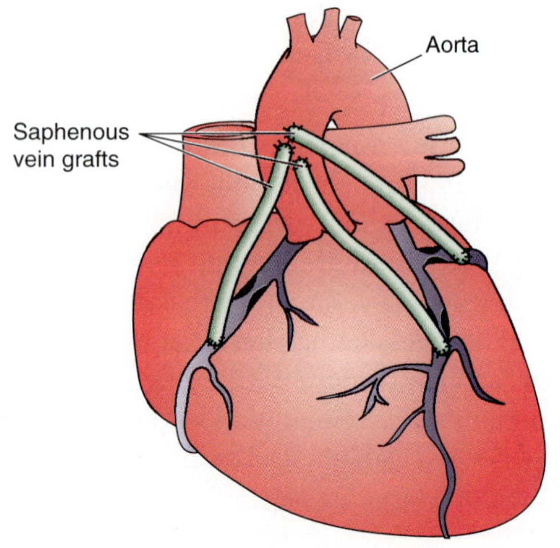

Figure 8–11 Coronary artery bypass graft (CABG).

Treatment of angina is to decrease workload on the heart by stopping the aggravating activity and to increase blood flow to the heart muscle. Vasodilatation of the coronary arteries or those that supply the heart muscle will improve blood flow and help relieve the oxygen deficit. Nitroglycerin (NTG) administered sublingually usually provides immediate relief. If the pain is not relieved with rest and three NTG tablets five minutes apart then the patient should notify EMS as she may be experiencing a myocardial infarction.

Myocardial Infarction. Myocardial infarction (MY-oh-**KAR**-dee-al in-FARK-shun) occurs when the heart muscle does not get adequate oxygen because of a decrease in blood supply, an increase in oxygen need, or a combination of both. The decrease in blood supply is most commonly caused by the atherosclerotic plaque of coronary artery disease. Any activity that increases oxygen need of the heart beyond the supply level may lead to a myocardial infarct. Activity may include shock, hemorrhage, stress, or excessive physical exertion.

Classic symptoms of a myocardial infarction include severe chest pain with diaphoresis (sweating), and nausea. Often the symptoms are not as obvious and may include referred pain in the left arm, neck, and jaw along with a discomfort similar to bad or unrelieved indigestion. Severity of symptoms may depend on the size of the infarction. If the area is small, symptoms may be mild. If the infarcted area is large, symptoms may include cardiogenic shock and subsequently death. Mortality from myocardial infarction is approximately thirty-five percent.

The main site involved in a myocardial infarction is the left ventricle. This is the hardest working area of the heart and has the greatest need for oxygen. Tissue changes that appear with an infarction depend on the degree or extent of oxygen deprivation suffered by the cells. Under microscopic examination, the infarcted area may take on a bull's eye appearance (Figure 8–13). The central core is made up of cells that are dead or necrotic. Severely damaged cells surround this core. These cells may regain function within a few weeks or they may die, thus extending the infarcted area. On the outer border of the bull's eye pattern are cells that suffered from ischemia. These cells usually live and may regain function.

Death of myocardial cells brings about a release of certain enzymes into the general circulation. Blood tests to measure the levels of these enzymes assist in determining the amount of dead or necrotic tissue and the severity and time of the attack. Blood enzyme levels along with an ECG (electrocardiography), history, and physical examination often confirm the diagnosis of myocardial infarction.

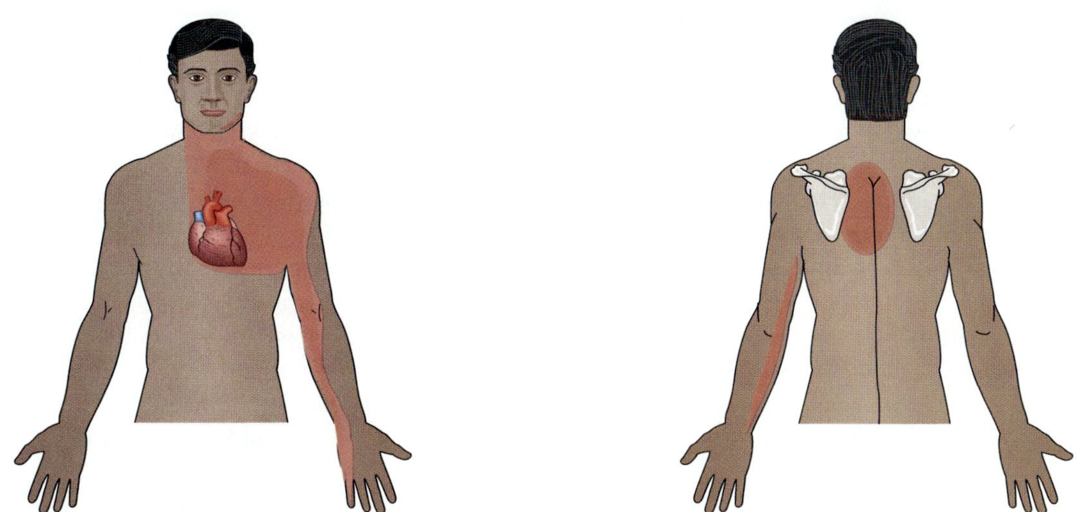

Figure 8–12 Patterns of angina.

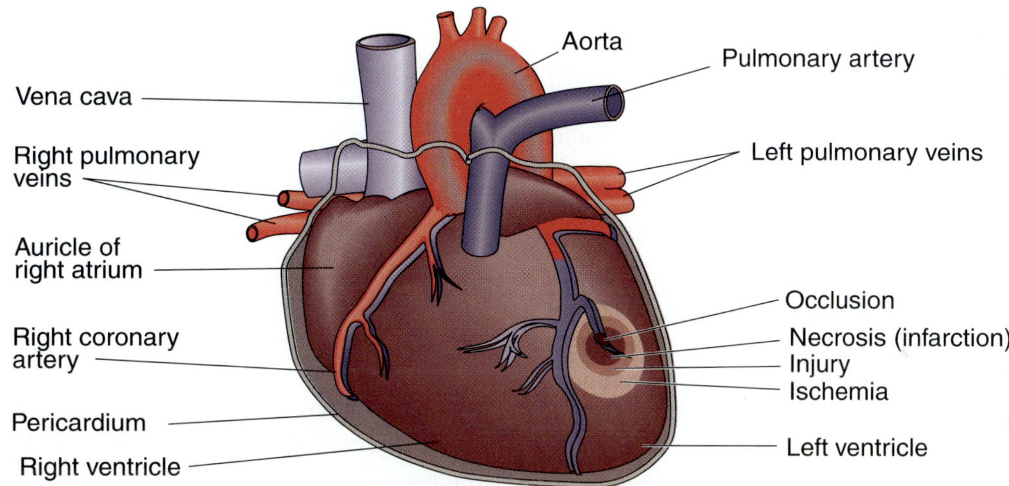

Figure 8–13 Myocardial infarction: areas of ischemia.

The area of infarction can be localized based upon which ECG leads show changes (Table 8–1).

The typical ECG findings of a myocardial infarction are not always present and the paramedic should keep

TABLE 8–1 Localizing Infarction or Ischemia by ECG Findings

Location	ST Elevation In:	Likely Occlusion
Septal	V_1 and V_2	Left anterior descending and/or posterior septal artery
Anterior Wall	V_3 and V_4	Left anterior descending artery
Lateral Wall	I, aVL, V_5 and V_6	Circumflex artery
Inferior Wall	II, III, aVF (perform right sided ECG to assess posterior wall)	Right marginal artery or right coronary artery
Posterior Wall	V_4R, II, III, aVF (or marked depression in V_1 through V_4)	Right coronary artery

the entire clinical picture in focus when evaluating a patient who presents with chest pain. The changes that occur do so because dead (infarcted) and ischemic cardiac cells conduct electricity differently than a normal cardiac cell. Ischemic tissue is tissue that is lacking in oxygen, but has not yet sustained injury. The ECG changes that occur in ischemia include ST-segment depression greater than 1 mm and peaked or inverted T-waves (Figure 8–14A).

If the ischemia continues for a relatively short period of time, the myocardial cells become damaged and change their electrical properties. At this point, the cells are damaged but not completely destroyed. The ECG change that occurs when cardiac cells are injured is ST-segment elevation greater than 1 mm, the typical ECG sign that occurs during an active MI (Figure 8–14B). This change must occur in two or more anatomically contiguous leads to be considered diagnostic of a myocardial infarction. These damaged cells do not contract properly, if at all. Because this area of the heart does not contract efficiently, the cardiac output and, indirectly, the blood pressure can be affected. If blood flow is restored to this area of myocardium quickly, then the cells may be saved and damage minimized.

If the injured cardiac tissue does not receive oxygenated blood within an hour, the cells begin to die. This cell death is called infarction, and is not reversible. The ECG change associated with infarction is an abnormal Q-wave. An abnormal Q-wave has a height greater than twenty-five percent of the R wave in the same complex (Figure 8–14C). Q-waves that do not meet the criteria may be normal for that patient. In the setting of an MI, Q-waves can develop as early as two hours into the infarct.

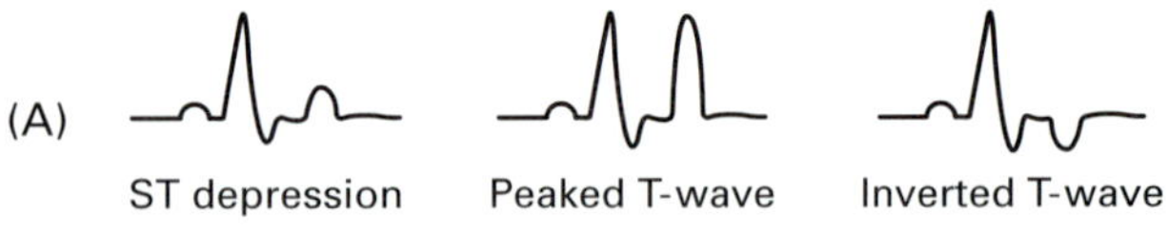

(B)

ST Elevation

(C)

Pathologic Q-wave

Figure 8–14 Typical ECG changes with A. ischemia, B. injury, and C. infarction.

Unless an old ECG is available to compare tracings, it is difficult to know if the pathologic Q-waves are from the current MI or an old MI, as Q-waves can be present for more than a year following an infarction. If they are present in combination with ST-segment elevations, then it is more likely that the Q-wave changes are from the current event.

Tissue infarction and injury naturally cause the inflammatory response. With this response comes an outpouring of PMNs (polymorphonuclear neutrophils) and macrophages. Within the first five to seven days, macrophages phagocytize the dead tissue often leaving a thin, weak myocardial layer. Possibility of rupture and sudden death is greatest at this time. Any activity that increases the workload of the heart or increases blood pressure should be avoided. Rest is essential during this time.

Within two weeks the infarcted area is healing with granulation tissue. This tissue is not made of muscle tissue; it is scar tissue. This scar or patch will not stretch or contract like muscle, and it will never function as normal heart tissue. The inability of this scarred area to function increases workload on the remaining heart muscle cells for the rest of the individual's life.

Risk factors for myocardial infarction are the same as coronary artery disease and primarily include hypertension, cigarette smoking, a sedentary lifestyle, obesity, and a high-cholesterol diet.

EMS management of a patient with a suspected MI includes assessing for adequate respirations and pulse, and initiating CPR and defibrillation as necessary. The ECG should be monitored continuously and a 12-lead ECG obtained if it is available in your system. IV access should be obtained as soon as possible. Initial treatment of MI follows the "*MONA*" memory aid for *M*orphine, *O*xygen, *N*itrates, and *A*spirin. Morphine, a narcotic analgesic, provides pain relief, relaxes the patient, causes the veins to dilate, and assists in dilating the arteries. This dilation of the veins reduces preload and the dilation of the arteries reduces afterload, both decreasing the amount of work the heart is performing, and reducing the oxygen requirement for the heart. Oxygen is administered to provide additional oxygen to the heart. Nitrates, for example nitroglycerine, act to dilate the coronary arteries, the systemic arterioles, and the systemic venoules, reducing heart work and allowing more oxygenated blood to flow through the coronary arteries. Aspirin acts to decrease the ability of platelets to form clots, acting to not allow the current thrombus to grow in addition to preventing new clot formation. These four interventions are the basic treatments for a patient with a suspected MI. Rapid transportation and early emergency department notification with 12-lead ECG transmission, if possible, allows the patient to gain the greatest chance of salvaging heart muscle.

Arrhythmias and shock are common complications of myocardial infarctions. EMS providers should refer to the Advanced Cardiac Life Support algorithms and local protocols for specific management of cardiac arrhythmias and shock secondary to MI.

In the emergency department, a fibrinolytic medication may be administered to patients who fit the criteria (Table 8–2). For patients who do not fit the criteria and are in a facility that has the capability, emergency angioplasty may be performed. The efficacy of fibrinolytic therapy in the field is still under evaluation. Current International Liaison Committee on Resuscitation (ILCOR) recommendations from the 2000 Emergency Cardiovascular Care Conference are for EMS fibrinolytic therapy only if a physician is present to interpret the ECG, with on-line medical control direction, or if transport time is greater than one hour.

Congestive Heart Failure. Congestive heart failure (CHF) is a condition in which the heart fails to pump an adequate amount of blood to meet the body's needs. The cardiopulmonary and general vascular system gradually become "congested." The individual experiences a gradual increase in dyspnea (dys = difficult, pnea = breathing). Tachycardia (tachy = rapid, cardia = heart) and tachypnea (TACH-ihp-**NEE**-ah; tachy = rapid, pnea = breathing) occur as the body tries to compensate for decreased blood flow.

TABLE 8–2 Criteria for Fibrinolytic Therapy in the Setting of MI

Chest discomfort:
More than 20 minutes
Less than 12 hours
Age greater than:
35 (males)
40 (females)
No history of stroke or TIA
No known bleeding disorder
No active internal bleeding in the past month
No surgery/trauma in past 3 weeks
No jaundice, hepatitis, or kidney failure
No use of anticoagulants
Blood pressure below 180/110

As CHF progresses, fluid builds up in the vascular system leading to neck vein distention and edema in the ankles and lower legs. Right-sided heart failure leads to congestion of the liver and spleen. Left-sided failure leads to congestion and edema of the lungs (pulmonary edema) (Figure 8–15).

Congestive heart failure develops slowly and usually follows any type of cardiac condition that increases the workload of the heart. Such diseases include myocardial infarction, hypertension, and coronary artery disease to name a few. Diagnosis is made after a thorough history and physical examination combined with chest X-ray and ECG. Treatment is aimed at decreasing the workload of the heart. Diuretic medications, low-salt diet, and fluid restrictions may be prescribed to increase urine output and limit fluid retention thus reducing blood fluid volume. Cardiac medications may be prescribed to strengthen and slow the heartbeat. Digitalis is a common medication given for this purpose.

CHF can worsen acutely for a variety of reasons, from ingesting too much salt to experiencing a myocardial infarction. This sudden exacerbation is typically left side heart failure leading to acute pulmonary edema and dyspnea. In fact, the patient's chief complaint may be

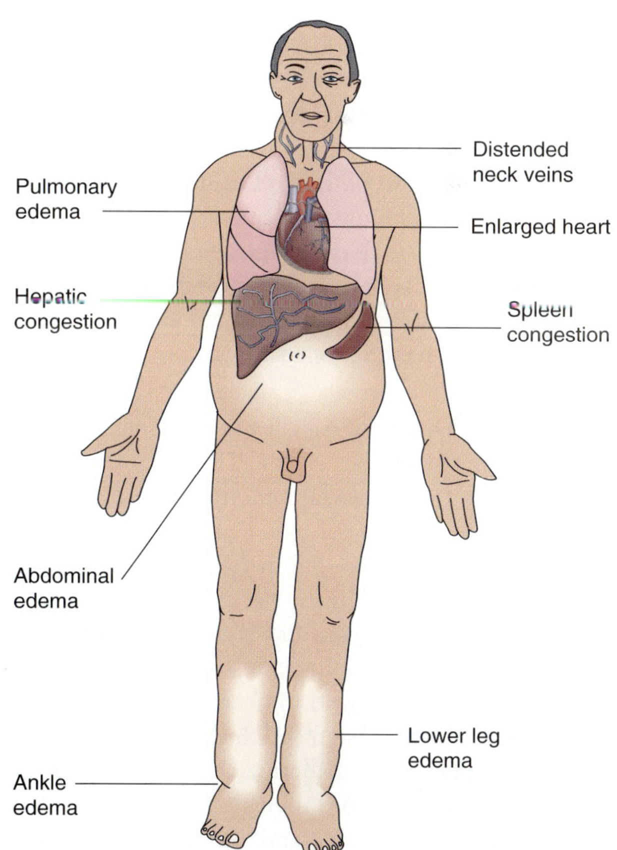

Figure 8–15 Signs of congestive heart failure.

dyspnea and only through EMS and emergency department evaluation is an MI uncovered. EMS treatment is aimed at supporting ventilations and decreasing the pulmonary edema. A helpful memory aid for CHF treatment is "*LMNOP*" which stands for *L*asix, *M*orphine, *N*itrates, *O*xygen, and vaso*P*ressors. The first four were discussed under treatment for MI. Vasopressors (e.g., dopamine, dobutamine) are sometimes required in order to support the blood pressure for a patient who is hypotensive. Morphine should be used with extreme caution as even slight respiratory depression from morphine can cause the patient to decompensate. The use of CPAP (continuous positive airway pressure) or BiPAP (bilevel positive airway pressure) to augment respirations is commonly employed in the Emergency Department to improve oxygenation and reduce the number of patients requiring intubation. The use of this modality in the prehospital setting is becoming more prevalent and may become commonplace in the EMS setting in the future.

Carditis. Carditis (kar-DYE-tis) is a general term describing inflammation of the heart. Forms of carditis include pericarditis, myocarditis, and endocarditis, depending on the area of the heart involved. Pericarditis affects the serous membrane on the outside of the heart as well as the pericardial sac. Myocarditis affects the heart muscle layer, while endocarditis affects the inside of the heart. All these inflammatory states may result from unknown causes, bacteria, and viruses or as a result of rheumatic fever. Carditis is often secondary to a respiratory tract, urinary tract, or skin infection. It may also be related to dental infections or diseases of other systems. Treatment for carditis generally includes bedrest to decrease the workload on the heart. Other treatments depend on the cause of the disease and may include antibiotics, analgesics, and antipyretics (anti = against, pyro = heat, or against fever).

Valvular Heart Disease. Valvular heart disease is related to malfunction of the heart valves. The purpose of a valve in the heart and the vascular system is to prevent backflow of blood. Backflow of blood causes extra workload on the heart, as it has to re-pump the blood. Malfunction of a valve may be caused by the valvular opening being too narrow (stenotic), or being too large to properly close (valvular insufficiency). Both of these problems may affect all the heart valves and lead to heart murmurs. A heart **murmur** is an abnormal sound in the heart or vascular system. One complication of all valve defects is the vascular tendency to form clots (thrombus) on the affected areas. If the thrombus breaks loose and becomes an embolus, it may occlude arteries leading to major organs such as the lungs, brain, liver, or kidneys. Another common problem of valvular heart disease is congestive heart failure caused by the increased workload on the heart. Common causes of valvular disease may be congenital anomalies or malformations, rheumatic fever, or endocarditis.

Dysrhythmias. The term dysrhythmia is used to describe an alteration in the normal cardiac electrical rhythm. This change in rhythm may produce outward signs and symptoms or may be benign, depending upon the rhythm and severity. Interpretation of dysrhythmias is beyond the scope of this text and I refer you to one of the many excellent texts on the subject of rhythm interpretation. Treatment of dysrhythmias will normally follow published Advanced Cardiovascular Life Support guidelines. As a reminder, ACLS treatment will be ineffective if basic CPR is performed poorly. All patients should receive supplemental oxygen, an intravenous line, and be placed on an ECG monitor.

Normal sinus rhythm is an electrical rhythm that is generated by the sinus node (see Figure 8–16) and travels in a normal fashion through the heart's electrical system. The intrinsic rate of the SA node is between 60 and 100 beats per minute. If the impulse is generated by the sinus node at a rate faster than 100 beats per minute but still travels down the normal pathway, the rhythm is called sinus tachycardia and if the impulse is generated at a rate slower than 60 beats per minute, then the rhythm is called sinus bradycardia. The only outward signs associated with these rhythm changes is an increased or decreased pulse rate. If no impulse is generated by the SA node, then this rhythm is called sinus arrest. In this situation, the cardiac output is reduced because of the loss of atrial contraction and the pulse quality may be decreased. In most cases the AV node or ventricular pathways take over and produce ventricular contractions at a slower rate than normal. Asystole is the absence of electrical activity and is observed as a "flat line" on the ECG monitor (Figure 8–17). With the exception of hypothermic individuals, patients who present in asystole and do not respond immediately to treatment have a very poor prognosis and resuscitation is typically terminated.

There are several dysrhythmias that originate in the atria and include premature atrial contractions, atrial fibrillation, atrial flutter, atrial tachycardia, and multifocal atrial tachycardia. Premature atrial contractions (PAC) are impulses generated from an irritable focus within the atria that occurs early in the cycle. PACs are typically benign. Atrial fibrillation occurs when the atria contract rapidly in an uncoordinated fashion. The ventricular response occurs in an *irregularly irregular* pattern, which

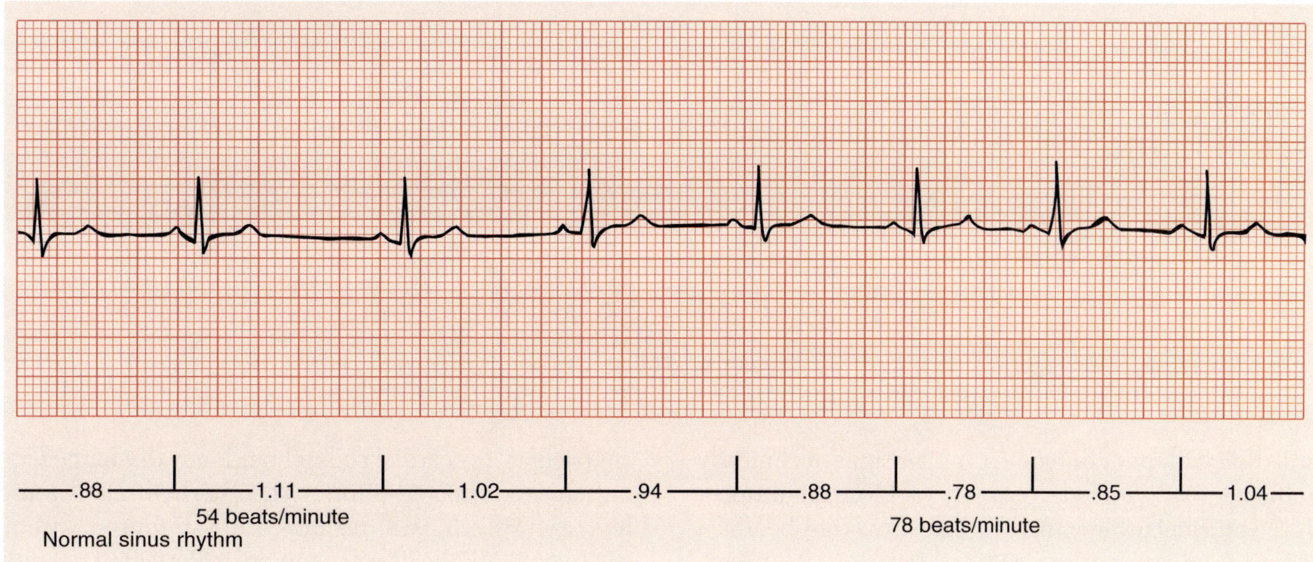

Figure 8–16 Normal sinus rhythm.

is one of the hallmarks of this rhythm. The other hallmark is an undulating wavy baseline and a loss of P-waves. One potential side effect of this rhythm is the development of a clot or thrombus in the atria caused by stagnant blood that can be flicked loose and occlude either a coronary artery and produce an MI or occlude a cerebral artery and produce a stroke. At times the ventricular response can be very rapid, up to 200 beats per minute or more, which reduces filling times and can produce hypotension. In these cases, DC cardioversion is indicated if the patient is unstable. If the patient is stable, then either calcium channel blockers or beta-blockers are used to control the rate. The patient is then evaluated to determine if it is safe to abolish the rhythm. If it is not safe, or the patient elects not to undergo cardioversion, then warfarin, an anticoagulant, is used to reduce the risk of a thrombus. Atrial flutter is a similar rhythm except there is one irritable atrial focus that fires at an extremely fast rate, upwards of 300 beats per minute. F-waves or flutter waves are often seen as a sawtooth pattern along the baseline instead of P-waves. Fortunately, in many cases the ventricular response remains in the normal range. However, the ventricular response can become increased with the same side effects as with atrial fibrillation. Treatment is the same as for atrial fibrillation. Atrial tachycardia and multifocal atrial tachycardia (MAT) differ in the number of foci involved in producing the tachycardia, with both capable of producing significant ventricular response rates. In order for a rhythm to be considered MAT, there must be at least three different P-wave morphologies indicating several foci. Initial treatment for a stable patient includes vagal maneuvers, administration of adenosine, and then either calcium channel blockers or beta-blockers for a patient with "normal" heart function or amiodarone for a patient with poor heart function. The unstable patient requires cardioversion and atrial tachycardia that does not respond to adenosine often responds to cardioversion.

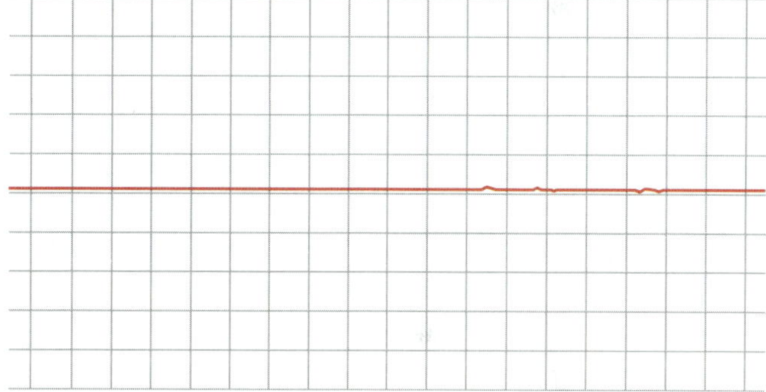

Figure 8–17 Asystole.

Dysrhythmias originating in the ventricles include premature ventricular complexes, ventricular tachycardia, ventricular fibrillation, idioventricular rhythm, and ventricular standstill. Premature ventricular complexes (PVCs), like PACs, are complexes indicating a premature discharge of the ventricles (Figure 8–18). Most PVCs are benign, however, they can become dangerous if they occur close to the relative refractory portion of the T-wave. If the PVC occurs during this time period, it can produce polymorphic ventricular tachycardia or ventricular

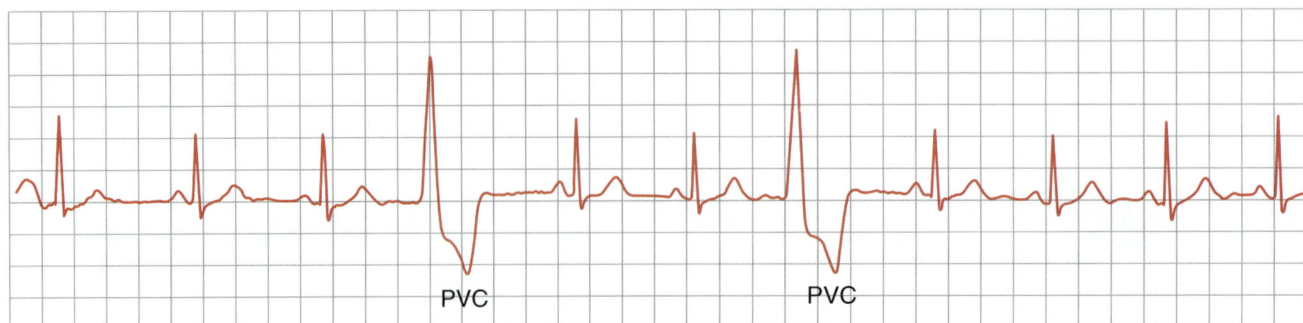

Figure 8–18 Monomorphic premature ventricular fibrillation.

fibrillation with poor outcomes. Other signs of clinically significant PVCs include couplets of PVCs, multiform PVCs, ventricular bigeminy where every other beat is a PVC, or frequent uniform PVCs. Ventricular tachycardia (VT), like atrial tachycardia, is caused by one irritable focus in the ventricles that produces a tachycardia (Figure 8–19). Patients with VT can still have a pulse, however, ventricular filling is decreased and individuals with prior heart disease generally cannot tolerate this rhythm well. Patients with preserved cardiac function may be able to tolerate this rhythm for up to a few hours, but most patients will deteriorate into a ventricular fibrillation or pulseless VT. Pulseless VT is treated identically to ventricular fibrillation as discussed below. If a pulse is present, treatment options include cardioversion for unstable patients and a choice between procainamide, amiodarone, or lidocaine for stable patients depending upon prior heart function. Polymorphic ventricular tachycardia, also known as torsades de pointes, is typically refractory to treatment but often responds to magnesium. Ventricular fibrillation (VF) is a lethal dysrhythmia that is most effectively treated by defibrillation. In VF, the ventricular myocardial cells all randomly discharge without any coordinated effort. This dysrhythmia is pulseless and death will occur within minutes without treatment. VF that is refractory to defibrillation is treated with epinephrine or vasopressin to increase systemic vascular resistance and improve coronary artery blood flow and one of several antiarrhythmics in an attempt to control the fibrillation. VF that is refractory to both defibrillation and medication is fatal and will eventually degenerate to asystole. An idioventricular rhythm is also known as an agonal rhythm and represents a slow and random discharge of the ventricles in the dying heart. Ventricular standstill is similar to sinus arrest in that the electrical impulse is not carried into the ventricles. Without immediate transcutaneous pacing or transvenous pacemaker insertion, these patients will not survive.

There are several dysrhythmias involving the AV node and ventricular conduction system. These dysrhythmias include heart blocks and junctional rhythms. As discussed earlier in the chapter, the atrioventricular node (AV node) produces a short pause in the transmission of the electrical impulse from the atria to the ventricles to allow the

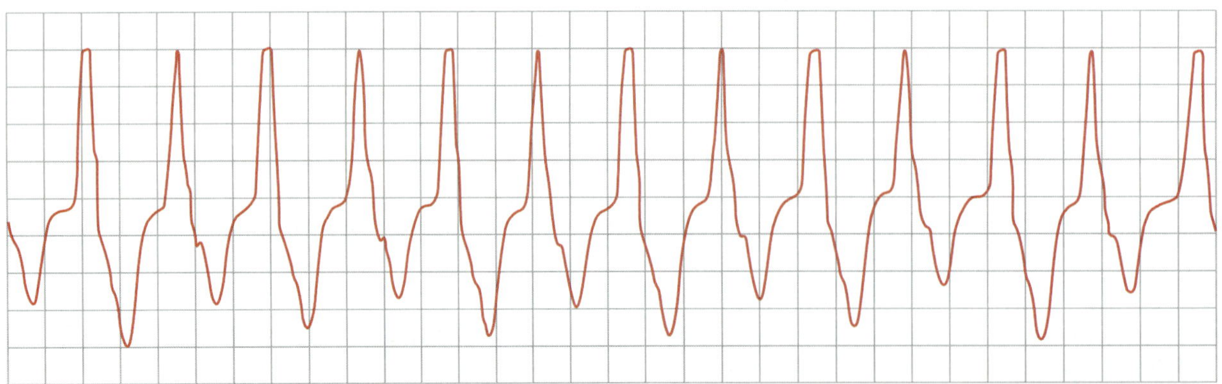

Figure 8–19 Ventricular tachycardia.

ventricles to fill completely prior to contraction. Several types of blocks can exist within this section of the conduction system that delay or impede impulse transmission. The most benign of the blocks is a first degree AV block and this involves a lengthening of the pause to a point where the PR Interval is greater than 0.2 seconds in duration. This lengthening is consistent and the PR intervals do not change. A second degree AV block involves periodic complete blocking of an impulse from the atria to the ventricles. A Mobitz Type I second degree block occurs when there is a progressive lengthening of the PR interval with a periodic nontransmitted impulse. After the "dropped beat," the mechanism resets and the PR interval returns to the starting point. A Mobitz Type II second degree block is a more ominous rhythm where the PR Interval remains constant, but there is a periodic blocked beat. A third degree AV block, also known as complete heart block, occurs when there is a total dissociation between the atria and ventricles. The atria contract at their own intrinsic rate, generally between 60 and 100, and the ventricles will contract at their intrinsic rate, either between 40 and 60 if originating in the AV node or between 20 and 40 if originating below the AV node. Second degree type II and third degree heart blocks are very ominous rhythms in patients who have compromised heart function caused by the loss in cardiac output. Either dysrhythmia can progress to ventricular standstill, and the EMS provider should be prepared to immediately apply a transcutaneous pacer if the patient becomes symptomatic. These rhythms typically have a widened QRS indicating the escape pacemaker is below the AV node and are not as responsive to atropine because the parasympathetic nervous system innervates the AV node and ventricles to a lesser extent than the sympathetic nervous system. Other blocks that can commonly occur include a bundle branch block where a block exists in one of the two bundle branches that run along the ventricular septum. In these blocks, the QRS is widened because of the longer impulse transmission time required to discharge the ventricles. Junctional rhythms that occur include premature junctional complexes and junctional tachycardia. Premature junctional complexes (PJCs) as with PACs and PVCs are premature complexes that originate from the AV node cells. PJCs, like PACs, have a narrow QRS, however the P-wave is absent, buried within the QRS, or occurs after the QRS. PJCs are generally benign. Junctional tachycardia is a tachycardic rhythm that looks similar to atrial tachycardia, however the P-waves are often absent or buried within the QRS. Junctional tachycardia can produce symptoms when the rate is increased above 140 beats per minute and is treated in the same manner as atrial tachycardia.

Diseases of the Veins

Diseases of the veins are more common in older adults. Age-related changes in the vessels and valves, along with other changes in the circulatory system, contribute to the overall general weakness of the vessels. Fluid often pools in the extremities causing edema. Disorders of the veins are usually more serious in individuals with other chronic disorders such as diabetes mellitus.

Thrombophlebitis. A complication of phlebitis is the development of a clot in the inflamed vessel. This condition is called thrombophlebitis. Clots in superficial veins rarely embolize (break loose and travel), but clots in deep veins often do, making this condition in a deep vein of serious concern. Thrombophlebitis in the deep veins is called deep vein thrombosis (DVT).

Deep Vein Thrombosis. Deep vein thrombosis (DVT) primarily occurs in the lower legs, thighs, and pelvis. Clots occurring in the femoral and pelvic veins commonly embolize. These clots are generally asymptomatic until embolization occurs, often causing a pulmonary embolism. Pulmonary embolism is often fatal. Risk factors for DVT include:

- Immobility—early postoperative ambulation (walking) is encouraged. Prolonged bedrest greatly increases risk
- Dehydration—increases blood viscosity (thickness) and increases risk of thrombus formation
- Varicose veins—veins already weakened with disease are more likely to develop a thrombus
- Leg or pelvic surgery, obesity and pregnancy —alter venous blood flow and increase risk

Treatment of DVT is aimed at reducing the formation of more clots and preventing embolization. Bedrest with elevation of the affected area is essential to improve blood flow. Anticoagulants are given to decrease potential thrombus formation; anticoagulants will not dissolve clots, only prevent formation of new ones.

TRAUMA

The cardiovascular system is affected in almost every trauma. Any injury to the body will produce bleeding, even the most minor injury. Long bone fractures (for example, the femur) and pelvic fractures can produce a substantial amount of bleeding. Other injuries, for example blunt cardiac injury, occur in eight to seventy-one percent of patients who receive blunt thoracic trauma, depending on the study. Conditions discussed below include hemorrhage, pericardial tamponade, blunt cardiac injury, and great vessel injury. Shock is discussed in detail in Chapter 6.

Hemorrhage

Hemorrhage (hemo = blood, orrhage = burst forth) is an abnormal loss of blood. Hemorrhagic blood loss may be external or internal. Blood loss may also be acute (sudden onset) or it may be chronic. Acute blood loss is usually related to trauma while chronic loss is more often related to disease processes.

External and internal blood loss, if severe enough, may lead to **exsanguination** (loss of circulating blood volume) and death. Internal blood loss may cause filling of body cavities. An example of internal bleeding into a cavity would be **hemothorax** (hemo = blood, thorax = chest, blood in the chest cavity). Internal bleeding may not be noticeable until a large amount of blood has been lost and the individual begins to show signs and symptoms of shock.

Hemorrhage may affect different vessels and thus have varying results. Hemorrhage of low-pressure vessels, the capillaries and veins, into the tissues leads to reddish to dark purple spots on the skin and mucosa. These discolorations are called petechiae, ecchymosis, or purpura, depending on the size or cause of the discoloration. Petechiae (pee-TEE-kee-ee) are small pinpoint hemorrhages. Ecchymosis (ECK-ih-**MOH**-sis) is a larger area of purplish color commonly called a bruise. Purpura (PUR-pew-rah) is spontaneous bleeding into the tissues related to a hemorrhagic disease that may be characterized by both petechiae and ecchymosis. Hemorrhage of the high-pressure vessels, the arteries, leads to forceful squirting of bright red (highly oxygenated) blood. The squirting of arterial blood is directly related to the beat of the heart.

Large venous and arterial hemorrhages, if not controlled, may be fatal. Blood volume varies with body size. The average adult has about five liters (approximately five quarts) of blood. Adults may lose approximately 500 ml (approximately one pint) of blood without any problems. This amount is equal to the amount given during a blood donation. Loss of one liter of blood may result in hypovolemic shock. Greater losses, 1500 ml and up, are usually lethal. Hemorrhaging in a closed cavity may also cause organ damage from increased pressure. For example, bleeding in the head may lead to brain tissue damage and/or death from the resulting increase in intercranial pressure.

Chronic hemorrhage, such as those occurring in the gastrointestinal and female reproductive tracts, commonly lead to anemia. Normal menstrual bleeding is approximately 70–80 ml. As discussed in Chapter 16, replacement of the lost iron may also lead to iron deficiency anemia.

Pericardial Tamponade

Pericardial tamponade occurs when fluid collects in the pericardium, the sac that surrounds the heart. While there is always a small amount of fluid present to allow the heart to glide smoothly as it expands and contracts, the amount is minimal. An increase in fluid can limit the ability for the heart to expand and fill. Tamponade can occur in trauma from a ruptured blood vessel or injured myocardium, or it can occur with a variety of medical conditions. Signs and symptoms of tamponade include heart sounds that are muffled, a narrowing pulse pressure (the difference between systolic blood pressure and diastolic blood pressure), distended neck veins, and in late stages, shock and cardiac arrest. Tamponade can be one reason a patient in cardiac arrest presents with PEA on the ECG. The patient requires support of the ABCs and rapid transport to the emergency department for a pericardiocentesis. The ED physician will pass a long needle into the pericardial sac and withdraw the blood or fluid to relieve the pressure.

Blunt Cardiac Injury

Blunt thoracic injury has the potential to cause significant damage to the heart and lungs (see Chapter 7). The secondary impact between the heart and the inside of the thoracic cage can cause injury or even infarction to the affected tissue. The coronary arteries or the valves can also be injured during this type of injury. Blunt cardiac injury (BCI) is a continuum from a minor bruise in the myocardium to a life-threatening rupture of a ventricle. Patients who have sustained a BCI can present with arrhythmias caused by myocardial damage, cardiac type chest pain resulting from the ischemia caused by a coronary artery rupture, shock, or cardiac arrest. All patients who sustain a significant blunt injury to the thorax should have their ECG monitored and have IV access available to allow the EMS provider to quickly treat hypotension should it occur.

Great Vessel Injury

Deceleration injuries to the thorax can also cause damage to the great vessels. The great vessels include the thoracic aorta, the superior and inferior vena cava, the pulmonary arteries, and pulmonary veins (see Figure 8–1). Rupture of any of these vessels can cause a significant hemorrhage and almost immediate death. Smaller leaks can cause hypotension, a hemothorax, or a pericardial tamponade. EMS treatment includes high flow oxygen and fluid resuscitation to treat shock, and rapid transport to a trauma center.

DEVELOPMENTAL DISEASES AND DISORDERS

The heart and its related great vessels are the most common sites of congenital defects. The defects may be small or quite large, thus consequences of these deformities may range from asymptomatic to life-threatening. Collectively these malformations of heart structure are called congenital heart defects. The cause of these defects is unknown but a genetic tendency is strongly suspected. Certain risk factors include maternal rubella, poor maternal nutrition, and alcoholism. Diagnosis is made by electrocardiogram, and physical examination including auscultation (listening to the chest with a stethoscope), which usually reveals heart murmurs (abnormal heart sounds) if present. Early diagnosis and surgical correction of these defects have improved drastically in recent years and have significantly reduced the mortality rate of infants born with heart defects.

Atrial Septal Defect

Atrial septal defect is an opening between the right and left atria (Figure 8–20A). This defect is commonly caused by the foramen ovale not closing at birth. The foramen ovale is a natural opening between the atria that allows blood to bypass the nonfunctional lungs during fetal life. Once the infant is born, the act of breathing causes a change in chest cavity pressure. This pressure change normally closes the foramen ovale. Atrial septal defects allow oxygenated blood to be pumped from the left atria to the right atria. This blood is again pumped to the right ventricle and to the lungs without ever circulating through the body. This repumping causes an increased workload on the right side of the heart. This defect occurs more commonly in girls than boys.

Ventricular Septal Defect

Ventricular septal defects are the most common heart defects, accounting for approximately twenty-five percent of all heart defects. As the name suggests, this defect is a hole between the right and left ventricle (Figure 8–20B) that allows blood from the left ventricle to flow into the right ventricle. Like the atrial septal defect, this oxygenated blood has to be repumped causing an increase in workload on the right side of the heart.

Patent Ductus Arteriosus

A ductus arteriosus is a connection between the pulmonary artery and the aorta of the normal fetal heart (Figure 8–20C). This structure allows blood to flow from the pulmonary artery to the aorta, thus bypassing the nonfunctional lungs. The ductus arteriosus, like the foramen ovale, normally closes off shortly after birth. If the structure does not close or remains "patent" the condition is called patent ductus arteriosus. With this condition, oxygenated blood shunts abnormally from the higher pressured aorta back to the pulmonary artery. Once in the pulmonary artery the blood is recirculated to the lungs. This condition causes an increased workload on the heart and pulmonary system. This condition occurs twice as frequently in girls as in boys.

Coarctation of the Aorta

Coarctation is a **stricture** or narrowing. A coarctation of the aorta is a narrowing of the descending or thoracic aorta (Figure 8–20D). This condition causes a high blood pressure proximal to the stricture and lower blood pressure distal to the stricture. Infants or children affected with coarctation of the aorta may have a high blood pressure in the arms but a lower blood pressure in the legs. Coarctation increases the workload on the heart as the heart attempts to pump blood through the narrowed vessels.

Tetralogy of Fallot

Tetralogy of Fallot is a combination of four (tetra) defects (Figure 8–20E) and is one of the most serious of congenital heart defects. The four defects are:

1. Pulmonary valve stenosis—the opening into the pulmonary artery is too small, restricting the amount of blood flow to the lungs
2. Right ventricle hypertrophy—caused by the increased workload on the right ventricle as it

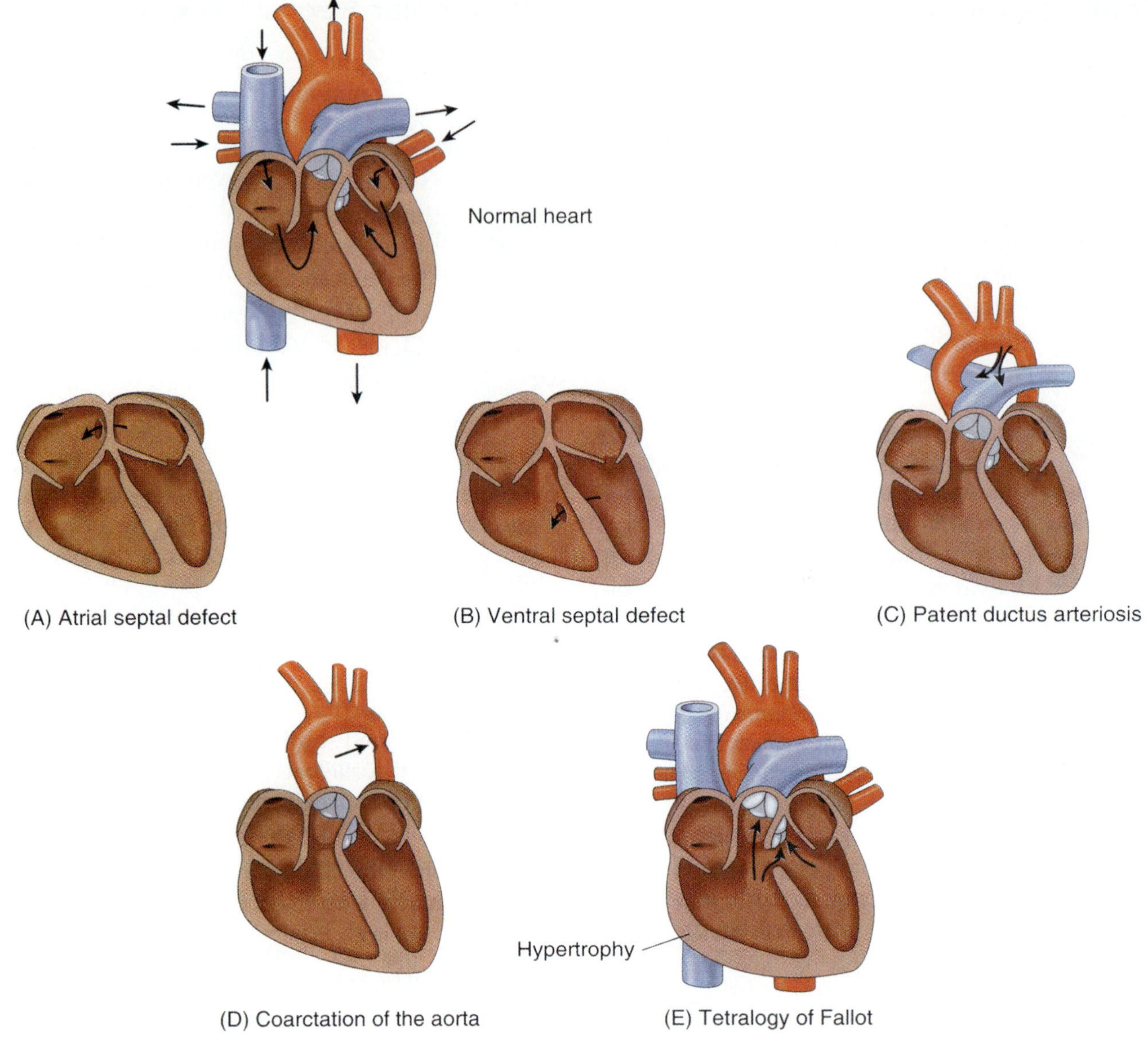

Figure 8-20 Congenital heart defects in tetralogy of Fallot.

attempts to pump blood through the stenotic valve

3. Ventricle septal defect—allowing oxygenated blood to flow from the left ventricle to the right
4. Abnormal placement of the aorta—the aorta opens over the ventricle septal defect allowing blood from both ventricles to be pumped into the aorta. The unoxygenated blood from the right ventricle enters the general circulation without passing through the lungs to become oxygenated. This unoxygenated blood from the right ventricle causes the tissues to become cyanotic or "blue."

Infants and children with tetralogy of Fallot are truly "blue babies." Cyanosis increases with age and clubbing of fingers and toes becomes evident. Older children will rest in a squatting position in order to breathe easier. This position also increases venous return. Other symptoms are growth retardation, severe dyspnea with exercise, and frequent respiratory infections. Surgical repair is the treatment of choice.

EFFECTS OF AGING ON THE SYSTEM

Heart and blood vessel diseases are a significant cause of death and disability in the older adult. As the individual ages, the heart muscle loses some of its contractility, causing a decreased cardiac output and/or an increased heart rate to compensate for the changes. The vessels lose elasticity, become more rigid and narrowed. The valves also lose some functioning, becoming thick and sclerotic. These changes add to the workload of the heart, increasing the heart rate and the blood pressure. The older adult may become tachycardic with minimal exercise. Although many of the changes in the system are caused by the normal aging process, other changes observed in the older adult result directly from lifestyle. Many individuals have smoked for years, been overweight, eaten a high-fat diet, endured a stressful job, and lived a fairly sedentary life. These modifiable behaviors contribute to the adverse changes in the cardiovascular system and increase the risk of chronic and acute problems in the system over time. Most older adults are at risk for hypertension, myocardial infarction, angina, arrhythmias, congestive heart failure, varicosities, and other cardiovascular problems.

With age, the arteries become more rigid, causing decreased blood flow to organs and distal body tissues. The vein valves lose some of their competency, reducing good blood flow even further. Decreased peripheral circulation often results in cool, pale extremities, improper healing, and pooling of fluid (edema) in the legs and feet. Medications may not be as efficiently transmitted to the body with these changes in circulation. This can affect the therapeutic regimen for the individual.

Many older adults have postural hypotension, which can be a significant safety problem. Postural hypotension is the decrease or drop in blood pressure that occurs when the individual raises to a sitting or standing position from a reclining position. The individual usually feels very dizzy upon rising and may fall. Prevention strategies should be in place to prevent injuries from postural hypotension.

SUMMARY

The cardiovascular system is responsible for pumping the blood throughout the body, delivering nutrients and oxygen to cells, and removing waste products. Cardiovascular disease affects over fifty-seven million Americans. It is a significant cause of mortality, especially in the older adult. The risk for developing many diseases of the system can be reduced by lifestyle behavioral changes. Common symptoms of cardiovascular disease include pain, fatigue, difficulty breathing, tachycardia, cyanosis, and edema. Some of the most common disorders of the system include hypertension, coronary artery disease, arteriosclerosis, and MI. Older adults are at greatest risk for developing heart disease. It is the number one cause of death in the elderly population.

REVIEW QUESTIONS

Multiple Choice

1. Which of the following risk factors are controllable or modifiable?
   a. heredity
   b. diet
   c. age
   d. stress
   e. smoking
   f. exercise
2. An aneurysm
   a. is a weakening and enlargement of the blood vessel that can lead to rupture.
   b. is often caused by atherosclerosis.
   c. can cause death from massive hemorrhage if it ruptures.
   d. all of the above.

3. Chest pain associated with angina:
   a. typically radiates down the right arm.
   b. is generally not relieved by rest.
   c. should be relieved by three NTG tablets; if not, it should be assumed the patient is having an MI.
   d. typically occurs at rest.

Short Answer

4. What are the functions of the cardiovascular system?

5. Which signs and symptoms are associated with common cardiovascular system disorders?

6. Describe the typical ECG findings associated with myocardial ischemia, injury, and infarction.

7. What symptoms are usually seen in congestive heart failure?

8. What is the most significant complication of a DVT?

9. What are the four parts to the Tetralogy of Fallot congenital defect?

10. What are some of the changes occurring in the cardiovascular system with age?

CASE STUDY

You are called to the home of Mr. Winston, a 72-year old gentleman who is complaining of chest pain radiating down his left arm which he has had for the past two hours. He states he is very nauseated, has been sweating profusely, and occasionally feels lightheaded. He has a history of hypertension, smoking, an MI ten years ago with bypass surgery, and an angioplasty three years ago. What is most likely wrong with Mr. Winston? If this were an MI, what would you expect to see on his 12-lead ECG? He states his pain feels similar to his MI ten years ago. His wife asks about fibrinolytic therapy because she saw a news report on it the other night on the national news. What can you tell her about its use in the pre-hospital environment?

BIBLIOGRAPHY

American Heart Association. (1999). *http://www.americanheart.org/hhf/index.html*
American Heart Association. (2000). *Handbook of Emergency Cardiovascular Care for Healthcare Providers.*
American Heart Association. (1997). *Advanced Cardiac Life Support.*
Aspirin lowers mortality in women with coronary artery disease. (1997). *Geriatrics, 52*(4), 100.
Barinaga, M. (May 30, 1997). How much pain for cardiac gain? *Science, 276,* 1324.
Basic heart disease prevention is best. (1997). *American Journal of Nursing, 97*(4), 10.

Beyond cholesterol. (1997). *Time, 150*, 48.

Centers for Disease Control and Prevention. (1997). *http://www. cdc.gov/nchswww/faq/deaths1.html*

Dajani, A. S. (June 11, 1997). Prevention of bacterial endocarditis: Recommendations by the American Heart Association. *Journal of the American Medical Association, 277*, 1794–1801.

Day, M. (June 7, 1997). Hunt for heart disease bug heats up. *New Scientist, 154*, 16.

Estrogen replacement to prevent heart disease: New insights developing. (1997). *Geriatrics, 52*(5), 83–84.

Fackelmann, K. (June 14, 1997). Can you catch heart disease? *Science News, 151*, 375.

Gore, J. M. (June 18, 1997). Cardiovascular disease. *Journal of the American Medical Association, 277*, 1845–1846.

Grady, D. (May 20, 1997). Study finds second-hand smoke doubles risk of heart disease. *New York Times*. p. A1.

Grundy, S. M. (May 1, 1997). Prevention of coronary heart disease through cholesterol reduction. *American Family Physician, 55*, 2250–2258.

Gutstein, D. (1997). Management of stable coronary artery disease. *American Family Physician, 56*(7), 99–106.

Hales, D. R. (1997). Women's health enemy number one. *Ladies' Home Journal, 114*(5), 110.

Heart Disease: How women can reduce their risk. (1997). *Consumer Reports, 62*(8), 56–57.

Killer Jobs. (1997). *New York Times*. p. C4.

Lewis, H. L. (1997). Penetrating the riddle of heart attack. *MITs Technology Review, 100*, 38–44.

Mandelbaum-Schmid, J. (1997). Stop heart disease before it starts. *McCall's, 124*(5), 76–78.

McGill, H. C. (1997). Childhood nutrition and adult cardiovascular disease. *Nutrition Reviews, 55*(1), S2–S11.

Mirich, T. M. (1997). Body fat and heart disease. *The Physician and Sports Medicine, 25*(6), 31–32.

Nestle, M. (1997). Alcohol guidelines for chronic disease prevention: From prohibition to moderation. *Nutrition Today, 32*(2), 86–92.

Older men with a 'short fuse' have a greater risk of coronary disease. (1997). *Geriatrics, 52*(4), 102–103.

Platt, D. (August 15, 1997). Malfunctioning hearts. *Commonwealth, 124*, 131.

Weighing hormone therapy's benefit. (1997). *Science News, 151*, 383.

When your heart sings the blues. (1997). *Psychology Today, 30*, 24.

CHAPTER

9

Neurological Diseases and Disorders

CONTENT OUTLINE

- Anatomy and Physiology
  - The Central Nervous System
  - The Peripheral Nervous System
- Common Signs and Symptoms
- Diagnostic Tests
- Common Diseases of the Nervous System
  - Infectious Diseases
  - Vascular Disorders
  - Functional Disorders
  - Dementia
  - Altered Mental Status
  - Tumors
- Trauma
  - Skull Fractures
  - Diffuse Axonal Injury
  - Focal Brain Injuries
  - Spinal Cord Injury
- Genetic and Developmental Disorders
  - Cerebral Palsy
  - Spina Bifida
- Effects of Aging on the System

KEY TERMS

Amnesia
Aura
Carotid endarterectomy
Cauterization
Cephalalgia
Chorea
Convulsion
Decompression
Dysphagia
Dysphasia
Epidural
Febrile seizure
Grand mal
Hemiparesis
Hydrophobia
Hypothermia
Intracranial pressure (ICP)
Jacksonian seizure
Nuchal rigidity
Paraplegia
Paresthesia
Partial seizure
Petit mal
Presyncope
Quadriplegia
Seizure
Status epilepticus
Subdural
Syncope

LEARNING OBJECTIVES

Upon completion of the chapter, the student should be able to:

1. Define the terminology common to the nervous system and the disorders of the system.
2. Identify common disorders of the nervous system.
3. Discuss the basic anatomy and physiology of the nervous system.
4. Identify the important signs and symptoms associated with common nervous system disorders.
5. Describe the common diagnostic tests used to determine type and/or cause of the nervous system disorder.
6. Describe the typical course and management of the common nervous system disorders.
7. Describe the effects of aging upon the nervous system and the common disorders of the system.

OVERVIEW

The nervous system is a complex system that provides communication from the brain to the rest of the body and from the body back to the brain. It is responsible for the individual's ability to reason, interact with other individuals, understand complex ideas, and to respond both intellectually and physically. Disorders of the system can affect any or all other normal functioning in the individual. Because brain and spinal cord injury often causes irreversible damage, the individual with a nervous system disorder may become a victim of severe permanent neurological deficits.

ANATOMY AND PHYSIOLOGY

The nervous system is composed of the brain, spinal cord, and nerves (Figure 9–1). It is divided into the central nervous system (CNS) and the peripheral nervous system (PNS). The CNS includes the brain and the spinal cord. The PNS includes the autonomic nervous system (ANS), the cranial nerves, and the spinal nerves. The central nervous system communicates with organs and other body systems via the peripheral nervous system.

The Central Nervous System (CNS)

The brain is a complex structure located within the protective covering of the skull. It is divided into the cerebrum, cerebellum, and brain stem. The cerebrum is divided into two hemispheres that can be further subdivided into lobes. Each of these lobes has a specialized function (Figure 9–2). The basal ganglia are a specific portion of the cerebrum that are involved in controlling motor function. Another part of the cerebrum is called the diencephalon. It is where the hypothalamus and thalamus are located. They are active in controlling the body's sleep/wake pattern and are involved in the actions of the pituitary gland. (See Chapter 11 for more information.) The thalamus is also involved in integrating sensory and motor information.

The cerebellum is located in the lower back part of the brain. It is important in coordination and fine motor movements.

The brain stem makes up the last part of the brain. It is subdivided into the midbrain, pons, and medulla. It contains nerve tracts and nuclei that are responsible for transmitting impulses that control respirations, swallowing, wakefulness, and other activities.

The spinal cord is a continuous structure running through the vertebral column from the medulla to the tailbone. The spinal cord is composed of both nerve cells and nerve axons. It has ascending and descending path-

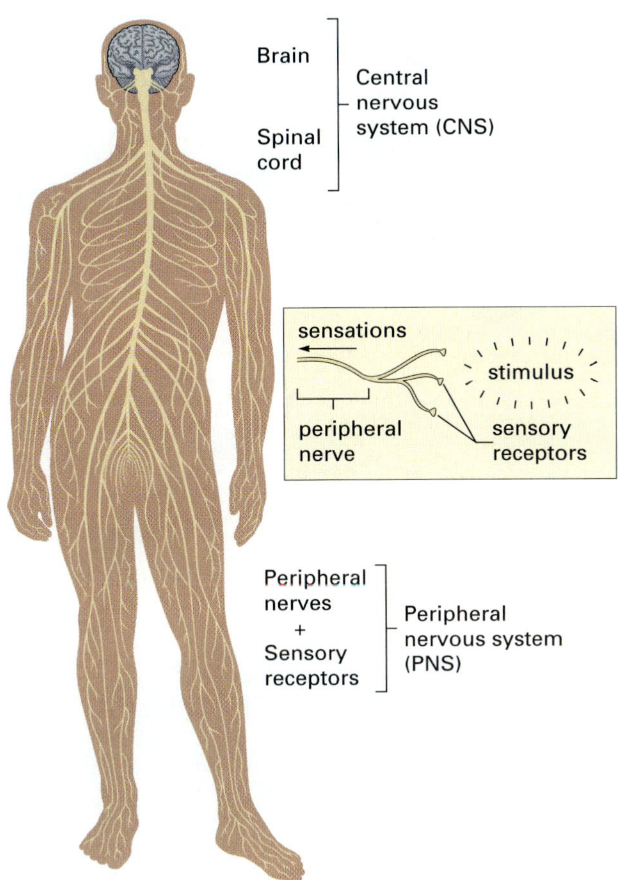

Figure 9–1 The nervous system.

ways that transmit impulses. Sensory impulses (pain, temperature, and touch) travel from the spinal cord to the brain. Motor impulses (for movement of muscles) travel from the brain to the spinal cord.

The meninges are membranes that cover the brain and spinal cord. The meninges are divided into three layers: the dura mater (outer cover), the arachnoid (middle layer), and the pia mater (inner layer). They provide protection, support, and nutrition for the system.

The spinal cord is organized into two functional areas (Figure 9–3). The butterfly shaped center section contains the nerve cell bodies that live within the spinal cord. The outer section contains the nerve tracts that relay information from the brain to the body (descending tracts) and the body to the brain (ascending tracts). These tracts are organized into areas that transmit specific types of information, both motor information in the descending tracts and sensory information in the ascending tracts.

The ascending nerve tracts (sensory information) are:

- Fasiculus gracilis and cuneatus carrying fine touch, vibration, and position information to the brain from the lower and upper extremity respectively. These fibers do not cross over at the spinal cord level.
- Spinothalamic tracts carrying pain, temperature, and crude touch information to the brain. These nerve fibers cross over at or near the level at which the sensory nerve enters the cord; for example the sensory nerves entering the cord at the T6 level cross over somewhere between T4 and T6 to the opposite side before heading to the brain.
- Spinocerebellar tracts that assist the cerebellum in coordinating body movements. These tracts provide feedback information to the cerebellum about motor information sent to the body from the motor cortex of the brain.

The descending nerve tracts (motor information) are:

- Lateral corticospinal tract which controls fine movements in the extremities. This nerve tract crosses over in midbrain.
- Reticulospinal tract, vestibulospinal tract, and ventral corticospinal tracts all work together to coordinate movements between the axial skeleton and

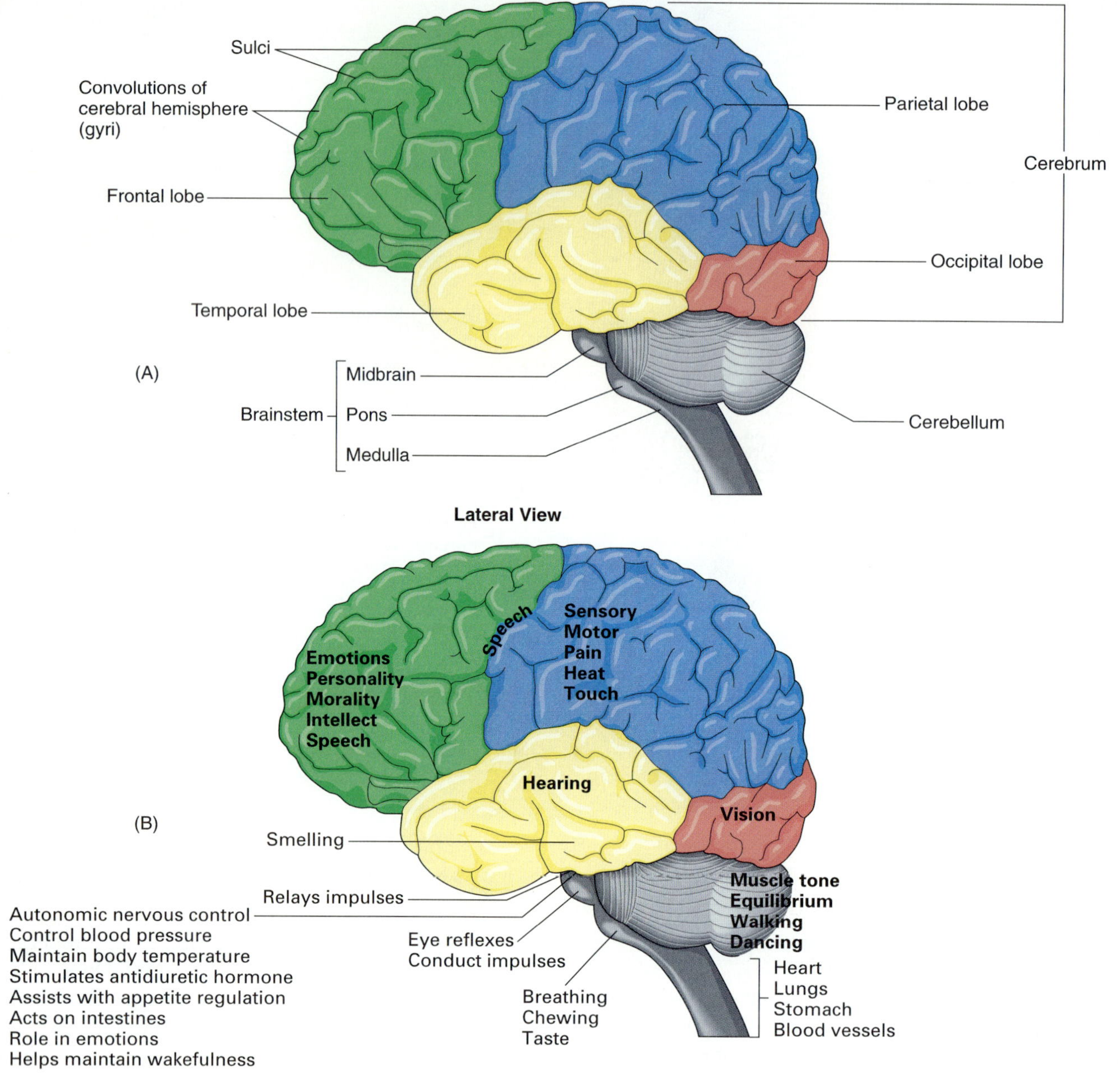

Figure 9–2 The cerebral lobes and their specialized functions.

the limbs. These tracts are responsible for controlling posture and gross movement.

- Rubrospinal tract controls the spinal neurons that relay movement information to the extremities so that movement begins and ends where the brain instructs the movement to begin and end.

The organization of the spinal cord can make it challenging to correctly diagnose incomplete spinal cord injuries. Common injury patterns are discussed later in this chapter.

The Peripheral Nervous System (PNS)

The autonomic nervous system controls the functions of the body's organs and innervates smooth muscle and cardiac muscle. It is divided into the parasympathetic and sympathetic systems. The parasympathetic system controls the "feed or breed" response and is primarily responsible for the movement of food through the digestive system. The sympathetic system controls the changes in the body needed to respond to stressors such as increasing

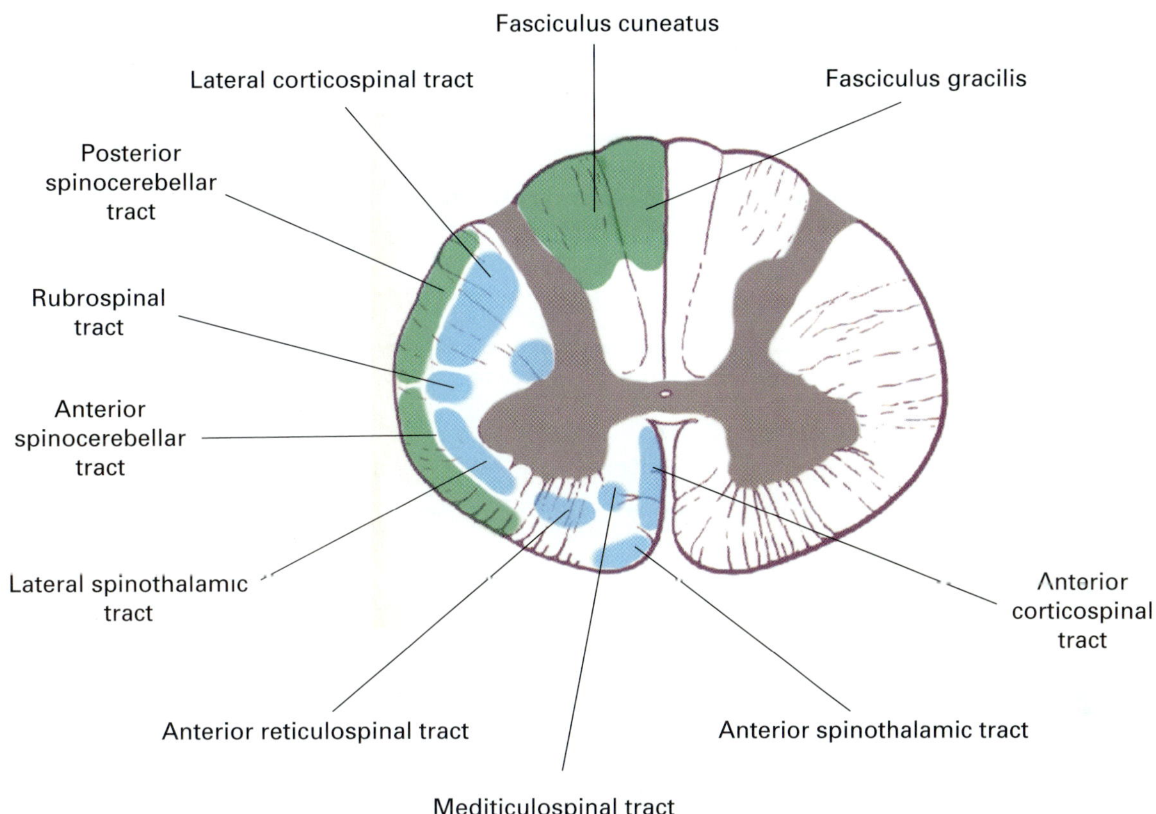

Figure 9–3 Major ascending and descending nerve tracts of the spinal cord.

the heart rate or blood pressure. This is often called the "fight or flight" response. The parasympathetic and sympathetic systems are in a constant balance that provides overall regulation of many of the body's systems. An example of this is the parasympathetic system returning the pulse rate and blood pressure to normal after heavy sympathetic activity, such as occurs after a scare or fright.

The autonomic nervous system also carries information about potentially painful stimuli back to the spinal cord and brain. The autonomic nervous system predominantly carries this information from visceral structures and is sometimes involved in upregulating or maintaining a painful condition. This phenomenon is called sympathetically mediated pain and may be present in patients with chronic pain complaints.

There are twelve pairs of cranial nerves that control sensation and movement in the area of the head and neck (Table 9–1). The thirty-one pairs of spinal nerves are divided into eight cervical, twelve thoracic, five lumbar, five sacral, and one coccygeal. Each spinal nerve innervates a designated area of the skin. These areas are called dermatomes (Figure 9–4). Each of the spinal nerves sends sensory impulses from the body surfaces and connective tissue to the spinal cord for transmission to the brain, and returns motor impulses from the brain to the spinal cord and then to the muscles.

COMMON SIGNS AND SYMPTOMS

Common signs and symptoms of nervous system disorders include headache, nausea, vomiting, weakness, mood swings, and fever. Symptoms specific to the nervous system include:

- Disturbance in motor function (or ability to move) including:
  1. stiffness in the neck, back, or extremities
  2. inability to move any part of the body
  3. seizures or convulsions
  4. paralysis
  5. myoclonus

TABLE 9-1 The Cranial Nerves

Cranial Nerve	Function
I Olfactory	Smell
II. Optic	Sight
III. Oculomotor	Movement of the eyeball, pupil, and eyelid and size of pupil
IV. Trochlear	Movement of eyeball
V. Trigeminal	Chewing; pain, temperature, and touch of face and mouth
VI. Abducens	Movement of eyeball
VII. Facial	Movement of face and secretion of tears and saliva; taste
VIII. Auditory	Hearing and balance
IX. Glossopharyngeal	Swallowing and secretion of saliva; taste and sensation in mouth and pharynx
X. Vagus	Sensation and movement in pharynx, larynx, thorax, and gastrointestinal system
XI. Accessory	Movement of head and shoulder
XII. Hypoglossal	Movement of tongue

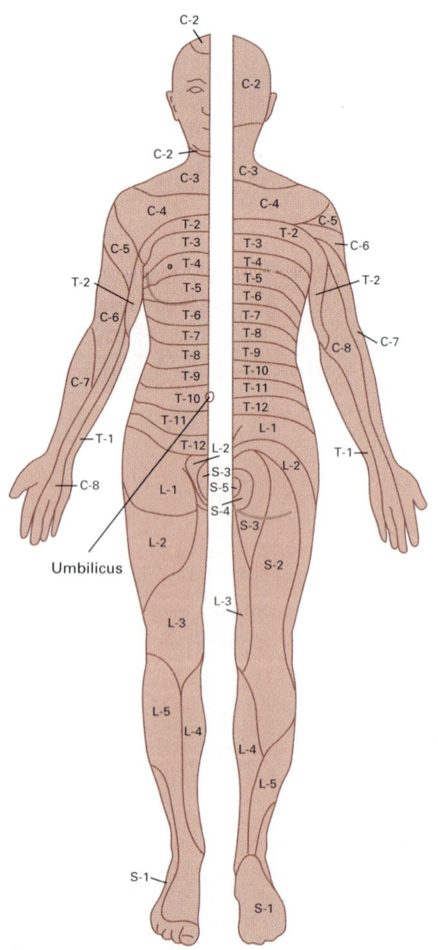

Figure 9-4 Spinal nerves and dermatomes.

- Disturbance in sensory function (or ability to sense or feel) including:
  1. visual difficulties
  2. inability to speak
  3. paralysis
- Alteration in mental alertness or cognitive function including:
  1. extreme or prolonged drowsiness
  2. stupor, unconsciousness/coma
  3. amnesia or extreme forgetfulness

DIAGNOSTIC TESTS

A neurologic examination includes testing motor, sensory, and mental functions. This examination is often performed on any individual presenting with an injury to the head, neck or spinal column, or exhibiting neurologic symptoms. Motor testing includes checking reflexes, gait, and posture. Sensory testing includes checking the ability to feel using pinprick or application of heat, cold, or vibration. Ability to see and smell may also be part of sensory testing. Testing of mental or cognitive function includes asking simple questions related to name, occupation, and location. Further testing may include simple math problems or questions about current events.

The cerebrospinal fluid (CSF) may be examined under a microscope to determine the presence of bacteria, leukocytes, red blood cells, neoplastic cells, and other microorganisms. In order to obtain this fluid, a lumbar puncture must be performed by inserting a spinal needle into the meningeal space around the spinal cord, and withdrawing CSF.

Radiologic examinations include X-rays of the skull and vertebral column for fractures and other abnormalities. A myelogram, or picture of the spinal cord, may be utilized for diagnosis of a herniated disk (HNP, herniated nucleus pulposus), tumor, or nerve root compression. Angiograms may help in determining vessel occlusion and hematomas in individuals exhibiting symptoms of cerebrovascular accident or stroke.

An electroencephalography (EEG) is a procedure to evaluate electrical brain activity. A damaged area of the brain may exhibit abnormal electrical activity as may occur with cerebrovascular accident (stroke) and epilepsy. EEG is also used to determine brain death.

Computerized tomography (CT or CAT scan) and magnetic resonance imaging (MRI) are both valuable tools to assess the anatomy of the brain and spinal cord and look for lesions caused by tumors, strokes, and abscesses.

COMMON DISEASES OF THE NERVOUS SYSTEM

The diseases of the nervous system can range from mild to severe depending on the particular condition. Age-related factors may influence the severity of the disease but many nervous system disorders can affect the individual at any age.

Infectious Diseases

Infections of the nervous system are more common in the young but can be found in older adults as well. Early diagnosis and treatment is essential to reduce the permanent neurologic deficits that may result from the infection.

Encephalitis. Encephalitis is an inflammation of the brain tissue. It is caused by a variety of microorganisms including bacteria and viruses, or as a complication of measles, chickenpox, or mumps. Viruses may be spread by mosquitoes and carried from animal to man or man to man. Symptoms include headache, elevated temperature, and a stiff neck and back, but may progress to lethargy, mental confusion, and even coma. Encephalitis is usually diagnosed by finding the causative agent in spinal fluid obtained by lumbar puncture. EMS treatment is supportive including maintaining a patent airway and supplementing ventilation as needed. Antiviral medication may be effective in some types of encephalitis. Prognosis is guarded, with some forms of encephalitis having a high mortality rate. Severe encephalitis may leave the individual with permanent neurologic impairment.

Meningitis. Meningitis is inflammation of the meninges, or covering of the brain and spinal cord. Meningitis may be caused by anything that causes an inflammatory response, including bacteria, virus, fungus, and toxins such as lead and arsenic. Some forms of meningitis are more contagious and more lethal than other forms of the disease. The most common cause of meningitis is bacterial invasion by *Neisseria meningitidis*. Bacteria and virus usually reach the meninges after invading and infecting other parts of the body such as the middle ear, sinuses, and upper respiratory tract, or they may be carried to the meninges in the blood as in septicemia.

Symptoms of meningitis often include a sudden onset of high fever, severe headache, photophobia, and a stiffness in the neck that resists bending the neck forward or sideways (**nuchal rigidity**). As the disease progresses, drowsiness, stupor, seizures, and coma may occur. Diagnosis is usually confirmed by finding the causative agent in the spinal fluid obtained by lumbar puncture. Antibiotic treatment of bacterial meningitis is usually effective in most cases. As with encephalitis, EMS treatment is focused toward protecting the airway and supporting ventilation and circulation.

Other treatments include antipyretics, anticonvulsive medications, and a quiet, dark environment. If untreated, meningitis can be fatal, especially in infants, children, and elderly individuals. Meningitis may cause permanent neurologic damage in children, leading to hearing loss, mental retardation, and epilepsy. Good hand washing practices can help in preventing the spread of the disease.

Central Nervous System Abscess. Abscesses within the central nervous system are often overlooked but can carry significant morbidity and mortality if left untreated or undertreated. Central nervous system abscesses occur in the brain and in the spinal cord, or in the dural layers surrounding these structures. Very rarely is an abscess caused by meningitis.

Abscess of the brain mainly occurs as an extension of severe upper respiratory disease or as metastatic seeding from another source. In only approximately ten percent of cases is the abscess caused by a direct infection, as in the case of a penetrating injury or skull fracture, and in almost twenty percent of cases the source is not identified. Severe infection of the sinuses, middle ear, or mastoid air cells can erode away at the bones and extend into the cranial vault to produce an abscess. Metastatic seeding of an infection from another source is responsible for approximately one-third of brain abscesses with endocarditis with vegetations on the heart valves (see Chapter 8, Cardiovascular System) and severe lung infections as the two most common sources.

The signs and symptoms of a brain abscess can vary depending upon its location. Headache is the most common presenting complaint and symptoms can be as severe as stupor or similar to a stroke. Fever is common early on, but the body temperature may return close to normal as the abscess becomes encapsulated. Signs and symptoms of an infection are commonly reported in the days to weeks preceding the neurological symptoms. Pre-hospital treatment will be similar to that for a suspected stroke: administering oxygen, providing airway support as required, initiating IV access, and treating other symptoms as appropriate.

Epidural spinal abscesses are also often missed, as the symptoms mimic other, more common conditions. Bacterial seeding can occur secondary to a penetrating injury to the tissues surrounding the spinal column, as an extension of osteomyelitis of the vertebrae, extension of an infection of the intervertebral disk, or via metastatic seeding from a wound or skin infection. One common cause of lumbar spine osteomyelitis and epidural spinal abscess is a piercing of the abdomen, which can easily become infected from clothing rubbing on the wound created by the piercing process.

Signs and symptoms of an epidural spinal abscess include fever and back pain that is typically localized and worsens with percussion over the infected segment. As the abscess grows, radicular pain may be present as the abscess begins to impinge spinal nerves as they exit the canal. The patient may also present with a headache and signs of meningeal irritation. As the condition worsens, the patient may undergo a rapidly progressing paresthesia and then paralysis as the abscess grows rapidly. This is a true surgical emergency and the patient requires immediate surgery to salvage the spinal cord. Abscess of the spinal cord itself is very rare and presents with the same symptoms as an epidural spinal abscess.

Pre-hospital treatment is often dictated by the specific patient presentation. If neurological deficit is present and trauma is a question, then the patient should be appropriately immobilized prior to transport. The EMS provider should be ready to treat for spinal shock, which can occur in patients who have a rapidly expanding abscess that disrupts sympathetic nervous system control from the cord. Supplemental oxygen may be beneficial in reducing cord ischemia. Other treatments should be directed at supporting the patient's airway, breathing, and circulation.

Poliomyelitis. Poliomyelitis is a viral infection affecting the brain and spinal cord. Polio was a major crippling and life-threatening disease affecting children prior to the development of a vaccine in the 1960s. Immunization programs since that time have virtually eliminated the disease in the United States. The poliomyelitis virus enters the body through the mouth and nose. It crosses the gastrointestinal tract into the blood then travels to the brain and spinal cord. The virus is spread by oropharyngeal secretions and by infected feces.

Symptoms of polio include muscle weakness, neck stiffness, and nausea and vomiting. As the disease progresses muscles atrophy and deteriorate. Muscles of the arms, legs, and respiratory system may become paralyzed. Diagnosis is made by clinical examination and confirmed by culturing the virus from the throat, feces, or spinal fluid. Treatment is supportive and includes analgesics and bed rest during the acute phase. Long-term physical therapy and use of braces may be needed. If the respiratory system is involved, mechanical ventilation may be necessary.

Tetanus. Tetanus is a highly fatal infection of nerve tissue caused by the bacteria *Clostridium tetani*. The effect of the toxin produced by this bacterium on the central nervous system leads to voluntary or skeletal muscle contraction. The first symptom is typically a stiffness of the jaw, commonly called "lockjaw," and is caused by strong jaw muscle contractions. One can see that this disease affects both the musculoskeletal system and the nervous system. More detailed information about tetanus is found in Chapter 10, Musculoskeletal System Diseases.

Rabies. Rabies is an often fatal encephalomyelitis caused by a virus. It primarily affects animals such as dogs, cats, foxes, raccoons, squirrels, and skunks, but can be transmitted to humans through a bite by an infected animal. Like tetanus, this virus travels slowly to the spinal cord and brain, so again the location of the bite is significant. Incubation time is from one to three months. Shorter incubation times are related to the position of the bite, making bites to the face and neck more serious than those to the extremities.

Symptoms of rabies include fever, pain, paralysis, convulsions, and rage. In animals, a change in temperament is often noticed. Wild animals may become friendly while family pets may become aggressive. Another classic symptom is spasm and paralysis of the muscles of swallowing. The sight of water or attempting to drink water causes throat spasms leading to **hydrophobia** (hydro = water, phobia = fear). Inability to swallow also causes a drooling of frothy saliva, an identifying symptom in animals.

Treatment of rabies includes immediate washing of the area with soap and water, followed by medical attention. A series of antirabies injections needs to be given before the virus has time to reach the brain. Any animal bite needs to be immediately investigated. The biting animal should be confined and placed under observation for symptoms of rabies and viral cultures should be obtained. If the animal cannot be captured and must be killed, care should be taken to not destroy the head since the brain must be examined for presence of disease. If the animal cannot be found, the injured individual will need to take the series of injections immediately.

There is no cure for rabies. Treatment is palliative and includes strong muscle relaxants to reduce convulsions. Untreated cases end with severe convulsions and respiratory arrest. Death usually occurs within two to five days after onset of symptoms. Prevention of rabies begins with vaccination of family pets and education of children in recognizing and avoiding animals with rabid symptoms.

Vascular Disorders

Vascular disorders of the nervous system can be quite severe, causing long-term debility. Some vascular disorders can be prevented or reduced in severity by lifestyle changes.

Cerebrovascular Accident (CVA or Stroke). Cerebrovascular accident, commonly called a stroke, is caused by poor blood supply to the brain. Strokes usually occur in people over fifty years of age and are a major cause of death in this age group. A common causative factor is arteriosclerosis. A CVA is to the brain what a heart attack is to the heart. Lack of blood flow to the brain causes brain tissue death. The three common causes of poor blood supply or lack of blood flow are:

- Cerebral thrombus is a clot in a brain artery and is the most common cause of vessel occlusion. Thrombus formation usually occurs in an area where the vessel is narrowed by arteriosclerosis. Symptoms usually appear gradually until blood flow is inadequate.
- Cerebral embolism is usually caused by a small piece of a thrombus or arterial plaque breaking loose and traveling in the artery until it wedges and occludes the vessel. Symptoms usually appear quite suddenly.
- Cerebral hemorrhage is the rupture of an artery filling the surrounding brain tissue with blood. Cerebral hemorrhage is usually caused by hypertension and arteriosclerosis (see Arteriosclerosis in Chapter 8). Hypertension and arteriosclerosis cause the vessel to weaken, tear, and hemorrhage. Another cause of cerebral hemorrhage is a weakened artery caused by a congenital aneurysm. Symptoms are very sudden with hemorrhage.

When an area of the brain loses blood supply, the individual suddenly loses consciousness and may die or have permanent neurologic disability. About one-third of individuals with a CVA will die. An equal number will live with and without disability (Figure 9–5). The symptoms of CVA are numerous depending on the area of the brain affected and the severity of the occlusion or hemorrhage. Common symptoms include **dysphasia** (dis-FAY-zee-ah; dys = difficulty, phasia = speaking), **dysphagia** (dis-FAY-jee-ah; dys = difficulty, phagia = swallowing), **hemiparesis** (HEM-ee-**PAR**-ee-sis; hemi = one half, paresis = paralysis), confusion, poor coordination, headache, and numbness.

Emergency department diagnosis of CVA is made and confirmed by physical examination and CT scan. One indicator of the location of brain damage is shown by the pattern of hemiparesis, if present. Hemiparesis affecting the left side is indicative of right-sided brain injury while

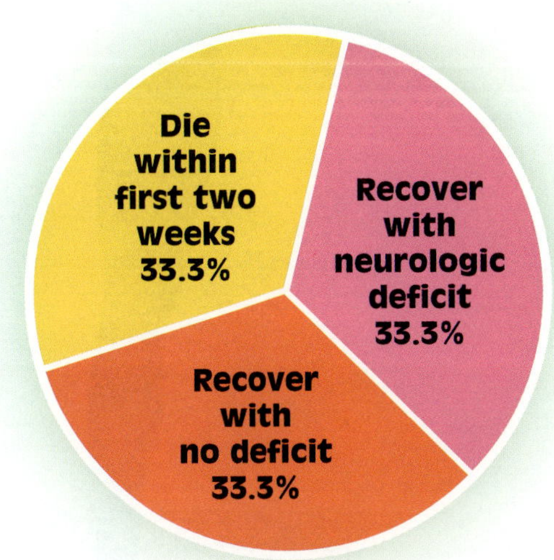

Figure 9–5 CVA—prognosis for individuals affected by CVA/stroke.

hemiparesis affecting the right side is indicative of left-sided brain injury. Symptoms of right and left side brain damage vary to some degree (Figure 9–6).

Treatment of CVA depends on the severity of the stroke and the symptoms. Field EMS assessment and treatment involves determining the exact time frame of symptom onset, as this will affect treatment options in the emergency department, and supporting the ABCs. Vascular access in the field may or may not be advised by the EMS provider's local protocols and should not involve administering a large amount of fluid unless the patient is hypotensive. Emergency department treatment includes anticoagulant and hypertensive medications given to control the formation of clots and to lower blood pressure. If the stroke is determined to be ischemic in nature, and the patient falls into time frame and disability criteria, then thrombolytic therapy may be initiated in the emergency department or intensive care unit. Thrombolytic therapy must be initiated within three hours to be effective, so prompt recognition and treatment is necessary.

Prevention of stroke is directed toward avoiding risk factors, which include:

1. Smoking
2. High fat diet
3. Obesity
4. Lack of exercise

These factors also play a role in arteriosclerosis, a main cause of CVA. Surgical intervention includes removal of

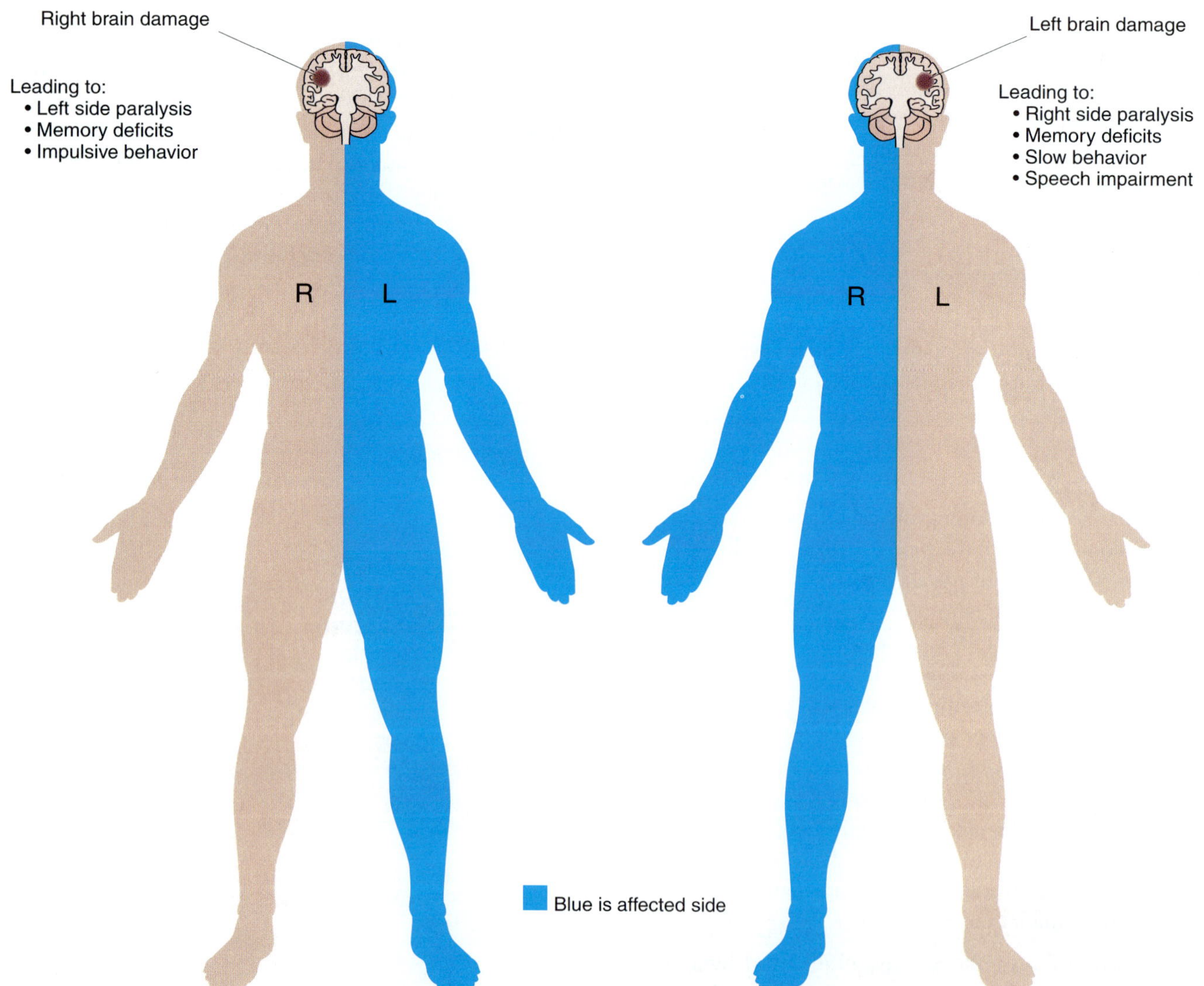

Figure 9–6 Symptoms of right and left CVA vary to some degree.

plaque in the carotid arteries to improve blood flow and reduce the risk of a thrombus. This surgical procedure is called a **carotid endarterectomy**. The heart is another source of clots and most patients who have atrial fibrillation are placed on anticoagulant therapy to decrease the risk of embolic stroke.

Transient Ischemic Attack (TIA). Transient ischemic attacks are sudden mild "mini strokes." They are caused by insufficient blood supply to the brain. They may serve as a warning of an impending stroke and are often caused by artery narrowing by arteriosclerotic plaque. Symptoms, like CVA, depend on the area of the brain that is affected. Some common symptoms are weakness of an arm and/or leg, dizziness, slurred speech, and a mild loss of consciousness. Total loss of consciousness usually does not occur. Symptoms usually subside within a few minutes to an hour. Diagnosis and treatment are similar to CVA. The more TIAs a patient has, the higher the risk for a major stroke. Preventive health measures and therapies may be helpful in certain patients to decrease their chance of a major stroke.

Functional Disorders

Functional disorders of the nervous system occur from alterations in the function of the nervous system. These conditions, although varying in severity, are some of the most common problems of the system. The cause of the disorder may be found, but in many cases it is unknown.

Headache. Headache, **cephalalgia** (SEF-ah-**LAL**-jee-ah; cephal = head, algia = pain) is one of the most common disorders of humans. It is usually a symptom of another disease rather than a disorder in and of itself. Disorders that typically include headache as a symptom may include sinusitis, meningitis, encephalitis, hypertension, anemia, constipation, premenstrual tension, and tumors, to name only a few. Most headaches are not related to disease but are caused by two mechanisms:

1. tension on the facial, neck, and scalp muscles
2. vascular changes in arterial size (dilation or constriction) of the vessels inside the head

Many factors produce headaches, including stress, noise, toxic fumes, lack of sleep, and alcohol consumption. Headaches may be acute or chronic, and may affect different areas of the head. The pain may range from mild to unbearable and incapacitating. Pain may be constant or intermittent and may be described as pressure, throbbing, or stabbing. Interestingly, brain tissue does not contain sensory nerves so the sense of pain must come from the pain receptors in the meninges, facial tissue, or scalp. Some of the more common types of headaches include:

- Tension—caused by stress, strain, and tension on the facial, neck, and scalp muscles. Pain is typically in the occipital area.
- Cluster—may be caused by stress, emotional trauma, or unknown reasons. These headaches occur at night after falling asleep. The pain is generally a severe, throbbing pain behind the nose and one eye. The skin in this area becomes reddened and the nose and eye water. The pain generally subsides after one or two hours but may recur several times during the night.
- Post lumbar puncture—a severe headache affecting up to forty percent of individuals following a lumbar puncture. It is thought to be caused by leakage of spinal fluid through the needle puncture site. This type of headache is often prevented by positioning the individual flat in bed without a pillow for two or three hours following this procedure.
- Migraine—a severe, incapacitating headache commonly accompanied by nausea, vomiting, and visual disturbances. Individuals affected by migraines may experience a visual **aura** or a sensation that precedes the event including flashing light, dim vision, or photophobia. Migraines can be severe enough to simulate some of the symptoms of a CVA, including unilateral blindness, weakness, and even hemiparesis. These symptoms typically resolve as the headache improves. This type of headache may begin in adolescence and diminish in intensity and frequency with age. Migraine headaches occur twice as often in women than men. The cause is still unknown although they tend to run in families suggesting some type of inheritance pattern. Some foods that trigger migraines are chocolate, wine, and cheese. It is also thought that these are vascular headaches caused by altered arterial blood flow and spasm of the arterioles in the brain.

Diagnosis of the cause of headache is dependent on individual history and physical examination. Testing in the emergency department may include X-ray, EEG, MRI, and CT scans to rule out hemorrhage or tumor. Treatment is dependent on cause. Treatment with analgesics and bed rest in a quiet, dark room is usually effective for most tension-type headaches. Muscle relaxants, muscle massage, warm baths, and biofeedback may also be effective. Vascular headaches may be relieved by the use of vasoconstrictor medication. A thorough neurological assessment should be performed to detect any deficit present that might indicate a more serious cause for the patient's headache.

Seizures. A **seizure** is abnormal electrical discharge within the brain that causes abnormal symptoms, for example a **convulsion** (abnormal muscle contraction), change in personailty, altered sensation, changes in autonomic nervous system control, or loss of consciousness. Seizures can result from several disease processes, including hypoxia, hypoglycemia, thyrotoxicosis, electrolyte imbalance, specifically hypocalcemia, toxic ingestion (including alcohol), sepsis or infection, tumor, head trauma, eclampsia, or epilepsy. **Febrile seizures** are common in the young pediatric population and are caused by a sudden rise or fall in body temperature. Febrile seizures typically resolve quickly and are benign, however they are very frightening for the parents.

Epilepsy is a chronic disease of the brain. It is characterized by intermittent episodes of abnormal electrical activity in the brain. This activity may be compared to an arrhythmia of the heart. The most noted symptom of epilepsy is a convulsive seizure. The cause of epilepsy may be brain tumors, neurologic disease, or scar tissue in the brain from trauma or stroke. More commonly, the cause cannot be determined during the individual's life or even upon autopsy.

The most common types of seizures are:

- **Grand mal** seizures are the type most often associated with epilepsy. These seizures are characterized by convulsions, loss of consciousness, urinary and fecal incontinence, and tongue biting. Epileptic individuals often have an aura with grand mal seizures allowing the individual time to lie down or call for support. Auras may include tingling of the fingers, ringing in the ears, and visual disturbances. Grand mal seizures often begin with a crying out as the contraction of the respiratory muscles forces exhalation. This is followed by generalized rhythmic contractions of the skeletal muscles of the body, arms, and legs. This stage is called the ictal stage and may last one to two minutes. Consciousness will return more slowly. The patient is often weak, drowsy, confused, and has no memory of the seizure event. This stage is called the postictal stage of the seizure.
- **Petit mal** seizures are also called absence seizures. These commonly occur in children and are often outgrown during puberty, but they may last a lifetime. These seizures consist of a brief change in the level of consciousness without convulsions. The involved individual may show symptoms of blank staring, blinking, and/or twitching of the eyes or mouth. The individual may remain seated or standing with loss of awareness of surroundings. Often the individual seated only appears to have a loss of attention or absentmindedness. Episodes often last only a few seconds but may occur multiple times during the day.
- **Partial seizures** are similar to grand mal seizures except the abnormal discharge is localized to a small portion of the brain. Partial seizures can be either simple or complex. Simple partial seizures involve localized abnormal motor, sensory, or psychiatric symptoms without an altered level of consciousness. The difference between simple and complex partial seizures is that the level of consciousness is altered with a complex partial seizure. A **Jacksonian seizure** is a partial seizure involving abnormal movement that starts in a very localized area, say one hand, and then spreads to other parts of the body as the abnormal electrical discharge spreads to and involves adjacent areas of the brain.

A life-threatening event is a state of continued convulsive seizure with no recovery of consciousness, called **status epilepticus**. This is a medical emergency as treatment is needed to prevent cerebral anoxia and possible death.

Field treatment of seizures includes loosening restrictive clothing, managing the airway, and assisting ventilation. Vascular access may be attempted if it is safe to do so. Diazepam will often be administered to a patient in a status seizure in an attempt to gain control of the seizure. Evaluation of the patient in the emergency department will often include a head CT for patients that do not have a prior seizure history to rule out hemorrhage or tumor. For patients who are on long-term anticonvulsants, blood medication levels will be checked to ensure they are in a proper range. Blood tests may be performed to indicate disorders of hypoglycemia and drug or alcohol toxicity.

Anti-convulsive medications, including Dilantin and Tegretol, are used in long-term treatment of epilepsy. Close monitoring and adjusting of medications are needed to get the best effect. Medications are effective in preventing or reducing seizures eighty percent of the time. Education and emotional support of the affected individual and family members are needed, as this disease is often feared because of lack of education.

Syncope. **Syncope** is a transient loss of consciousness that the lay public calls "passing out" or "blacking out." The patient will typically collapse to a supine position after which the patient will undergo a rapid return to full consciousness. **Presyncope** is basically the same condition, except that consciousness is never completely lost. Both conditions can signal an ominous underlying condition and are evaluated in a similar manner.

There are many conditions that can cause syncope. In approximately fifty percent of cases, the history and physical exam will be normal and the cause attributed to autonomic nervous system dysregulation. This is most apparent when the syncopal episode occurs after a rapid change in position from a seated or supine position to standing in a patient whose autonomic nervous system is unable to compensate quickly for the normal drop in blood pressure. The four most deadly underlying conditions that can present with syncope are dysrhythmias, MI, cardiac valve rupture, and pulmonary embolus. Other causes of syncope include seizure, CVA, hypoglycemia, and medications.

Evaluation of the patient includes a targeted cardiovascular, pulmonary, and neurological history and physical exam. The classic triad associated with a pulmonary embolus is hemoptysis (blood tinged sputum), syncope, and tachypnea. New murmurs can be indicative of valve disease. Palpitations may indicate an arrhythmia. The patient should receive supplemental oxygen, intravenous access, ECG monitor, and blood glucose reading by finger stick. Treatment is directed at the underlying cause, with almost half of the patients who experience a syncopal episode having an undefined cause. The EMS provider should have a high index of suspicion for the four deadly causes of syncope and evaluate the patient in light of those conditions.

Bell's Palsy. Bell's palsy is a disease affecting the facial nerve (seventh cranial nerve) causing unilateral (one-sided) paralysis of the face. It commonly occurs in individuals twenty to sixty years of age. This disease is idiopathic, but possible causes include autoimmune problems and viral disease. Symptoms include a drooping weakness of the eye and mouth, with inability to close the affected eye and drooling of saliva. The affected individual is unable to whistle or smile and has a distorted facial appearance (Figure 9–7). Diagnosis is made on the basis of clinical history and symptoms. Treatment includes analgesics and anti-inflammatory medications. If the individual is unable to close the affected eye, protection of the eye with a patch and artificial tear medication may be needed. Warm, moist heat, electrical nerve stimulation, and massage may be prescribed to prevent facial muscle atrophy. Prognosis for Bell's palsy is good with most cases resolving spontaneously in two to eight weeks. Plastic surgery may be prescribed to correct the facial deformities caused by chronic disease.

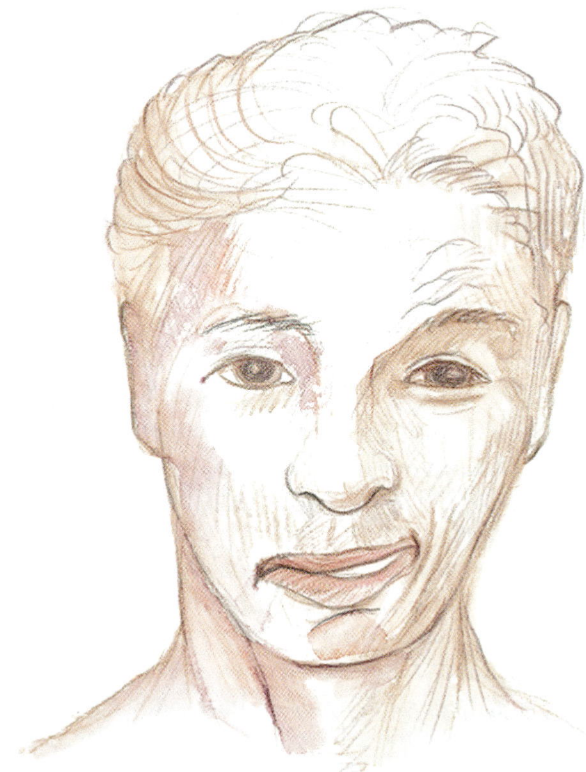

Figure 9–7 Facial appearance of Bell's Palsy.

Dystonia. Dystonia is a functional neurological disorder where muscles are involuntarily held in an abnormal state of contraction that leads to an abnormal position or posture. This posture is persistent and may worsen with movement of the affected muscles. Muscles of the extremities, neck, and the face are commonly affected. There are several rare genetic disorders that can cause congenital dystonia, however it is more commonly seen as a side effect of certain neurological diseases or medication use. Dystonia is commonly seen in Parkinson's disease, Huntington's chorea, hypoxia, and other less common neurological diseases. Certain medications, especially phenothiazines, butyrophenones, or metoclopramide, can produce dystonia as an acute side effect. Dystonia resulting from a medication side effect commonly responds to treatment with intravenous diphenhydramine.

Amyotrophic Lateral Sclerosis (ALS). Amyotrophic lateral sclerosis, also known as Lou Gehrig's disease, is a destructive disease of the motor or movement neurons. The cause of ALS is unknown, although genetic and viral-immune factors have been suggested. ALS is characterized by atrophy of the muscles leading to a progressive loss of movement of the hands, arms, and legs. As the disease progresses, loss of muscle function in the face and chest area leads to difficulty in talking, chewing, swallowing, and breathing. Eventually, the loss of motor function causes quadriplegia. One distinguishing factor of ALS is there is not a loss of sensory neurons, thus the individual can feel the extremities, but movement is impaired. Mental function is unaffected, thus the affected individual is aware of the condition and may take an active role in planning care. ALS usually affects men twice as often as women, with onset of the disease after age fifty. Management of respiratory complications is vital as most individuals affected with ALS die of respiratory failure. Acute respiratory failure is generally caused by a respiratory illness, such as pneumonia; however, a patient who is gradually progressing toward respiratory failure caused by weakness may present with altered mental status secondary to hypoxia. Emergency treatment is generally aimed at improving respiratory function and may include supplemental oxygen, bronchodilators, steroids, and intubation and mechanical ventilation as appropriate. ALS is eventually fatal.

Guillain-Barré Syndrome. Guillain-Barré Syndrome is an acute, progressive disease affecting the spinal nerves. The cause of this disease is unknown, but an autoimmune disorder has been suggested as the symptoms usually begin ten to twenty-one days after a febrile illness, such as a respiratory infection or gastroenteritis. Early symptoms include nausea, fever, and malaise. Within twenty-four to seventy-two hours, **paresthesia** (PAR-es-**THEE**-see-ah; abnormal sensation, burning, tingling, or numbness), muscle weakness, and paralysis usually begin. These symptoms generally begin in the legs and move upward, but may also start in the face and arms and move downward. A classic sign of Guillain-Barré is the absence of reflexes in the affected extremities. Guillain-Barré Syndrome becomes life-threatening if respiratory muscles are involved. Symptoms may progress for several days to weeks. Once progression ceases, recovery begins and may require three to twelve months. Treatment is supportive and the patient may require supplemental oxygen and ventilatory assistance. Recovery is usually complete.

Huntington's Chorea. Huntington's chorea is an inherited disease. It is a dominant gene disorder affecting fifty percent of all children in families where one parent has Huntington's. This disorder does not appear until middle age, so children are often grown before the parent shows symptoms. Huntington's is a progressive degeneration of the brain characterized by loss of muscle control and **chorea**, a constant, jerky uncontrollable movement. The disease also leads to mental deterioration with symptoms of personality change, moody behavior, and loss of memory. Over a period of years, dementia (dee-MEN-she-ah; total mental incapacitation) occurs. There is no cure for Huntington's chorea. Treatment is supportive and protective with institutionalization often necessary to provide the needed care. Genetic counseling is needed in families with this inheritance pattern.

Multiple Sclerosis (MS). Multiple sclerosis is a disease that causes demyelination of the nerves of the central nervous system. Myelin, as one will recall, acts as an "insulator" around nerves much like the insulation around an electric cord. Demyelination allows information to "leak" from the nerve pathway leading to poor or absent nerve transmission. The cause of MS is not clear. It is thought that a genetic predisposition plays some part, since it is fifteen times more likely to occur in first degree relatives of affected persons. It is also believed that the immune system and viral infection play a part.

Symptoms caused by demyelinating lesions are muscle weakness, lack of coordination, paresthesia, speech difficulty, loss of bladder function, and visual disturbance, especially diplopia (double vision). Symptoms are varied depending on the location of the lesions, making diagnosis difficult.

The complaints a patient with MS may present to EMS can vary and include abdominal pain secondary to constipation or urinary retention, flank pain from pyelonephritis (kidney infection, see Chapter 14), dyspnea secondary to a respiratory infection, or high fever. Treatment is directed at the cause of the chief complaint as there is no specific EMS treatment for MS.

MS usually affects young adults between the ages of twenty to forty years. It is characterized by periods of remission and exacerbation usually over a period of several years. Physical therapy and muscle relaxants may be helpful to maintain muscle tone and reduce spastic movement. The severity of the disease varies from individual to individual, but generally speaking, most affected individuals live a normal life span.

Parkinson's Disease. Parkinson's disease is a slow, progressive brain degeneration usually developing in individuals in their late fifties and sixties. Parkinson's affects men more often than women. The cause is unknown, but individuals with Parkinson's have been found to have a deficiency of the neurotransmitter dopamine in the brain. Classic symptoms include:

- Rigidity and immobility of the hands and a very slow speech pattern
- A fine tremor in the hands described as a "pill rolling" motion of the fingers
- An expressionless facial appearance with a fixed stare and infrequent blinking called Parkinson's facies
- An abnormal "bent forward" posture that includes a bowed head and flexed arms (Figure 9–8)
- A peculiar gait of short, fast-running steps caused by the abnormal posture that makes the individual tend to stumble forward leading to frequent falls

Treatment of Parkinson's is symptomatic. Dopamine replacement medications may be utilized in the long-term treatment of Parkinson's. These medications do not stop the progression of the disease, but may help with symptoms. Physical therapy for muscle soreness and psychological support are also helpful. A patient with Parkinson's disease may present to EMS with medication toxicity. Medication toxicity in patients with Parkinson's disease can cause psychiatric disturbances, for example, hallucinations or psychosis, cardiac arrhythmias, and orthostatic hypotension. The patient may also present to EMS after falling, either from the changes in gait and balance that normally accompany the disease or from a syncopal episode secondary to orthostatic hypotension. EMS treatment should be directed at the presenting symptoms.

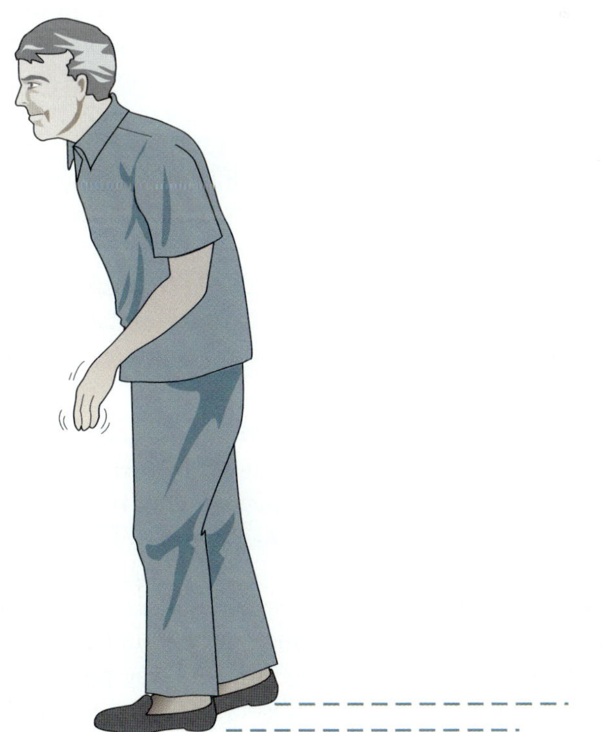

Figure 9–8 Parkinson's Disease.

Peripheral Neuropathy. A peripheral neuropathy is a general term for any condition that causes a problem with the function of a peripheral nerve. There may be sensory changes, motor changes, or changes in both sensation and motor function. A classic example of chronic change is the peripheral neuropathy that occurs in patients with a long history of diabetes. This specific type of peripheral neuropathy will present over time with a loss of sensation bilaterally in a stocking or glove distribution. The motor nerves are not affected. Other types of peripheral neuropathy can be caused by metabolic or immune problems, as discussed above in Guillain-Barré. Peripheral neuropathy can also be caused by direct trauma to a nerve or nerve plexus, as can happen with birth or other trauma. The EMS provider may be the first health care provider to discover a peripheral neuropathy, especially in a patient with diabetes.

Trigeminal Neuralgia. Trigeminal neuralgia is an extremely painful disorder that involves the sensory branches of the trigeminal nerve, which is the fifth cranial nerve. This condition is sometimes referred to as tic douloureax. The patient often complains that the pain has an electric quality. The pain is typically unilateral and confined to one of the specific areas covered by the nerve, covering the jaw, the cheek, or the forehead. The pain can be severe and can mimic an abscessed tooth, or sinus infection or headache.

Dementia

Dementia (dee-MEN-she-ah) is a loss of mental ability resulting from the loss of neurons or brain cells. Dementia may be caused in several ways. One of the most common dementias is senile dementia and is related to degeneration of cells with aging. The most common cause of senile dementia is Alzheimer's disease. For this reason, Alzheimer's and senile dementia are often used synonymously, but in reality an individual may have senile dementia without Alzheimer's. Vascular dementia may also be considered a form of senile dementia as it tends to occur in older individuals. Most patients will not present to EMS acutely with a complaint related to dementia, but patients with dementia may present with other complaints or for interfacility transfer.

Alzheimer's Disease. Alzheimer's (ALTZ-high-merz) disease is a form of dementia characterized by the death of neurons and replacement of these neurons by microscopic plaques. It is the most common cause of dementia in the elderly. The disease usually affects individuals seventy years old and older. The number of cases increases with age with an estimated fifty percent of individuals over age eighty-five being affected. The cause of Alzheimer's disease is unknown, but factors being considered are heredity, viral infection, autoimmunity, and aluminum toxicity. Research also shows a higher rate of Alzheimer's in individuals with a history of head trauma. Symptoms of the disease begin with mild mental impairment characterized by loss of short-term memory, inability to concentrate, and slight changes in personality. As the disease progresses, the affected individual struggles with communication skills, uses meaningless words, and cannot form sentences. Increased forgetfulness along with the difficulties in communication lead to irritability and agitation. In the final stages, which may take five to ten years to develop, the affected individual's mental and physical capabilities are severely affected. The affected individual becomes restless, disoriented, incontinent, hostile, and combative, and is totally dependent on a caregiver. Death is usually from a secondary cause such as infection.

Diagnosis cannot be positively made until after death with autopsy. Initially, a diagnosis may be made on the basis of symptoms after ruling out other brain diseases. In the final stage of the disease, CT or MRI may reveal the characteristic brain atrophy and microscopic plaques. Treatment is supportive, as there is no known cure for Alzheimer's disease. As the individual's capabilities decline, care is focused on safety and maintaining adequate nutrition, hydration, and personal hygiene. Mobility and mental capabilities are supported for as long as possible. Emotional support of family members and caregivers is of primary concern.

Vascular Dementia. Vascular dementia is caused by atrophy and death of brain cells resulting from decreased blood flow. Atherosclerotic plaque is the common cause of decreased blood flow and is common with aging. As the atherosclerotic plaques develop slowly, so do symptoms. Symptoms progress so slowly that they often go unnoticed by family members until they become quite severe. Symptoms include changes in memory, personality, and judgment. Irritability, depression, and sleeplessness may also occur. Personal hygiene is lacking and is often the sign that alerts family members to the condition. The affected individual may become disoriented and become lost in familiar surroundings. Diagnosis is made on the basis of a history and physical and blood flow testing. Treatment is aimed at increasing blood flow to the brain. If the cerebral arteries are involved or narrowed, medications may help improve blood flow. Carotid artery plaques can be surgically cleaned by a carotid endarterectomy (END-ar-ter-**ECK**-toh-me; endo = inside, arter = artery, ectomy = excision of). Prognosis depends on the effectiveness of treatment and the amount of brain cell death. If treatment is not possible or effective, or if a large amount of brain tissue has been lost, the affected individual will become progressively more demented and may need institutionalization for care.

Head Trauma Dementia. Head trauma dementia is caused by death of brain cells related to head trauma. A type of head trauma dementia is Boxer's dementia, and is caused by repeated blows to the head, as in the sport of boxing. Other types of trauma may be those sustained in accidents, especially motor vehicle accidents and sports-related activities. The death of brain cells may be caused by the injury itself or edema and increased intracranial pressure. This increase in pressure decreases or halts blood flow to brain cells, leading to cell death. Symptoms of head trauma dementia include a decrease in mental intellect and cognitive function. The affected individual may be unable to perform activities that were easily completed prior to the injury. Diagnosis is made on the basis of history, cranial X-rays, MRI, and CT. Treatment is aimed at correcting the damage if possible, preventing further damage, and maintaining the existing healthy tissue. Dead brain cells cannot be replaced so damage is permanent. Therapy and rehabilitation is needed to regain as much function as possible. Individuals suffering severe head trauma may need institutionalization for long-term care.

Substance Induced Dementia. Substance induced dementia is brain cell death caused by toxicity of drugs and toxins. This type of dementia may be caused by repeated exposure to, or use of, or abuse of certain substances. Commonly those substances include alcohol, cocaine, heroine, lead, mercury, and fumes of paints, paint thinners, nitrous oxide or "laughing gas," and insecticides to name only a few. Brain cell death often persists long after the exposure to the substance ends. Symptoms of mental impairment and decreased cognitive ability are permanent and often worsen over a period of time.

Altered Mental Status

Alteration of mental status is a common presenting complaint to EMS. Many disease processes can induce a change in mental status. Even something as benign as a change in medications can result in an alteration of mental status. A useful way to remember some of the common causes is AEIOU-TIPS (Table 9–2). One additional cause that the EMS provider should always keep in mind is hypoxia.

EMS management of the patient with altered mental status is focused on managing the airway and ventilatory and circulatory support. Specific treatment is based upon the underlying cause, for example, administering D50 to a hypoglycemic patient or fluids to a patient in shock.

Tumors

Brain tumors may be classified as primary or secondary. Primary tumors start in the brain tissue while secondary tumors occur in other areas and metastasize to the brain. The ratio of primary versus secondary tumor is about 50/50. Common sites of primary tumor that metastasize to the brain include breast and lung. Tumors may also be classified as benign and malignant (see Chapter 3). Benign tumors of the brain are often malignant if surgical removal is not possible. The growth of benign tumors in the confined space of the skull places pressure on the brain tissue and blood vessels leading to loss of function and death of normal tissue. Tumors may occur in any area of the brain.

Symptoms are varied depending on the area involved and include headache, vomiting, seizures, mood and personality changes, visual disturbances, and loss of memory. Diagnosis is made on the basis of clinical history, symptoms, X-ray examinations, CT, MRI, and biopsy. A biopsy is the most definitive study to determine the type of tumor and thus assist with treatment and prognosis. Further studies may be needed to determine the primary location of metastatic brain tumors. Treatment may include surgery, radiation, and chemotherapy. Treatment and prognosis are dependent on the type and location of the tumor. The most common reason a patient with a brain tumor will present to EMS is seizure. A new onset seizure disorder in an adult may be the first sign of a brain tumor. EMS treatment priorities include airway management, supplemental oxygen and ventilatory assistance, and the use of diazepam to stop the seizure.

TABLE 9-2 Common Causes of Altered Mental Status

A	Alcohol
E	Epilepsy, electrolytes, environmental, endocrine
I	Insulin
O	Overdose
U	Uremia
T	Trauma, tumor
I	Infection
P	Poisoning, psychosis
S	Seizure, stroke, shock

TRAUMA

Injuries to the brain, neck, and spinal cord are a main cause of disability and death nationwide. Trauma to the head can cause edema, increased intracranial pressure, hemorrhage, and infection resulting in brain damage. Injury to the neck and spinal cord may lead to temporary or permanent paralysis.

Skull Fractures

The greatest danger of a skull fracture is the resulting brain tissue damage (Figure 9–9). Bony fragments may cut into the brain tissue severing a vessel and causing a

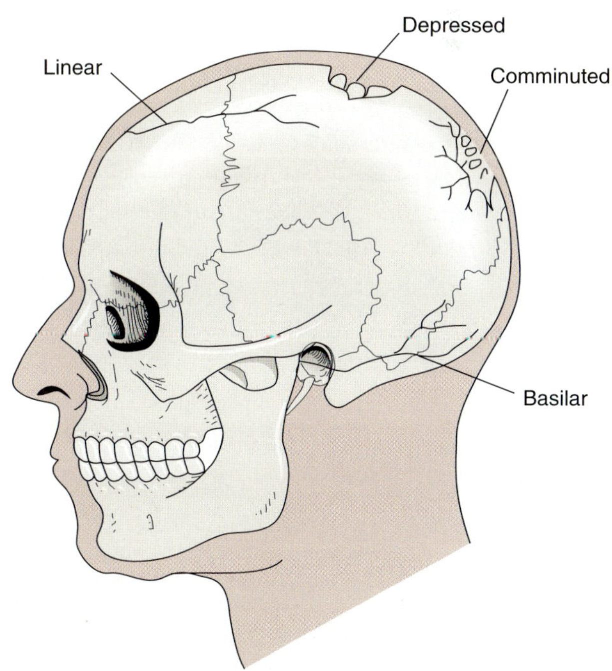

Figure 9-9 Common sites and types of skull fractures.

hematoma. Brain injury may cause temporary or permanent damage. The position of the fracture may cause a variety of symptoms. A fracture near the base of the skull may injure the respiratory center of the brain causing the individual to stop breathing. Fractures in other positions may lead to hemiparesis and seizures.

Another potential problem is infection of the brain tissue through the fracture site. Diagnosis is made on the basis of clinical history, physical examination, cranial X-rays, and CT scan. Treatment is dependent on the type and position of the fracture. A craniotomy (cranio = skull, otomy = incision) may be performed to relieve intracranial pressure from swelling. Surgical repair of the fracture may be performed if the fractured bone is pressing on the brain tissue. Protective headgear may be needed until the fracture site is healed.

Brain injury may be diffuse or focal in nature. Diffuse injury can range from a mild concussion to severe generalized edema. Focal injuries include contusions and hematomas, which are collections of blood that can be life-threatening.

The mechanism of injury can be direct or indirect. Direct injury is caused by penetration into the brain, either from an external object (e.g., bullet) or a bone fragment. Indirect injury is caused by the brain striking against the inside of the skull, which can lead to damage directly at the impact site or tearing of blood vessels from the shear forces applied to the brain. This injury can be described as a coup or contracoup injury. Coup injury (Figure 9–10) occurs on the section of brain adjacent to the impact site. Contracoup injury (Figure 9–10) occurs when the head rebounds and the brain strikes the inner surface of the skull opposite the primary impact site.

Diffuse Axonal Injury

Diffuse axonal injury (DAI) is a term used to describe a generalized form of brain injury. DAI is a shearing, stretching, or tearing of nerve fibers that cause some degree of damage to the nerve axons. This damage can vary from mild to severe and may affect nerve transmission. DAI is divided into three categories, mild, moderate, and severe, each with a slightly different presentation and different prognosis.

Mild DAI, the least severe category, is also known as a concussion or "ding." Mild DAI is the most common result of blunt head trauma. There is very little anatomic damage to the nerve axons, but the nerve cell physiology is temporarily altered. Typically, there is a transient episode of dysfunction and a rapid return to the patient's baseline mental status and function. Symptoms associated with mild DAI are confusion, disorientation,

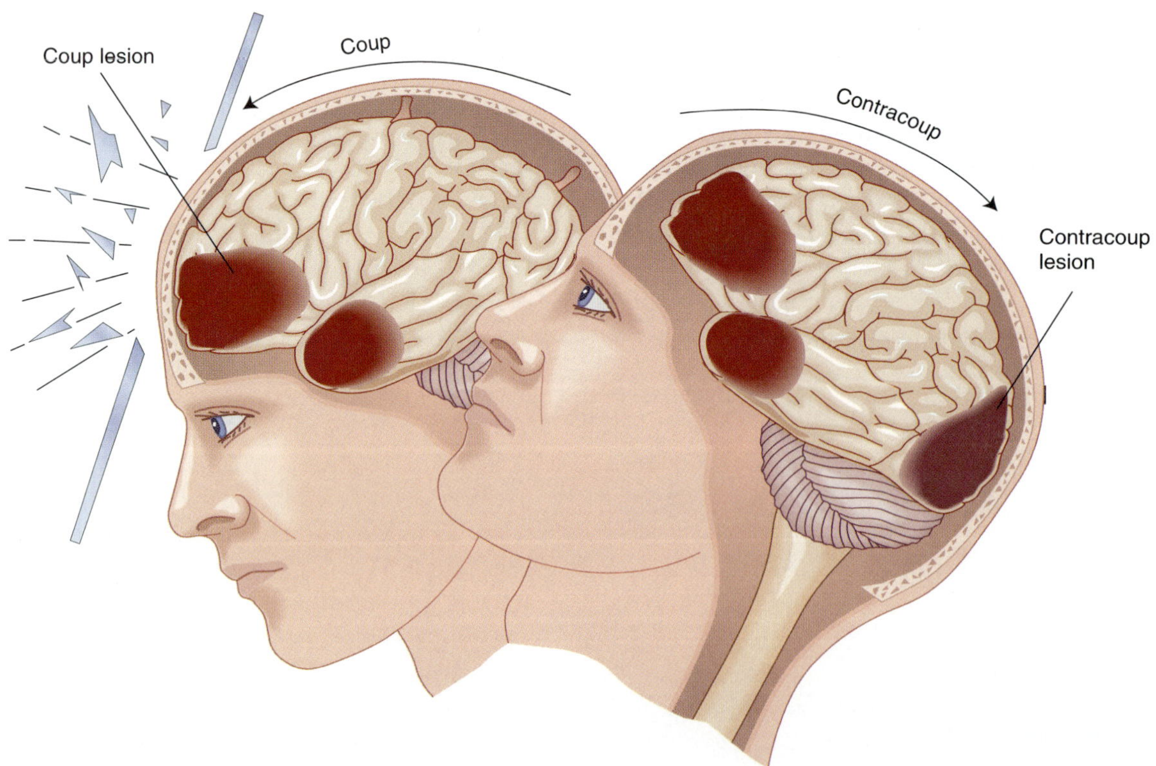

Figure 9–10 Coup-contracoup lesions.

and event **amnesia**, or an inability to remember the event. Some patients with mild DAI have a brief period of unconsciousness; however, unconsciousness is generally associated with moderate or severe DAI.

In moderate DAI, there is a generalized, minute bruising of nerve tissue. This occurs in approximately twenty percent of all severely head injured patients. Moderate DAI is commonly associated with a basilar skull fracture. Some degree of residual neurological impairment is common and most patients will survive this level of injury. The residual deficit may be focal, psychiatric, personality, sensory, or motor in nature. If the brain stem or the reticular activating system is involved, the patient may be unconscious. The sign that differentiates moderate DAI from mild DAI is the presence of either immediate unconsciousness or persistent confusion. Other signs and symptoms of moderate DAI include disorientation and moment to moment amnesia where the patient repeatedly asks what happened and does not remember what the EMS provider tells them about the event.

Severe DAI occurs in approximately sixteen percent of severely head injured patients and involves a significant disruption of many axons in both cerebral hemispheres and the brain stem. The presenting sign that usually differentiates severe DAI from the less severe categories is prolonged unconsciousness. The patient may also be postured with the arms rigidly flexed or rigidly extended and have other signs of increased intracranial pressure (see discussion later in this chapter). If the patient survives, a significant neurological deficit will be present.

EMS treatment of DAI is similar for all three classifications. During the initial assessment, the EMS provider needs to focus on airway management and ventilatory support. In the focused exam, a thorough neurological examination should be performed and other injuries prioritized and treated. Increased intracranial pressure should be treated, if present. As with any significant blunt trauma, the patient should be fully immobilized and cervical spine precautions used throughout EMS care. If possible, the patient should be transported in a quiet and calm manner to minimize CNS stimulation.

Focal Brain Injuries

Unlike diffuse axonal injury, which is a generalized process, focal injuries typically are localized to one area of the brain. Common types of focal injuries caused by trauma include brain contusion, epidural hematoma, and subdural hematoma.

A brain contusion is an area where a small amount of bleeding has occurred within the brain tissue and is similar to a bruise on the skin. The bleeding will generally stop without intervention but can occasionally continue to bleed and form a hematoma. Brain contusions are relatively common in patients who have a prolonged period of confusion after blunt head injury. The injury may be either coup or contracoup as discussed earlier. Brain contusions are often associated with moderate DAI and the patient will present differently depending upon the area of the brain affected by the injury.

EMS management includes assessing for signs of increased intracranial pressure (see section later in this chapter), maintaining adequate ventilation, and maintaining a stable cervical spine. As with DAI, the patient should be kept warm and comfortable and transported quietly.

A blow to the head is the common cause of an **epidural** (EP-ih-**DOO**-ral; epi = above, dural = dura, outer meninges) hematoma. Such a blow may be obtained in a fight or accident. Blood vessels are ruptured and hemorrhage or seep blood between the bony skull and the first or outer meninges, the dura mater (Figure 9–11A). The most common site of blood vessel rupture is along the middle meningeal artery. This artery contributes a significant amount of blood flow to many structures within the skull and lies directly against the inner surface of the skull. The point where it is most vulnerable is where it passes beneath the temple, the thinnest section of the bony skull. This artery can rupture from seemingly minor head trauma, causing a fatal bleed. Blood usually collects rapidly over a period of hours pushing the dura away from the inner bony skull. Symptoms of an epidural hematoma initially include headache, dilated pupils, nausea, vomiting, and dizziness. As the hematoma grows, the individual may lose consciousness and develop an increase in intracranial pressure. The textbook presentation includes immediate unconsciousness, recovery and consciousness for a period of time followed by a rapid decline in level of consciousness.

A **subdural** (SUB-**DOO**-ral) hematoma is a collection of blood between the dura (outer meningeal layer) and arachnoid (middle meningeal layer) as depicted in Figure 9–11B. Subdural hematomas are often caused by the tearing of the veins that bridge between the dural layers and the brain cortex. This generally occurs in acceleration / deceleration injuries when the vessels are suddenly stretched. Subdural hematomas generally develop more slowly over a period of days, although a significant amount of bleeding can be present and cause a rapid loss of consciousness. Symptoms are caused by increased intracranial pressure and often mimic a stroke. Symptoms may include hemiparesis, nausea, vomiting, dizziness, convulsions, and loss of consciousness.

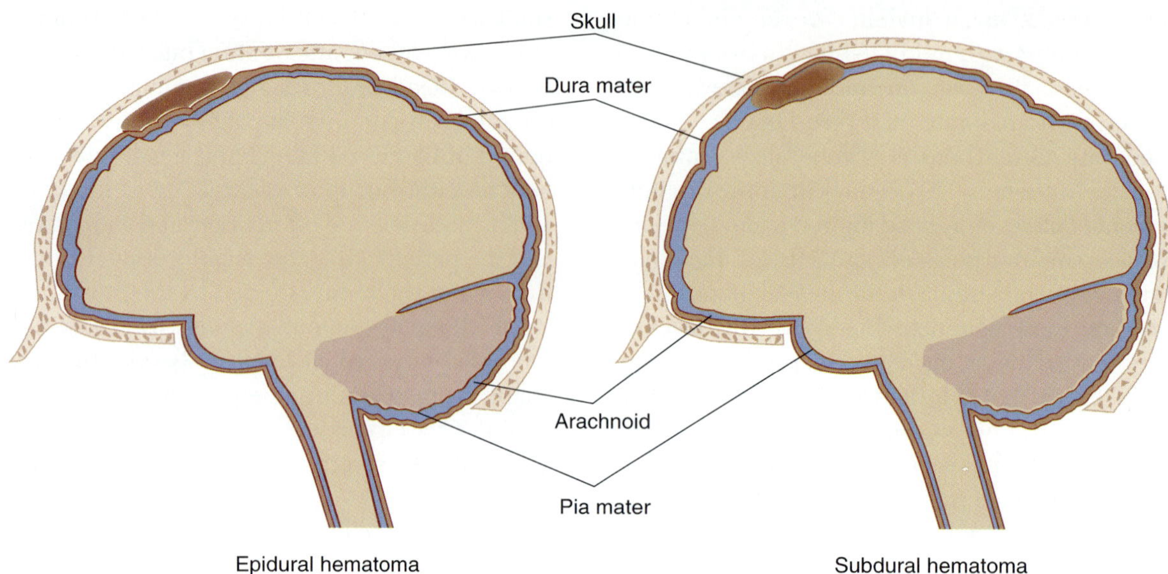

Figure 9–11 A. Epidural hematoma. B. Subdural hematoma.

Diagnosis of a cerebral hematoma is made on the basis of clinical history, physical examination, and, in the emergency department, head CT. The EMS provider must have a high index of suspicion, especially for subdural hematomas, which may only present with subtle initial findings. Field management includes appropriate triage to a trauma facility, management of the airway and maintaining adequate ventilation. The EMS provider should also assess and treat for increased intracranial pressure. Emergency department treatment is aimed at decreasing intracranial pressure. Pressure may be relieved by craniotomy called "bur holes" to drain the blood and **cauterization** (KAW-ter-eye-**ZAY**-shun; electrical burning of tissue) to stop the bleeding. If intracranial pressure is treated promptly, prognosis is good. Untreated, increased intracranial pressure is fatal.

Effect of Increased Intracranial Pressure. The most significant result of any trauma to the head is an increased pressure inside the skull, otherwise known as an increased **intracranial pressure** (ICP). The ICP is important for two reasons. Because of the relatively rigid skull, buildup of pressure inside the skull cannot be relieved by changing the shape of the skull. This increase in ICP has the potential to compress and damage brain tissue. ICP also plays an important role in allowing the flow of blood to the brain. The cerebral perfusion pressure (CPP) is the minimum pressure required to move blood into the brain, and is approximately 60 mmHg in an average adult without brain injury. The CPP is related to the mean arterial blood pressure (MAP) and the ICP by the equation: CPP = MAP – ICP. Once the ICP rises above a certain point, the blood pressure also has to increase and the cerebral arteries dilate to maintain blood flow to the brain. When the MAP increases to compensate for decreased cerebral blood flow, the flow of blood to the brain increases, causing the ICP to also rise. This turns into a vicious spiral as the ICP rises, causing another increase in MAP and so on.

ICP can increase as a result of edema, hematoma, hypotension, and hypercarbia. As previously discussed, swelling of the brain tissue from an injury will increase the ICP because of the rigidity of the skull. A subdural or epidural hematoma will also cause an increase in ICP as the hematoma compresses the brain. Hypotension will cause an increase in ICP as a response to the drop in CPP that occurs. Reviewing the relationship between CPP, MAP, and ICP above, as the MAP decreases because of hypotension, CPP will also decrease. This causes a dilation of the cerebral blood vessels and an increase of blood flow to the brain. This increased blood flow to the brain causes an increase in ICP. A large enough increase in ICP can set off the vicious spiral described above. Hypercarbia is an increase in the carbon dioxide (CO_2) level in the blood. Higher than normal CO_2 levels cause brain tissue to swell, again increasing ICP. The effects of hypercarbia on brain tissue is the reason severe head injury patients are initially hyperventilated. The increased tidal volume and rate increases the amount of oxygen and decreases the amount of CO_2 in the blood, reducing cerebral edema. However, lowering the CO_2 level too much, which can easily happen with overzealous hyperventilation, may cause cerebral vasoconstriction and reduce the amount of blood and oxygen flowing to the brain. This reduction in blood flow can possibly harm brain tissue that is only mildly injured and would otherwise recover. For this reason, hyperventilation of head injured patients is only recommended for a short period of time if a sudden change in neurologic status occurs. The EMS provider's goal in treatment of the head injured patient is to ensure the patient does not become hypoxic.

Glasgow Coma Scale. The Glasgow Coma Scale (GCS) is a quick and easy way to assess neurological function and has been correlated with outcomes from brain injury. The GCS score is determined by assessing the patient in three key areas, eye opening, verbal response, and motor response (see Table 9–3). These three areas are assessed and the scores added together to compute the GCS. As described in Table 9–3, the GCS score ranges from 3 to 15, and is divided into mild brain injury (GCS = 13–15), moderate brain injury (GCS = 9–12) and severe brain injury (GCS ≤8). The EMS provider should consider intubation and aggressive airway management for patients who have a GCS ≤8, as these patients have a severe injury and will not be able to protect their airway. There is a subset of patients in the mild brain injury category (GCS = 13–15) that suddenly deteriorate, sometimes while in EMS care. The EMS provider should be prepared to take aggressive action in the event of a sudden decline in neurological status.

The initial GCS score has been related to mortality. An initial GCS > 10 is associated with very low mortality except when a sudden neurological decline occurs that puts the patient into the severe head injury category. Overall mortality for a patient with an initial GCS of between 3 and 5 is approximately sixty percent, which drops to twelve percent for patients with an initial GCS between 6 and 8, and only two percent for patients with an initial GCS between 9 and 12. When combined with an acute subdural hematoma, a patient with an initial GCS of between 3 and 5 has a seventy-five percent

TABLE 9-3 Glasgow Coma Scale

	Adult	Pediatric (< 5 years old)
Eye Opening	4. Spontaneous	4. Spontaneous
	3. Voice	3. To shout / voice
	2. Pain stimulus	2. Pain stimulus
	1. None	1. None
Verbal	5. Oriented	5. Normal cry, smile, coo, or appropriate words for age
	4. Disoriented	4. Cries or inappropriate words for age
	3. Inappropriate words	3. Inappropriate cry or scream
	2. Incomprehensible	2. Grunts
	1. None	1. None
Motor	6. Obeys	6. Spontaneous
	5. Localizes pain	5. Localizes pain
	4. Flexion / withdrawal	4. Flexion / withdrawal
	3. Decorticate posturing	3. Decorticate posturing
	2. Decerebrate posturing	2. Decerebrate posturing
	1. None	1. None
Total	3–15	3–15
Interpretation		
Mild	13–15 (Observe for rapid decline)	
Moderate	9–12	
Severe	Less than 8 (consider intubation)	

mortality and less than a ten percent chance of a favorable recovery. In contrast, a patient who has DAI without a mass and a GCS of between 6 and 8 has only a ten percent mortality and a sixty-seven percent chance of good recovery. The initial GCS is a good indicator of the patient's prognosis.

Spinal Cord Injury

The spinal cord is protected by the bony vertebral column. When this column is fractured or injured, the spinal cord may also suffer injury. The spinal cord may be injured at any level, but the mobility of the neck causes this area to be the most vulnerable. The site of the injury, the type of trauma, and the degree of injury will all play a role in determining whether paralysis will occur and whether it will be temporary or permanent. Injury to the spinal cord may result in varying degrees of loss of movement and feeling below the area of injury. (Refer to Figure 9–12 while reading the following material for a better understanding of spinal cord injuries and preventive measures.)

Complete Spinal Cord Injury. Injury to the neck is common in automobile accidents and sports accidents Automobile accidents commonly lead to injury in the form of whiplash injury. Injury to the highest level of the cervical spine (C1–C3) is usually fatal. Injuries to the cervical spine or neck area (C1–C4) may lead to **quadriplegia** (KWAD-rih-**PLEE**-jee-ah; quadri = four, plegia = paralysis). Quadriplegia is the loss of movement and feeling in the trunk and all four extremities with the accompanying loss of bowel, bladder, and sexual function. Other life-threatening symptoms include hypotension, **hypothermia** (hypo = low, thermia = heat or temperature), bradycardia, and respiratory problems. In some cases, respirations must be permanently assisted with mechanical ventilation. Injury to the lower cervical spine (C5–C7) may lead to varying degrees of paralysis of the arms and shoulders.

Injury to the thoracic or lumbar section of the spinal cord may lead to **paraplegia** (PARA-ah-**PLEE**-jee-ah; para = beyond or two like parts, plegia = paralysis). Paraplegia is a loss of movement and feeling in the trunk and both legs. Loss of bladder, bowel, and sexual function are common. Paraplegia is often the result of a fall or an injury resulting in compression to the lower spine.

EMS treatment of a patient with a suspected spinal cord injury includes managing the airway while protecting the cervical spine, assisting ventilations, and assessing for and treating shock. The patient should be fully immobilized using a cervical collar and secured to a long spine board. A neurological assessment should be performed before and after immobilization to document baseline status. Administration of an IV steroid may be ordered by medical control to help reduce swelling and limit additional cord injury.

Diagnosis in the emergency department is made on the basis of history of injury, neurologic examination, spinal X-rays, MRI, and CT scan. Treatment includes realignment and stabilization of the bony spinal column and **decompresssion** or release of pressure on the spinal cord. Treatment may include surgery and medications. Much of the early treatment is aimed at preventing further spinal cord injury. Generally, the earlier the treatment is begun the better the prognosis. If the damage to the spinal cord is severe, there is little or no hope for regaining movement and feeling. Paralysis, initially, results in the inability to move the extremities, but with time reflex functions may return leading to spastic movements. Early and intensive rehabilitation is necessary for the best prognosis.

Incomplete Spinal Cord Injury. In contrast to a complete spinal cord transsection, partial injury to the cord can occur. Partial injuries can be easily overlooked by a cursory neurologic exam. Four common partial cord injury syndromes are the anterior cord syndrome, the central cord syndrome, the Brown-Sequard syndrome, and the cauda equina syndrome.

Anterior Cord Syndrome. The anterior cord syndrome involves either direct injury to the anterior (front) portion of the cord or injury to the small spinal artery that supplies the anterior portion of the cord. This is generally caused by a hyperflexion mechanism of injury. As the motor tracts are primarily affected; however, there is a complete loss of motor below the injury. Pain and temperature sensation below the level of injury is also affected; however, the sense of touch and position sense are maintained. This injury is most likely to require surgery to manage the injury.

Central Cord Syndrome. The central cord syndrome involves injury to the more central sections of the cord and is generally caused by a hyperextension injury. With the central cord syndrome, there is motor weakness in the hands and arms, but the legs are typically spared. Sensory changes are variable, but minor in most cases. The prognosis is good and surgery is not always required.

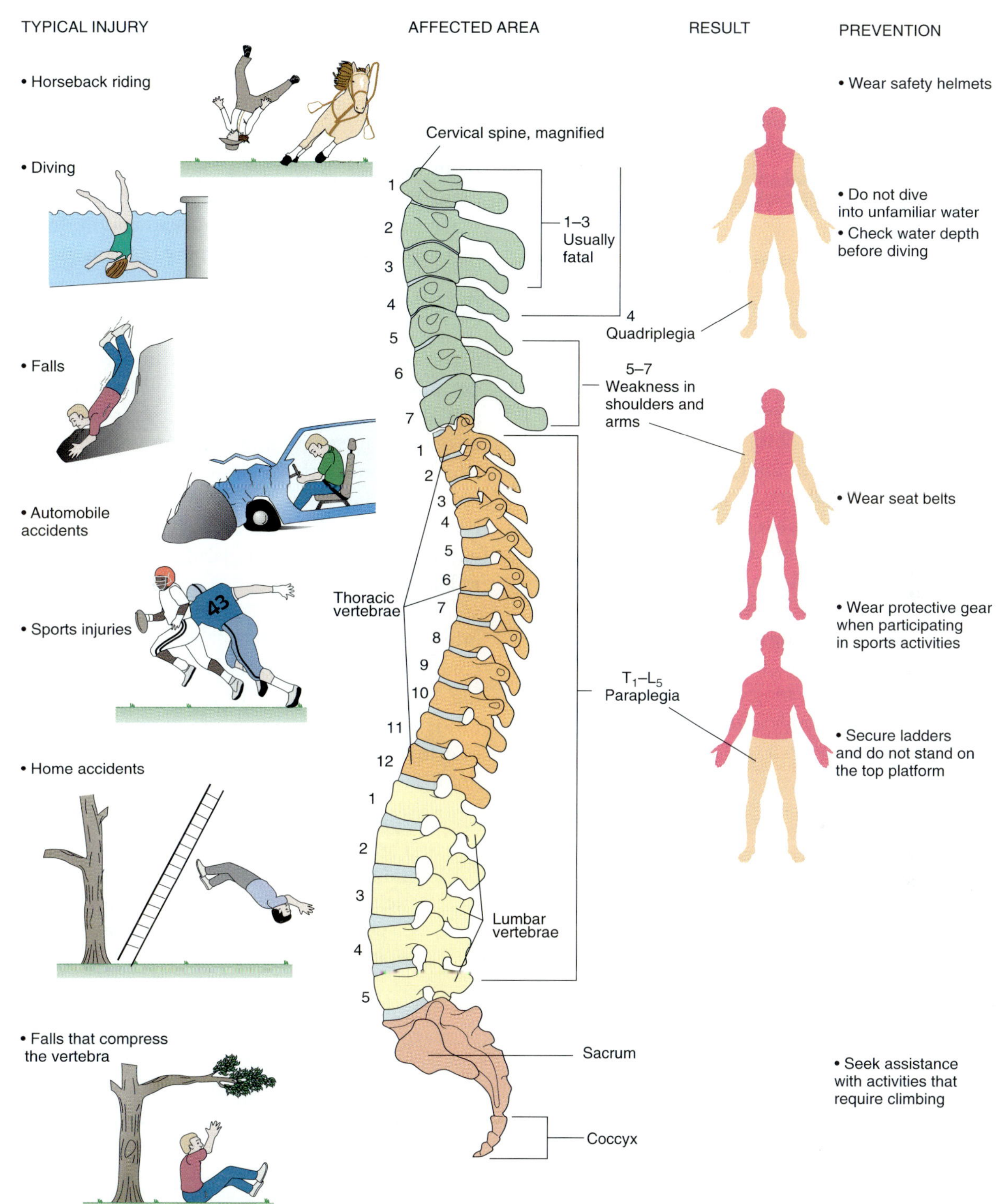

Figure 9–12 Spinal cord injuries.

Brown-Sequard Syndrome. The Brown-Sequard syndrome is a hemisection of the spinal cord, most often caused by a knife or other penetrating trauma to the spinal cord. With this type of spinal injury, there is weakness and loss of position sense on the same side as and below the injury and loss of pain and temperature on the side opposite the injury. This loss of pain and temperature opposite the injury occurs because these nerve fibers cross over to the opposite side of the spinal cord very close to where they enter the spine.

Cauda Equina Syndrome. The cauda eqina, or horse's tail, syndrome is a compression of the lumbar portion of the spinal cord, generally caused by a ruptured intervertebral disc or spinal cord tumor. The name originates from the spinal cord's appearance similar to a horse's tail. This syndrome involves back pain, loss of reflexes in the lower extremities and loss of bowel and/or bladder function. This is a significant emergency and emergency surgery is often carried out to alleviate pressure on the cord.

Autonomic Hyperreflexia. Autonomic hyperreflexia syndrome is associated with chronic spinal cord injury patients who have lost their ability to control the autonomic nervous system balance. The sympathetic nervous system becomes stimulated, and this stimulus is amplified, producing an extreme cardiovascular response that is not compensated. This cardiovascular response can include extreme hypertension (SBP up to 300 mmHg), severe headache, blurred vision, sweating with flushed skin, nasal congestion, nausea, and bradycardia. The stimulus can be something as innocuous as a full bladder or rectum. Autonomic hyperreflexia can be life-threatening for patients with a spinal cord injury above the level of T6.

GENETIC AND DEVELOPMENTAL DISORDERS

Genetic and developmental neurologic disorders are some of the most severe because of their long-term debilitating effects.

Cerebral Palsy

Cerebral palsy (SER-eh-bral PAWL-zee) is a congenital bilateral paralysis that results from inadequate blood or oxygen supply to the brain during fetal development, the birthing process, or in infancy. Causes of CP include maternal rubella, toxemia, birthing difficulties such as prolonged labor, anoxia, hypoxemia, asphyxia from the umbilical cord being wrapped around the infant's neck, head trauma, and meningitis. Often the cause of CP is unknown. Cerebral palsy is the most common crippler of children and more often affects premature infants and males. This disorder usually affects motor or muscle performance and may be noticed if the infant has difficulty sucking or swallowing. Other complications include visual and hearing deficits, seizure activity, and mental retardation. Cerebral palsy is characterized by hyperactive reflexes, rapid muscle contraction, and muscle weakness. The affected child commonly has a "scissors gait" exhibited by toe walking and crossing one foot over the other with each step. There is no cure for cerebral palsy. Treatment involves physical therapy, speech therapy, orthopedic cast, braces, and often surgery to help the child reach full potential. Anticonvulsant and muscle relaxant medications may also be of some benefit.

Spina Bifida

Spina bifida (SPY-nah BIF-ih-dah) is a congenital disorder in which one or more of the vertebrae of the bony spinal column fails to close over the spinal cord leaving an opening in the column. *Bifid* means split in two parts, which describes the vertebra in this condition. Development of the spinal cord and column occurs during the first trimester of pregnancy. The cause of this malformation is unknown but risk factors include maternal radiation, virus, and genetic factors as children born with spina bifida are more often born to mothers who have other children with this defect. There are several other conditions that tend to accompany spina bifida, including hydrocephalus, cleft palate, and club foot. Spina bifida can be seen on X-ray examination. There are several forms of spina bifida (Figure 9–13). These forms are described as:

1. Spina Bifida Occulta—the most common form. There is a spina bifida but it is asymptomatic and hidden (occulta). Signs of the malformation often include a dimpling of the skin, and a tuft of hair or port wine nevus on the skin surface above the defect.
2. Meningocele—occurs when the meninges of the spinal cord protrude through the opening in the vertebral column forming a fluid-filled sac on the skin surface. Since nerve tissue is not involved, the infant usually does not have neurologic problems. Surgical intervention to correct the condition is usually performed in the first twenty-four to forty-eight hours of life.
3. Myelomeningocele—the most serious spina bifida. The meninges and a portion of the spinal cord protrude through the opening in the vertebral column causing neurologic symptoms. Common symptoms include skeletal malformation, deformed joints, paralysis of the legs, and bowel and bladder incontinence. Surgical intervention to correct the condition is usually performed in the first twenty-four hours of life. Additional procedures may be needed as the child grows. Some of these children

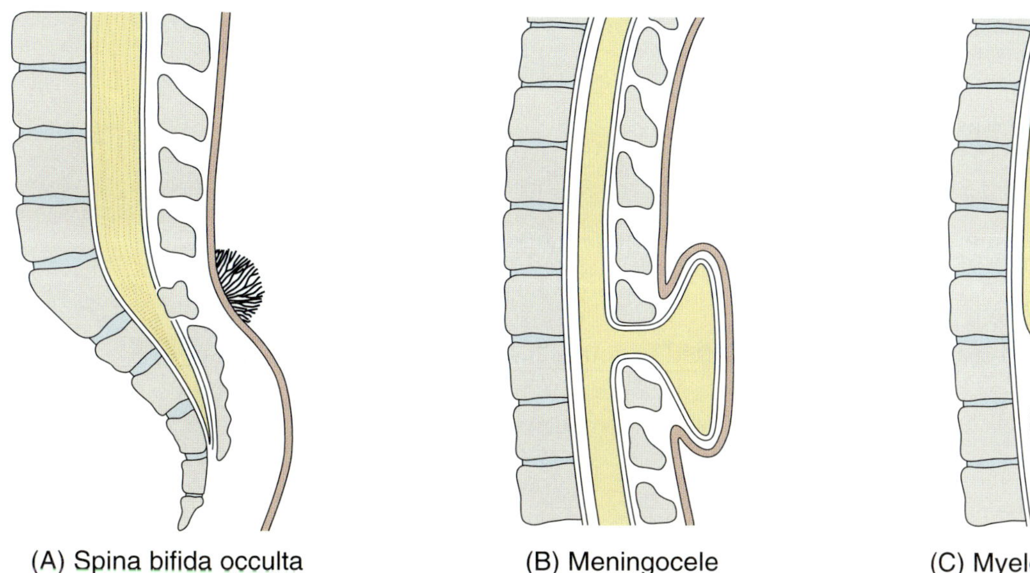

Figure 9–13 Types of spina bifida.

are unable to walk and may die before the age of two or three years.

EFFECTS OF AGING ON THE SYSTEM

The effects of aging on the nervous system are some of the most noticeable to the older adult. Along with aging there is a decrease in nervous system activity in the brain and spinal cord. This is caused by a loss of neurons and the shrinking of the hypothalamus. Research has shown that continued active use of the brain decreases this process to some extent, but some changes still occur. With these changes in the brain and spinal cord come many changes in the individual's functioning. As the individual ages, there is a loss in short-term memory, but not in long-term memory. There is also a slower general reaction time. The elderly may also have difficulty completing fine motor skills. General touch perception is somewhat diminished too, so the individual may have difficulty distinguishing temperature changes and pain stimuli.

Vision ability is one of the first changes the individual often notices. There is a loss of visual acuity, and a decrease in peripheral vision. Some individuals also become intolerant to very bright light and have difficulty adapting to changes in light from dark to bright. Some hearing loss is a subtle process that occurs at different levels in individuals. Taste sensation may also diminish over time.

Sleep patterns are usually affected in the aging process. Generally, the older adult does not sleep as well at night but makes up for this deficit by taking short naps throughout the day or in the early evening.

SUMMARY

The nervous system is a highly complex system responsible for the individual's ability to reason, interact with other individuals, understand complex ideas, and to respond both intellectually and physically. Disorders of the system usually result in symptoms involving many other systems.

Injuries to the brain, neck, and spinal cord are a main cause of disability and death nationwide. Permanent neurologic deficits are common in brain and spinal cord injuries.

Changes in the nervous system with aging result in some of the most commonly seen symptoms. Losses in the senses are the most noticeable problems seen in the older adult. Changes in vision and hearing are some of the earliest symptoms realized by the middle-aged individual. Alzheimer's disease is one of the most common disorders of the nervous system diagnosed today.

REVIEW QUESTIONS

Short Answer

1. What are the functions of the nervous system?

2. Which signs and symptoms are associated with common nervous system disorders?

3. Which diagnostic tests are most commonly used to determine type and/or cause of the nervous system disorder?

Matching

4. Match the disorders listed in the left column with the correct description in the right column:

_____ Encephalitis
_____ Tetanus
_____ Meningitis
_____ Transient ischemic attack
_____ Cephalalgia
_____ Concussion
_____ Contusion
_____ Subdural hematoma
_____ Alzheimer's disease
_____ Amyotrophic lateral sclerosis
_____ Multiple sclerosis
_____ Bell's palsy

a. inflammation of the covering of the brain/spinal cord
b. a disorder affecting the seventh cranial nerve
c. disruption in the electrical activity of the brain causing unconsciousness
d. blood collection between the dura mater and arachnoid layer of the brain
e. physical bruising of the brain
f. infection of nerve tissue
g. disease characterized by the demyelination of nerves of the CNS
h. inflammation of brain tissue
i. headache
j. a neurodegenerative disease characterized by cognitive dysfunction
k. destructive disease of the motor neurons
l. mild stroke

CASE STUDY

You are transporting Mr. Speed, a 57-year-old male patient who sustained a spinal cord injury at the level of T2 several weeks ago. You are bringing him to a rehab facility so he can continue his rehabilitation. Mr. Speed is discussing his passion for model railroads with you when you notice he suddenly becomes flushed and diaphoretic. At about the same time he states that he has a sudden headache and feels a little dizzy. You take a quick set of vital signs and find his pulse rate to be 64 and bounding and his blood pressure to be 250/130. What do you think is going on with Mr. Speed? What could be the source of his sudden hypertension and other signs? What would you do next?

BIBLIOGRAPHY

A president fades into a world apart. (October 5, 1997). *New York Times*, A1.

Alzheimer's disease: a multidisciplinary challenge. (1997). *Geriatric*, 52(8), S1–S58.

Boswell, B. B. (1997). Exploring quality of life of adults with spinal cord injuries. *Perceptual and Motor Skills*, *84*(6) pt. 2, F2.

Breakthroughs in neuromuscular diseases. (1997). *Current Health, 24*(10), 28–29.

Cantu, R. C. (1997). Stingers, transient quadriplegia, and cervical spinal stenosis: Return to play criteria. *Medicine and Science in Sports and Exercise, 29*(7), S233–S235.

Ciol, M. A. (1996). An assessment of surgery for spinal stenosis: Time trends, geographic variations, complications, and reoperations. *Journal of the American Geriatric Society, 44*(3), 285.

Dobkin, B. H. (1996). The player: Diagnosis of meningioma, a tumor of the spinal cord. *Discover, 17*(11), 45–49.

Dryden, M.S. (August 31, 1996). Lyme myelitis mimicking neurological malignancy. *Lancet, 348*, 624.

Fighting to fund an "absolute necessity." (1996). *Newsweek, 128*, 56.

Grady, D. (September 30, 1997). Spine researchers seek recipe for regeneration. *New York Times*, F1+.

Herbert, B. (July 4, 1997). A chance to survive. *New York Times*, A19.

Huffman, G. B. (November 1, 1997). Updated treatments for acute spinal cord injury. *American Family Physician, 56*, 1845+.

Ijaz, T. (March 13, 1997). Intermedullary spinal cord metastases. *The New England Journal of Medicine, 336*, 768.

Lang, D. (1997). Seizure disorders and physical activity. *The Physician and Sports Medicine, 25*(10), 24e–24f.

Leary, W. E. (July 12, 1997). Fetal tissue injected into injured spinal cord. *New York Times*, p. 9.

Loughrey, L. (1997). Nina was flirting with disaster. *Nursing 97, 27*(8), 56–58.

Raloff, J. (December 13, 1997). From fleas to brain tumors. *Science News, 152*, 375.

Roush, W. (June 27, 1997). Are pushy axons a key to spinal cord repair? *Science, 276*, 971–972.

Safire, W. (May 18, 1995). Using our brains. *New York Times*, A23.

Secrets of the brain. (1996). *Maclean's, 109*, 44–51.

Seymour, J. (January 27, 1996). Virtually real, really sick: Neurological disorders associated with virtual reality games. *New Scientist, 149*, 34–37.

Shua-Haim, J. R. (1997). Bell's palsy (seventh nerve palsy). *Geriatrics, 52*(12), 61.

The tumor war: Work of brain surgeon K. Black. (1997). *Time, Special fall issue, 150*, 46–48.

Young, W. (September 26, 1997). Fear of hope. *Science, 277*, 1907.

Zamula, E. (1977). Reasons for brain tumor increases not black and white. *FDA Consumer, 31* (5/6), 26–32.

Zoroya, G. (1997). Ray of hope. *Washingtonian, 32*(6), 161–166.

CHAPTER

10

Musculoskeletal Diseases and Disorders

CONTENT OUTLINE

- Anatomy and Physiology
- Common Signs and Symptoms
- Diagnostic Tests
- Common Diseases of the Musculoskeletal System
  - Diseases of Bone
  - Diseases of Joints
  - Diseases of Muscle and Connective Tissue
  - Neoplasms
- Trauma
  - Fracture
  - Strains and Sprains
  - Dislocations and Subluxations
  - Crush Injury
  - Compartment Syndrome
  - Low Back Pain (LBP)
  - Bursitis
  - Tendonitis
  - Torn Rotator Cuff
  - Torn Meniscus
  - Cruciate Ligament Tears
  - Shin Splints
- Developmental and Genetic Disorders
  - Muscular Dystrophy
  - Osteogenesis Imperfecta
- Effects of Aging on the System

KEY TERMS

Anaerobic
Computerized Axial Tomography
Densitometry
Discectomy
Dowager's hump
Electromyography
Interphalangeal
Laminectomy
Magnetic Resonance Imaging
Metacarpophalangeal
Metatarsophalangeal
Myelogram
ORIF
Radiologic
RICE
Sciatica
Spasms
Tetany
Tophi

Types of Fractures

angulated
articular
avulsion
closed
Colles'
comminuted
complete
compound
compression
displaced
extracapsular
femoral neck
greenstick
impacted
incomplete
intertrochanteric
intracapsular
longitudinal
non-displaced
oblique
open
pathologic
Pott's
simple
spiral
stellate
stress
subcapital
transverse

LEARNING OBJECTIVES

Upon completion of the chapter, the student should be able to:

1. Define the terminology common to the musculoskeletal system and the disorders of the system.
2. Identify the common disorders of the musculoskeletal system.
3. Discuss the basic anatomy and physiology of the musculoskeletal system.
4. Identify the important signs and symptoms associated with common musculoskeletal system disorders.
5. Describe the common diagnostic tests used to determine type and/or cause of the musculoskeletal system disorder.
6. Describe the typical course and management of the common musculoskeletal system disorders.
7. Describe the effects of aging upon the musculoskeletal system and the common disorders of the system.

OVERVIEW

The musculoskeletal system provides the structure and movement function for the individual. Because the muscles and bones run throughout the body, disorders of the system may affect any other system, and disorders of other systems frequently affect the musculoskeletal system. The system includes bones, joints, ligaments, muscles, and tendons. Each of these has a unique function but also interacts with the other components of the system to support the person and provide for mobility. Problems with the musculo-skeletal system frequently affect the individual's independence and, thus, the quality of life.

ANATOMY AND PHYSIOLOGY

The skeletal component of the musculoskeletal system is made up of bones and joints. The bones are responsible for providing the framework for support of the body. They also produce blood cells, store fat and minerals, protect soft tissues (like the brain), and help create body motion. Bones are very vascular. Blood circulates through bone picking up or storing body minerals such as calcium, phosphorus, magnesium, and sodium. Osteoblasts are active bone-building cells, osteoclasts are cells that reabsorb bone, and osteocytes are mature bone cells.

Bones are often classified by shape and composition. For example, the skeletal system is composed of long bones such as the femur in the leg, short bones such as the metacarpal bones in the fingers, flat bones such as the sternum or skull, and irregular bones such as the vertebrae or pelvic bones (Figure 10–1). The composition of bone is either cortical or cancellous. Cortical bone is dense, smooth, and compact while cancellous bone is spongy, with many open spaces throughout. The ligaments are fibrous connective tissue that connect bones to other bones and joints.

Bone can be damaged and can repair itself. The steps of bone repair include (1) bleeding at the site of injury with clot and granulation tissue formation; (2) proliferation of cells at the site forming a callus (soft bony deposit) over the injury or fracture; (3) cells become bone (osteoblasts) or cartilage at the site; (4) the bone becomes calcified (hardened) by the deposit of inorganic salts at the site; and (5) the bone "remodels" or eventually becomes the shape necessary to complete the designated function of the bone. Bone repair is dependent on many factors. The general health status of the individual will affect the healing process, as well as age, degree

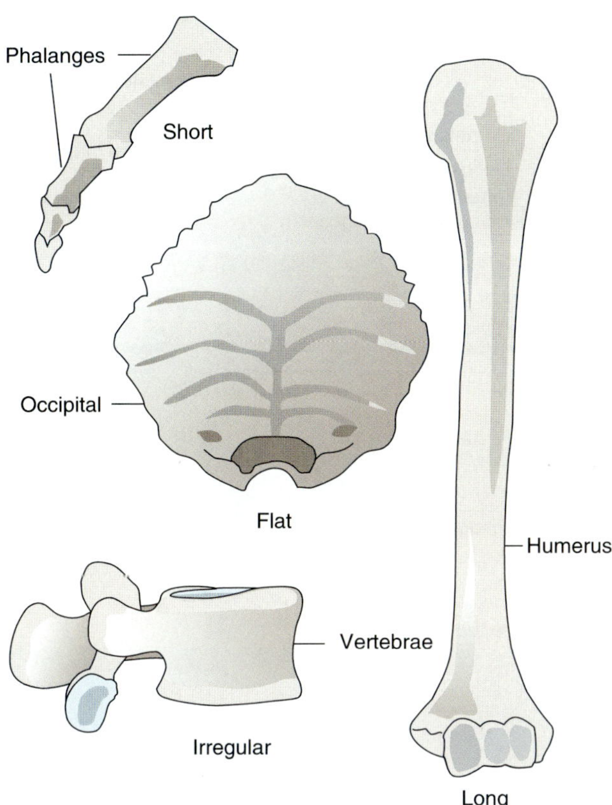

Figure 10–1 Examples of types of bones.

of injury, circulation to the site, and presence of other diseases or infection.

The joints are where two or more bones meet. They are usually classified as to the amount of movement of the joint, but they may also be classified by their structure. The classification of joints by movement is described in Table 10–1. Classification of joints by structure includes fibrous, such as the joints of the skull, cartilaginous, such as the joints of the vertebrae, and synovial, such as the joints of the knee. The synovial joints are those separated by a fluid-filled cavity.

The major movements of joints are flexion (bending), extension (reaching out or spreading out), abduction (away from the body), adduction (toward the body), rotation (turning on an axis), circumduction (circular movement), and elevation (lifting).

Cartilage is collagen tissue that supports articulating (adjoining) bones. It provides protection and a cushion to prevent friction between bones. Cartilage also acts like a shock absorber and distributes the load to reduce stress on the bone surface.

The functions of the muscles of the body are to provide structure, movement, and produce heat (Figure 10–2). The muscles of the musculoskeletal system are called "striated" because they look striped or banded under a microscope. They are also called voluntary muscles because most are moved by conscious control as opposed to other muscles, like cardiac, that move involuntarily. Skeletal muscles move in response to signals from the central nervous system. Connective tissue holds the muscle fibers together. Tendons are long, fibrous, non-elastic connective tissues that attach muscle to bone.

COMMON SIGNS AND SYMPTOMS

The most common signs and symptoms of bone and joint disease are pain, swelling, decreased mobility, and deformity. Most fractures are associated with pain caused by a disruption of the periosteum and related sensory nerves. Many fractures are easy to recognize because of the obvious displacement and related deformity. **Non-displaced** (not out of place or position) fractures are not as easy to recognize, but may cause pain just the same.

Weakness is the most common sign or symptom of muscle disorders. Weakness may be related to a primary disease of the muscle or it may be secondary to a neurologic disorder. Muscle tissue will atrophy if weakness persists for an extended length of time. On the other hand, just the reverse may occur, and muscle atrophy may lead to muscle weakness.

The "six Ps" of musculoskeletal assessment examine for many of these symptoms and signs. The six Ps are pain, pallor, paresthesia, pulses, paralysis, and pressure. Pain can occur either during palpation, with motion, or present continuously. Pallor is assessed during visual examination, pulses are assessed by palpating distal to the injury. Pallor or a loss of distal pulse may be the result of circulatory compromise. Paresthesia and paralysis can

TABLE 10–1 Classification of Joints by Movement

Classification	Amount of Movement	Example of Joint
Synarthrosis	No movement	Suture of the skull
Amphiarthrosis	Some movement but very limited	Pelvis
Diarthrosis	Complete movement	Knee, hip, elbow

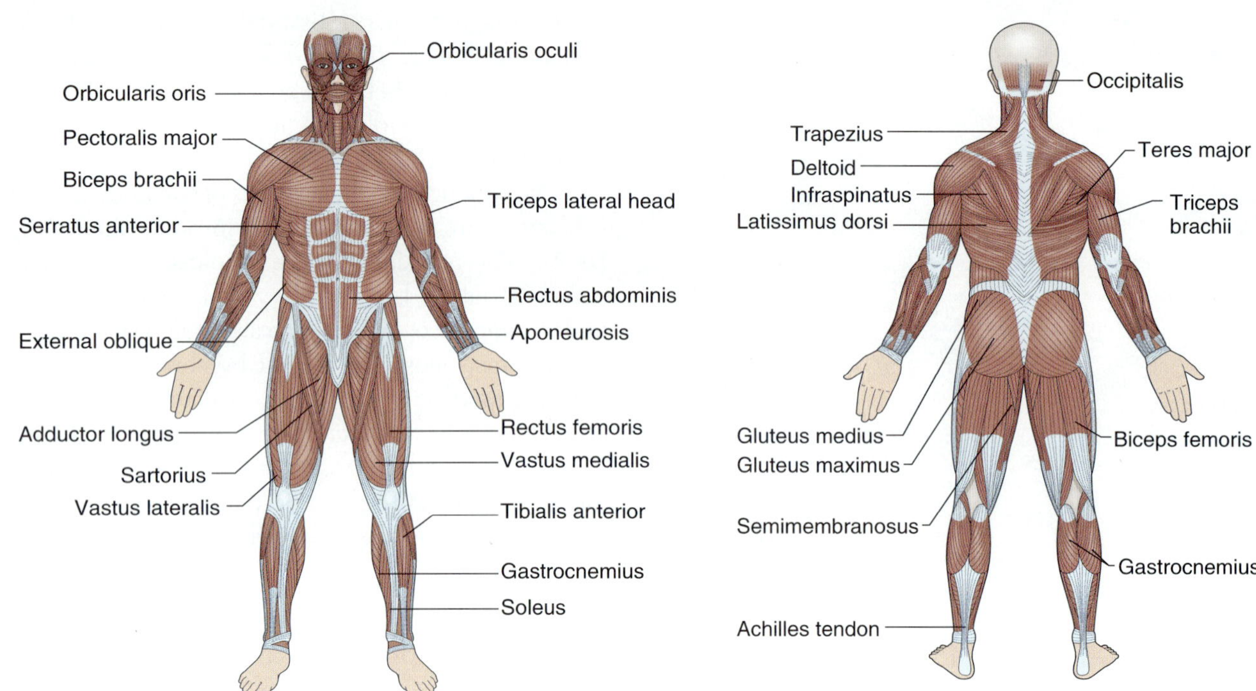

Figure 10–2 The skeletal muscles.

result from nerve irritation or compression and may be assessed during the neurological examination. Pressure may result from tissue swelling and be reported as a symptom or noticed during the physical assessment as an increase in edema, or swelling.

DIAGNOSTIC TESTS

Radiologic examinations (X-rays) are the primary tool utilized in diagnosing bone and joint disorders. **Computerized Axial Tomography** (CAT or CT scan) and **Magnetic Resonance Imaging** (MRI) may be needed for more detailed studies.

Computerized Axial Tomography involves taking specialized X-rays of the affected individual in a tube-like scanner. The individual must be able to lie still for between five and thirty minutes. The results are detailed X-ray type pictures that appear to cut the area of consideration into slices, thus the name tomogram (tomo = cutting, gram = picture) (Figure 10–3).

Magnetic Resonance Imaging is another detailed examination that utilizes a large magnet to produce the images. Individuals must be able to lie still and must not wear any type of metal to the test. MRI is more expensive to perform but makes more detailed images of soft tissue than CT scanning.

Blood studies including calcium, phosphorus, and the enzyme alkaline phosphatase may also prove helpful with metabolic disorders. Infectious disorders may be cultured. Often the specimen for culture is obtained during surgical procedures like débridement.

Muscle disorders are often evaluated by **electromyography** (EMG). This is accomplished by inserting a small needle into muscle tissue and recording the electrical activity. Electromyography can assist in determining if the disorder is muscular or neurologic in nature. Muscle tissue biopsy may be performed on difficult cases. Biopsy is the most definitive means of determining cause of muscle disorder. Biopsy is also the most reliable test for tumors of the musculoskeletal system.

COMMON DISEASES OF THE MUSCULOSKELETAL SYSTEM

Musculoskeletal injuries are commonly seen by EMS providers and can involve sports, recreation activities, workplace incidents, or motor vehicle crashes. Musculoskeletal system diseases and disorders affect almost every individual. In the younger age groups, musculoskeletal injuries, including fractures, sprains, and strains, are common, especially among active athletes. As we age, bone mass is lost leading to osteoporosis, increasing the likelihood of stress fractures. Low back pain is

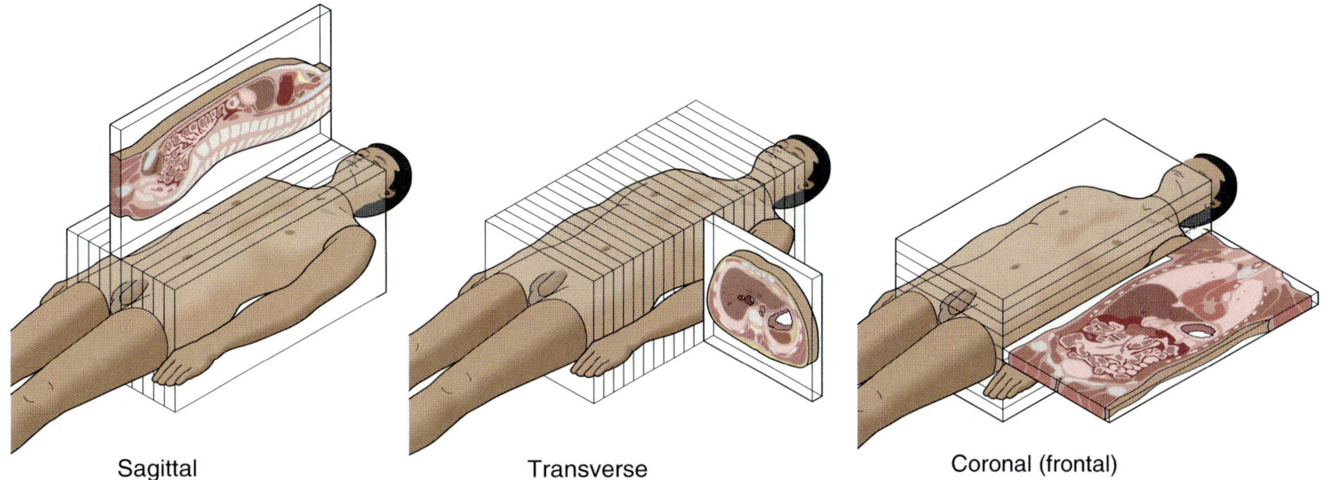

Figure 10–3 CT scan.

a very common condition in Western society with some studies estimating the lifetime prevalence as high as eighty-four percent. These conditions involve bone, joints, and muscles.

Diseases of Bone

Diseases of the bone may range from mild to severe with the most serious causing extreme deformity or disability. Many of the disorders are more common in the older adult as changes in the system may lead to increased risk for skeletal problems. Individuals with bone disease frequently need assistive devices such as crutches, walkers, or canes to maintain mobility. Internal devices such as artificial joints, pins, and braces may also be necessary.

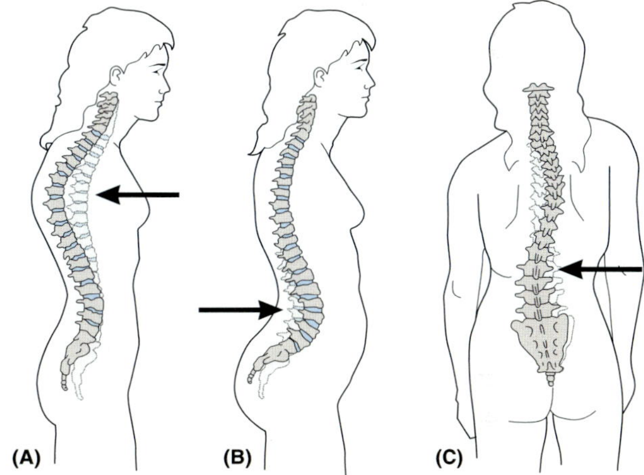

Figure 10–4 Spinal deformities: kyphosis, lordosis, and scoliosis.

Spinal Deformities. Spinal deformities may be caused by a variety of factors including congenital defects, poor posture, bone disease, and growth disorders. Deformities may be very obvious at onset as with congenital defects, but more commonly they progress slowly and are unnoticed until symptoms arise. Symptoms commonly include back pain and fatigue. Diagnosis is generally confirmed by X-ray and clinical examination. Treatment includes eliminating or treating causative factors, bracing, and spinal surgery. Untreated spinal deformities may progress to life-threatening conditions when cardiac and respiratory function are compromised.

Kyphosis (kie-FOE-sis) is an exaggerated curvature of the thoracic spine, commonly called humpback or hunchback (Figure 10–4A). Kyphosis often appears in postmenopausal osteoporitic females.

Lordosis (lor-DOE-sis) is an exaggerated anterior or inward curve of the lumbar spine and is also called swayback (Figure 10–4B). It normally occurs with pregnancy as the woman compensates for the increased size of the abdomen. When compared to the normal spine, lordosis results in a protruding abdomen and buttocks and a swayed lower back. Obesity is a common cause of lordosis.

Scoliosis (SKOLE-lee-**OH**-sis) is a lateral curvature of the spine (Figure 10–4C). It affects both sexes, but girls usually have more severe curvatures and account for approximately ninety percent of the cases. Scoliosis may occur at any age but is usually noticed during the early teen years when growth rate is accelerated. Treatment often includes bracing. Compliance with brace wearing for female adolescents is often poor leading to need for further treatment. Scoliosis screening in school-aged children was initiated in the 1960s and is now mandated by law in some states. Screening involves observation of the spine as the individual bends forward. Scoliosis is suspected if the spine curves to the side and the scapula shifts upward.

Osteoporosis. Osteoporosis (OS-tee-oh-por-**OH**-sis) is a metabolic bone disease that causes a porosity or Swiss cheese appearance of the bone leading to a decrease in bone mass. It is the most prevalent bone disease worldwide. It is estimated that osteoporosis causes major orthopedic problems in approximately one-third of the women in the United States.

There are many causative factors that play a part in osteoporosis. Age-related osteoporosis affects both men and women equally and is caused by normal age-related bone loss. Osteoporosis occurs secondary to diseases that affect mobility. For example, quadriplegia may lead to a loss of thirty to forty percent of bone mass after six months of immobility. The most common type of osteoporosis is seen in women who are postmenopausal and estrogen-deficient. It is believed that this osteoporosis is caused by a combination of factors, including a decrease in estrogen, calcium, and exercise.

Osteoporosis is a slow progressive disease that robs skeletal bone of its mass and strength. It may be decades before the bone becomes weak enough to fracture. Most fractures in women over age fifty are related to osteoporosis. Diagnosis may be confirmed by clinical examination, X-rays, CT scan, and bone **densitometry** (measurement of bone thickness).

Early signs of osteoporosis include **compression** (bone mashed down on itself, common in vertebra) fractures of the spine and pathologic wrist fractures. Compression fractures of the spine lead to a decrease in height and pain in the thoracic and lumbar spine. Over a period of time the individual may lose four to five inches of height, decreasing the thoracic and abdominal cavity size. This decrease in chest cavity size leads to decreased activity tolerance caused by shortness of breath. A decrease in the abdominal cavity size leads to feelings of fullness after eating only small amounts of food and a constant bloated feeling. Other symptoms are kyphosis and the appearance of a **Dowager's hump** (abnormal curvature in the upper thoracic spine (Figure 10–5). Wrist fractures, especially of the distal radius, commonly occur in osteoporitic individuals with just a slight fall. As the disease progresses, the individual has an increased risk for fracturing a hip. More than one million hip fractures occur annually in the United States. Hip fractures in frail, elderly women often lead to complications that result in significant mortality in the year following the fracture (Figure 10–6).

Currently there is no treatment to reverse osteoporosis because bone mass is not replaced in older adults. The progression of osteoporosis can be slowed and bone

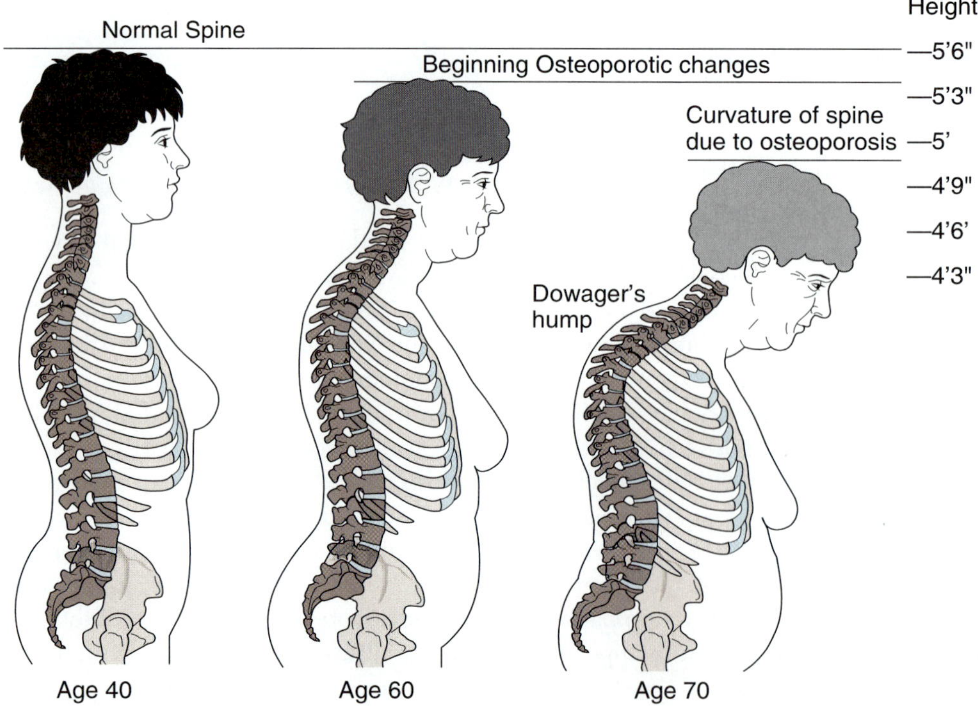

Figure 10–5 Osteoporosis: loss in height and the Dowager's hump.

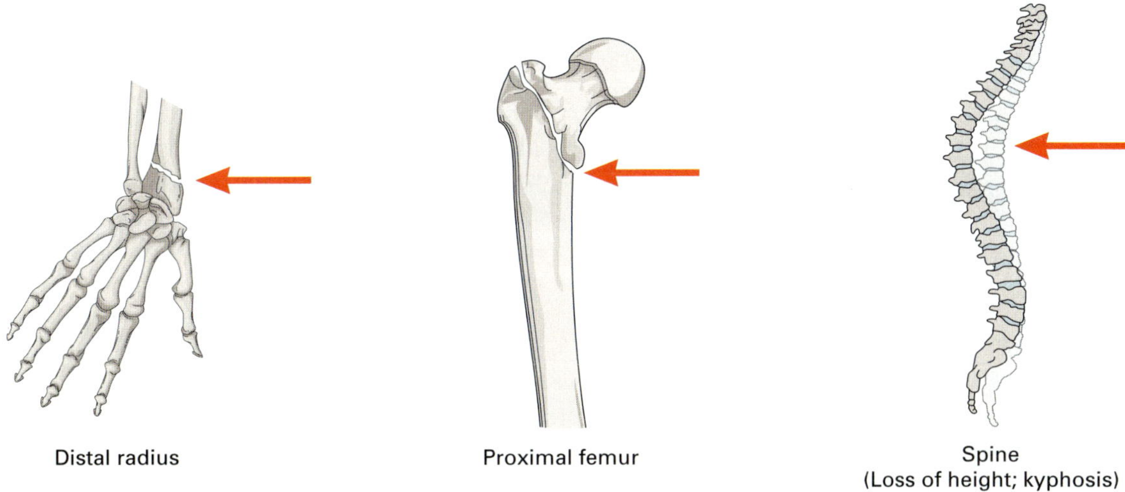

Figure 10–6 Fracture sites related to osteoporosis.

mass levels maintained by a combination of therapies. Prevention, by reducing risk factors, is the best treatment (Table 10–2). Preventive measures for osteoporosis need to begin early as bone mass is built prior to age thirty. Young women should be encouraged to exercise daily, eat a balanced diet, quit smoking, and limit caffeine and alcohol consumption. Entering menopausal years with good bone mass and maintaining as much of the bone as possible is the best weapon against osteoporosis.

Osteomyelitis. Osteomyelitis (OS-tee-oh-MY-ull-**LIE**-tis; osteo = bone, myel = marrow, itis = inflammation) is an inflammation of the bone commonly caused by infection. *Staphylococcus aureus* is the responsible organism in approximately ninety percent of the cases. This bacterium may enter the bone through a wound, spread from an infection nearby, or come from a skin or throat infection. Osteomyelitis usually affects the long bones of the arms and legs. It most often occurs in children and adolescents as a result of a throat infection. In severe cases it may affect the growth plate of the bones leading to shortening of the limb.

Symptoms of osteomyelitis may include sudden onset of high fever, chills, tenderness over the affected bone, leukocytosis (leuko = white, cyto = cell, osis = condition of increase), and bacteremia (bacteria = microscopic organisms, emia = blood, bacteria in the blood). In adults, osteomyelitis often occurs following a traumatic accident involving the bone or following bone surgery, especially when implants such as screws, plates, or other hardware are needed.

Treatment for osteomyelitis is aggressive intravenous antibiotic therapy. Affected bone is often débrided surgically in order to speed the healing process. Surgical hardware is often removed for this same reason. Acute osteomyelitis, if not treated effectively, may become chronic and lead to a lifetime of problems for the affected individual.

TABLE 10–2 Risk Factors for Osteoporosis

The following are considered factors that would increase the risk of developing osteoporosis:
• Family history of osteoporosis
• Age—risk increases with age
• Medications—tetracycline, corticosteroids, aluminum antacids, some diuretics, some anticonvulsants may increase risk
• Female, white or Asian
• Lack of exercise
• Lack of calcium in diet or supplements
• Oophorectomy (removal of ovaries)—risk increases post-surgery

Diseases of Joints

Most of the diseases of joints occur as a slow degenerative process, so they tend to be more common with age. As with diseases of bones, diseases of the joints often result in the individual requiring assistive devices or artificial parts to maintain mobility. Frequently, damage to joints occurring during youth is not apparent until middle or older adulthood.

Arthritis. Arthritis (arthro = joint, itis = inflammation) and rheumatism are terms commonly used to describe a variety of conditions that cause pain and stiffness in the musculoskeletal system. Both are terms that cover a broad group of conditions but arthritis is a condition of inflammation in a joint, whereas rheumatism is a condition of stiffness. Arthritis is any inflammation of a joint. Everyone at some time or another has had arthritis; for example, a sprained ankle or jammed finger are arthritic conditions. Arthritis can be divided into two main groups: osteoarthritis and rheumatoid arthritis. Osteoarthritis is the most common form of arthritis, but rheumatoid arthritis is the more serious and debilitating type.

Osteoarthritis or Degenerative Joint Disease. Osteoarthritis is a degenerative process or a "wearing out" of a joint. It may begin in the early twenties, with ninety percent of all adults showing some radiologic changes. The amount or degree of wear is associated with several factors (Table 10–3). Sports injuries speed the "wear and tear" on the joints leading to osteoarthritis at a younger age.

Older adults are usually symptomatic with this type of arthritis. It often affects frequently used joints such as those in the hands, and joints that are weight bearing such as those of the spine, hip, and knee. Affected joints of the hands often swell and are painful. The distal and proximal **interphalangeal** (inter = between, phalangeal = finger bones) joints are often affected and may lead to a crooked deformity of the fingers. The **metacarpophalangeal** (meta = beyond, carpo = wrist, phalangeal = finger bones) joints are usually not affected (Figure 10–7).

TABLE 10–3 Risk Factors for Osteoarthritis

The following are considered factors that would increase the risk of developing osteoarthritis:
• Family history of osteoarthritis
• Excessive wear and tear or injury to joints
• Obesity
• Age—risk increases with age
• Female

Osteoarthritis that affects weight-bearing joints often affects the spine, hips, and knees. As the joints of the spinal column are affected with arthritis, individuals may become symptomatic with back pain. Osteoarthritis affects the hips and knees by wearing away the **articular** (are-TICK-you-lar) cartilage at the end of the long bones where bones articulate or meet. Eventually the entire surface of the cartilage may be worn away exposing areas of raw bone. When this occurs, new bone forms in and around the joint causing the bone ends to thicken. Fragments of this new bone are called osteophyte, or bone spurs, and often lead to a decrease in joint motion. X-ray examination may reveal the spurs and only small patches of cartilage on the bone ends. This is called a "bone on bone" condition. Osteoarthritis peaks in the fifth to sixth decade of life with approximately eighty percent of individuals showing symptoms by age seventy.

Treatment for osteoarthritis includes rest, non-weight-bearing exercise such as swimming and biking, heat, and use of analgesics and anti-inflammatory medications. Severe osteoarthritis may be treated by steroid injections into the joint capsule to relieve pain. Total surgical joint replacement may be recommended.

Rheumatoid Arthritis. Rheumatoid arthritis is discussed in Chapter 12 as an autoimmune disorder that not only affects the joints, but also affects the connective tissues of the entire body. Rheumatoid arthritis often affects the lungs, heart, and blood vessels causing the individual to appear chronically ill. This type of arthritis often affects people in the prime of life and affects women more often than men. It is a debilitating chronic disease that destroys the joints. A noticeable difference in the way osteoarthritis and rheumatoid arthritis affect the joints can be observed in joints of the hand. Osteoarthritis, as discussed, affects the working joints of the hand (primarily the distal and proximal interphalangeal joints) causing swelling and pain. All joints of the hand may be affected in the hand of rheumatoid individuals often with noticeable deformity and destruction in the metacarpophalangeal joints (see Figure 10–7). Also, refer to Chapter 12 for more information on rheumatoid arthritis.

Gout. Gout is often called gouty arthritis as this condition leads to inflammation of the affected joints. Gout is caused by a metabolic error in the breakdown of certain protein foods. Individuals with gout deposit uric acid crystals in joints of the body. The primary joint that is affected is the **metatarsophalangeal** (meta = between, tarso =

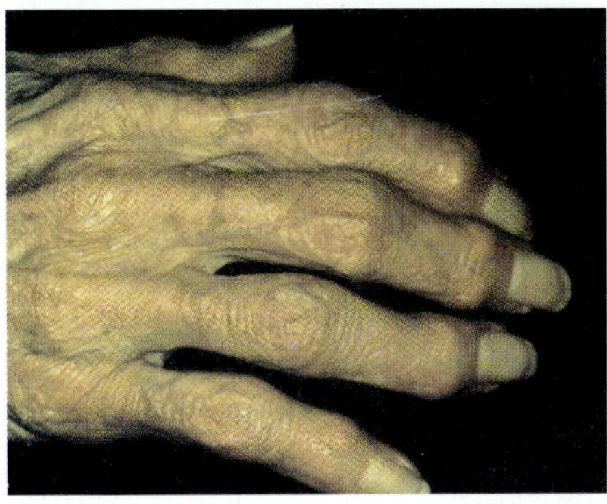

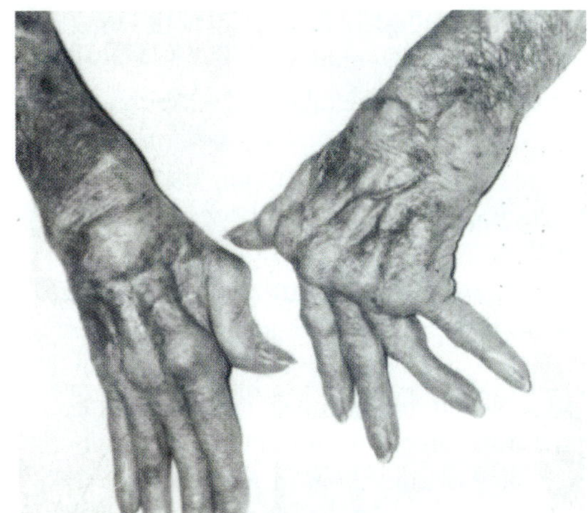

Figure 10–7 Comparison of (A) osteoarthritis and (B) rheumatoid arthritis: hands and joints.

foot, phalangeal = toe bones) joint of the big toe. These uric acid crystals have razor sharp edges that irritate the joint causing an acute inflammatory response. Symptoms are redness, heat, swelling, and pain in the joint.

Gout affects primarily males with approximately ninety-five percent of gout patients being male. Onset is usually after age thirty. Chronic gout may be characterized by uric acid deposited in subcutaneous tissue as well. These deposits appear as small whitish nodules called **tophi** and are commonly seen in the soft tissue of the ear (Figure 10–8). Kidney dysfunction and an increase in the occurrence of kidney stones is common with chronic gout. Treatment may include dietary adjustments to decrease the amount of protein consumed and anti-gout medication. Weight loss in obese patients may also be beneficial.

Diseases of Muscle and Connective Tissue

Diseases of muscle and connective tissue, unlike many of the bone disorders, are quite common in the very young or young adult individuals. Some of these disorders, such as the muscular dystrophies, are chronic, progressive, and devastating to families as they usually result in early death. Other disorders of the muscle and connective tissue are considered to be rather minor and may be treated medically or surgically.

Muscular Dystrophy (MD). Muscular dystrophy is an inherited genetic disorder that affects skeletal muscle. This condition is discussed later in this chapter under Developmental and Genetic Disorders.

Myasthenia Gravis. Myasthenia gravis (MY-uh-**STHEE**-nee-uh GRAV-iss) is an autoimmune disorder characterized by muscle weakness and fatigue that is somewhat relieved with rest. The problem is related to blocking of the neurotransmitter, acetylcholine, by antibodies in the neuromuscular junction. Myasthenia gravis is reviewed in detail in Chapter 12.

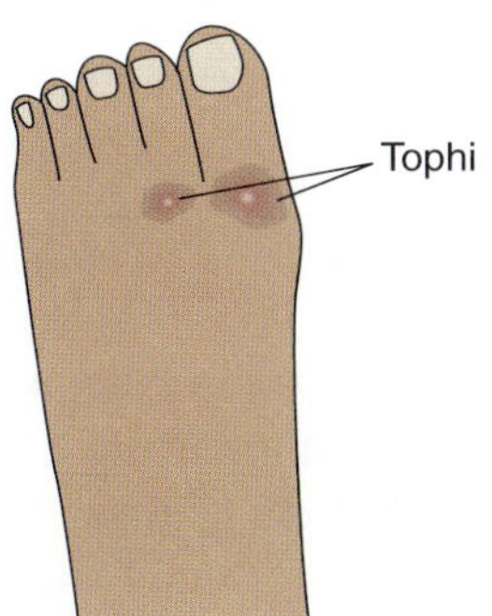

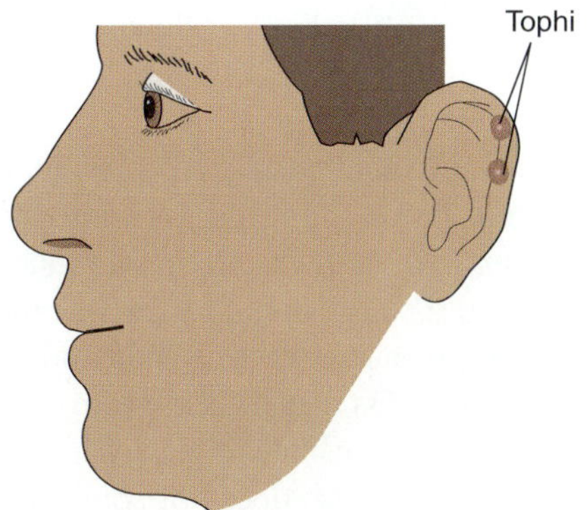

Figure 10–8 Sites affected by gout.

Tetanus. Tetanus, also called lockjaw, is an acute, infectious, life-threatening disease characterized by painful, uncontrolled contractions of skeletal muscle. A toxin produced by the bacillus bacterium, *Clostridium tetani*, causes tetanus. This bacterium is commonly found in animal feces, and when excreted lives as spores in the soil. The number of these spores is especially high in barnyards, pastures, or garden areas fertilized with animal manure. When this infectious bacterium enters the body in an **anaerobic** (ana = without, erobic = air) wound, such as that provided in a puncture wound, it multiplies and produces a dangerous toxin. This toxin travels in the blood and attaches to motor or muscle neurons, where it irritates the nerve producing the stimulus for skeletal muscle contraction.

The bacterial toxin affects the nervous system rather slowly. The further the distance between the wound and the spinal cord the slower the progression. One to three weeks may pass before the onset of symptoms. The jaw muscles are often the first muscles affected with **tetany** (TET-ah-nee) or rigid muscle contraction. The individual may not be able to open the mouth, hence the term "lockjaw." Eventually, muscles of the esophagus, neck, back, arms, and legs are affected. Other symptoms are a high fever, tachycardia (rapid pulse rate), dysphagia (difficulty swallowing), and intense pain.

Treatment is a prompt and immediate cleansing of wounds, with special consideration given to puncture-type wounds. Immunization may be needed depending on the individual's immunization history. If the individual has not received a tetanus toxoid injection in the past five years, an antitoxin may be given. Tetanus toxoid injection will cause the immune system to build antibodies. Tetanus toxoid should initially be administered to children as part of basic immunization with DPT (diphtheria, pertussis, and tetanus). Tetanus antibodies need to be "boosted" approximately every seven to ten years throughout life. An antitoxin may be given to prevent tetanus following an injury, as the body does not have time to build up its own antibodies. Following this episode, it is usually recommended that the individual follow up with the proper tetanus toxoid booster.

Care of an individual with tetanus includes symptomatic treatment, primarily respiratory, nutritional, and hydration support. Antibiotics and muscle relaxants may also be administered. Even with the best of care, tetanus can be fatal from respiratory failure. If the individual survives, the disease process usually lasts six to eight weeks. Surprisingly, the disease usually does not leave any permanent disability, but it also does not confer any lasting immunity to tetanus.

Rhabdomyolysis. Rhabdomyolysis is any event that results in muscle necrosis or damage. Events that can cause rhabdomyolysis include direct trauma, third and fourth degree burns, severe muscle ischemia (e.g., from acute compartment syndrome), medications, infections, and genetic defects. When the muscle tissue is damaged, water, sodium chloride (NaCl), and calcium enter the cells. Potassium, phosphate, lactic acid, myoglobin, and creatinine are among the materials that leave the damaged muscle cells in large quantities. This increase in circulating waste products tends to overload the kidneys, inducing acute kidney failure. Additionally, the resulting hypovolemia, hypocalcemia, and hyperkalemia are cardiotoxic and may produce arrhythmias and cardiac ischemia. Metabolic acidosis (Chapter 5) and disseminated intravascular coagulation (DIC, discussed in Chapter 16) can also occur as a result of rhabdomyolysis.

Symptoms of rhabdomyolysis may include a history of drug ingestion, trauma, shock, or infection, and reddish–brown colored urine caused by myoglobin in the urine. Signs of rhabdomyolysis may include an elevated body temperature, evidence of trauma or infection, dehydration, muscle weakness or swelling, and elevation of the electrolyte levels discussed above. Signs of metabolic acidosis, DIC, and renal failure (Chapter 14) may also be present. Treatment includes vigorous fluid replacement with the goal of maintaining good urine output. Mannitol or furosemide may be administered to assist in diuresis, and the urine may be alkalinized with sodium bicarbonate in patients who are not producing urine. Significant hyperkalemia may require dialysis treatment to decrease blood potassium concentration. If the patient is symptomatic or ECG changes are present (see Figure 10–9), medical control may direct treatment with calcium chloride or calcium gluconate to protect the heart; insulin and glucose to assist in moving potassium back into the cells; furosemide to help excrete potassium via the kidneys; and sodium bicarbonate to treat acidosis. Because of the electrolyte changes, the patient's ECG should be continuously monitored. The inciting event also requires treatment, for example, surgical treatment of a compartment syndrome or antimicrobial treatment of sepsis.

Neoplasms

Primary neoplasms of the musculoskeletal system are uncommon. Typically, neoplasms of this system are secondary, metastasizing from the lungs, breast, and prostate. The most common primary tumor of bone is osteosarcoma. Primary tumors of the bone marrow include myeloma or multiple myeloma, and Ewing's sar-

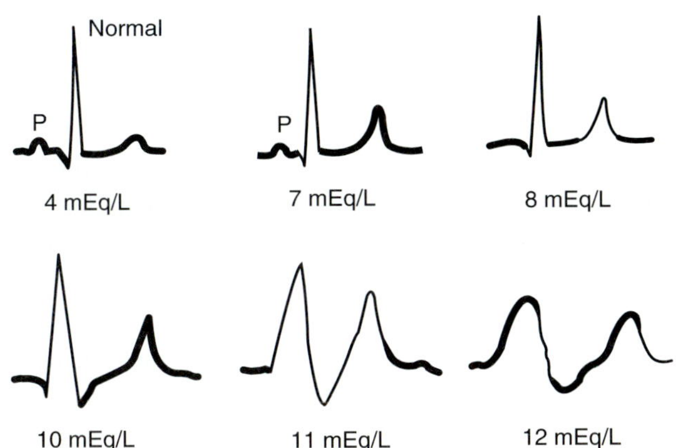

Figure 10–9 ECG tracing in a patient with the progressive changes in the QRS complex associated with specific serum potassium levels.

coma. Myeloma is the most common marrow tumor. It affects the pelvis, vertebra, and long bones of adults. Ewing's sarcoma affects primarily long bones in children and teens. It is highly malignant and quickly metastasizes to nearly every organ of the body. Kaposi's sarcoma affects soft tissue of primarily immunosuppressed individuals. Rhabdomyosarcoma is a very rare, but highly malignant, tumor of skeletal muscle.

Symptoms of musculoskeletal tumors may include pathologic fracture and bone pain. Clinical examination followed by radiologic studies, CT scan, blood studies, and biopsy often confirm the diagnosis. Treatment of malignant tumors of the musculoskeletal system may include radiation, chemotherapy, and surgery. Surgical procedures often involve excision and amputation. Even with aggressive therapy, prognosis for these malignant neoplasms is often very poor.

TRAUMA

Trauma is the main cause of problems in the musculoskeletal system. Fractures are by far the most common and frequent injury to bone. Tennis elbow is the most frequent ailment of the upper body. Treatment for sprains and strains are among the top ten reasons that patients seek medical attention for acute disease. Low back pain is in the top ten for chronic disease.

Fracture

A fracture is any discontinuity of a bone. A fracture and a "break" are synonymous, although a **stress** (related to too much weight bearing or pressure) fracture or incomplete fracture may not "break" the bone in two. Fractures may be caused by trauma (injury) or may be **pathologic** (caused by weakness from another disease).

Types of Fractures. Fractures may be classified in a number of ways. One method of classification is based on the condition of the overlying skin. If the bone has protruded through the skin or an object has punctured the skin making an opening through the skin to the fracture site, it is an **open** fracture. Open fractures are also called **compound** fractures, because the fracture plus the open skin is compounding the problem. An open fracture is always an emergency, because of the high risk of infection. Patients with open fractures are taken to surgery for cleaning and débridement. If there is no opening in the skin, it is called a **closed** or **simple** fracture.

Another method of classification considers the condition of the bone. If the fracture goes completely through the bone, it is a **complete** fracture. If the bone is fractured but not in two, it is an **incomplete** fracture. A common incomplete fracture that occurs in children is called a **greenstick** fracture, because it appears to have broken partially like a sap-filled green stick.

Fractures may also be described by the number of fragments or the position of the fragments. A **displaced** fracture is one in which fragments are out of position, while non-displaced means the fragments are still in correct position. An **angulated** fracture is a fracture of a long bone that is positioned such that the bone is bent out of place. If there are more than two ends or fragments, the break is a **comminuted** fracture. Bone appearing to be mashed down is a compression fracture. A common site of a compression fracture is in the vertebrae. An **impacted** fracture is one characterized as a bone end forced over the other end. **Avulsion** fracture describes a separation of a small bone fragment from the bone where a tendon or ligament is attached.

The position of the fracture line as compared to bone position may also describe the fracture. A **longitudinal** fracture runs the length of the bone, while a **transverse** fracture runs across or at a 90 degree angle. **Oblique** fractures run transversely at less than 90 degrees, while **spiral** fractures twist around the bone. **Stellate** fractures form a star-like pattern, commonly seen on the skull or patella.

Location may be used to describe the fracture. An articular fracture involves a joint surface. **Intracapsular** and **extracapsular** describe fractures inside or outside the joint capsule. **Intertrochanteric** describes fractures in the trochanter of the femur, while **femoral neck** and **subcapital** fractures describe fractures located on the femur. Finally, fractures may be named by the physician who first described them, for example, **Colle's** and **Pott's** fractures (Figure 10–10).

To be very specific, a fracture may be more clearly defined by using several descriptive names. For example, a diagnosis of a "closed fracture" is a broad diagnosis covering many different fractures. A more descriptive diagnosis would be a "closed, comminuted fracture." An even clearer diagnosis would be a "closed, comminuted femoral neck fracture."

Sites and causes of fractures vary by age and gender. Children commonly fracture their arms during falls. Teen males commonly have long bone fractures related to MVAs (motor vehicle accidents) or sports injuries. Elderly females suffer with hip fractures generally related to falls and osteoporosis.

Treatment of Fractures. Treatment of fractures involves splinting the affected body part in a manner that immobilizes the fracture ends but does not affect circulation and neurologic function distal to the fracture. In general, suspected fractures of the shaft of the bone require immobilization of the joints above and below the fracture site. Suspected fractures involving a joint require immobilization of the bones on either side of the joint. Patients with suspected spinal fractures can be immobilized with a cervical collar and long backboard, and pneumatic anti-shock garment / military anti-shock trousers (PASG / MAST) can be used to immobilize a suspected pelvic fracture. Regardless of the location of the suspected fracture, the EMS provider must assess distal motor, neurologic, and circulatory function prior to immobilization and after immobilization.

Angulated fractures generally require slightly different treatment. Depending upon your local protocol, angulated fractures should be splinted in the anatomical position of the bone to provide a more stable immobilization, better vascular supply, and reduce additional tissue injury during transport. Some protocols only allow EMS providers to straighten angulated fractures if the distal pulse is absent and others only allow one attempt to straighten the bone. As with any fracture, assess and document distal motor and neurovascular function before and after splinting.

Mid-shaft femur fractures in hemodynamically stable patients may be immobilized with a traction splint. When the femur is fractured, the leg muscles may go into spasm and displace the fractured ends, shortening the bone. Traction may be applied to stretch the leg muscles and return the femur ends to a normal position. This will generally reduce the spasm and pain associated with a femur fracture. In the case of a hemodynamically unstable patient (i.e., those in uncompensated shock) or a multiple trauma patient, the femur fracture may be immobilized by using the PASG/MAST or by immobilizing the femur to the long spine board.

At the hospital, the fracture may require reduction. If this can be accomplished without a surgical incision it is called a closed reduction. Closed reduction is common in fractures of the extremities. Radiography is utilized to confirm proper position of the bones. If the fracture cannot be reduced without internal manipulation, the area is surgically opened or incised and an open reduction is performed. Open reductions commonly require some type of internal fixation or holding device such as pins, plates, screws, or rods. This procedure is an **ORIF** (open reduction, internal fixation). Open fractures require surgical intervention to clean and débride the involved tissue. An open fracture site is usually cleansed with copious (excessive) amounts of fluid in an effort to prevent infection and osteomyelitis.

Complications of Fractures. Complications of fractures include hemorrhage, mal-union, non-union, avascular necrosis, and infection. Blood loss from long bone fractures can be significant. Fractures of the tibia and fibula can involve the loss of up to 550 cubic centimeters (cc) of blood. Patients with a femur fracture can lose one liter of blood, while a patient with a pelvic fracture can lose up to two liters of blood. All patients who have suspected fractures require repeated assessment for shock. Malunion is the healing of the fracture in an abnormal or nonfunctional position. Non-union is the failure of the bone to heal. The complication of avascular necroses occurs when the blood supply to the bone is not adequate to maintain bone health and the bone tissue dies of necrosis. Infection of the bone was discussed in detail as osteomyelitis.

Strains and Sprains

A strain is an injury from overstretching a muscle leading to soreness, pain, and tenderness. Individuals commonly have lumbar strains from lifting too much weight, lifting improperly, or lifting repetitively. Strained backs are common after a weekend of activity by an individual not in proper condition. Treatment includes rest, moist heat, and the use of analgesics and anti-inflammatory medications. A strain is less serious than a sprain.

A sprain is a traumatic injury to a joint with partial or complete tearing of ligaments (Figure 10–11). The ankle joint is commonly affected and may become so painful that the joint cannot be used. The degree of

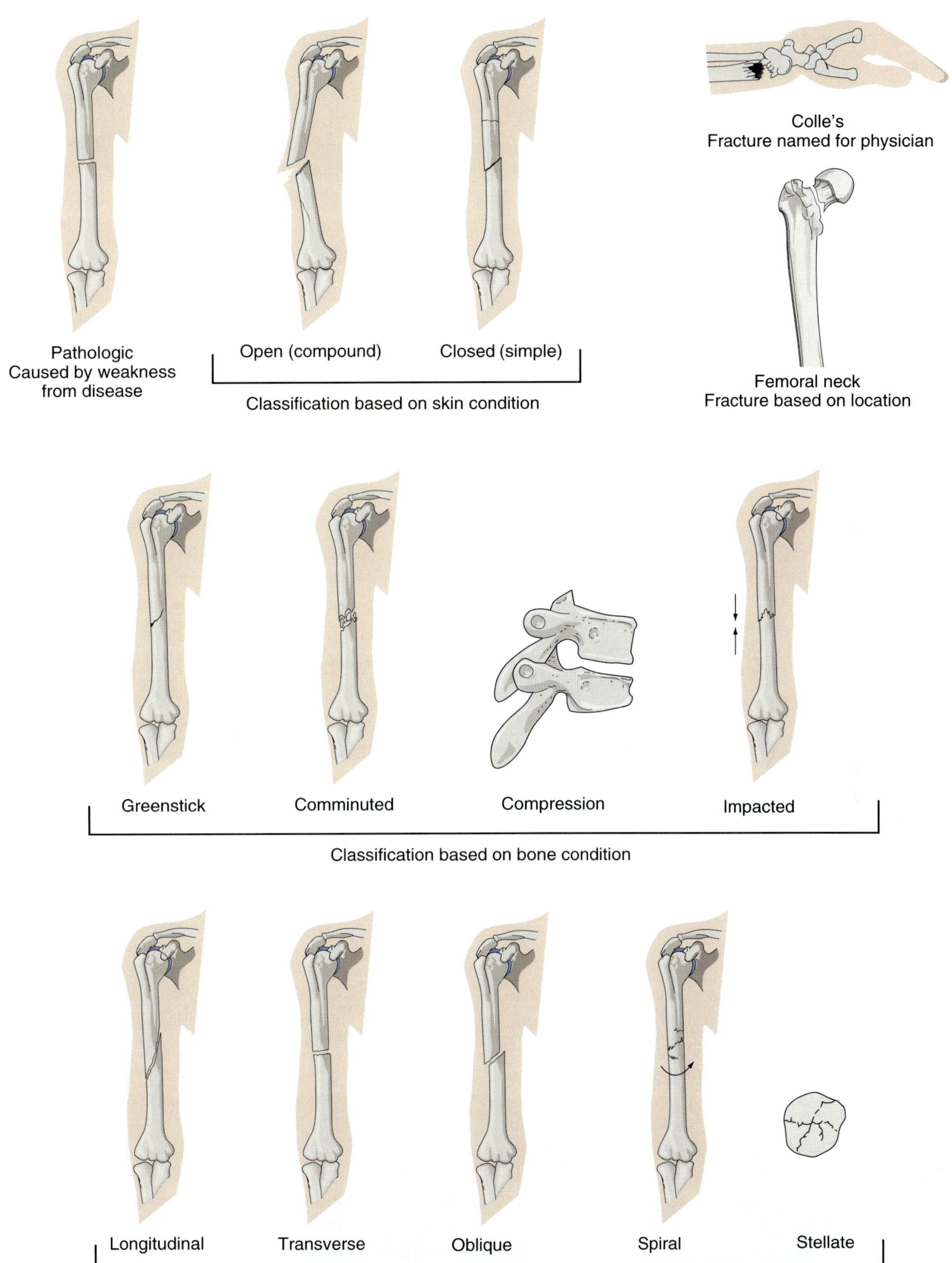

Figure 10–10 Types of fractures.

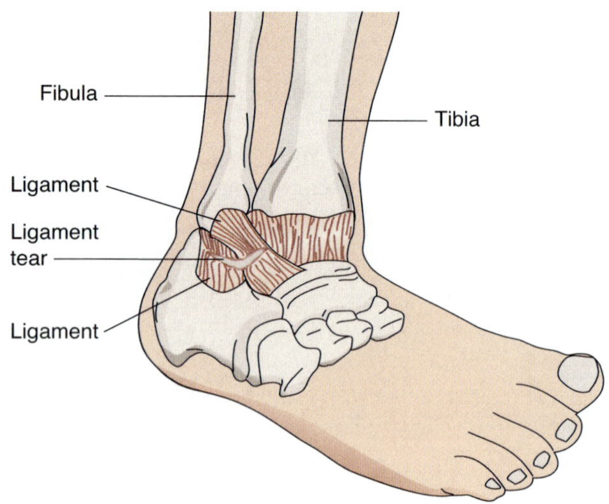

Figure 10–11 Sprained ankle.

ligament tearing plus involvement of associated tendons, muscles, and blood vessels determines the degree of injury. Sprains are classified into three different types based upon the amount of damage. A first degree sprain involves microscopic tears of the ligament. This causes some swelling and more localized tenderness but the joint is still stable. A second degree sprain involves a severe stretch and partial tear of the ligament. Typically there is moderate tenderness and swelling, mild bruising, and some pain while bearing weight on the joint. A second degree sprain also involves a minor loss of function or stability in the joint. A third degree sprain involves the complete rupture of the ligament, causing severe pain, moderate swelling, bruising, and an inability to bear weight. While there is no bony deformity present or fracture on a radiograph, the joint is generally unstable because of ligament rupture.

Treatment for sprains includes the concepts of "**RICE**," rest, ice, compression, and elevation (Healthy Highlight 10–1). Treatment in the field will generally also involve immobilization of the affected joint in the same manner as if a fracture were suspected. In the emergency department, some suspected sprains will be evaluated with an X-ray exam to determine if an underlying fracture is present. For ankle sprains, this will involve patients who are unable to walk unassisted four steps, those with tenderness over their medial or lateral malleoli (the two "bumps" just above the ankle), or tenderness over the proximal portion of the fifth metatarsal.

HEALTHY HIGHLIGHT 10-1

RICE

RICE, an acronym for **R**est, **I**ce, **C**ompression, **E**levation can be used effectively for almost all types of injury from a sprained ankle to a broken bone. When an injury occurs, RICE should be followed for the first twenty-four hours.

REST—Immediate non-weight bearing rest will prevent further damage. Rest includes use of splints, slings, and crutches.

ICE—Application of ice slows bleeding and swelling by causing vasoconstriction. The more blood that collects in an area, the longer the healing time. Ice should not be applied directly to the skin. Wrap the ice pack in a towel before application. Alternate ice treatment, 30 minutes on and 15 minutes off, is a general rule. Heat is applied after twenty-four hours to improve vascular flow and carry away tissue debris.

COMPRESSION—Application of a compression stocking or ace wrap will provide support and limit swelling, speeding healing time. Compression devices should be snug but not so tight as to cut off circulation leading to increased pain and numbness.

ELEVATION—Place the injured area at a height above the heart to allow gravity to assist venous flow to further reduce swelling.

Dislocations and Subluxations

Dislocation is the complete separation of a bone end from its normal position in a joint. A subluxation is a partial separation (Figure 10-12). Dislocations occur with major traumatic injuries such as MVAs, contact sports, or falls. A dislocation injury may also cause a fracture. Dislocations may also be related to joint abnormalities or disease. In the case of disease, the dislocation may occur frequently and without cause.

Dislocation causes acute pain and obvious joint deformity. In ball and socket joints, the ball may be totally anterior or posterior to the socket. The joint tissue rapidly swells making reduction difficult. For this reason, a dislocated joint should be reduced or repositioned by a physician immediately. If protocol and training allows, some EMS providers may reduce uncomplicated dislocations in the field to reduce discomfort and facilitate trans-

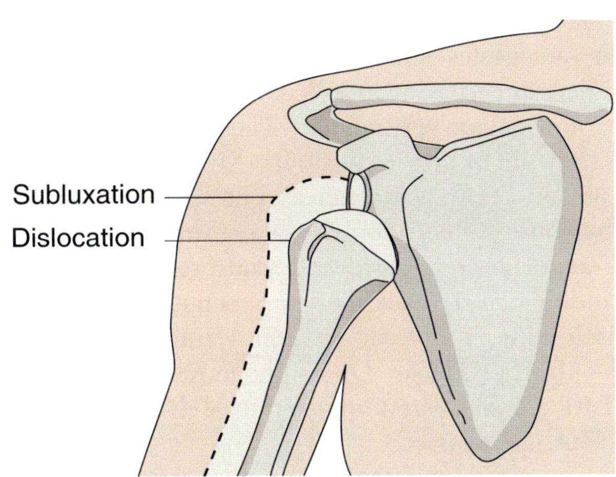

Figure 10-12 Dislocation and subluxation.

portation. Even with emergency treatment, general anesthesia may be needed for the reduction procedure. If the joint ligaments become weakened with repeated dislocations, surgery may be necessary to tighten the ligaments thereby strengthening the joint.

Crush Injury

A crush injury is an injury sustained from a compressive force that is large enough to interfere with the normal function of the affected tissue. A crush injury may involve an extremity or the entire body. Common complications of a crush injury include compromise of neurovascular function distal to the injury caused by direct damage to the blood and nerve supply; compartment syndrome caused by bleeding into an extremity compartment; rhabdomyolysis and electrolyte and acid-base disturbances caused by the products released when muscle cells die; shock; acute renal failure; and death.

A crush injury to an extremity should be treated similarly to a fracture. Any hemorrhage should be controlled and neurovascular and motor function should be assessed before and after immobilization of the affected extremity. For pelvic crush injuries, the PASG/MAST may be used to stabilize the fracture and assist in hemorrhage control. Crush injuries to the head, chest, abdomen, and pelvis carry high mortality rates. Crush injuries to the extremities typically require extensive reconstruction or amputation and long-term rehabilitation.

Compartment Syndrome

Compartment syndrome results from an increase in compartment pressure in an extremity and can cause neurovascular compromise and ischemia. In the upper and lower extremities, layers of fascia surround muscle groups forming compartments. Within these compartments lie the blood and nerve supply in addition to the muscles. If the pressure within the compartment increases to a level above the capillary pressure in the compartment, then no exchange of oxygen and nutrients will occur in the cells within that compartment, resulting in cell death.

Classic symptoms of compartment syndrome follow the "Five Ps." The five classic symptoms of compartment syndrome are *pain*, *pallor*, *pulselessness*, *paresthesias*, and *puffiness*. The pain from compartment syndrome can range from a dull ache to excruciating pain over a muscular area of the extremity. Pallor and pulselessness are caused by vascular compromise and decreased blood flow into that extremity. Paresthesia is a sense of "pins and needles" caused by nerve compression or irritation. The complaint of paresthesia may be located over the compartment or may be in an area distal to the compartment. The puffiness is caused by muscle swelling and vascular and lymphatic congestion. The swelling may also be assessed by the EMS provider when comparing the affected leg to the unaffected leg. Compartment pressure, sometimes called the sixth "P," is assessed in the emergency department directly by placing a needle attached to a gauge into the compartment and reading the pressure.

Compartment syndrome can be divided into acute and chronic. Chronic compartment syndrome is typically caused by overuse of the muscles within the compartment. The muscles swell from overuse, and are used again before they can repair themselves. This swelling over time can put pressure on the neurovascular structures within the compartment and decrease the amount of oxygen delivered to them. Acute compartment syndrome occurs as a result of trauma, for example, a crush injury, or as a result of a sudden overuse, as in the example of a patient who is generally sedentary and runs several miles on the first run. Acute compartment syndrome is serious in that neurovascular function within the compartment is compromised and the structures within the compartment have approximately four to six hours before tissue death begins to occur. Aggressive treatment is necessary in order to save function of the affected extremity.

Treatment of compartment syndrome is different if it is chronic or acute. Chronic compartment syndrome can be responsive to rest, ice, and elevation, all aimed to reduce swelling and allow repair. The patient can perform this at home before and after a competition or vigorous exercise to reduce swelling. Because of the severity of acute compartment syndrome, these patients often require surgery to correct the neurovascular compromise associated with acute compartment syndrome. This surgery, called a fasciotomy, involves making an incision in the fascial layer that covers the compartment, allowing the pressure to release, and restoring neurovascular function to the extremity.

Low Back Pain (LBP)

Low back pain is a very common disorder of the musculoskeletal system. This pain may be acute and resolve in a few days or it may be a chronic discomfort that lasts a lifetime. The low back or lumbar area of the spine is very susceptible to stress or strain. This stress may be increased by such factors as obesity, poor posture, weak abdominal muscles, and constant or improper lifting. These factors are more likely to cause low back pain in individuals who have spinal deformities or diseases affecting the spine.

Some disorders that affect the spine and often lead to LBP include spinal deformities, osteoarthritis, rheumatoid arthritis, osteoporosis, and bone cancer to name just a few. X-ray examinations are usually helpful in determining the cause of LBP, but further detailed study with CT scan or MRI may be needed.

Treatment of acute LBP is usually rest, warm moist heat, analgesics and anti-inflammatory medications. Lumbar **spasms** (uncontrolled muscle contractions) are common and are very painful. These spasms often twist the back out of normal position. Muscle relaxants may be prescribed for acute attacks, but rest and application of heat are usually adequate to control spasms. Once the acute attack subsides, a daily exercise program including aerobic walking is very beneficial in building muscle tone, increasing flexibility, and decreasing the risk of further attacks. One of the most common causes of LBP is a herniated intervertebral disc or herniated nucleus pulposus.

Herniated Nucleus Pulposus (HNP). HNP is commonly called herniated disc, ruptured disc, slipped disc, or bulging disc. All these different terms are very similar. The problem is the protrusion of the soft center (nucleus pulposus) of a disc on the spinal cord or spinal nerve (Figure 10–13). Pressure on the spinal nerve may cause pain in the distribution of the sciatic nerve, called **sciatica**, which radiates down the backside of the leg.

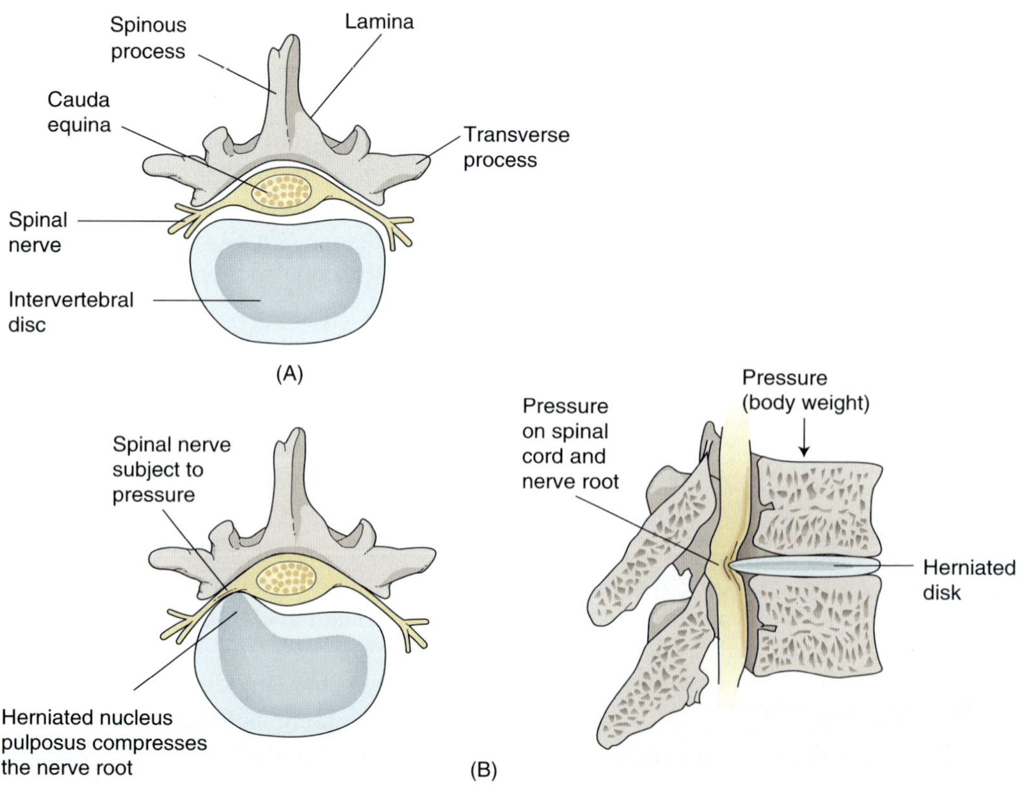

Figure 10–13 (A) Normal intervertebral disc (B) Two views of a herniated disc.

Diagnosis involves physical examination often confirmed by CT scan, MRI, or **myelogram**. A myelogram involves injecting dye into the spinal canal and taking pictures to reveal compression on the spinal cord or spinal nerves.

Treatment of HNP is often the same as for LBP. Extensive exercise therapy may reduce the size of the protrusion and relieve the associated LBP. If pain persists after therapy or if the disc is found to be causing severe spinal cord or spinal nerve compression, surgery for disc removal may be needed. Cauda equina syndrome is a neurologic emergency where a lumbar disc is compressing the distal end of the spinal cord to the point where the patient loses bowel and bladder continence. The patient may also complain of pins and needles or a loss of feeling between his legs. Emergency surgery is performed to relieve pressure from the cord in the hope of restoring nerve function. Surgery to remove the disc or to cut away vertebra to open the area around the nerve is called a **discectomy** or **laminectomy**, respectively.

Bursitis

Bursitis (ber-SIE-tis) is the inflammation of a bursa or small fluid-filled sacs that surround joints. Bursae help to reduce friction during movement. Repetitive motions often lead to irritation of the bursa resulting in bursitis. Any joint may be affected, but bursitis of the shoulder is the most common type. Bursitis affecting the knee and elbow is also common.

Symptoms include severe pain that limits motion in the joint. Rest, application of moist heat, and use of analgesics and anti-inflammatory medications will usually resolve the condition. If bursitis persists, further treatment of the bursa includes injection with corticosteroids, draining, and surgical excision. Active range-of-motion exercises are needed after pain subsides to regain and maintain joint motion.

Tendonitis

Tendonitis is inflammation of a tendon, or the connective tissue that attaches muscle to bone. Tendonitis may occur in any tendon, but most often it affects the shoulder. It may be caused by calcium deposits or repetitive motion injury. Athletes in baseball, basketball, swimming, and tennis are often affected. Tendonitis may also be in association with bursitis. Treatment is rest, application of ice (which may irritate bursitis), and use of analgesics and anti-inflammatory medications. Active range-of-motion exercises may be initiated once the pain subsides in order to restore motion. If joint adhesions have developed, surgical intervention may be necessary to free the joint and restore mobility.

Torn Rotator Cuff

The rotator cuff is a group of muscles that hold the head of the humerus in the shoulder socket area. Tears in the tendons that hold these muscles to the bone produce a snapping sound followed by acute pain and the inability of the individual to abduct (move away from midline) or raise the arm. Tears are commonly traumatic injuries of baseball, basketball, and tennis.

Diagnosis is made by physical examination and may be confirmed with an MRI. Acute rotator cuff tears are surgically repaired to restore motion of the shoulder. Active rehabilitation exercise is needed postoperatively to restore shoulder function.

Torn Meniscus

There are two semilunar cartilages in each knee joint that form a lateral and medial meniscus. The meniscus (meh-NIS-cuss) is attached to the top of the tibia and provides cushion for the distal femur. Athletes participating in football, baseball, soccer, and tennis commonly injure a meniscus. The tear usually results from a sudden twisting of the leg while the knee is flexed (Figure 10–14A).

Symptoms include acute pain with weight bearing on the affected knee. The individual may feel that the knee is "locking or giving." Full flexion or extension of the knee may not be possible because of increased pain or swelling. X-ray or MRI may be needed to confirm the diagnosis. Treatment is immobilization, elevation, and application of ice to decrease inflammation and pain. Analgesics and anti-inflammatory medications may also be needed. If surgical treatment is needed, it is commonly done arthroscopically or with the use of a scope to look into the knee. An extensive exercise rehabilitation program is begun postoperatively.

Cruciate Ligament Tears

Cruciate (shaped like a cross) ligaments are located inside the knee joint (Figure 10–14B). They work as a pair; the anterior cruciate ligament and the posterior cruciate ligament form a cross giving the knee front to back and rotary stability. These ligaments are often injured when the leg is twisted or hit from the front or back while in a planted or weight-bearing position. Diagnosis involves clinical examination, joint stability testing, and possible CT scanning. Treatment depends on the degree of injury and may vary from immobilization to surgical intervention.

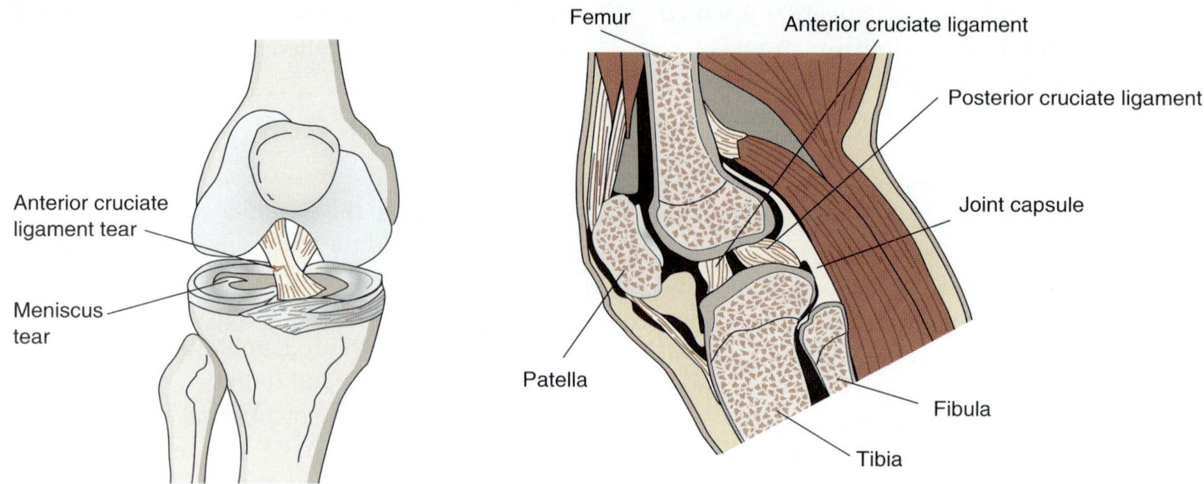

Figure 10–14 (A) Meniscus and anterior cruciate ligament tear (B) cruciate ligaments.

Shin Splints

Shin splints is a term used to describe an overuse injury to the periosteum and extensor muscles of the lower leg. Pain and tenderness along the inner aspect of the tibia which worsen with exercise and disappear with rest are common symptoms. Shin splints occur routinely with a sudden increase in activity or a new exercise routine. This disorder commonly occurs in runners, joggers, and high-impact aerobics enthusiasts. Running on hard surfaces may also cause the problem. Diagnosis is usually based on clinical examination, but X-ray examination may be utilized to rule out a stress fracture.

Rest, analgesics, anti-inflammatory medications, and alternating ice and heat treatments are usually beneficial. Proper conditioning, stretching exercises, and padded exercise shoes assist in preventing this disorder.

GENETIC AND DEVELOPMENTAL DISORDERS

Genetic and developmental musculoskeletal disorders are some of the more familiar severe disorders. The severity of the disease varies with the particular disorder, and other problems the individual may have.

Muscular Dystrophy (MD)

Muscular dystrophy (dys = abnormal, trophic = nourishment, growth) is a group of genetically inherited diseases characterized by degeneration or weakening of the muscles. The affected muscles are unable to store needed protein. Malnourished muscle fibers die and are replaced with fat and connective tissue. Fat and connective tissue fibers are unable to contract and function like muscle fibers resulting in progressive weakness. Over a period of time the muscle digresses from weak to useless. The most common type of muscular dystrophy is Duchenne's MD. Duchenne's is also called pseudohypertrophic (pseudo = false, hyper = excessive, trophic = nourishment, growth) MD because the affected muscle appears healthy and bulging when in reality the muscle is bulking up in size from fat deposits. This bulking of muscle mass is especially noticeable in the calf muscle. Duchenne's MD is a sex-linked disorder generally passed from mother to son. Onset is usually between the ages of two to five years of age. The pelvic and leg muscles are usually affected first, leading to a characteristic waddling gait, toe walking, lordosis, and Gower's maneuver (a characteristic way of getting up from a squatting position that demonstrates the weakness of the pelvic muscles) (Figure 10–15). Affected children are usually confined to a wheelchair by age nine. Life expectancy is usually in the late teens or early twenties with death caused by respiratory or cardiac complications. Diagnosis is made on the basis of physical examination, muscle biopsy, and electromyography. Although there is no cure for MD, physical therapy, orthopedic appliances such as leg braces, and exercise are quite effective in maintaining mobility and quality of life.

Osteogenesis Imperfecta

Osteogenesis (osteo = bone, genesis = beginning) imperfecta (not perfect or normal) is an inherited condition characterized by abnormally brittle bones often leading to frequent fractures. Undiagnosed children affected with osteogenesis imperfecta may be suspected as victims of child abuse because of the frequency of

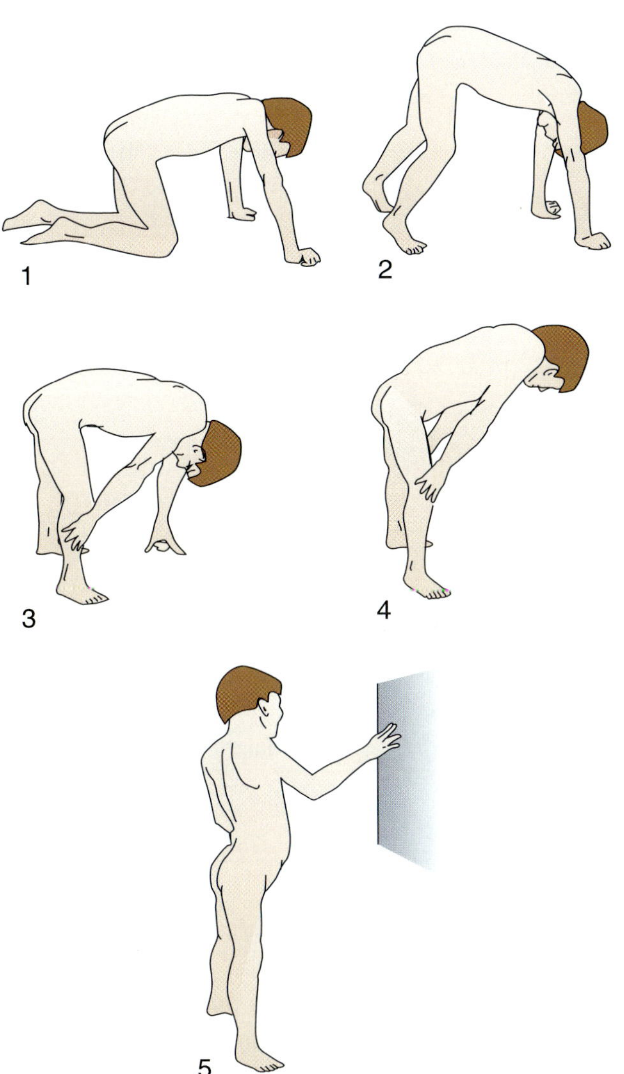

Figure 10-15 Gower's maneuver.

bone fractures. Other significant signs are an abnormally blue coloration of the sclera of the eyes, otosclerotic deafness, translucent skin, and thin dental enamel of the teeth. There is no cure for osteogenesis imperfecta but the tendency to fracture decreases with age and often disappears by adulthood.

EFFECTS OF AGING ON THE SYSTEM

Normal changes that occur in bones, joints, and muscles cause a variety of problems in the older adult. Bone density decreases with age as calcium is reabsorbed from the bone. This causes greater brittleness of the bone with increased risks for fractures. Osteoporosis is a common problem in the older adult, especially in older females because of its association with decreasing estrogen levels in the blood.

As the individual ages, muscles decrease in strength and mass. Some muscle cells atrophy and decrease in total number. Arm and leg muscles lose tone and become somewhat flaccid and flabby appearing.

Changes in height and curvature of the spine occur from changes in the vertebral discs and compression of the vertebrae. The water content of the vertebral discs decreases, causing them to become less flexible, contributing to the normal one-half to three-quarter inch loss in height. As muscles waste and joints stiffen, some loss of flexibility and agility is also common, along with an overall decreased mobility. New research is demonstrating the benefits of weight training and exercise classes for the older adult to prevent some of this muscle wasting, decrease in bone density, and loss of flexibility.

Musculoskeletal diseases, especially the debilitating ones such as arthritis, are extremely difficult for the older adult. Healing, for example, after a fracture, is slower and often impaired by other chronic disorders common to the older adult. Pain associated with these disorders and changes in the system tend to decrease the individual's mobility and independence even more. Safety issues are of utmost importance when musculoskeletal system disorders are present, as falls are one of the most common causes of injury in the older adult.

SUMMARY

The musculoskeletal system consists of bones, joints, muscles, ligaments, and tendons. It is the body's main framework and is responsible for all movements. Movements are the result of contraction and relaxation of the muscle fibers. The muscles are stimulated by responses from the nervous system. Most muscle movements are voluntary movements. The most common symptoms of musculoskeletal system disorders are pain, immobility, and disability. Diagnosis of a musculoskeletal system problem is usually made by assessment and X-ray or magnetic resonance imaging (MRI). However, other specific tests such as bone scans or arthroscopy may also be utilized. Fractures, sprains, and low back injuries are the most common musculoskeletal system complaints that the EMS provider will encounter. Changes in the musculoskeletal system in the older adult often lead to increased risk for fractures and disability.

REVIEW QUESTIONS

Short Answer

1. What are the major functions of the musculoskeletal system?

2. What are the common signs and symptoms associated with musculoskeletal system disorders?

3. What are the most common tests used to diagnose musculoskeletal system disorders?

Fill in the Blank

Fill in the blanks in the following statements:

4. A _______________ involves damage to a ligament.
5. _______________ attach muscle to bone.
6. When caring for a suspected fracture of the tibia/fibula, you should immobilize the fracture site and _______________.
7. An angulated fracture should be immobilized _______________.
8. Low back pain associated with loss of bowel and/or bladder function is a surgical emergency called _______________.
9. _______________ is a condition where muscle tissue is destroyed, causing electrolyte imbalance, myoglobin in the urine, and possible renal failure.

Matching

10. Match the fracture-related term in the left column with the appropriate description in the right column.

_____ Comminuted	a. Bone fragments are in correct position
_____ Non-displaced	b. One bone end is forced over another
_____ Transverse	c. More than two ends or fragments present
_____ Greenstick	d. Bone has protruded through the skin
_____ Stress	e. An incomplete fracture common in children
_____ Impacted	f. Fracture runs across or at a 90-degree angle
_____ Compound	g. Caused by too much weight bearing or pressure

CASE STUDY

You respond to the house of Estella Gore, a 76-year-old woman whom you have seen before for cardiac issues. Today, a neighbor called EMS because he found Ms. Gore on the floor after falling during the night. She is complaining of pain in the area of her right hip and proximal femur and was unable to get herself up from the floor. What factors would put Ms. Gore at an increased risk for fractures? How can you immobilize her hip? How can you assess her for complications of her suspected fracture?

BIBLIOGRAPHY

A death foretold. (1996). *People Weekly, 45*, 89–90+.

Aldous, P. (August 10, 1997). Adding exercise to injury. *New Scientist, 151*, 17.

Brander, V. A., Stulberg S. D., & Chang, R. W. (1994). Rehabilitation following hip and knee arthroplasty. *Joint Disease, 5(4)*, 815.

Buck, M., & Paice, J. (1994). Pharmacologic management of acute pain in the orthopaedic patient. *Orthopaedic Nursing, 13(6)*, 14.

Buckwalter, J. A. (December 21–28, 1996 supp). Healing of bones, cartilages, tendons, and ligaments: A new era. *Lancet, 348, psII*, 118.

Cohen, P. (June 22, 1996). Broken bones heal better with DNA. *New Scientist, 150*, 14.

Cummings, S. R. (December 26, 1996). Hip fracture. *The New England Journal of Medicine, 335*, 1994–1996.

Deathe, A., & Hayes, K. (Winter 1993). The biomechanics of canes, crutches, and walkers. *Critical Reviews in Physical and Rehabilitation Medicine, 5(1)*, 15.

Dubowitz, V. (February 27, 1997). The muscular dystrophies—clarity or chaos? *The New England Journal of Medicine, 336*, 650–651.

Eiff, M. P. (1997). Management of clavicle fractures. *American Family Physician, 55(1)*, 121–128.

Farley, D. (1996). New ways to heal broken bones. *FDA Consumer, 30(4)*, 14-18.

Ham, R., & deTrafford, J. (1994). Patterns of recovery for lower limb amputation. *Clinical Rehabilitation, 8(4)*, 320.

Hayes, K. (1993). Heat and cold in the management of arthritis. *Arthritis Care and Research, 6(3)*, 156.

Holden, C. (August 6, 1996). Multiple sclerosis: A multigene disease. *Science, 273*, 741.

Jones-Walton, P. (1994). Orthopaedic health promotion 2000. *Orthopaedic Nursing, 3(3)*, 29.

Kaul M., & Herring, S. (1994). Superficial heat and cold. *The Physician and Sportsmedicine, 22(12)*, 65.

Loney, P. L. & Stratford, P.W. (1999). The prevalence of low back pain in adults: A methodological review of the literature. *Physical Therapy, 79*(4), 384–396.

Lyth, H. (1995). Invisible problem. *Nursing Times, 91(19)*, 38.

Maher, A. B., Salmond, S.W., & Pellino, T.A. (1994). *Orthopaedic nursing*. Philadelphia: W.B. Saunders Company.

McCabe, M. P. (1996). The impact of multiple sclerosis on sexuality and relationships. *The Journal of Sex Research, 33(3)*, 241–248.

Meissner, J. E. (1994). Caring for patients with multiple sclerosis. *Nursing 94, 24(8)*, 60–61.

Moriarty, L., & Rothman, N. L. (1994). Transitional home care after joint arthroplasty. *Home Healthcare Nurse, 12(1)*, 31.

Mourad, L., & Droste, M. (1993). *The nursing process in the care of adults with orthopaedic conditions* (3rd ed.). Albany: Delmar Publishers.

Rothman, N. L. (1994). Establishing a home care protocol for early discharge of patients with hip and knee arthroplasties. *Home Healthcare Nurse 12(1)*, 24.

Sadovnick, A. D. (June 22, 1996). Evidence for a genetic basis of multiple sclerosis. *Lancet, 347*, 1728–1730.

Salmond, S., Mooney, N., & Verdisco, L. (1996). *National Association of Orthopaedic Nurses Core Curriculum for Orthopaedic Nursing*. NJ: Anthony J. Jannetti, Pitman.

Shu, Y. (1995). A study on functioning for independent living among the elderly in the community. *Public Health Nursing, 12(1)*, 31.

Women with previous fractures benefit from alendronate therapy. (1997). *Geriatrics, 52(2)*, 27.

Worton, R. (November 3, 1997). Muscular dystrophies: Diseases of the dystrophin-glycoprotein complex. *Science, 270*, 755–756.

Yandrich, T. (1995). Preventing infection in total joint replacement surgery. *Orthopaedic Nursing, 14(2)*, 15.

Zuckerman, J. D. (1993). Enhancing independence in the older hip fracture patient. *Geriatrics, 48(5)*, 76–78+.

CHAPTER 11

Endocrine Diseases and Disorders

CONTENT OUTLINE

- Anatomy and Physiology
- Common Signs and Symptoms
- Diagnostic Tests
- Common Diseases of the Endocrine System
  - Thyroid Gland Diseases
  - Adrenal Gland Diseases
  - Disorders of Glucose Metabolism
- Trauma
- Effects of Aging on the System

KEY TERMS

Adenoma
Androgens
Cortisol
Diabetic retinopathy
Estrogen
Exophthalmos
Glucagon
Glucocorticoids
Glycogen
Glycosuria
Goiter
Hyperglycemia
Hypoglycemia
Insulin
Islets of Langerhans
Ketoacidosis
Ketones
Lipids
Mineralocorticoids
Myxedema
Progesterone
Striae
Thyroid storm
Vasopressin

LEARNING OBJECTIVES

Upon completion of the chapter, the student should be able to:

1. Define the terminology common to the endocrine system and the disorders of the system.
2. Identify common disorders of the endocrine system.
3. Discuss the basic anatomy and physiology of the endocrine system.
4. Identify the important signs and symptoms associated with common endocrine system disorders.
5. Describe the common diagnostic tests used to determine type and/or cause of the endocrine system disorder.
6. Describe the typical course and management of the common endocrine system disorders.
7. Describe the effects of aging upon the endocrine system and the common disorders of the system.

OVERVIEW

The endocrine system is a highly complex system of glands that secrete important hormones for a variety of body functions. The glands of the system work in harmony discharging the hormones into the bloodstream as needed. The disorders of the system may be caused by problems in the primary gland or from problems in another gland whose secretions control the primary gland. Disorders of the endocrine system may be related to oversecretion of the gland's hormones or undersecretion of its hormones. Some disorders are chronic and controlled, while some can be acutely life-threatening.

ANATOMY AND PHYSIOLOGY

The endocrine system consists of many glands located throughout the body (Figure 11–1). It includes the following glands:

1. hypothalamus—located beneath the thalamus in the area of the third ventricle of the brain
2. pituitary or hypophysis—located at the base of the brain
3. pineal—located behind the midbrain
4. thymus—located in the mediastinal cavity under the sternum, near the heart
5. thyroid—located in the neck on each side of the trachea
6. parathyroids—usually four glands, imbedded in the posterior part of the thyroid
7. adrenals—two glands, one on top of each kidney
8. pancreatic islets—imbedded in the pancreas
9. ovaries (female) and testes (male)—one ovary on each side of the uterus or one testis in each side of the scrotal sac

Each of these glands has a unique function and delivers its secretion as needed into the bloodstream. Table 11–1 lists the glands, their hormones, and the functions of each hormone. The mechanism known as "negative feedback" controls the amount of hormones secreted into the bloodstream. In the negative feedback system, levels of the particular hormone in the bloodstream trigger the release of the hormone as needed. If the concentration of the hormone in the blood is low, the sequence of events stimulates the gland to secrete more hormones. In a similar manner, if the concentration of the hormone in the blood is higher than normal, the feedback mechanism triggers the gland to suppress the release of more hormones.

The hypothalamus, located in the third ventricle area of the brain, contains neurosecretory cells that secrete

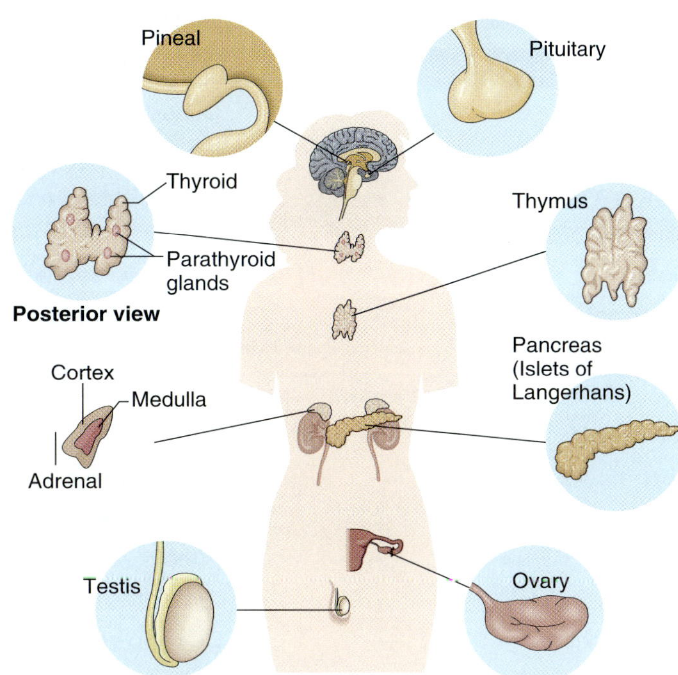

Figure 11–1 The endocrine system.

TABLE 11–1 The Endocrine Glands: Their Hormones and Hormone Functions

Endocrine Gland	Hormone	Hormone Function
Hypothalamus	Inhibiting hormones and Releasing hormones	Inhibits or releases hormones from the anterior pituitary
Hypophysis (Pituitary)	Adrenocorticotropin hormone (ACTH)	Stimulates release of adrenal cortex hormones
Adenohypophysis (Anterior Pituitary)	Thyrotropin hormone (TSH)	Stimulates release of thyroid gland hormones
	Somatotropin hormone (STH)	Stimulates growth
	Melanocyte stimulating hormone (MSH)	Stimulates melanin production
	Lactogenic hormone (prolactin)	Stimulates mammary gland and lactation
	Follicle-stimulating hormone (FSH)	Stimulates estrogen secretion
	Luteinizing hormone (LH; also called interstitial cell-stimulating hormone, ICSH).	Induces ovulation in females and testosterone secretion in males
Neurohypophysis (Posterior Pituitary)	Antidiuretic hormone (ADH)	Increases reabsorption of water in the distal tubules of the kidneys
	Oxytocin	Stimulates uterine contraction and the initiation of breast milk flow in females and increases the ejection of sperm into the seminal fluid in males
Pineal	Melatonin	Affects circadian rhythms

(continues)

TABLE 11-1 The Endocrine Glands: Their Hormones and Hormone Functions (continued).

Endocrine	Gland Hormone	Hormone Function
Thymus	Thymopoietin	Causes immune response development in the newborn and maintains it in the adult
Thyroid	Triiodothyronine (T_3) Thyroxine (T_4)	Stimulates growth and development and regulates metabolism
	Calcitonin	Increases calcium deposits into the bones
Parathyroid	Parathormone (PTH)	Regulates calcium and phosphate levels and increases reabsorption of calcium from the bones
Adrenals		
Adrenal Cortex	Glucocorticoids	Affects stress reactions; Promotes protein and fat use to raise blood sugar Affects sodium and water reabsorption
	Mineralocorticoids	Promotes sodium and water reabsorption
	Sex hormones	Develops secondary sex characteristics
Adrenal Medulla	Epinephrine	Fight or flight response Increases blood pressure and metabolism
	Norepinephrine	Causes vasoconstriction and increases blood pressure
Pancreas Islets		
Alpha cells	Glucagon	Increases blood glucose levels and is counterregulatory to insulin
Beta cells	Insulin	Regulates protein, carbohydrate, and fat metabolism
Delta cells	Somatostatin	Counterregulatory to insulin, glucagon, and somatotropin (STH)
Ovaries	Estrogen Progesterone	Regulates development, maturation, secondary sex characteristics and the reproductive cycle in females
Testes	Testosterone	Regulates growth and development, maturation, secondary sex characteristics and the reproductive system in males

hypothalamic hormones. These hormones regulate the function of the anterior pituitary gland. The hypothalamus also produces the two hormones stored in the neurohypophysis or posterior pituitary gland.

The pituitary gland, also known as the hypophysis gland, is divided into two distinct parts. The adenohypophysis, or anterior part of the gland, produces several hormones that affect other endocrine glands. These include adrenocorticotropin hormone (ACTH), thyrotropin hormone (TSH), somatotropin hormone (STH), melanocyte stimulating hormone (MSH), lactogenic hormone (prolactin), follicle-stimulating hormone (FSH), and luteinizing hormone (LH; also called interstitial cell-stimulating hormone, ICSH).

The posterior pituitary, also called the neurohypophysis, stores two hormones that are secreted by the hypothalamus. Oxytocin (pitocin) helps the progress of labor in the pregnant female, and causes uterine contractions after childbirth. It also affects the cells in the breasts causing a release of milk during lactation. The antidiuretic hormone (ADH; also known as **vasopressin**) is also released from the neurohypophysis. It affects the reabsorption of water from the renal tubules.

The pineal gland, located behind the midbrain, secretes melatonin. It may also secrete other hormones that interact with the hypothalamus and the pituitary gland to cause the secretion of hormones from other glands.

The thymus gland, located just behind the upper part of the sternum, secretes thymopoietin, a hormone that stimulates the development of lymphocytes. Lymphocytes are important for immunity development and prevention of infections. The thymus gland is prominent in infants and young children and decreases significantly in size by adulthood.

The thyroid gland, located in the neck on either side of the trachea, secretes thyroxine (T_4), triiodothyronine (T_3), and calcitonin. These hormones are released as needed in response to the thyroid-stimulating hormone secreted by the pituitary gland. Thyroxine and triiodothyronine increase metabolic activity. Calcitonin affects the regulation of calcium and works in opposition to the hormone secreted by the parathyroid gland.

Imbedded in the posterior part of the thyroid gland are the parathyroid glands. There are usually four parathyroid glands, but there can be more. The parathyroid glands secrete parathormone, important in the regulation of calcium and phosphorus in the body.

The adrenal glands, located on top of each kidney, have two distinct parts. The cortex, the outer part, secretes **mineralocorticoids**, **glucocorticoids**, and **androgens**. The mineralocorticoids promote sodium retention. The glucocorticoids affect the metabolism of protein, glucose, and fats. **Cortisol** is the main glucocorticoid and is important for metabolism of carbohydrates. The androgens enhance masculinization. The most common androgen hormone is testosterone. The adrenal medulla or middle section secretes epinephrine and norepinephrine.

The beta cells located in the pancreas secrete **insulin**, another important hormone. Insulin is most important in the metabolism of glucose, but it also promotes fatty acid synthesis and amino acid entry into cells. Insulin secretion is regulated by the feedback mechanism and by counterregulatory hormones such as **glucagon**, cortisol, epinephrine, and the growth hormone.

The ovaries and testes secrete the sex hormones, as they are commonly known. The ovaries secrete **estrogen** and **progesterone**, important for development and maturation, and maintaining the functions of the reproductive system. The testes secrete testosterone, important for growth and development, secondary sex characteristics, and maintaining the reproductive system functions. See Chapter 21 for more information about the reproductive system.

COMMON SIGNS AND SYMPTOMS

Most endocrine disorders are caused by hypo- or hypersecretion by the gland. Diagnosis is dependent on matching the signs and symptoms with the hormone dysfunction. The difficulty in diagnosing endocrine disorders is related to tracking the problem to the correct source. Some common signs and symptoms of endocrine system disorders include mental abnormalities, lethargy or fatigue, and tissue atrophy. Specific signs and symptoms are included in discussions of specific diseases.

DIAGNOSTIC TESTS

The only endocrine glands that can be physically examined are the thyroid glands and testes. Enlargement or atrophy of these glands can be felt. Severe enlargement can also be seen. Assessment of proper function of the endocrine organs can be accomplished with blood or urine testing for the hormones they produce. Computerized tomography (CT) and magnetic resonance imaging (MRI) may be utilized to check for presence of tumors or alteration in organ size. EMS providers may suspect endocrine diseases based upon the patient's history, signs and symptoms, and medications. Most endocrine disorders are chronic in nature with periodic exacerbations of the disease that may require EMS intervention.

COMMON DISEASES OF THE ENDOCRINE SYSTEM

Endocrine diseases are the result of abnormally high or low hormone secretion by endocrine glands. Abnormal secretion may be caused by the size of the gland. Abnormally large or hypertrophied glands tend to produce abnormally high hormone levels while abnormally small or atrophied glands tend to produce abnormally low levels. Abnormal gland size may be the result of injury to the gland by surgery, trauma, infection, or radiation. Abnormal function of endocrine glands leads to many different physical and mental abnormalities. Abnormalities vary with the amount of hormone secreted (hypersecretion or hyposecretion) by the gland and the age of the individual involved. In this section we will cover the endocrine diseases most applicable to the EMS provider in the emergency care setting.

Thyroid Gland Diseases

The activity of the thyroid gland affects the entire body. The hormone released by the thyroid gland (thyroxine) regulates metabolism, or the rate that calories are used. In this way, thyroxine also regulates body heat, ensuring that the body is kept warm even in a cold environment. Thyroxine also stimulates the gastrointestinal system by increasing gastric secretions and peristalsis. In order to make thyroxine, the thyroid gland uses iodine. Without iodine, thyroxine cannot be produced. Diseases of the thyroid gland are primarily those of hypersecretion and hyposecretion.

Hyperthyroidism. Hyperthyroidism occurs when the thyroid gland secretes excessive thyroxine. This condition is caused by an **adenoma** (AD-eh-**NO**-ma; adeno = gland, oma = tumor) on the thyroid. This growth on the thyroid produces a characteristic **goiter** (GOI-ter) or noticeable protrusion of the thyroid gland (Figure 11–2). Overproduction of thyroxine increases metabolism, leading to symptoms of tachycardia, nervousness, hyperactivity, and excessive excitability. The individual has a tremendous appetite but loses weight to the point of extreme thinness. Diarrhea is common since thyroxine speeds up peristalsis of the gastrointestinal tract. High metabolic rate causes high heat production leading to excessive sweating and an intolerance of heat. The skin is always moist and the individual has extreme thirst because of this water loss. Medications to reduce thyroxine production are often effective. In some cases surgery may be needed to reduce the size of the thyroid and decrease thyroxine production.

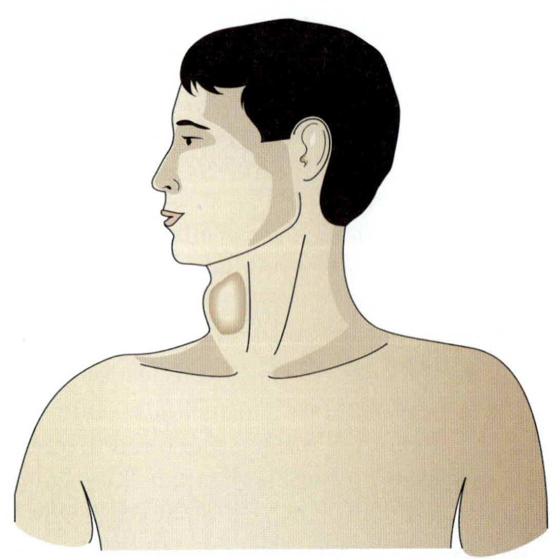

Figure 11–2 Goiter.

Hyperthyroidism caused by an autoimmune condition is called Graves' disease. Antibodies stimulate the thyroid leading to glandular hypertrophy. Graves' disease commonly affects young women. Symptoms include those previously discussed. One very distinguishing characteristic of Graves' disease is a stare in the eyes caused by **exophthalmos** (ECK-sof-**THAL**-mos; abnormal protrusion of the eyeballs). This protrusion of the eyeballs is caused by edema in the tissues behind the eye. Exophthalmos may be so severe that the eyelids will not close. Unfortunately, this condition does not resolve when the hyperthyroidism is corrected. Graves' disease may be treated with medication, radiation of the thyroid, or surgical removal of all or part of the gland. If the entire gland is removed, hormonal supplement will be needed for the life of the individual.

A sudden life-threatening exacerbation of all symptoms of hyperthyroidism is called **thyroid storm**. This generally occurs in patients who have a history of Graves' disease or during the immediate postoperative period following a thyroidectomy (ectomy = excision or removal of). Symptoms of thyroid storm include severe tachycardia with heart rates reaching 200 beats per minute, tachypnea, loss of temperature regulation characterized by a rapid and steady increase in body temperature, a widened pulse pressure, and delirium, seizures, or coma. Atrial fibrillation and premature ventricular contractions (PVCs) may occur, although sinus tachycardia is the most common rhythym.

EMS management includes maintaining the airway and ventilation, administering supplemental oxygen if appropriate, monitoring the ECG and initiating IV access. Pharmacologic intervention may include a beta-adrenergic blocker to combat the tachycardia and arrythmias depending upon local protocol and medical control direction. In the emergency department, antithyroid medication may be administered to block the effect of the thyroid hormones.

Hypothyroidism. Hypothyroidism is the decrease in normal thyroxine production. This condition occurs more frequently in women and is usually caused by thyroid gland dysfunction rather than pituitary dysfunction. Hypothyroidism is often the result of surgical or radiation treatments to cure hyperthyroidism. Symptoms of hypothyroidism are just the opposite of hyperthyroidism. The affected individual is fatigued, drowsy, sensitive to cold temperature, has thin nails, brittle hair, and gains excessive weight. The individual becomes sluggish, mentally and physically. Diagnosis is confirmed by clinical history and blood hormone tests. Treatment with thyroid hormone replacement is usually rapid and effective. Regardless of cause, the symptoms, diagnosis, and treatment plan for hypothyroidism are quite similar.

The most common natural cause of hypothyroidism is an autoimmune disorder called Hashimoto's disease. It is believed that lymphocytes react with thyroid tissue leading to atrophy and destruction of the thyroid gland tissue.

Advanced hypothyroidism in an adult is called **myxedema** (MICK-seh-**DEE**-mah). Myxedema commonly occurs in middle-aged women. Symptoms of myxedema include those previously mentioned with hypothyroidism, plus a characteristic swelling or bloating of the facial tissue, thickened tongue, and puffy eyelids (Figure 11–3).

Myxedema coma is a severe manifestation of hypothyroidism and includes a decreased mental status, hypotension, bradycardia, and respiratory failure. Psychosis occasionally occurs. EMS treatment includes managing the airway, supporting ventilation mechanically or with supplemental oxygen, and initiating IV access. Hypotensive patients may require fluid replacement and severe hypotension may require vasopressors to maintain an adequate blood pressure.

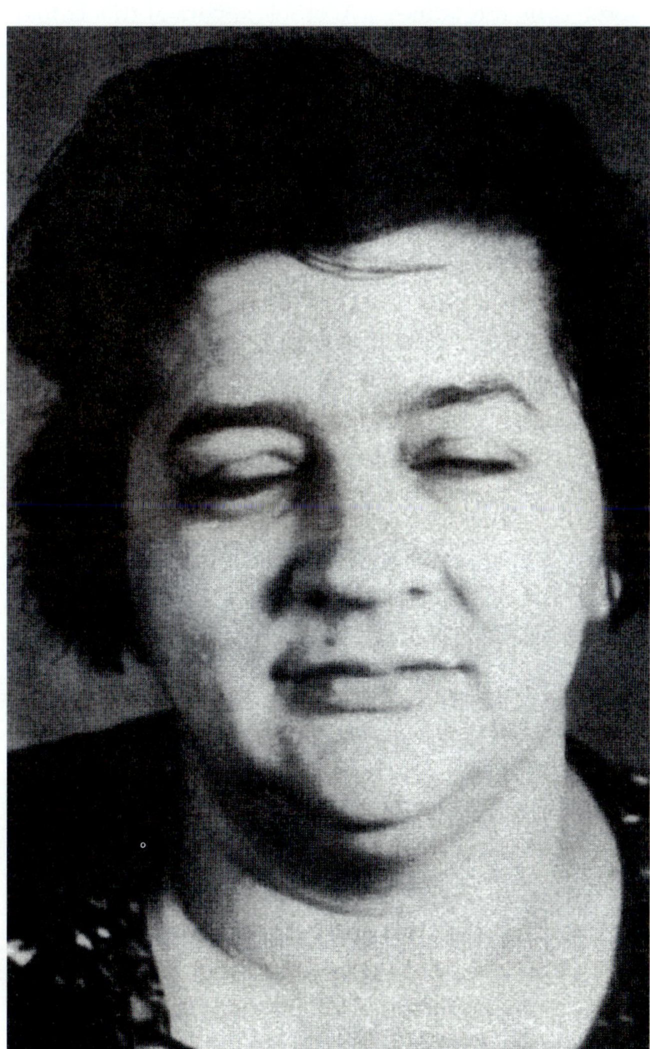

Figure 11–3 Myxedema.

Adrenal Gland Diseases

The adrenal glands sit atop the kidneys and have two distinct parts that function quite differently. The inner part, called the medulla, releases two hormones, epinephrine (adrenalin) and norepinephrine, when stimulated by the nervous system. These hormones have a direct effect on the vascular system and are known as *fight or flight* hormones. The cortex, or outer part of the adrenal gland, is controlled by the pituitary gland's release of adrenocorticotropic hormone (ACTH). The adrenal cortex secretes several hormones.

1. Mineralocorticoids, the primary hormone being aldosterone, regulate salt balance.
2. Glucocorticoids, the primary hormone being cortisol (cortisone) or hydrocortisone, regulate carbohydrate metabolism.
3. Sex hormones, the primary ones being androgens and estrogens, provide male and female characteristics respectively. Males and females have both of these androgenic sex hormones.

Cortisone is a hormone frequently used to treat inflammatory diseases such as arthritis since it acts as an anti-inflammatory agent. Cortisone does not cure the inflammatory condition; it only relieves the inflammation and the associated pain. Prolonged use of cortisone is avoided when possible as it has some very detrimental side effects. Side effects of prolonged cortisone use include hypertension, ulcers, puffy face called "moon face," and drowsiness. The anti-inflammatory properties of cortisone reduce the body's inflammatory response. This alteration in the immune system may mask the symptoms of an infection, allowing it to go unnoticed until it is in advanced stages. This side effect of prolonged cortisone use can be potentially life-threatening. Long-term steroid use may also decrease the ability for the adrenal glands to produce natural corticosteroids.

Hyperadrenalism. Hyperadrenalism is the oversecretion of hormones by the adrenal cortex. The specific forms of hyperadrenalism depend on which hormones are secreted in excess.

Cushing's syndrome is caused by an overproduction of the glucocorticoid, cortisol. Cushing's syndrome may be caused by a tumor on the pituitary gland or on the adrenal cortex. Classic symptoms include a round "moon-shaped" face and a "buffalo hump" on the upper back. Other symptoms include poor wound healing, a rotund abdomen with pencil thin arms and legs, hypertension, and **striae** (stretch marks) on the skin. Cushing's syndrome may develop in individuals receiving long-term glucocorticoid steroids. These individuals need to be carefully monitored for symptoms of Cushing's syndrome. In general, patients with Cushing's syndrome will not require emergency treatment for the disease. However, patients on long-term corticosteroid therapy who abruptly stop taking their steroid medication may require emergent treatment for adrenal insufficiency.

Hypoadrenalism. Hypoadrenalism, or adrenal insufficiency, is an uncommon undersecretion of hormones by the adrenal cortex called Addison's disease. Causes of Addison's disease include an autoimmune disorder, tumor of the pituitary gland, tuberculosis, and prolonged steroid hormone therapy. As much as ninety percent of the adrenal cortex may be destroyed before hyposecretion occurs. Symptoms of Addison's disease may be mild to life-threatening. Lack of mineralocorticoids allows depletion of sodium, leading to diarrhea and dehydration. Deficiency in glucocorticoids affects blood sugar levels, leading to **hypoglycemia** (HIGH-poh-gly-**SEE**-me-ah; hypo = decreased, glyc = glucose, emia = blood). Increased ACTH levels by the pituitary lead to a hyperpigmentation, or increased skin coloring, ranging from yellow to dark brown. This increased skin color affects the palms, elbows, scars, skin folds, and the areola of the nipples. Hormone blood levels can be measured to confirm the diagnosis.

Adrenal crisis is a severe and life-threatening form of adrenal insufficiency. Patients lose their ability to compensate for external stressors against the body, resulting in shock and altered mental status. Adrenal crisis can be precipitated in a patient with a history of adrenal insufficiency by external stress, including infection, MI, surgery, or traumatic injury. The patient may be bradycardic or may have a pulse rate in the normal range instead of mounting a tachycardic response to shock. Emergency treatment includes managing the airway, supporting ventilation, and intravenous fluids to support circulation. Intravenous steroids and vasopressors may be ordered by medical control.

Disorders of Glucose Metabolism

The pancreas is both an exocrine and endocrine gland. As an exocrine gland, it secretes digestive juices by way of ducts into the digestive system. As an endocrine, it secretes two hormones, insulin and glucagon, directly into the blood. Both of these hormones are secreted by specialized tissue called **islets of Langerhans** which are scattered throughout the pancreas. Insulin and glucagon have an antagonistic relationship. Insulin lowers blood sugar while glucagon raises it. The overall effect of these hormones is maintaining a normal blood sugar level of between 70 and 120 mg/dl.

When blood sugar levels rise after a meal, insulin is secreted. Insulin assists in moving sugar out of the blood and into the tissues, thus decreasing the blood sugar level (Figure 11–4). Without adequate insulin, the blood sugar level rises and the tissues are depleted of sugar.

Sugar, or glucose, is the primary source of energy for all tissue cells. Without glucose, cells must burn fats and proteins for energy. When tissue cells burn fats and proteins, they produce waste products called **ketones**. Ketones are picked up by the blood to be filtered and excreted by the kidneys. Acetone, a part of this ketone waste, is excreted by the respiratory system, giving the affected individual a "fruity or sweet" smelling breath. This condition of having ketones in the blood, breath, and urine is called ketosis. Chemically, a large part of ketones are acid in nature, which leads to metabolic acidosis, or a low pH in the body tissues. For this reason, ketosis is often called **ketoacidosis**.

When carbohydrates or sugars are eaten, the extra sugar, the amount not needed for immediate energy, is stored primarily in the liver as **glycogen**. If blood sugar levels drop, for instance, during exercise, the pancreas secretes glucagon. Glucagon circulates in the blood and stimulates the liver to release glycogen in the form of glucose, thus raising the blood sugar to normal.

Diabetes Mellitus. Diabetes mellitus is a chronic disease affecting carbohydrate or sugar utilization caused by inadequate production of insulin by the pancreatic islets of Langerhans. This is the most common and major disease of the endocrine pancreas and is commonly known simply as "diabetes." Diabetes is characterized by symptoms of polyuria, excessive urination, polydipsia, excessive thirst, and polyphagia, excessive eating. **Glycosuria** (GLYE-koh-**SOO**-ree-ah; glyco = glycogen or sugar, uria = urine) or the "spilling of sugar in the urine" is also a common symptom. The excessive sugar in the blood, known as **hyperglycemia** (hyper = excessive, glyc = glycogen or glucose, emia = blood), causes the kidney to filter out part of the excess resulting in glycosuria. Hyperglycemia indicates that sugar is not being pulled into the tissues, and cells are using fat for energy, resulting in the formation of

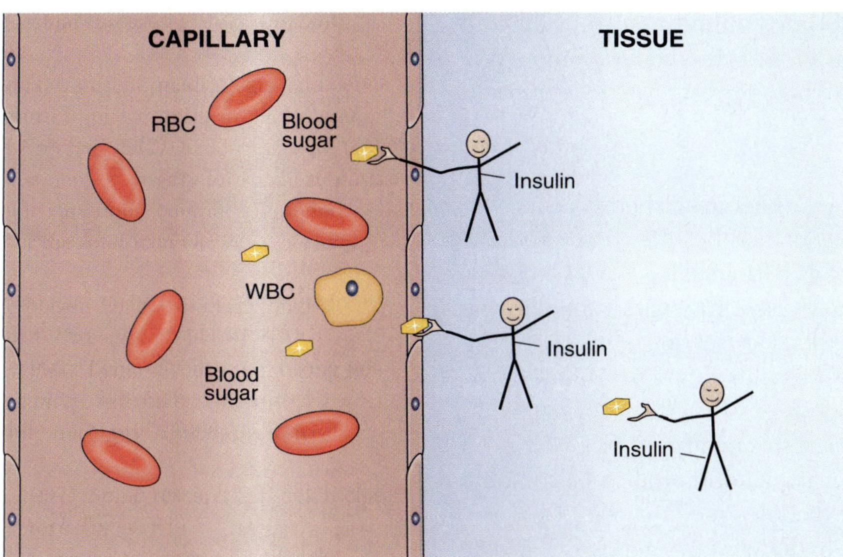

Figure 11–4 Effect of insulin on blood glucose. Insulin assists in moving sugar out of the blood and into the tissues thus decreasing blood glucose levels. If insulin is not present, glucose remains in the blood, resulting in an elevated blood glucose level.

ketones, the waste products of fat metabolism. Ketones can be found in the blood and urine, and smelled on the breath.

There are two types of diabetes mellitus:

1. Type 1, formerly known as insulin dependent diabetes mellitus (IDDM) or juvenile onset diabetes. This form of diabetes is the most serious. It usually occurs quite suddenly and affects children and young adults before age twenty-five. This form of diabetes requires daily injections of insulin. Type 1 is thought to be caused by an autoimmune disorder. It is thought that affected individuals inherit a genetic tendency for the disease. The immune system, when triggered by a virus or some other stressor, develops antibodies and begins war against the islets of Langerhans, thereby destroying the insulin-secreting cells. Affected individuals generally do not secrete any insulin, making regulation of blood glucose levels quite difficult. Individuals with Type 1 must follow a strict diet, monitor blood sugar levels, and administer the needed amounts of insulin. Exercise and stress can alter insulin needs and must be considered as part of the treatment plan.
2. Type 2, formerly known as non-insulin-dependent diabetes mellitus (NIDDM) or adult onset diabetes. This is the more common form of diabetes mellitus. It usually has a gradual onset and occurs most often in obese females over age forty. This form of diabetes is thought to be caused by a "wearing out" of the pancreatic islets of Langerhans. It is believed that excessive carbohydrate consumption for the life of the individual places such a heavy demand on the pancreas to produce the needed insulin that over an extended period of time this increased demand literally "wears out" the pancreatic cells leading to Type 2. Insulin injections are rarely needed as Type 2 is usually controlled with diet, exercise, and oral medications that stimulate insulin secretion.

Long-term complications of diabetes usually appear gradually after many years. With improper carbohydrate metabolism, **lipids** or fats are pulled into the bloodstream to be utilized for cellular energy. This increase in lipids in the vascular system leads to atherosclerosis. Atherosclerosis leads to a variety of complications, including myocardial infarction, cerebrovascular accidents or strokes, and peripheral vascular disease. The poor circulation caused by peripheral vascular disease is the cause of diabetic gangrene in the feet and legs, which may lead to amputation. Poor circulation also leads to poor wound healing. Atherosclerosis also affects the vessels of the eyes and kidneys. The retinas of the eyes become damaged, causing **diabetic retinopathy** (retino = retina, opathy = disease) and leading to blindness. Damage to the kidney leads to kidney failure, a frequent cause of death in individuals affected with diabetes.

Diagnosis is confirmed by a positive history of symptoms along with blood glucose testing. Diabetes cannot be cured. Management of the disease is dependent on education and a lifetime commitment to following the treatment regimen of diet, medication, and exercise. The long-term goal is to prevent the development of complications.

Gestational Diabetes. Gestational diabetes occurs during pregnancy. The condition may be either asymptomatic or the same symptoms of diabetes mellitus may occur. This type of diabetes is usually discovered with routine urine testing during prenatal visits. Destruction of insulin by the placenta and blocking of insulin action by elevated levels of estrogen and progesterone lead to gestational diabetes. It is important that this condition be discovered as it may lead to fetal or neonatal mortality. Gestational diabetes is treated like diabetes mellitus, with exercise, dietary control of carbohydrate intake, and medications. Injectable insulin may be needed to control blood sugar levels. Oral hypoglycemic medications are contraindicated as these pass across the placenta and may lead to fetal birth defects or hypoglycemia. Gestational diabetes usually disappears after delivery. If this condition does not disappear with delivery, the affected individual will need to continue diabetic management. Women affected with gestational diabetes are often affected later in life by adult onset diabetes.

Hyperglycemia. Hyperglycemia occurs when there is insufficient insulin available to transport glucose into the cells. This process generally occurs insidiously over a period of days to weeks. Hyperglycemia is the typical initial presentation for adult patients who develop diabetes. The two common hyperglycemic presentations are diabetic ketoacidosis, known to the lay public as diabetic coma, and hyperosmolar hyperglycemic nonketotic syndrome.

Diabetic ketoacidosis (DKA) is a state where blood glucose is high, the patient's insulin is low, and ketones have developed and are present in the patient's blood and urine. DKA often occurs in patients with a history of type II diabetes who have an infection or stress to their cardiovascular system. The patient typically has a period of polyuria caused by increased blood glucose, polydipsia caused by increased urination, and polyphagia because the body thinks that it requires more glucose at the cellular level. This increased urination results in a loss of many electrolytes. As the ketones in the blood build up, the patient develops a metabolic acidosis. This metabolic acidosis causes the patient to become tachypnic and to hyperventilate in an effort to decrease the amount of acidosis in the blood. This tachypnea and hyperventilation are called Kussmaul's respirations (see Chapter 7). The ketones in the blood may also produce the fruity, acetone breath commonly associated with DKA. The patient may also present with altered mental status or unconsciousness, nausea, vomiting, or abdominal pain.

Hyperosmolar hyperglycemia nonketotic syndrome (HHNS) is similar to DKA in that the patient has an elevated blood glucose level; however, ketones are not present in the patient's blood. HHNS is the common presentation for patients with new onset diabetes. The signs and symptoms are similar to DKA, however Kussmaul's respirations and acetone breath are not present because of the lack of ketones. It may be difficult to differentiate between the two entities in the field as the diagnosis is usually made by analyzing the patient's blood.

Treatment of hyperglycemia in the field includes managing the airway and supporting ventilation, checking blood glucose level with a glucometer if available, and initiating IV access. Patients with DKA or HHNS may become profoundly dehydrated because of their polyuria, so intravenous administration of two liters of normal saline may be warranted. In the emergency department, insulin will be started, electrolytes will be replaced, and a solution containing D5 will be started at the appropriate time.

Hypoglycemia. Hypoglycemia (HIGH-poh-gly-**SEE**-me-ah; hypo = decreased, glyc = glucose, emia = blood) is an abnormally low blood sugar. Hypoglycemia occurs any time the blood glucose level drops below 60 mg/dl, although individuals may become symptomatic at different blood glucose levels. Some individuals tolerate unusually low blood glucose levels while others do not.

Symptoms include lightheadedness, diaphoresis, and trembling. If untreated, symptoms may progress to include mental confusion and coma. Most individuals have had an episode of hypoglycemia at one time or another. Some common causes of hypoglycemia are fasting, skipping meals, and excessive exercise. Hypoglycemia is also caused by administration of too much insulin, as previously discussed. Other causes of hypoglycemia include pancreatic adenoma, gastrointestinal disorders, and some hereditary disorders. Diagnosis is confirmed by a positive clinical history and blood glucose testing.

EMS treatment of hypoglycemia includes managing the airway, supporting ventilation, initiating IV access, and assessing the blood glucose level with a glucometer if available. An IV bolus of D50 can be administered to treat hypoglycemia, and the patient will often quickly respond after one or two 25 gram D50 boluses. If IV access is difficult, then glucagon can be administered intramuscularly to help mobilize glucose from available liver stores. If the patient is alert enough to protect his own airway, then oral glucose, in the form of either a commercial paste or liquid, for example orange juice, can be administered. Some EMS systems allow EMS providers to release the patient if the patient is alert and oriented at the scene after treatment and does not require further care. EMS providers should follow local protocols and medical control direction in the treatment and release of this group of patients.

TRAUMA

Head injury can result in multiple organ dysfunction if the pituitary is involved. Hypersecretion and hyposecretion may occur with injury to any of the individual organs. Organ destruction and failure can be life-threatening when the pituitary, pancreas, and adrenal glands are involved.

EFFECTS OF AGING ON THE SYSTEM

As the individual ages there are changes that occur in the endocrine glands. Decreases in the secretions from the glands alter the body's ability to respond to stressors, diseases, and other changes that occur from aging. The older adult is at high risk for hypoglycemic reactions and excessive fluid loss caused by reduced levels of glucocorticoids and aldosterone. Digestive and metabolism problems are common because of reduced secretions of pancreatic and thyroid hormones. The secretions from the gonads are reduced, resulting in changes in secondary sex characteristics. Since glucose tolerance lessens with age, the serum glucose levels tend to be higher in the older adult. Diabetes mellitus is common in the elderly population, but it usually can be regulated by dietary adjustments. With all the other changes that occur during the aging process, diabetes becomes a very serious condition, adversely affecting many systems.

SUMMARY

The endocrine system is a very complex system of many glands located throughout the body. Each of the glands has a unique function and delivers its hormones into the bloodstream. The hormones help the body's growth, regulation, and metabolism. Overproduction or underproduction of any one gland can cause dysfunction in other systems. If the gland malfunctions in childhood, the result is a different disorder than if the gland malfunctions in adulthood. The most common endocrine disorder overall is diabetes mellitus. The older adult with an endocrine disorder is at risk for other systemic problems. Secretions from the endocrine glands decrease slowly with age.

REVIEW QUESTIONS

Short Answer

1. What are the functions of the endocrine system?

2. Which signs and symptoms are associated with common endocrine system disorders?

3. What is the difference between an endocrine gland and an exocrine gland?

Multiple Choice

4. Which of the following is not an endocrine gland?

   a. Pituitary c. Liver
   b. Adrenal d. Ovary

5. What function(s) do glucocorticoid hormones perform?
   a. Promote absorption of calcium in the bones
   b. Stimulate the thyroid to produce its hormones
   c. Affect stress reaction
   d. Raise blood sugar
   e. Both c and d
6. Thyroid storm is:
   a. a severe manifestation of hyperthyroidism.
   b. an abnormal increase in the activity of the pituitary gland.
   c. a result of too little thyroid hormone production.
   d. associated with bradycardia.
7. Myxedema coma:
   a. is an extreme form of hypothyroidism.
   b. includes decreased mental status, hypotension, and bradycardia.
   c. may present with all of the above.
8. Hypoadrenalism is also known as which of the following disorders?
   a. Acromegaly
   b. Myxedema
   c. Cushing's syndrome
   d. Addison's disease
9. In Type 1 diabetes mellitus the individual needs replacement of which of the following?
   a. Steroids
   b. Antidiuretic hormone
   c. Insulin
   d. Estrogen
10. The individual affected by Type 2 diabetes mellitus can usually control the disorder by:
   a. Insulin injections
   b. Diet and oral medications
   c. Replacement hormones
   d. Steroid therapy

MATCHING

11. Match the hormone in the left column with its gland in the right column. Some glands may be used more than once.

_____ ACTH	a. anterior pituitary
_____ triiodothyronine	b. posterior pituitary
_____ oxytocin	c. pineal
_____ mineralocorticoids	d. thyroid
_____ melatonin	f. adrenals
_____ estrogen	g. testes or ovaries
_____ insulin	h. pancreatic islets
_____ norepinephrine	
_____ ADH	
_____ calcitonin	

CASE STUDY

You respond to a call for a middle aged female who is complaining of "a flutter in my heart." She states she is very restless and she is wearing only a T-shirt when other family members in her home are wearing sweatshirts. Her family members also state she has had periods recently where "she wasn't all there." She states she was recently told by her family physician that she has Graves' disease and asks you about the disease. What can you tell her? What is the most likely diagnosis for this patient? What possible rhythms may be found on the ECG monitor? What treatments can you initiate?

BIBLIOGRAPHY

Bhatara, V. S. (1996). Learning disorders and the thyroid. *Journal of the American Academy of Child and Adolescent Psychiatry, 35*(4), 406–407.

Brewer, K. W. (July 17, 1997). Screening patients with insulin-dependent diabetes mellitus for adrenal insufficiency. *The New England Journal of Medicine, 337*, 202.

Bromberg, J. S. (April 10, 1997). Adrenal insufficiency. *The New England Journal of Medicine, 336*, 1005–1007.

Drinka, P. J. (1996). Low TSH levels in nursing home residents not taking thyroid hormone. *Journal of the American Geriatrics Society, 44*(5), 573–577.

Johnson, J. (August 11, 1997). Higher cancer rate from U.S. bomb tests. *Chemical and Engineering News, 75*, 10.

Leo, R. J. (1997). Utility of thyroid function screening in adolescent psychiatric inpatients. *Journal of the American Academy of Child and Adolescent Psychiatry, 36*(1), 103–111.

Oelkers, W. (October 17, 1996). Current concepts: Adrenal insufficiency. *The New England Journal of Medicine* 335, 1206–1212.

Porte, D. (May 3, 1996). Diabetes complications; why is glucose potentially toxic? *Science, 272*, 699–700.

Travis, J. (October 4, 1997). Hidden virus suspected in diabetes. *Science News, 152*, 218

Will, J. C. (1997). Diabetes mellitus among Navajo Indians: Findings from the Navajo Health and Nutrition Survey. *The Journal of Nutrition, 127*(10), 2106s–2113s.

Wooldridge, J. (1996). Preventing diabetic foot disease: Lessons from the Medicare therapeutic shoe demonstration. *American Journal of Public Health, 86*(7), 935–938.

CHAPTER 12

Immune and Lymphatic Diseases and Disorders

CONTENT OUTLINE

- Anatomy and Physiology
- Common Signs and Symptoms
- Diagnostic Tests
- Common Diseases of the Immune System
  - Hypersensitivity Disorders
  - Immune Deficiency Disorders
- Common Diseases of the Lymphatic System
  - Lymphadenitis
  - Lymphangitis
  - Lymphedema
  - Lymphoma
  - Mononucleosis
- Trauma
- Effects of Aging on the Immune System

KEY TERMS

Allergen(s)
Allergy
Anaphylaxis
Antigen(s)
Autoimmune
Bronchospasm
Corticosteroid(s)
Cytotoxic
Hemolytic
Hypersensitivity
Immunodeficiency
Isoimmune
Kaposi's sarcoma
Lymph
Lymphadenopathy
Lymphangiography
Lymphangiopathy
Lymphocytes
Lymphocytopenia
Lymphocytosis
Pneumocystis carinii
Prophylactic
Self-antigen
Status asthmaticus
Streptococcal
Urticaria

LEARNING OBJECTIVES

Upon completion of the chapter, the student should be able to:

1. Define the terminology common to the immune and lymphatic systems and the common disorders of these systems.
2. Identify disorders of the immune and lymphatic systems.
3. Discuss the basic anatomy and physiology of the immune and lymphatic systems.
4. Identify the important signs and symptoms associated with common immune and lymphatic system disorders.
5. Describe the common diagnostic tests used to determine type and/or cause of the immune and lymphatic system disorder.
6. Describe the typical course and management of the common immune system disorders.
7. Describe the effects of aging upon the immune and lymphatic systems and the common disorders of the systems.

OVERVIEW

The immune system provides protection for the body through the processes of defense, attack, and removal of pathogens. The immune system also helps the body by removing aged or dead cells and other debris. Diseases or disorders of the immune system may range from mild to severe. Many of the disorders of the system are extremely debilitating and require long-term therapy. Immune diseases can affect individuals of any age, race, or gender. If the immune system is not functioning properly because of disease or other linfluencing factors, the result may be a secondary disease of the body resulting from the compromised immune system. The lymphatic system is the infection fighting system of the body. It works with the immune system to play an important role in preventing infection and maintaining one's immunity. The lymphatic system includes the lymph nodes, lymph vessels, and fluid lymph. It is a special vascular system that picks up excess tissue fluid and returns it to the blood. Disorders of the system include inflammatory conditions and neoplasms. The lymphatic system is also closely related to the hematologic system (Chapter 16) and the cardiovascular system (Chapter 8).

ANATOMY AND PHYSIOLOGY

The immune system is made up of a complex group of cells and organs that are found throughout the body. The system includes primary organs such as the thymus gland and the bone marrow, and secondary organs such as the lymph nodes, spleen, liver, and the tonsils (Figure 12–1). The lymphocytes, the major cells of the immune system, arise and develop in the primary organs. The secondary organs are responsible for filtering foreign substances and for providing the space for antigen reactions.

The cells of the immune system include four types of leukocytes: polymorphonuclear leukocytes, monocytes, macrophages, and lymphocytes. The polymorphonuclear leukocytes, also known as granulocytes and PMNs, are active in the inflammatory process. Some leukocytes react when infection threatens the body, while others respond when there is an allergic reaction preventing damage to cells and tissues. The monocytes and macrophages become phagocytic in the presence of pathogens and foreign substances. The lymphocytes are the major players in the immune response (Table 12–1).

Lymphocytes are formed in the bone marrow. Those remaining and maturing in the bone marrow become B lymphocytes. Others migrate and mature in the thymus and become T lymphocytes. Once mature, both B and T lymphocytes enter the blood and circulate and colonize the lymphatic organs—predominately the spleen and lymph nodes.

T lymphocytes are responsible for the cell-mediated response. These cells destroy microorganisms that invade the body. These reactions do not require antibodies produced by the B cells because the T cells have been previously sensitized by circulating antigens. There are several different types of T cells functioning to stimulate

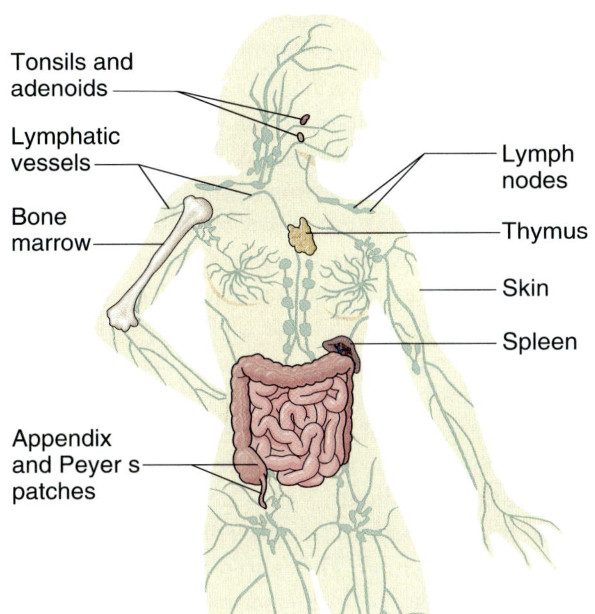

Figure 12–1 Organs of the immune system.

B cells to produce antibodies, destroy foreign cells in the body, stop the immune response, and remember previous exposure to antigens.

B lymphocytes are responsible for humoral immunity. Humoral immunity is associated with circulating antibodies, in contrast to cell-mediated immunity. The B lymphocytes enlarge and divide to become mature plasma cells. The plasma cells secrete antibodies into the blood and lymph to protect the body against infections and toxins produced by microorganisms.

There are two types of immune responses in the body: specific and non-specific. Specific immune response is associated with antigens and the antibody reaction. It is the body's watch-guard system for foreign invaders. The antibody response occurs after exposure to an antigen. Antibodies may neutralize, kill, or cause clumping of the foreign microorganism. The complement system also works with the antibodies to destroy the invader. The complement system is a group of proteins that are formed in the liver and circulate in the serum. They enhance the work of the antibodies in destroying foreign cells.

The non-specific immune response includes inflammation, phagocytosis, physical barriers (the skin and mucous membranes), and chemical barriers (acids and other secretions). These immune response defenses are the body's first line of protection against foreign invaders.

There are several ways to classify types of immunity, but the most common method used is to divide immunity into passive and active, and natural and artificial. Table 12–2 outlines the types of immunity and examples of each. In addition, some classification systems use the term "natural resistance" when describing immunity. Natural resistance is the inherited immunity the individual may possess because of race, species, or ethnic background. Some races, species, or particular groups of populations are naturally resistant to certain diseases, just as some are more susceptible to certain diseases.

The lymphatic system includes lymph vessels, ducts, and nodes (Figure 12–2). It is important in protecting the body from infection. It is responsible for filtering bacterial and non-bacterial products resulting from the inflammatory process. The goal of the system is to prevent

TABLE 12–1 Types and Functions of Leukocytes

Type	Function
Polymorphonuclear leukocytes:	
Neutrophils	Phagocytosis
Eosinophils	Allergic responses
Basophils	Release histamine
Monocytes	Become macrophages (phagocytosis)
Macrophages	Phagocytosis
Lymphocytes:	
T lymphocytes	Cell-mediated immunity
B lymphocytes	Humoral immunity
Plasma Cells	Antibody production

TABLE 12–2 Types of Immunity

Type of Immunity	Example
Active natural immunity	Having the disease (like mumps)
Active artificial immunity	Receiving a vaccination (like MMR)
Passive natural immunity	Antibodies produced by self or received from maternal-fetus transmission
Passive artificial immunity	Injection of antibodies

these waste products from entering the general circulation. This activity may cause some inflammation of the node filtering the waste products causing swelling and redness of the involved node.

The lymphatic system is dependent, to some extent, on the vascular system. The lymphatic system returns its fluids and other matters to the vascular system. There is diffusion of fluid between the lymphatic vessels, the interstitial spaces, and the blood capillaries.

The fluid in the lymphatic is called **lymph**. Lymph is a clear liquid similar to plasma and contains many white cells. The conducting vessels of the lymphatic system include the capillaries, the smallest vessels, and the larger lymph vessels, which have valves much like the veins in the cardiovascular system. In the lymph vessels, the direction of flow is toward the thoracic cavity. The vessels meet in the right lymphatic duct or the left lymphatic duct, which drain into the venous system. The right lymphatic duct drains the lymph from the right half of the head, upper torso, and right arm. The rest of the lymph vessels in the body drain into the left lymphatic duct, also called the thoracic duct.

The lymph vessels have other functions besides the transportation of lymph. They also return important nutrients, such as proteins and large particulate matter that have leaked out into the capillaries, to the blood vessels (Figure 12–3). In the course of a day, approximately three liters of extra fluid is leaked into the tissue and not picked up by

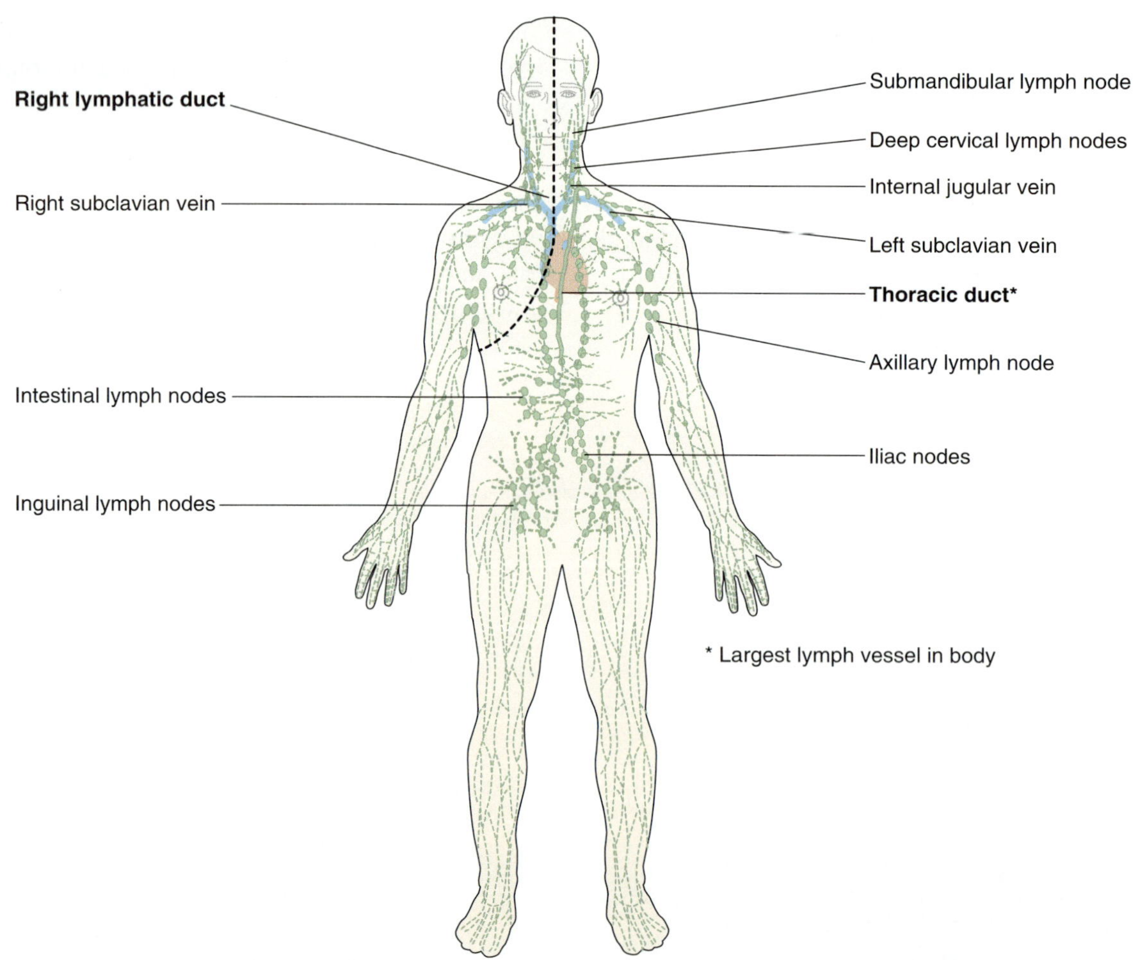

Figure 12–2 The lymphatic system.

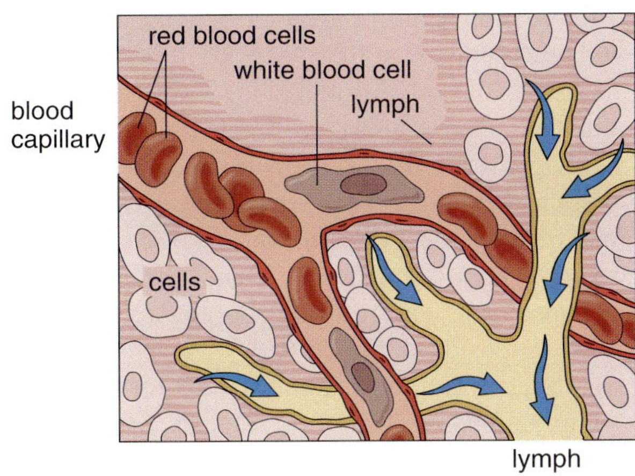

Figure 12–3 Exchange of fluids between the lymph and blood vessels.

the venous system. The lymphatic system picks up this extra fluid and returns it to the blood. In addition, the lymph vessels transport toxic substances to the nodes for filtration. In the digestive process, the vessels are important in the absorption of fats. The nodes are important in the filtering process, but they also produce lymphocytes and protect the body by developing immunity to some diseases.

Organs related to the lymph system are the tonsils, thymus gland, and spleen and were discussed earlier.

COMMON SIGNS AND SYMPTOMS

The common signs and symptoms related to the various immune system diseases are quite varied depending on the organ or organ system that is affected. Symptoms common to allergic reactions include local or systemic inflammatory responses (redness, heat, swelling, and itching) and respiratory symptoms (runny nose, coughing, sneezing, and nasal congestion).

The classic clinical problem with immune deficiency disorders is the development of unusual and severe infections such as pneumonia, meningitis, or septicemia, to name just a few. Also the development of infections by microorganisms that are not usually pathogenic (opportunistic infections) may be indicative of an **immunodeficiency** (lack of immunity) disorder. The common signs and symptoms related to the various **autoimmune** (immunity against self) and **isoimmune** (immunity against other humans) disorders are quite varied depending on the organ or organ system that is affected, and the invading pathogen. For this reason, signs and symptoms of these diseases are identified in the discussion of the specific disease.

Enlargement of the lymph glands or nodes is common and is usually caused by infection somewhere in the body. Infection stimulates activity of the nodes and glands to produce more **lymphocytes** (white cells created in the lymphatic system). Fever, fatigue, and weight loss are common with lymphatic diseases.

Most disorders of the lymphatic system are related to diseases of other systems. **Lymphocytosis** (lympho = lymph, cyto = cell, osis = increase or an abnormal increase in lymphocytes) and **lymphocytopenia** (lymphocyte = lymph cell, penia = decrease or an abnormal decrease in lymphocytes) in blood and tissue may accompany diseases of the immune system as well as the lymphatic system.

DIAGNOSTIC TESTS

Determining the cause of an allergic reaction may be quite difficult. There are hundreds of possible **antigens** (**allergens**) that cause allergic reactions. Some of the more common allergens are: house dust, pet hair, chocolate, ragweed, cigarette smoke, pollen, seafood, nickel, plants, paints, dyes, and chemical cleaners.

One type of test for diagnosing allergies is the skin test. A skin test may be performed by intradermal injection of a small amount of the suspected antigen under the skin. A skin patch test utilizes placement of a small antigen soaked patch against the individual's skin. Another skin test is a scratch test, performed by placing a small amount of suspected antigen in a small scratch. All three types of tests are used to identify an allergen.

Allergy to the antigen is positive if an inflammatory response or wheal occurs at the injection site. The size of the wheal is usually indicative of the individual's sensitivity to the allergen. There are hundreds of allergic antigens that may be used in skin testing.

Hypersensitivity reactions to blood cells is usually identified by a blood count indicating low levels of red cells, white cells, and platelets. Antibodies may form against all these blood elements leading to anemia, leukopenia, and thrombocytopenia, respectively.

A Coombs' test will indicate the formation of antibodies on the red blood cell. This test can be used to determine blood type and diagnose certain **hemolytic** (HE-moh-**LIT**-ick; hemo = blood, lytic = destroying) anemias. A Coombs' test may also indicate the presence of maternal antibodies against the fetal blood type as occurs in erythroblastosis fetalis.

Autoimmune disorders may be diagnosed utilizing blood tests that measure for specific diseases. For example, individuals with systemic lupus erythematosus will have a positive ANA or antinuclear antibody test.

Rheumatoid factor (RF) in the blood is often indicative of rheumatoid arthritis.

Immunodeficiency disorders are usually diagnosed by blood testing revealing low white cell counts, specifically B and T lymphocytes. Presence of an antibody in the blood against a causative pathogen may also be utilized. Finding an antibody against the human immunodeficiency virus (HIV) is indicative of exposure to AIDS.

A complete blood count with white cell differential may assist in determination of inflammation or infectious diseases of the lymphatic system.

Lymphangiography (lim-FAN-jee-**OG**-rah-fee; lymph = lymph, angio = vessel, graphy = procedure) consists of injecting a contrast dye and taking X-rays. This procedure may be helpful in diagnosing vessel conditions. Magnetic resonance imaging (MRI) and computerized tomography (CT) may also be utilized.

Biopsy of lymph glands and nodes may assist in determination of lymphoma. For example, a special connective tissue cell called a Reed-Sternberg cell confirms a diagnosis of Hodgkin's disease.

COMMON DISEASES OF THE IMMUNE SYSTEM

Diseases of the immune system may be divided into two main groups: hypersensitivity disorders and immune deficiency disorders. There are several specific diseases within each grouping. Each of these has some unique problems associated with the disease, but some of the signs and symptoms may be quite similar.

Hypersensitivity Disorders

Hypersensitivity disorders are the result of an overreaction of the immune system to an antigen or allergen. Hypersensitivity disorders may be further classified as those related to allergy, autoimmunity, and isoimmunity (Figure 12–4).

Allergies. Allergies are among the most prevalent types of hypersensitivity problems. Millions of people suffer from some type of allergy. Hay fever, asthma (AZ-ma), **urticaria** (UR-tih-**KAR**-ree-ah; a reaction characterized by intense wheals and itching), and contact dermatitis are common allergic reactions. These reactions are usually just bothersome, but they can be a serious health threat. Severe asthma, for example, may be life-threatening. Food allergies are also common in some populations, but may be difficult to diagnose.

Allergy is an acquired hypersensitivity. The individual with an allergy must first be exposed or sensitized to the antigen. Subsequent or repeated exposure leads to the reaction by the immune system identified as an allergy or an allergic reaction. Allergens may cause an immediate response such as those identified with hay fever, asthma, or food allergy. Delayed response allergies are slower to react and usually less harmful. An example of delayed response allergy would be contact dermatitis, caused by exposure to poison ivy.

Signs and symptoms of allergies include local or systemic inflammatory responses such as redness, heat, swelling, and often itching of the tissues involved. Respiratory symptoms may include runny nose, coughing, sneezing, wheezing, and nasal congestion.

Asthma. This chronic allergic condition is also known as bronchial asthma. It affects five to ten percent of children, making it the leading cause of chronic illness in childhood. Male children have asthma twice as often as girls prior to puberty. After puberty the rate is more equal.

When exposed to an allergen, the hypersensitive individual has episodes of wheezing caused by **bronchospasm** (**BRONG**-ko-SPA-zm) or muscularconstriction of the bronchi of the respiratory tract. The individual appears perfectly normal between episodes. Symptoms of an attack are extreme shortness of breath, difficulty breathing, wheezing, and anxiety. Attacks vary in severity from mild to almost suffocating. Coughing during the attack usually begins with a mild dry cough but progresses to production of large amounts of mucus as the attack continues. Skin may be pale and moist in mild attacks, with cyanosis of the nail beds and lips occurring in more severe attacks. During an attack, patients often assume a sitting position, leaning forward with hands resting on the knees. This position helps the patient breathe by utilizing all the respiratory muscles (Figure 12–5). A severe asthma attack that is associated with extreme dyspnea and does not respond to typical first line treatment of inhaled bronchodilators is called **status asthmaticus** (**AZ**-MAH-ti-kus). This is a life-threatening medical emergency that requires aggressive pre-hospital and emergency department treatment and may take several weeks for the patient to finally recover.

Asthma may be caused by allergens in the environment such as pollen, dust, pet dander, smoke, or various fumes. Other causes of asthma are non-allergic and include events that produce stress. Triggers for non-allergic asthma include respiratory infections like the common cold, changes in temperature and humidity, exercise, and emotional stress.

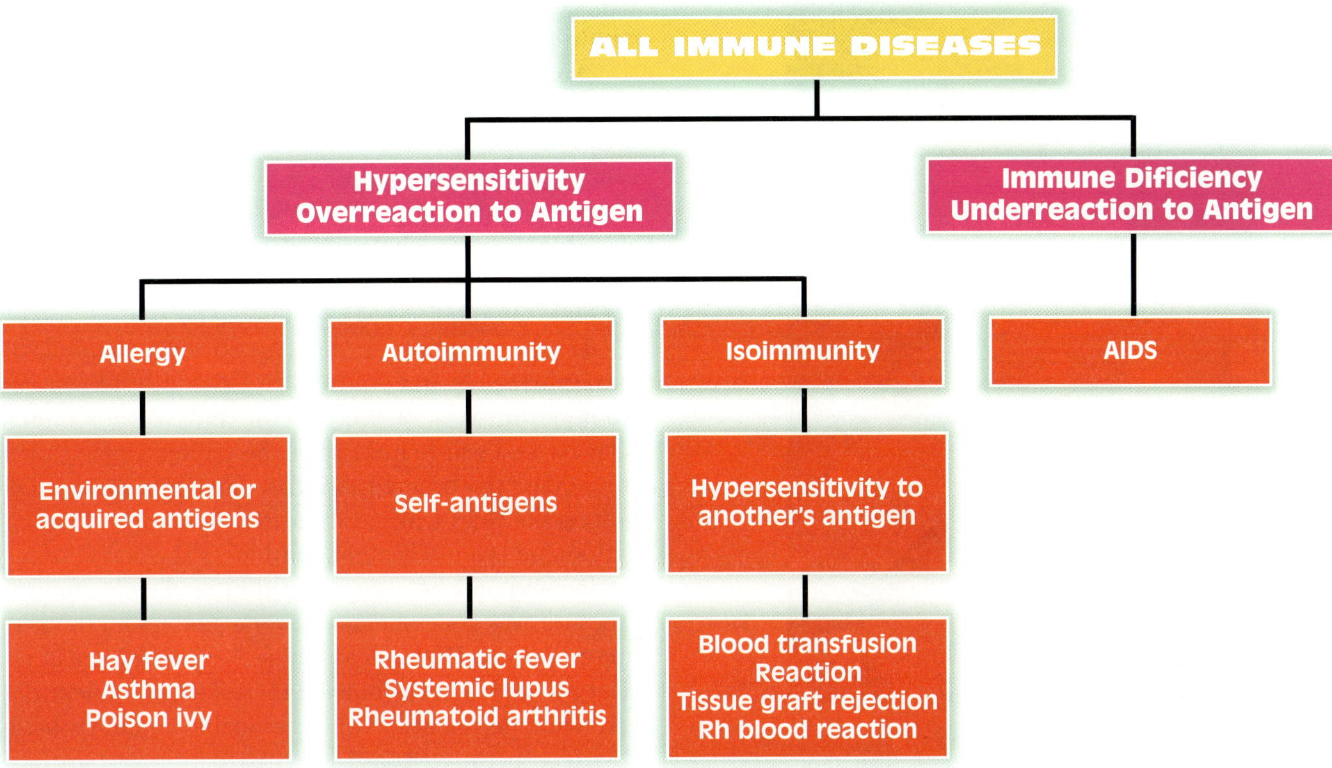

Figure 12–4 Classification of hypersensitivity disorders.

Emergency treatment for a patient experiencing an asthma attack includes supplemental oxygen and inhaled bronchodilators. Intravenous steroids and magnesium sulfate may also be administered in more severe attacks. Some patients may require intubation and ventilation if they tire and progress into respiratory failure. Patients should be educated to avoid causative allergens, quit smoking, and remain compliant with their medications. Many patients are given a handheld spirometer that they can use to assess their peak flows with instructions to call their physician if their peak flow falls below a certain level into their yellow zone, and to call EMS if the peak flow falls into the red zone.

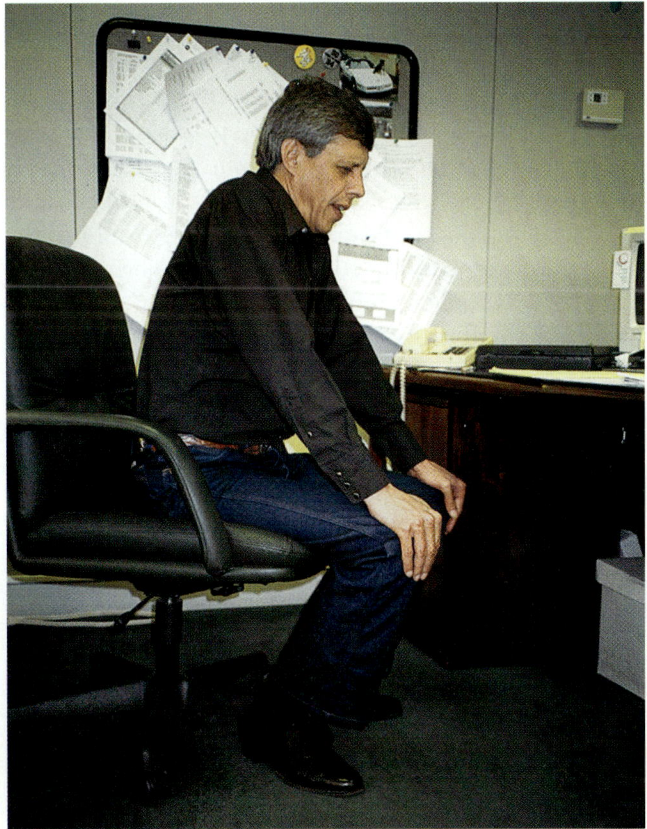

Figure 12–5 Positioning in an asthma attack.

Urticaria. Commonly called hives or nettle rash, urticaria is a vascular reaction of the skin. It is characterized by slightly elevated lesions that are redder or paler than the surrounding skin and is associated with severe itching. The elevated areas are called wheals or hives. Scratching or rubbing the hypersensitive area may lead to formation of larger or additional wheals (Figure 12–6). This condition is caused by contact with an external irritant, such as insect bites, pollen, drugs, food, or plants. Treatment includes antihistamines and avoidance of the allergen.

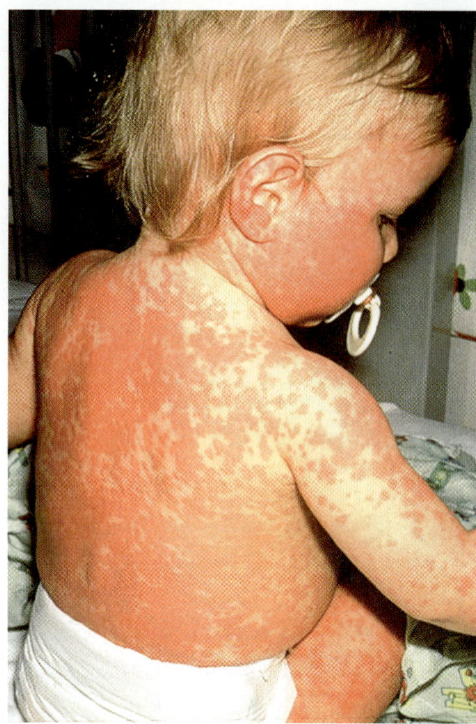

Figure 12–6 Urticaria. (Courtesy of Robert A. Silverman, MD, Clinical Associate Professor, Department of Pediatrics, Georgetown University.)

Anaphylaxis. This is a severe allergic response to an allergen that often leads to anaphylactic shock without intervention. **Anaphylaxis** (AN-ah-fih-**LACK**-sis), also known as an anaphylactic reaction, is caused by absorption of the antigen into the blood directly or through the mucous membranes. Substances that commonly cause anaphylaxis include: antibiotics, anesthetics, codeine, insulin, hormones, iodinated X-ray contrast media, vaccines, antitoxins, foods, pollen, mold, animal dander, latex, and insect venom of wasps, bees, or hornets.

A local anaphylactic reaction may be mild and produce generalized itching, swelling, and urticaria. This reaction should be closely monitored as it may rapidly progress to systemic anaphylaxis. Systemic anaphylaxis is a true medical emergency involving the release of histamine from MAST cells throughout body tissues. The signs and symptoms of anaphylaxis are caused by the release of histamine, which dilates blood vessels and causes the capillary walls to become leaky. Within minutes, the individual feels itching of the throat, tongue, and scalp. Edema or swelling of the face and airways leads to difficulty in breathing. The individual suffers a huge drop in blood pressure (shock) and body temperature. Unconsciousness usually occurs with the drop in blood pressure. If these symptoms are not reversed with medical attention, death from respiratory and cardiac arrest may occur within fifteen to twenty minutes.

Airway management is a key concern in a patient experiencing anaphylaxis. The edema in the tongue and upper airway combined with the bronchospasm significantly limit the amount of air available for ventilation. Supplemental oxygen will increase the amount of oxygen available during each breath. Intubation or surgical airway, depending upon the EMS provider's scope of practice, may be required to maintain an airway.

If the patient is having severe anaphylaxis, epinephrine is generally the first line treatment. Epinephrine is a vasoconstrictor and smooth muscle relaxant and will help to raise the patient's blood pressure, dilate the bronchi, decrease laryngeal spasms, and reduce the fluid leakage from the capillaries. Diphenhydramine is a medication that blocks the action of histamine and may be administered immediately after the exposure, as it generally takes several minutes for the reaction to occur. Diphenhydramine is often administered after epinephrine to enhance the effect of epinephrine and decrease the effect of additional histamine release. **Corticosteroids** (**KORT**-ti-ko-STEHR-oyds) are also given to stabilize MAST cell membranes and decrease histamine production.

Follow-up treatment would include identifying the allergen. The patient is taught to identify and avoid the allergen and recognize the onset of a reaction. These patients should wear an allergy identification necklace or bracelet. Patients who experience this severe reaction should always carry an allergy kit containing Benadryl (an antihistamine) and a prescription autoinjector of epinephrine that can be self-administered immediately after exposure to a known allergen. The patient and family members should understand and practice the appropriate steps in treatment of a reaction.

Autoimmune Disorders. Autoimmune disorders are hypersensitivities in which the body fails to recognize its own antigens or **self-antigen**. An individual's body cells have specific antigen on the cell surfaces. Failure to recognize this antigen as a self-antigen leads to the body attacking and destroying its own tissues. Several theories exist as to the cause of this type of disorder but currently the cause for autoimmune disorders is unknown. The autoimmune disorders include rheumatic fever, rheumatoid arthritis, myasthenia gravis, systemic lupus erythematosus, and multiple sclerosis.

Rheumatic Fever. Rheumatic (ROO-**MAT**-ik) fever occurs in a small number of individuals following a group A

streptococcal (**STREHP**-toh-KAHK-al) infection, usually strep throat. In this select number of individuals the proteins in their heart and other connective tissue are similar to the protein of the strep bacteria. For this reason, rheumatic fever tends to run in families. Exposure to strep bacteria causes the immune system to make antibodies to fight the bacteria. These antibodies also attack the tissues of the heart and joints as they are similar to the surface markers on the bacteria. Rheumatic fever is characterized by myocarditis (myo = muscle, cardi = heart, itis = inflammation) and arthritis.

Rheumatic fever usually occurs one to four weeks after a streptococcal infection. Children and adolescents are most commonly affected. Onset of the disease may be sudden or gradual and includes symptoms of fever, malaise, and joint pain. The first occurrence of rheumatic fever may be mild and resolve without any permanent damage. Further episodes are usually more severe and may lead to permanent scarring and deformity of the heart valves (Figure 12–7). Deformity of the mitral and aortic valve may eventually lead to heart failure.

Prompt and accurate diagnosis and treatment of group A streptococcal infections is the best preventive measure against rheumatic fever. Culturing for strep infections and prolonged treatment (at least ten days) with antibiotics is most effective. **Prophylactic** (pro-fil-LACK-tic; works to prevent) antibiotics may be given to susceptible individuals before dental and other outpatient procedures. Surgical replacement of the heart valves may be necessary for individuals with severe valve deformity.

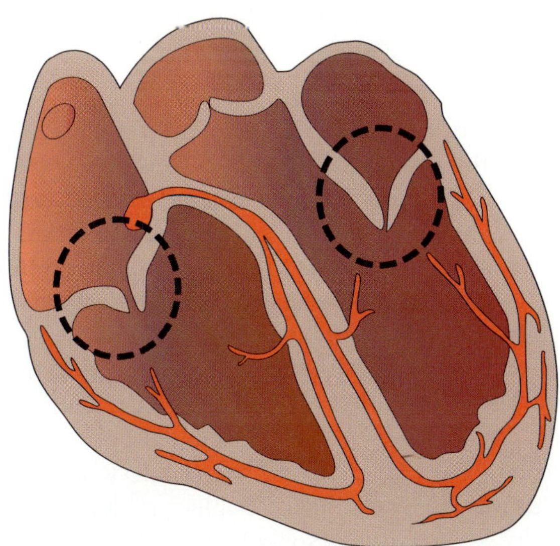

Figure 12–7 Valvulitis.

Rheumatoid Arthritis. Rheumatoid arthritis is an autoimmune disease that causes chronic inflammation of connective tissue. Joint tissue is primarily affected, but any connective tissue of the body may be involved. The exact cause of rheumatoid arthritis is unknown, but it is associated with the production of an abnormal antibody that attacks or attaches to the body's own cells and tissues. Presence of the antibody called rheumatoid factor (RF) in the affected individual's blood is usually indicative of the disease.

Commonly, metacarpophalangeal joints of the hands are initially affected with rheumatoid arthritis. This leads to a classic sign of rheumatoid arthritis called ulnar deviation of the fingers (Figure 12–8). As the disease progresses, involvement of other synovial joints may occur. Joints affected may include those of the fingers, wrists, elbows, feet, ankles, and knees. Symptoms of rheumatoid arthritis may vary in severity from mild to severe, and may go through periods of remission and exacerbation.

Rheumatoid arthritis begins with inflammation of the synovial lining of the joint leading to pain, stiffness, and joint deformity. Eventually the cartilage of the joint is destroyed and replaced with a granulation tissue called pannus (PAN-nus). As the disease progresses, the entire joint surface is destroyed and replaced with fibrous tissue making the joint less movable. Fusion or total loss of joint function is called ankylosis (ANG-kih-**LOH**-sis) (Figure 12–9).

In addition to joint changes the individual may also have lesions in the collagen of the lungs, blood vessels, heart, and eyes leading to pleuritis (PLOO-**RIGH**-tis; pleura = pleura or lining of the lung, itis = inflammation), anemia, valvulitis (VAL-view-**LYE**-tis; valvu = valve, itis = inflammation), and glaucoma (glaw-KOH-mah), respectively. Rheumatoid nodules characteristically appear in the subcutaneous tissue around the fingers, toes, and

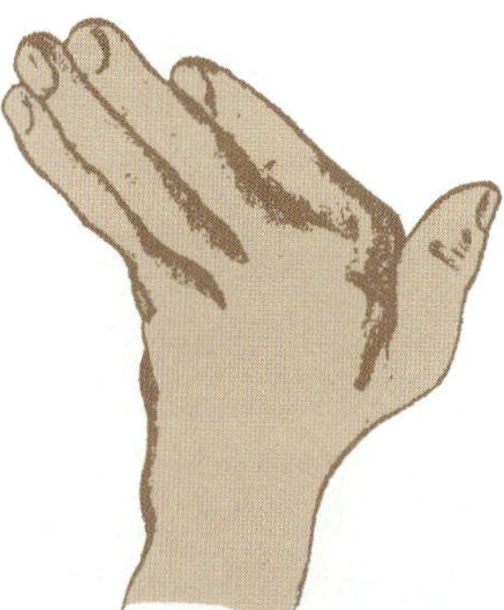

Figure 12–8 Ulnar deviation from rheumatoid arthritis.

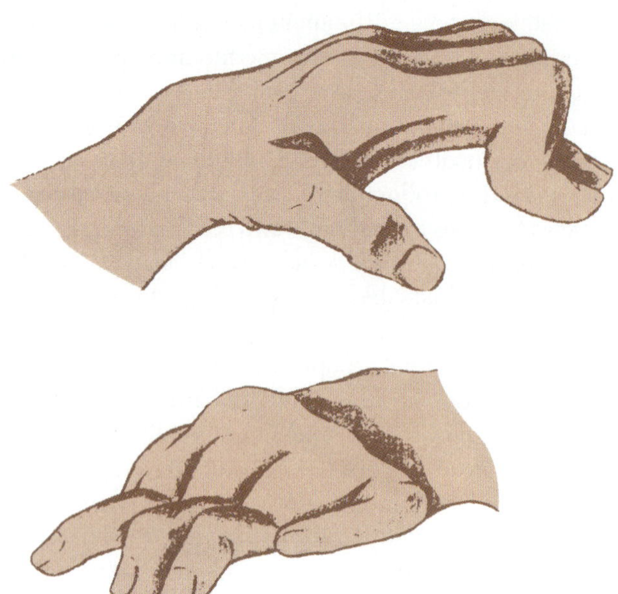

Figure 12–9 Joint changes form rheumatoid arthritis.

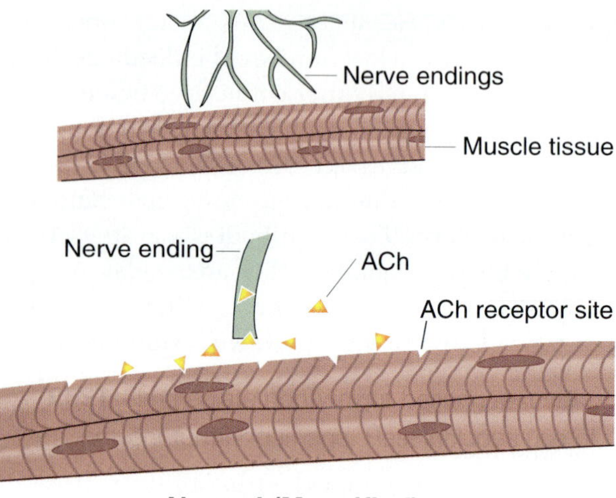

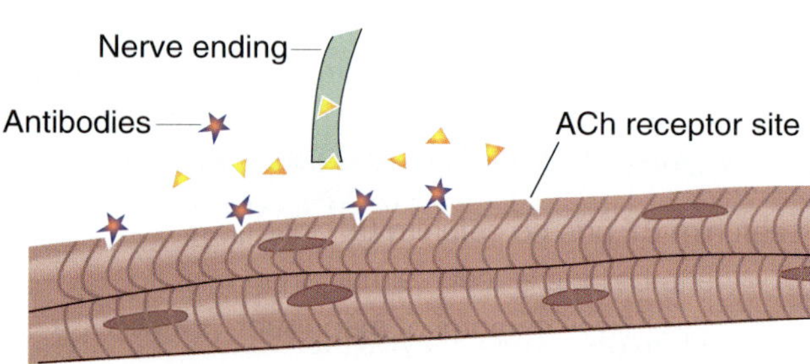

Myasthenia Gravis (Magnified)

Nerves do not touch muscle tissue to stimulate movement. Nerve endings secrete a neurotransmitter, acetylcholine (ACh), that sticks to muscle tissue receptor sites causing muscle contraction.

Antibodies produced with myasthenia gravis block these receptor sites thus blocking muscle stimulus and movement.

Figure 12–10 Blocking of receptor sites in myasthenia gravis.

elbows. Individuals with rheumatoid arthritis often appear frail and chronically ill. Anemia and infection are common secondary problems.

This chronic disease affects both sexes and all ages, but onset is most common in women between the ages of twenty and forty. Women are affected three times more often than men. Rheumatoid arthritis in children usually affects infants to children aged sixteen. It may be very severe and is called juvenile rheumatoid arthritis or Still's disease.

Rheumatoid arthritis, like other autoimmune disorders, cannot be cured. Treatment includes use of anti-inflammatory medications and analgesics. An exercise and rest routine is developed to maintain joint function. Corticosteroids may be prescribed for short terms during periods of exacerbation. Surgical joint replacement may also be beneficial.

Myasthenia Gravis. Myasthenia gravis (MY-uh-**STHEE**-nee-uh GRAV-iss) is characterized by severe muscle fatigue. This disease affects the transmission of nerve signals to muscle at the neuromuscular junction. There is no muscle or nerve tissue disease. Nerve impulses are carried to the muscle by the neurotransmitter acetylcholine (ah-SEE-til-**KOH**-leen). These impulses are sent by the nerve, but are not properly received by the muscle. This error in transmission is caused by antibodies attacking the muscle receptors, which blocks the transmission by acetylcholine (Figure 12–10). This poor transmission of information to the muscle leads to weak muscle contractions and fatigue.

There are approximately 100,000 Americans affected with myasthenia gravis. The incidence is only about one in 10,000 individuals so it is considered to be a fairly rare disorder (The Myasthenia Gravis Foundation of America, 1997). Myasthenia gravis can be categorized as an autoimmune, musculoskeletal, or neurologic disease as it has characteristics of problems in each of these systems. Onset of the disease is usually slow and diagnosis may be difficult as it may affect any muscle of the body. Commonly, facial muscles are the ones initially affected leading to diplopia (dip-PLOHP-ee-ah; double vision), ptosis (TOE sis; drooping eyelids), dysphagia (dys-FAY-jee-ah; difficulty swallowing), dysphonia (dys-FOH-nee-ah; difficulty talking), and difficulty with facial expressions, which may leave the individual with an expressionless facial appearance. Other symptoms relate to fatigue of all voluntary muscles and include difficulty rising from a sitting position, lifting the arms, standing, and walking.

The degree of weakness varies with the time of day and activities. Generally these individuals feel stronger in the morning because of a buildup of acetylcholine and become weaker as the day progresses because acetylcholine stores diminish. Short rest periods are necessary to help restore muscle function.

Periods of exacerbation and remission do occur. During exacerbation, complete bed rest may be necessary.

Treatment may include cholinergic medications such as Mestinon that do not allow the normal breakdown of the neurotransmitter acetylcholine. These drugs allow a buildup of the neurotransmitter thus improving neuromuscular transmission. Plasma exchange to remove the circulating antibodies provides some improvement in the condition. Myasthenia gravis may progress over a period of years, but it is ultimately fatal. Death is usually caused by muscle weakness leading to respiratory failure.

Type 1 Diabetes Mellitus (Insulin-dependent Diabetes Mellitus). Type 1 diabetes mellitus, formerly known as insulin-dependent diabetes mellitus or IDDM, is a disease that alters the body's carbohydrate or sugar metabolism. It is believed to be caused by an autoimmune disorder triggered by a viral infection. The most common viral infections that may lead to diabetes include rubella, mumps, and influenza. The infecting virus inflames insulin-producing beta cells of the pancreas. The inflammatory process, for reasons that remain yet unclear, seems to stimulate the beta cells to produce an abnormal cell antigen. Lymphocytes recognize the abnormal antigen as non-self and destroy it along with the beta cells. Without insulin-producing beta cells, the individual becomes dependent on insulin injections to manage carbohydrate utilization.

The normal antigens in the cells of the pancreas are HLAs (histocompatibility locus antigens). Individuals genetically inherit the HLAs of the pancreas. The tendency to develop an autoimmune response, and thus diabetes mellitus, is considered hereditary in nature.

There are other types of diabetes that are not caused by autoimmunity. As all types of diabetes affect the endocrine system they are discussed and compared in detail in Chapter 11.

Isoimmune Disorders. Isoimmunity refers to a hypersensitivity of one individual to another individual's tissues. Examples include blood type reactions, tissue rejections, and maternal/fetal reactions.

Blood Transfusion Reaction. All body cells have a specific antigen that identifies them. Red blood cells have surface antigens. Transfusion of blood from one individual to another is a type of tissue transplant. RBCs have to be typed and crossmatched to properly identify antigens and prevent rejection.

The blood types are identified by antigens and can be divided into four groups: A, B, AB, and O. Types O and A are the most common. Each red blood cell has an antigen and a corresponding antibody. Blood type A has an A antigen and anti-B antibody. B type has a B antigen and anti-A antibody. O has no antigen and both anti-A and anti-B antibody. AB has an A and B antigen and no antibody. These antigen-antibody patterns make type O the universal blood donor and type AB the universal blood recipient (Figure 12–11).

If a blood type with an antigen is given to a type that has antibodies against that antigen, the antibodies will attack the antigen and break down the donor RBCs. For example, if type A (with antigen A and anti-B antibody) is given to type B (with antigen B and anti-A antibody), the anti-A antibody in the B type recipient's blood will attack the A antigen and break down the type A donor blood (see Figure 12–11).

As antibodies react with the antigen, they also cause clumping of the blood leading to microthrombi (microscopic sized blood clots). These microthrombi can lead to multiple organ emboli and thus have fatal consequences. Symptoms of transfusion reaction include chills, shivering, and fever. The transfusion must be discontinued immediately to avoid fatality.

Erythroblastosis Fetalis. Erythroblastosis fetalis (eh-RITH-roh-blas-**TOH**-sis feh-TAH-lis) is an isoimmune condition where antibodies in a mother's blood attack and destroy the antigen on the baby's red blood cells, ultimately killing the unborn fetus. This condition is also known as hemolytic (hemo = blood, lytic = breaking or crushing) disease of the newborn.

Antigens on the red blood cells give each type of cell a special identity. In addition to antigens that determine blood type, eighty-five percent of Americans have another antigen called the Rh factor. This group is collectively called Rh positive (Rh+) since they have the factor or antigen. Those who do not have the factor, approximately fifteen percent of the population, are Rh negative (Rh-). Crossmatching for transfusions must not only match an appropriate type, but also a compatible factor. The common rule is that "those who don't have it don't want it, those that have it don't care." So in other words, Rh- individuals cannot receive Rh+ blood. On the other

Type	Percent of Population with Type	Antigen	Antibody	Color Jar Example	Donate Blood To:	Receive Blood From:
A	41	A	B	RED	A and AB	A and O
B	12	B	A	BLUE	B and AB	B and O
O	44	None	A and B	CLEAR	A, B, AB, O	O
AB	3	A and B	None	PURPLE	AB	A, B, AB, O

To understand the concept of transfusion reaction with antigen and antibodies, consider this example. The particular blood type can give blood to any type that does not change the color in the jar and receive blood from any type that does not change the color in the jar. For example, A can give blood to AB because adding red to purple will not change the purple color. However, A cannot give to B because giving red to blue will change the color. Since O is in the clear jar, it can give to all types but could not receive from anything but O or the clear color would change.

Figure 12–11 Blood types for donors and recipients.

hand, Rh+ individuals "don't care" so they can receive Rh+ or Rh- blood. Blood type and factor are genetically determined or received from an individual's mother or father.

Because blood type and factor is determined by one's mother or father it is possible for a mother to be pregnant with a baby of different blood type and factor (received from the father) (Figure 12–12). Mothers pregnant with babies of different blood types do not have a problem as red blood cells do not cross the placenta. Oxygen and nutrients simply diffuse across placental membranes to nourish the baby. RBCs do not normally exchange between the mother and the infant. Mothers who are Rh- and "don't want" Rh+ factor may have difficulty with Rh+ babies.

Rh- mothers pregnant with Rh+ babies usually do not have a problem with the first baby. During the first pregnancy the mother's blood has not had the opportunity to identify the antigen because there has been no exchange of blood cells or antigens. However, there may be some slight mixing of blood during the birthing process. As this blood intermingles, the Rh+ antigen is picked up by the mother's blood. The mother's immune system recognizes this antigen as a foreign invader and builds antibodies to destroy it. Subsequent Rh+ babies can be affected by these antibodies.

If this Rh- mother becomes pregnant with another Rh+ baby, antibodies against the Rh factor that she has built up in her blood do cross the placental membranes. These antibodies attack the blood of the unborn child breaking down the RBCs leading to anemia and possibly death of the baby.

This condition only affects Rh+ babies carried by Rh- mothers. Rh+ mothers have the antigen so they do not build up antibodies against it.

Treatment for erythroblastosis fetalis is exchange transfusion of the baby's blood with Rh- blood at birth. This treatment stops the destruction of the baby's red blood cells. Over a period of time the transfused Rh- blood is replaced by the baby's own blood. If erythroblastosis fetalis is a possibility in Rh- mother, the baby's condition may be monitored by amniocentesis. Babies who are mildly affected may be allowed to be carried to full term. Severe cases may indicate the need to induce labor and premature delivery of the baby in order to begin lifesaving treatment.

Erythroblastosis fetalis rarely occurs in the modern world. The development of RhoGAM, a special immune globulin, has halted this condition. RhoGAM is an injectable medication given to Rh- females to prevent the development of antibodies against Rh+ factor. This medication is given prophylactically after the delivery of the first fetus.

Organ Rejection. Organs such as the liver, kidney, heart, and lungs could be easily transplanted if it were not for the human immune system. The immune system recognizes transplanted tissue as foreign and attacks it. This

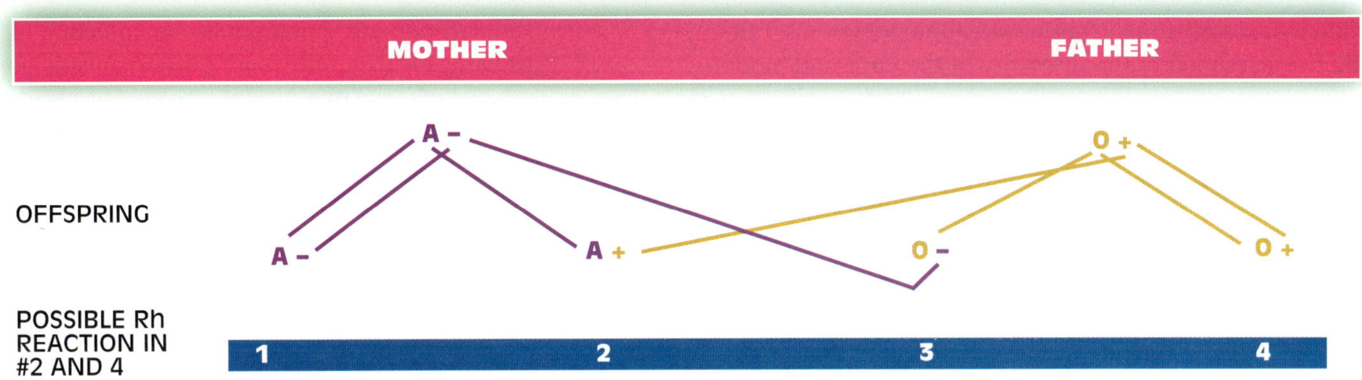

The offspring of this mother and father have the possibility of four different blood types. As this is an Rh– mother, there is a possibility of an Rh reaction with the two Rh+ children. If the father was also Rh–, all offspring would be Rh– and no reaction would occur in any of the children. If the mother were Rh+ no Rh reaction could occur in any of the offspring as Rh+ mothers are not sensitive to the Rh antigen.

Figure 12–12 Blood type in inheritance patterns and identification of possible Rh reactions.

attack by lymphocytes brings about donor tissue destruction recognized as tissue or organ rejection.

Donated organs are matched to possible recipients. The closer the donor antigen matches that of the recipient the less chance the organ will be rejected. Administration of immunosuppression medications also decreases the possibility of rejection. Immunosuppression medications must be taken prior to transplantation surgery and for the remainder of the organ recipient's life. These medications suppress or decrease the body's ability to destroy the donor tissue.

Transplant rejection may be hyperacute in nature and actually occur during the surgical procedure. Acute rejection occurs within the first few weeks while chronic rejection occurs over a period of time, usually months to years. Chronic rejection occurs slowly and is caused by vessel damage that decreases blood flow to the donor tissue. Decreased blood flow causes chronic ischemia and ultimately death of the donor organ.

Immune Deficiency Disorders

The second classification of immune disorders is immunodeficiency. These disorders represent an inability of the immune system to protect the individual against disease. This deficiency may be congenital, caused by a genetic disorder, or it may be acquired during the individual's lifetime. Acquired disorders are the most common type and may be caused by disease therapies. Chemotherapy and radiation treatments often lead to immunodeficiency by suppressing bone marrow, thus decreasing leukocyte production. Medications given to organ transplant recipients purposefully suppress the immune system. The most common and fatal disorder is acquired immunodeficiency syndrome (AIDS).

The classic clinical problem with immunodeficiency disorders is the development of unusual and severe infections such as pneumonia, meningitis, or septicemia to name a few. Also, the development of infections by microorganisms that are not usually pathogenic (opportunistic infections) may be indicative of an immunodeficiency disorder. Other signs and symptoms are numerous and varied depending on the organs or organ systems affected and the invading pathogen. Specific signs and symptoms will be included in the discussion of the specific disorder.

Acquired Immunodeficiency Syndrome (AIDS). The name of this disease briefly describes its pathology. It is an acquired disease that causes the immune system to be deficient in its ability to protect the body, leading to a syndrome of symptoms or secondary diseases. The cause of AIDS is a virus called human immunodeficiency virus or HIV.

The wicked characteristic about HIV is that its battle plan is to wipe out the individual's lymphocytes, thus leaving the body defenseless against attack by all pathogenic organisms. The primary target is the T lymphocyte, but macrophages are affected as well. HIV is **cytotoxic** (cyto = cell, toxic = killing). Ultimately the HIV infected individual will have a low T lymphocyte cell count, indicative of a positive diagnosis of AIDS.

AIDS was first diagnosed in the United States in the early 1980s. The first diagnosed cases were a group of homosexual men who became ill with a series of opportunistic diseases and eventually died. These individuals had surprisingly suppressed immune systems. Further research led to the discovery of the virus and mode of transmission.

Previously, HIV was staged as four separate clinical presentations. Those stages were Asymptomatic carrier, Latency, AIDS Related Complex (ARC), and Full-blown AIDS. Currently HIV infection is known to be a continuous disease process. Staging this disease may be helpful for medical intervention. The new stages of HIV infection are acute infection, asymptomatic HIV, symptomatic HIV, and advanced disease.

1. Acute infection—This stage begins about one to three weeks after initial infection. During this time the virus undergoes massive replication. Signs and symptoms include fever, sore throat, headache, and malaise. At this stage, HIV infection may be misdiagnosed as influenza.
2. Asymptomatic HIV—No chronic signs or symptoms are displayed during this stage. Lymphadenopathy (lymph = lymphatic, adeno = gland, opathy = disease) and headache may occur intermittently. If blood testing is utilized during this stage, the T lymphocyte count may be dropping by 40 to 80 cells per microliter per year (normal T cell count is 750–1000 cells per microliter). T cell count is a useful indicator of disease progression. This count is utilized in studying the effects of antiviral drugs and predicting the potential for opportunistic infections. This stage may last for ten to twelve years depending on drug therapy and individual resistance.
3. Symptomatic HIV—This stage is divided into *early* and *late* phases. During the early phase, the individual becomes symptomatic with a variety of symptoms or diseases affecting any or all of the body organs. Fever is a common symptom along with oral *Candida albicans*, recurrent herpes simplex lesions, and night sweats. The chronic diarrhea of this phase leads to dehydration and cachexia. Individuals are considered to be in the late phase when their T cell count drops below 200 cells per microliter. At this point the individual has met the criteria set by CDC for a diagnosis of AIDS. Common diseases and disorders experienced during this phase include gastric ulcer, esophagitis, colitis, hepatitis, pancreatitis, fungal infections, neurologic disorders, herpes zoster, dermatitis, nausea, and vomiting, to name just a few. In this phase, the individual experiences severe weight loss, weakness, persistent diarrhea, and usually at least one opportunistic disease. These opportunistic infections include:
   - **Pneumocystis carinii** (NEW-moh-**SIS**-tis kah-RYE-nee-eye) pneumonia—an infection of the lungs with a protozoan. This organism has never been documented as a cause of pneumonia in persons with normal immune systems.
   - **Kaposi's sarcoma** (KAP-oh-seez sar-KOH-mah)—a blood vessel cancer that causes reddish-purple skin lesions (Figure 12–13).
4. Advanced HIV— This stage is determined by a T cell count of fewer than 50 cells per microliter. In this stage, mortality increases significantly. Commonly, more virulent and persistent infections occur that are more resistant to treatment. Symptoms at this stage include seizures, confusion, urinary and fecal incontinence, blindness, hemiparesis (hemi = one side, paresis = weakness), and coma.

Once AIDS is diagnosed, life expectancy is approximately three to five years. Currently AIDS is 100 percent fatal. Life can be extended by vigorous treatment of infections. In late-stage AIDS, every possible symptom or disease may be present as the individual's immune system is crumbling and incapacitated (Figure 12–14). Ultimately, super infections and massive diarrhea may be the cause of death. Anti-viral medication such as zidovudine (AZT) may slow HIV replication and thus slow the progression of the disease to some extent.

Transmission of AIDS. HIV is transmitted from one individual to another through intimate contact and sharing of body fluids. The virus must enter the body and bloodstream in order to infect the individual. The human immunodeficiency virus is a fragile virus that is easily killed by temperature changes. There are many misconceptions and

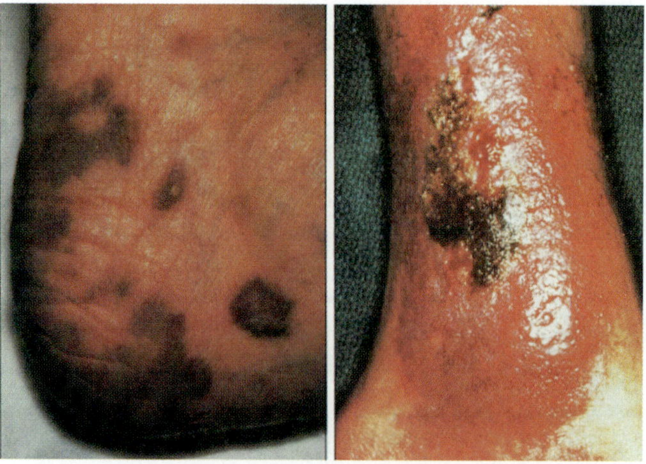

Figure 12–13 Kaposi's sarcoma.

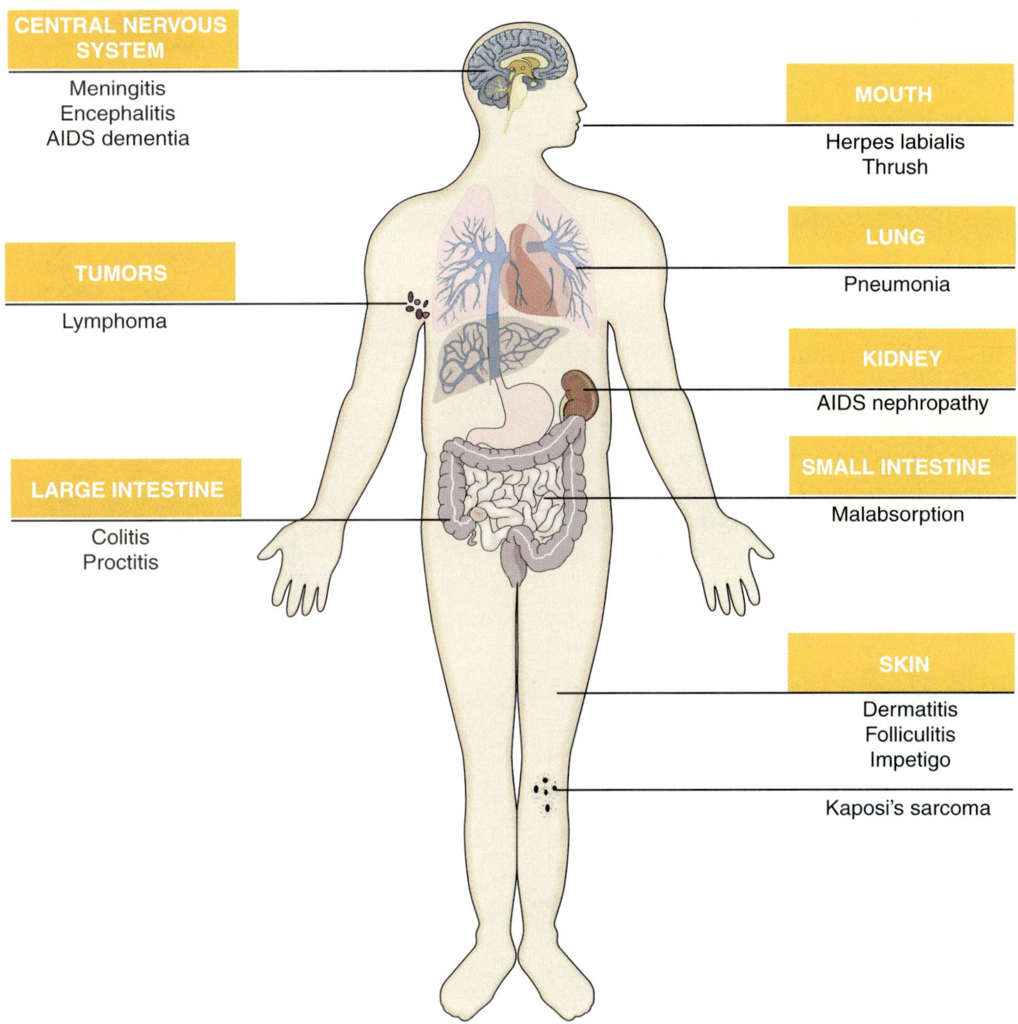

Figure 12–14 Pathologies associated with AIDS.

fears about the transmission of AIDS still prevalent in society today. An individual *cannot* get HIV infection from toilet seats, doorknobs, furniture, water fountains, and other objects. An individual *cannot* get HIV from social kissing, coughing, sneezing, even sharing eating utensils. HIV is *not* transmitted through air, food, urine, feces, or water. HIV is primarily transmitted or spread in three ways:

1. Sexual intercourse—semen and vaginal secretions carry HIV. Transmission rate is higher from male to female because females may have microscopic vaginal tears during intercourse. Transmission rate is very high with anal intercourse as the internal lining of the rectum is very thin. Approximately seventy-five percent of infected individuals in the United States contract AIDS through sexual intercourse.
2. Sharing of hypodermic needles—HIV infected blood is injected into the body by the sharing of needles. This type of transmission accounts for eighteen to twenty-five percent of infected individuals in the United States.
3. In utero from infected mother to unborn child—HIV passes across the placenta to infect the baby. This accounts for one to three percent of AIDS cases.

Transmission of HIV through blood transfusions has been virtually eliminated due to effective screening methods. Health professionals following appropriate precautions are at very little risk of contracting HIV.

COMMON DISEASES OF THE LYMPHATIC SYSTEM

Diseases of the lymphatic system commonly include inflammatory conditions. Often diseases of this system are the result of disease in another system. Disease of lymph glands may be collectively called **lymphadenopathy** (lim-FAD-eh-**NOP**-ah-thee; lymph = lymph, adeno = gland, opathy = disease). **Lymphangiopathy** (lim-FAN-jee-**OP**-ah-thee; lymph = lymph, angio = vessel, opathy = disease) is a general term to describe any disease of the lymph vessels.

Lymphadenitis

Lymphadenitis (lim-FAD-eh-**NIGH**-tis; lymph = lymph, adeno = gland, itis = inflammation) is characterized by swelling of the lymph gland and/or nodes. Swelling, pain, and tenderness of the gland or node are common. Lymphadenitis is usually caused by infection somewhere in the body. Drainage of bacteria or toxic substances may cause the swelling. The location of the affected nodes may assist in determination of cause. Antibiotic treatment is helpful with bacterial infections.

Lymphangitis

Lymphangitis (lymph = lymph, angi = vessel, itis = inflammation) is a condition of swelling of the lymph vessel caused by inflammation. This inflammation is commonly caused by infection with streptococcal bacteria following a trauma. Lymphangitis is often characterized by a red streak at the site of bacterial entry that extends to the area lymph nodes. Other symptoms include fever, chills, and malaise. Cellulitis (inflammation of cellular or connective tissue) and leukocytosis may also be present. Lymphangitis is commonly treated with antibiotics. Warm, moist packs and elevation of the affected area are also helpful.

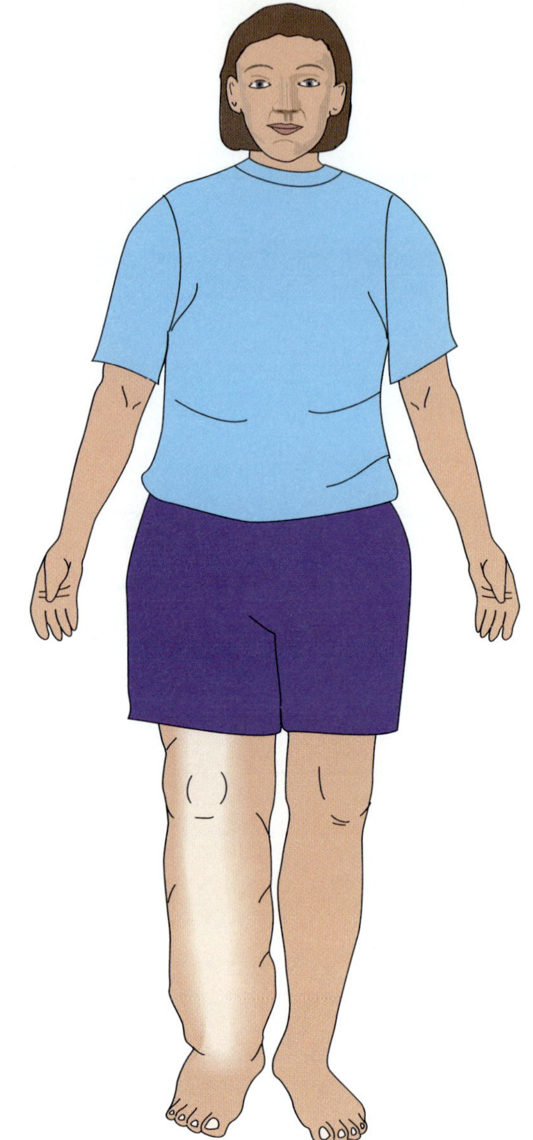

Figure 12–15 Lymphedema.

Lymphedema

Lymphedema (lymph = lymph, edema = swelling) is an abnormal collection of lymph fluid usually observed in the extremities (Figure 12–15). Causes may include:

- obstruction of a lymphatic vessel
- abnormal uptake of fluid by the lymphatic capillaries because of injury
- overproduction of interstitial fluid because of increased capillary blood pressure

Lymphatic vessels may be occluded or obstructed by inflammation or by tumors. Pressure on the vessels decreases lymphatic flow. Diagnosis may be confirmed by lymphangiography. Treatment may include antibiotics or surgical intervention depending on cause.

Abnormal uptake of fluid by the lymphatic capillaries caused by injury may be the result of surgery or radiation of tissues. Breast surgery and radiation may lead to a chronic lymphedema of the arm on the affected side. Placing the affected arm above the heart while resting and exercise to increase lymph flow may decrease the edema. Procedures such as obtaining blood pressure and drawing blood samples should not be performed on the affected side as affected tissue is more prone to infection.

Pregnancy and constrictive clothing often cause an increase in venous pressure. This increase in venous pressure results in an increase in capillary pressure and thus an overproduction of interstitial fluid commonly observed in the ankles and feet. Decreasing venous pressure in these cases will relieve lymphedema. To reduce venous pressure in the pregnant female, lying on the left side helps improve venous flow as the inferior vena cava is to the right of midline. Resting with the legs above heart level will also reduce edema. Constrictive clothing should be removed or loosened when lymphedema is observed.

Lymphoma

Lymphoma refers to several types of neoplasms that affect lymphoid tissue (lymph nodes, tonsils, spleen, and lymph fluid). There are many types of lymphoma but all affect normal lymphocyte production leading to an impaired immunity. Symptoms include night sweats, fever, and weight loss. Treatment is dependent on type of lymphoma and stage of the disease. Treatment may include surgery, chemotherapy, radiation, and bone marrow transplantation. Lymphoma is discussed in more detail in Chapter 16 under the heading "Disorders of White Blood Cells."

Mononucleosis

Mononucleosis is a viral infection that affects primarily children and young adults. It is somewhat contagious and is commonly called "kissing disease." This disease is discussed in more detail in Chapter 16 under the heading "Disorders of White Blood Cells."

TRAUMA

Trauma to the immune system is generally limited to treatments or medications that suppress the system. Chemotherapy and radiation treatments often lead to immunosuppression. Individuals on corticosteroid medications often have undetected infections as this medication suppresses the protective inflammatory response. Graft and organ recipients take immunosuppression medications to purposefully traumatize the system in hopes of protecting the transplanted graft or organ.

EFFECTS OF AGING ON THE IMMUNE SYSTEM

Presently, not all age-related changes in the immune system are well understood. It is known that the thymus gland degenerates with age. The thymus reaches its maximum size in early childhood and then slowly decreases in size after puberty. As the gland decreases in size, so do the number of T cells as they originate in the cortex of the thymus. The remaining T cells do not function as well, increasing the chance of developing invasive diseases (like cancer) as the individual ages. There also are some defects in lymph cells that occur in the aging process.

The B cell levels remain stable throughout the age of the individual but the antibodies may not function as well as in younger years. Thus, infections are common in the elderly population. The antibodies are more likely to attack the body's own tissue (autoantibodies) as a result of loss of tolerance to self-antigens. General resistance to disease seems to decrease with age but this may be caused by many other factors, such as general nutrition, exercise, medications, and psychosocial influences rather than changes in the immune system.

As the individual ages, there is decreased ability to produce antibodies, leading to decreases in the normal immune response. This interferes with the normal ability to ward off infections. If other chronic diseases are also present, the individual may be at an even higher risk for poor healing and development of infections. In addition, as the immune response becomes less effective, the individual is more susceptible to autoimmune disorders. Many diseases of the older adult have some direct relationship to the decreased immune response. Because the lymphatic system is dependent for some of its functions on the vascular system, additional problems arise in the elderly who have impaired circulation or other vascular system diseases.

SUMMARY

The immune system consists of organs such as the thymus gland, bone marrow, lymph nodes, spleen, liver, and tonsils, and major cells such as the lymphocytes. The immune system is an important defense system for the body. A malfunctioning or compromised immune system leaves the body with weakened defense against invading microorganisms. Many secondary disorders such as infections are caused by a compromised immune response. Primary diseases or disorders of the immune system are categorized as hypersensitivity disorders or immune deficiency disorders. Hypersensitivity disorders include allergies, autoimmune disorders, and isoimmune disorders. The immune deficiency disease AIDS is one of the most common and debilitating fatal conditions of the immune system. Diagnostic testing for immune disorders includes skin testing, complete blood cell counts, and some specific antibody studies. Treatment for immune disorders varies with the specific problem. Some immune disorders are quite mild while others are severe and require long-term therapy. The lymphatic system plays an important role in the body's ability to fight infection and in immunity. The system is composed of lymph, lymph nodes, and vessels to transport the lymph. The lymphatic system also transports fluid that has leaked into the interstitial areas to the blood vessels. Diseases of the system are usually caused by infections or neoplasms and can range from mild to severe. Treatment varies with the particular type of disease. Common symptoms include fever, fatigue, weight loss, and enlarged lymph nodes.

REVIEW QUESTIONS

Short Answer

1. What are the functions of the immune system?

2. Which signs and symptoms are associated with common immune system disorders?

3. What are the three main functions of the lymphatic system?

4. Name the four signs and symptoms associated with common lymphatic system disorders.

Matching

5. Match the disorders listed in the left column with the correct category of the immune system diseases in the right column. (Right hand column categories may be used more than once.)

____	Hay fever	a. allergies
____	AIDS	b. autoimmune disorders
____	Anaphylaxis	c. isoimmune disorders
____	Rheumatic fever	d. immune deficiency disorders
____	Erythroblastosis fetalis	
____	Organ rejection	

Multiple Choice

6. Which of the following behaviors may contribute to increasing the risk for HIV transmission?
   a. Donating blood
   b. Sharing intravenous needles
   c. Failure to wash hands after toileting
   d. Unprotected sex
   e. Sharing eating utensils
   f. Direct contact with body fluids
   g. Frequent use of laxatives and enemas

True or False

7. T F The immune system is the body's only defense system against invading organisms.
8. T F Signs and symptoms of hypersensitivity disorders may include rash, redness, heat, swelling, nasal congestion, coughing, and sneezing.
9. T F The Coombs' test is used to detect certain antibodies in the blood.
10. T F Autoimmune disorders are hyposensitivities in which the body fails to recognize its own antigens.
11. T F The effects of aging put the older adult at an increased risk for immune system problems.
12. T F Diseases of the lymphatic system commonly include inflammatory conditions.
13. T F Lymphangiography is a biopsy of a lymph node or several nodes.
14. T F Lymphadenitis is characterized by a swelling of the lymph nodes.
15. T F Lymphangitis is a condition of swelling of lymph vessels caused by inflammation.
16. T F Lymphedema is always caused by obstruction of a lymphatic vessel.
17. T F Mononucleosis is a bacterial infection that usually affects children and young adults.
18. T F Lymphoma affects lymphocyte production and impairs immunity.

CASE STUDY

You are called to the home of Mr. Stevens, a 26-year-old male patient who is HIV positive that you have transported before for periodic respiratory infections. Today he is complaining of dyspnea and a productive cough that is blood tinged. What do you remember about the transmission of HIV? What are the modes of transmission? Are there any special precautions that should be taken during this transport?

BIBLIOGRAPHY

Altman, L. K. (December 30, 1996). Stanford researchers report promising results in test of a treatment for lymphoma. *New York Times*, p. 9.

Altman, L. K. (January 21, 1997). Tsongas's legacy: Checking health of candidates. *New York Times*. p. C3.

Another meaty link to cancer. (1996). *Science News, 149*, 365.

As winter comes. (1995). *People Weekly, 44*, 73–74.

Balakrishnan, K., & Adams, L. (1995). The role of the lymphocyte in an immune response. *Immunological Investigations, 24*(1-2), 233.

Boss and guinea pig. (1997). *People Weekly, 47*, 121–124.

Cann, S. A. (September 30, 1995). Role of lymphagenesis in neovasculation. *Lancet, 346*, 903.

DeLandazuri, M. O. (1996). Immunology research. *Clinical Science, 90*(3), 148.

Dobbing, E. A. (1993). Preventing transference of bloodborne pathogens in the workplace: Reducing your risk of contracting HIV/HBV. *Point of View, 30*(2), 8–13.

Frank, M. M., Austen, K. F., Claman, H., & Unanue, E. R. (1995). *Samter's immunologic diseases* (Vol. I). Boston: Little, Brown and Company.

Frank, M. M., Austen, K. F., Claman, H., & Unanue, E. R. (1995). *Samter's immunologic diseases* (Vol. II). Boston: Little, Brown and Company.

Fraser, V. J. & Powderly, W. G .(1995). Risks of HIV infection in the health care setting. *Annual Review of Medicine, 46*, 203–211.

Gautam, A. M. (1994). Immunology: Why does the human immune system sometimes attack itself? *Today's Life Science, 6*(12), 28.

Health care workers at risk: An interview with Patricia Wetzel, MD. (1995). *Asepsis, The Infection Prevention Forum, 17*(1), 10–13.

Hibberd, P. L. (1995). Patients, needles, and healthcare workers: Understanding the epidemiology, pathophysiology, and transmission of the human immunodeficiency virus, hepatitis B and C, and cytomegalovirus. *Journal of Intravenous Nursing, 18*(6s), S22–31.

Hochhauser, D. (December 21-28, 1996). Sparing the lymph nodes but saving the patient. *Lancet, 348*, 1723.

Immunology web links. (1996). *Immunology Today, 17*(2), 51.

Lawlor, G. J., Fischer, T. J., & Adelman, D. C. (1995). *Manual of allergy and immunology*. Boston: Little, Brown and Company.

Magic bullets for lymphoma. (1995). *Forbes, 156*, 206+.

McCarthy, M. (April 12, 1997). Cytomegalovirus hoodwinks the immune system. *Lancet, 349*, 1074.

Meal bonus. (1995). *Prevention, 47*(12), 28.

Morris, K. (May 10, 1997). Never say never to a cure for HIV-1 infection. *Lancet, 349,* 1371.

Mullins, J. I. (June 27, 1997). Curtailing the AIDS pandemic. *Science, 276,* 1955–1957.

The Myasthenia Foundation of America. (September 11, 1997), MGFA@aol.com.

Patlak, M. (1996). Non-Hodgkin's lymphoma becomes more common, more treatable. *FDA Consumer, 30*(12), 20–24.

PCBs linked to rise in lymph cancer. (1997). *Science News, 152,* 85.

Searight, H. R. (1997). Behavioral and psychiatric aspects of HIV infection. *American Family Physician, 55*(3), 1227–1237.

Snow, R. L. (February 13, 1997). 24-year old woman with cervical lymphadenopathy, fever, and leukopenia. *The New England Journal of Medicine, 336,* 492–499.

Stites, D. P., Abba, I. T., & Parslow, T. G. (1994). *Basic & clinical immunology*. Norwalk: Appleton & Lange.

Swartz, M. A. (1996). Transport in lymphatic capillaries. *American Journal of Physiology 270*(1), H324–H329.

Tizard, I. R. (1995). *Immunology: An introduction.* Philadelphia: WB Saunders.

CHAPTER 13

Gastroenterologic Diseases and Disorders

CONTENT OUTLINE

- Anatomy and Physiology
- Common Signs and Symptoms
- Assessment
- Common Diseases and Disorders
    - Diseases of the Mouth
    - Diseases of the Throat and Esophagus
    - Diseases of the Stomach
    - Diseases of the Small Intestine
    - Diseases of the Colon
    - Diseases of the Rectum
    - Gastrointestinal Bleeding
    - Diseases of the Liver
    - Diseases of the Gallbladder
    - Diseases of the Pancreas
- Trauma
    - Solid Organ Trauma
    - Hollow Organ Trauma
- Evaluation of Abdominal Pain
- Developmental and Genetic Disorders
    - Developmental Malformations
    - Cleft Lip and Palate
    - Pyloric Stenosis
    - Hirschsprung's Disease
- Effects of Aging on System

KEY TERMS

Abdominocentesis
Achlorhydria
Adhesions
Albumin
Amylase
Ascites
Asymptomatic
Atresia
Autodigestion
Caput medusae
Cholecystectomy
Cirrhosis
Defecate
Delirium tremens
Dental caries
Esophageal varices
Exacerbation
Fulminant
Gynecomastia
Hematemesis
Hematochezia
Hepatomegaly
Ileus
Intrinsic factor
Intussusception
Jaundice
Malaise
Melena
Motility
Occult blood
Ova and Parasite (O&P)
Palmar erythema
Paralytic obstruction
Perforation
Peristalsis
Peritonitis
Peritonsillar abscess
Portal hypertension
Pyloromyotomy
Rebound tenderness
Referred pain
Remission
Retropharyngeal abscess
Septicemia
Somatic pain
Spider angiomas
Splenomegaly
Stool
Strangulated hernia
Strep throat
Vermiform
Virulent
Visceral pain
Volvulus

LEARNING OBJECTIVES

Upon completion of the chapter, the student should be able to:

1. Define the terminology common to the digestive system and the disorders of the system.
2. Identify the common disorders of the digestive system.
3. Discuss the basic anatomy and physiology of the digestive system.
4. Identify the important signs and symptoms associated with common digestive system disorders.
5. Describe the common diagnostic tests used to determine type and/or cause of the digestive system disorders.
6. Describe the typical course and management of the common digestive system disorders.
7. Describe the effects of aging upon the digestive system and the common disorders of the system.

OVERVIEW

The digestive system provides nutrients for the body through the processes of ingestion, digestion, and absorption, and eliminates waste products from the system. Diseases or disorders of the digestive system are some of the most common medical problems. Because there are many differences in eating patterns, lifestyle behaviors, and inherited traits, digestive system problems vary considerably among individuals. Some digestive system problems are caused by poor nutritional habits, while others may be caused by structural problems or a particular disease process.

The liver, gallbladder, and pancreas are the accessory organs of digestion. Although these organs are not considered part of the digestive system, they have important roles in the digestive process, as well as having many other functions in the body. Disorders of the liver, gallbladder, or pancreas can cause serious digestive problems and many other systemic disorders.

ANATOMY AND PHYSIOLOGY

The digestive system has been described as a long tube running through the body. It has two main purposes: 1) changing the food we eat into simpler substances in order for them to be absorbed into the blood and carried to all cells of the body, and 2) eliminating waste products from the body. The two major parts of the digestive system are the alimentary canal and the accessory organs, including the tongue, teeth, salivary glands, gallbladder, pancreas, and liver.

The alimentary canal (Figure 13–1) is a continuous tube running from the mouth to the anus. The term "gastrointestinal (GI)" tract technically refers only to the stomach and intestines, but is often used as a synonym for the alimentary canal. The alimentary canal is approximately thirty feet or nine meters in length, but most of it is coiled up in the abdomen surrounded by the peritoneum. The peritoneum is a large serous membrane covering the organs in the abdomen and lining the walls of the abdominal cavity. It secretes fluid to prevent friction between organs in the abdomen as they move during the process of digestion. The alimentary canal starts at the mouth where ingested food begins to be broken down to supply the body with needed nourishment. The teeth begin the process by breaking the food into smaller parts. The tongue, the organ of taste, assists the process by helping move the food in the mouth. The salivary glands, located outside the mouth with ducts leading from the glands to the mouth, secrete about 1500 milliliters of saliva per day. The saliva continues the process of breaking down food and moistening it to make it easier to swallow. At the back of the mouth lies the pharynx, the channel for food to pass from the mouth to the esophagus.

The esophagus (see Figure 13–1) is a tube (about nine inches in length) which extends from the pharynx to the stomach. The walls of the esophagus are very muscular. Movement of these muscles is called peristaltic contraction. These contractions, the process called **peristalsis**, moves the food from the pharynx to the stomach.

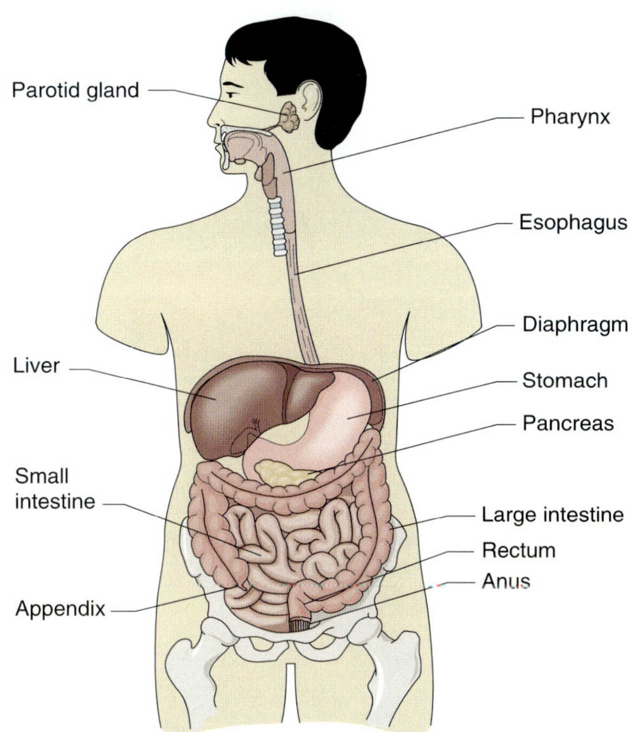

Figure 13–1 The digestive system.

The stomach is a sac-like organ that lies just under the diaphragm in the upper abdomen (see Figure 13–1). The esophagus connects to the stomach at the cardiac orifice (opening). A thick ring of smooth muscle, called the cardiac or gastroesophageal sphincter, surrounds this opening. The upper portion of the stomach, at the cardiac orifice end, is called the fundus, while the middle portion of the stomach is called the body. Food is broken down in the stomach by a process of chemical changes from the action of pepsin, an enzyme, and hydrochloric acid secreted by cells in the stomach. Food is mixed with these chemicals by the contractions of the stomach. The lining of the stomach also secretes a substance called the **intrinsic factor,** which is necessary for the absorption of vitamin B_{12}. At the lower portion of the stomach, called the pyloric region, the stomach is connected to the first part of the small intestine, called the duodenum. The opening at this end of the stomach is the pyloric orifice, which is surrounded by the pyloric sphincter. The sphincter muscles control the flow of fluid into and out of the stomach.

The small intestine (see Figure 13–1) extends from the pyloric orifice to the ileocecal valve at the beginning of the large intestine. It is divided into three sections. The first section, the duodenum, is about ten inches or twenty-five centimeters in length. It is the shortest of the three sections. The duodenum receives bile from the liver and pancreatic juices from the pancreas, which aid in the digestive process. The duodenum connects the stomach to the jejunum on the left side of the upper abdomen. The jejunum is the second section of the small intestine. The jejunum extends from the duodenum to the ileum. It is about seven and one-half feet or two meters in length and is coiled throughout the abdomen. The ileum is the third section of the small intestine, attaching to the jejunum at its beginning and ending at the ileocecal valve, the beginning of the large intestine.

The major function of the small intestine is digestion and absorption of food and fluids. Material is moved through the small intestine by muscular action (peristalsis). Most of digestion takes place in the small intestine. Finger-like projections called villi are located on the inside surface of the intestine. These projections contain lymph vessels and blood capillaries. Additional extensions called microvilli cover the villi forming a velvety surface, which greatly increases the surface area of the small intestine. As a result of this increased surface area, nutrient absorption is greatly increased. Nutrients pass into the vascular capillaries to be delivered to the body cells.

The large intestine connects to the small intestine at the ileocecal valve in the right lower portion of the abdomen. The first section of the colon is called the cecum. The appendix is attached to the cecum near the ileocecal valve. The large intestine, also called the colon, is about five feet or one and one-half meters in length. Each section of the colon is named according to its anatomical position. The colon (see Figure 13–1) begins in the lower right quadrant of the abdomen (cecum), rises to the mid-level (ascending colon), crosses the abdomen at the umbilicus level (transverse colon), and descends on the left side (descending colon), into the pelvic cavity where it is called the sigmoid colon. The sigmoid colon forms an s-shaped tube that extends into the lower pelvic region ending at the rectum and anus. The process of digestion and absorption continues in the large intestine. The most important function of the large intestine is the absorption of water and electrolytes and the elimination of feces, the material not absorbed by the intestines.

The liver is the largest solid organ of the body. This organ takes second place only to the skin as the largest organ overall (Figure 13–2). The liver has many functions, most of which are related to its chemical actions. The liver plays a role in digestion, absorption, metabolism, blood clotting, the manufacture of important chemicals, and storage of nutrients. The liver is composed of two lobes, weighs about three and a half pounds, and lies in the right upper quadrant of the abdomen. Some of the most important functions of the liver include:

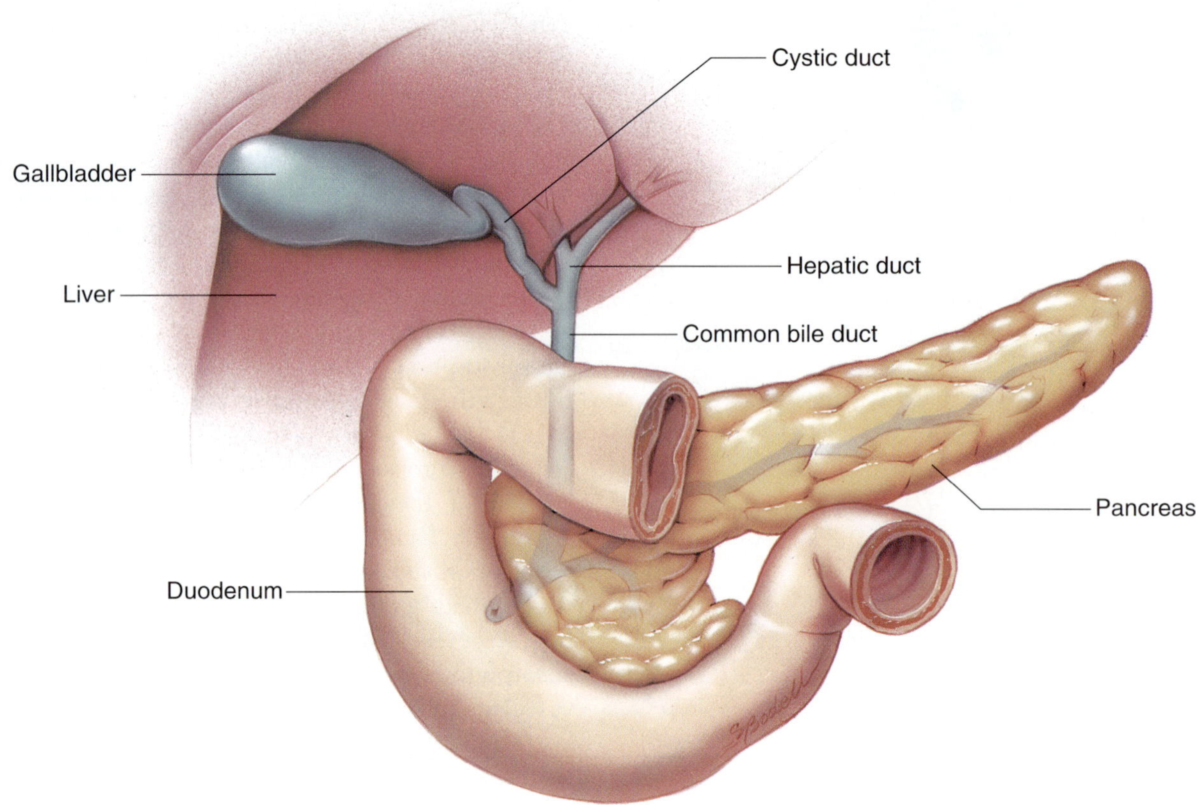

Figure 13–2 The liver, gallbladder, and pancreas.

- production and secretion of bile used for fat digestion
- production of cholesterol
- oxidation of fatty acids and glycerol used for body energy
- metabolism of carbohydrates, fats, and protein
- conversion of glucose to glycogen for storage and the reverse process for energy
- synthesis of amino acids
- detoxification of many drugs and other toxins
- storage of vitamins and other minerals
- production of fibrinogen and prothrombin for blood clotting

The liver receives blood from the portal system via the portal vein and the hepatic artery. About 1,450 ml of blood flows through the liver every minute. The blood returns to the circulatory system via the hepatic vein to the inferior vena cava.

Bile is continually produced in the liver. It is used to emulsify or break down lipids in the intestine. The hepatic duct connects the liver to the duodenum. When bile is not needed in the digestive process, excess bile is stored in the gallbladder.

The gallbladder is a small pear-shaped organ lying just under the liver (see Figure 13–2). Bile is stored here until needed by the intestine in the digestive process. Bile travels from the gallbladder to the duodenum via the cystic duct and the common bile duct.

The pancreas lies in the abdomen behind the stomach between the duodenum and the spleen (see Figure 13–2). It is both an endocrine gland (the islet cells secrete hormones) and an exocrine gland, producing and secreting most of the digestive enzymes. The pancreas secretes intestinal juices consisting of chymotrypsin and trypsin, which break down proteins; amylase, which breaks down starch; and lipase, which breaks down fats. The pancreatic juices exit the gland by way of the pancreatic duct to the duodenum.

COMMON SIGNS AND SYMPTOMS

Diseases of this system usually result in signs and symptoms related to hemorrhage, **perforation**, and altered **motility** (movement) in the system. Hemorrhage may be mild or severe and may originate at any site along the system. Terms identifying bleeding are **hematemesis** (HEM-ah-**TEM**-eh-sis; hemat = blood, emesis = vomiting), **hematochezia** (HEM-at-toe-**KEE**-zee-ah) bright red blood in the feces) and **melena** (meh-LEE-nah), dark tarry **stool** (feces), caused by the presence of blood. The term "coffee grounds" is sometimes used to describe blood that has been digested. This blood is often vomited, but may also be defecated.

Perforation in any area of the tract can be life-threatening because of the bacteria present in the tract and the ease of spread in the abdominal cavity. Perforation in the stomach or intestines allows spillage of contents into the abdominal cavity causing **peritonitis** (PER-ih-toe-**NIGH**-tis; an inflammation of the peritoneum). Pain and rebound tenderness are common symptoms of peritonitis. Peritonitis may also be caused by bleeding within the peritoneal cavity. Gastric contents that are spilled are high in gastric acid and thus corrosive to abdominal organs. Intestinal contents have a normally high bacterial count. Spilling of intestinal contents into the abdominal cavity causes infection, which may lead to **septicemia** (SEP-tih-**SEE**-me-ah; septic = dirty, emia = blood or bacteria in the bloodstream). Causes of perforation may include peptic ulcer, injury such as gunshot or stab wounds, and untreated appendicitis.

Alteration in motility or movement of food along the tract commonly leads to a variety of symptoms including nausea, vomiting, diarrhea, or constipation. Diarrhea is a disorder characterized by frequent watery stools. Irritability of the intestinal lining causes hyperactivity of muscle contractions (peristalsis), causing a rushing of the watery contents in the small intestine through the large intestine. This rushing does not allow the large intestine the time needed to reabsorb the water. The primary concern with diarrhea, especially in young children and the elderly, is loss of fluids leading to dehydration. Causes of diarrhea include a sudden increase in stress or nervous condition, bacterial or viral infection, or food poisoning.

Constipation is the opposite of diarrhea. The stool in the colon remains for an extended period of time, too much water is reabsorbed and the stool becomes hard, dry, and difficult to pass. Constipation is commonly caused by poor dietary and elimination habits. Avoiding the urge to **defecate** (have a bowel movement) increases the amount of time the stool remains in the colon and thus increases constipation.

Jaundice (JAWN-dis, a yellowish discoloration of the skin) is an obvious symptom of liver disease. Jaundice may also be secondary to gallbladder disease. If a bile duct is blocked, the bile backs up into the liver and leads to jaundice.

Jaundice is caused by high levels of bilirubin in the blood. Bilirubin is a byproduct of the breakdown of heme, the main component of hemoglobin in red blood cells. The liver filters bilirubin out of the blood and excretes it in bile. If the liver is unable to filter bilirubin and excrete it, hyperbilirubinemia (hyper = too much, bilirubin, emia = blood) or excessive bilirubin in the blood occurs. Excessive bilirubin leaks into the tissues and the individual's skin, mucosa, and sclera (white part of the eye) become yellowish in color. Bilirubin can be broken down in the skin by exposure to sunlight or direct lighting. This explains the use of "bili lights" to clear bilirubin in a jaundiced newborn infant. Excessive bilirubin is also filtered out of the blood by the kidneys, causing dark brown urine.

Pain is a common symptom of gallbladder disease, pancreatitis, and end stage pancreatic cancer. With gallbladder disease, right-sided abdominal pain commonly occurs following a meal containing fat. Acute abdominal pain occurs with pancreatitis and end stage pancreatic cancer.

ASSESSMENT

In the field, the EMS provider may use the techniques of inspection, auscultation, palpation, and percussion to assess the abdomen. One should visually inspect the abdomen to look at its shape, discolorations, injuries, and scars, and use a stethoscope to auscultate the abdomen for bowel sounds. This may be difficult to do in noisy environments. Bowel sounds that are present are typically heard within a short period of time, but one cannot report for certain that bowel sounds are absent unless the EMS provider has listened for five minutes. A high pitched sound similar to water dripping may indicate an obstruction. Palpation is used to detect masses and elicit pain. Pain that occurs when the EMS provider quickly releases pressure on the abdomen is called **rebound tenderness** and indicates that the peritoneum is irritated. Percussion can also be used to elicit signs of peritoneal irritation. A hyperresonant sound may indicate an obstruction or constipation.

Diagnostic tests used by the physician to evaluate the digestive system vary depending upon the area of concern and may involve X-ray or Computed Axial Tomography (CAT or CT) evaluation, ultrasound, endoscopy (visualizing a body cavity with a lighted scope), biopsy, blood tests, or stool cultures.

X-ray evaluation may include plain film, upper GI series, or lower GI series films. In a plain film, an X-ray is taken of the abdomen and the physician observes the air and fluid patterns to determine if there is an obstruction of the large or small intestine. Radiopaque dye can be swallowed or instilled in the rectum to assess the upper and lower sections of the gastrointestinal tract. Dye can also be injected directly into the gall bladder or biliary tree (cholecystogram and cholangiogram, respectively) to show the presence of gallstones, tumors, and function of the gallbladder. A similar dye can be injected intravenously and excreted from the liver into the biliary tree to perform the same studies.

Computed axial tomography scans may be performed to visualize the liver, gallbladder, and pancreas. Visualization of these structures aids in the diagnosis of hepatic and pancreatic cancer, and may assist in diagnosing gallstones obstructing or partially obstructing the common bile duct.

Ultrasound examination is commonly used to evaluate the liver, gallbladder, and pancreas for size, shape, and position. It is also commonly used to look for evidence of bile duct blockage in patients who present with right upper quadrant pain. Ultrasound can also be utilized to evaluate the hepatic portal system for direction and volume of blood flow and can be useful to assess the effects of hepatic disease on a patient.

Endoscopic examination allows the physician to look directly into the digestive organs by use of a lighted scope (Figure 13–3). The name of each procedure is identified by naming the organ that is being scoped. Examples of this include: stomach = gastroscopy, colon = colonoscopy, sigmoid colon = sigmoidoscopy, entire upper GI area = esophagogastroduodenoscopy (EGD). The physician may decide to biopsy the tissue in the digestive tract in order to aid in diagnosis. During an endoscopic examination, the physician may obtain a biopsy to determine the presence of a neoplasm or other disease process. A liver needle biopsy can be performed using CT guidance to assist in locating the target tissue for biopsy. The liver biopsy is the most reliable test for chronic hepatitis, cirrhosis, and cancer.

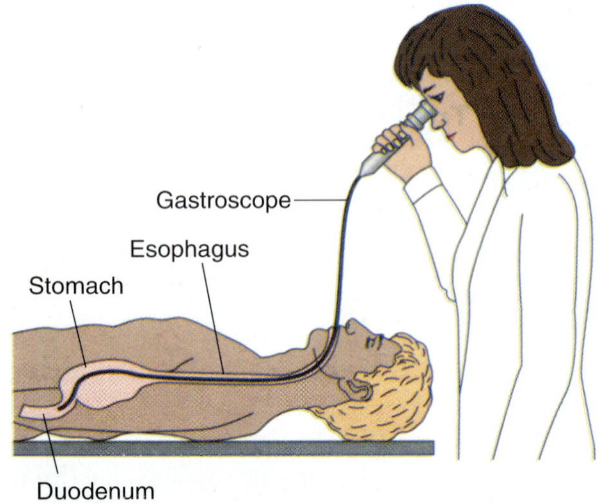

Figure 13–3 EGD.

Several laboratory tests may be performed to assist in the diagnosing of digestive system diseases. One of these is the hemoccult or stool for **occult** (hidden) **blood**. This is an examination of stool content for hidden blood. A positive Hemoccult may be indicative of colon cancer.

Another laboratory test is an **ova and parasite** (O&P). This is an examination of a stool specimen for the presence of adult parasites or their eggs (ova). Parasites identified by an O&P may include roundworms, tapeworms, pinworms, hookworms, and protozoa. Stool or fecal cultures may be utilized to determine bacterial infections in the colon.

Blood tests to evaluate liver function include bilirubin, albumin (blood protein), alkaline phosphatase (enzyme), aspartate aminotransferase (AST), and alanine aminotransferase (ALT) levels. Damage to liver cells will elevate the AST and ALT. Elevated bilirubin and alkaline phosphatase may indicate problems with the gall bladder, cystic duct, and common bile duct. In many disease states and malnutrition, the albumin level will be low. Additionally, the PT, a coagulation test, is used to evaluate the effects of hepatic disease on the liver's production of clotting factors.

Blood tests to evaluate pancreatic function include serum amylase and lipase. Amylase and lipase are digestive enzymes produced by the pancreas that break down carbohydrates and fats, respectively. These values are significantly elevated in pancreatitis, and may be somewhat elevated if a gallstone is lodged in the common bile duct at the junction with the pancreatic duct.

COMMON DISEASES AND DISORDERS

Disease and disorders of the digestive system range from minor disorders, for example, pharyngitis, to life-threatening disorders, for example, bowel obstruction. Conditions that affect the digestive system may be easily confused with problems in other systems. For example, gastritis or peptic ulcer disease can cause pain in the lower chest directly in the center and may be difficult to distinguish from pain caused by a myocardial infarction. Assessment of the GI system can be challenging as many of these conditions require imaging or lab studies not available in the pre-hospital arena. A thorough history and physical examination by the EMS provider can help narrow down the differential between the possible diagnoses and further direct emergency department management of the patient.

Diseases of the Mouth

The primary function of the mouth is to begin the breakdown of food into smaller particles. Diseases of the mouth include those related to inflammation and tumors.

Tooth Pain. Tooth pain may develop for a number of reasons that may vary from minor to serious. The majority of dental pain is caused by **dental caries** (cavities), and may range from minor pain to excruciating pain that interrupts sleep. The pain caused by dental caries is generally localized and can be a sharp to a dull throbbing pain that is aggravated by temperature changes. It may refer to other areas of the mouth and even to the jaw on the other side of the mouth. The source of the pain may be confirmed by percussing, or tapping, the tooth with a tongue blade, reproducing the pain. A periodontal abscess is an infection that extends into the space between the gingiva and tooth (Figure 13–4) and is considered a dental emergency. Tooth pain may also be caused by referred pain from oral lesions, such as herpes zoster ("shingles") or herpes simplex. Finally, lower jaw pain in the absence of localized findings should cause the EMS provider to consider referred pain from a myocardial infarction as its source and include a thorough cardiovascular and respiratory history and physical exam.

Diseases of the Throat and Esophagus

There are many diseases of the throat and esophagus. They range from mild to severe and acute to chronic. Infections and inflammatory conditions are the most common. Pharyngitis is often categorized as a respiratory problem as the pharynx is common to both the respiratory system and the digestive system.

Pharyngitis. Pharyngitis is commonly called a "sore throat." Pharyngitis may be caused by viral or bacterial microorganisms. The most frequent and earliest symptom of pharyngitis is a sore throat. Visual examination reveals redness in the area. A common type of pharyngitis is an inflammation of the tonsils called tonsillitis. In

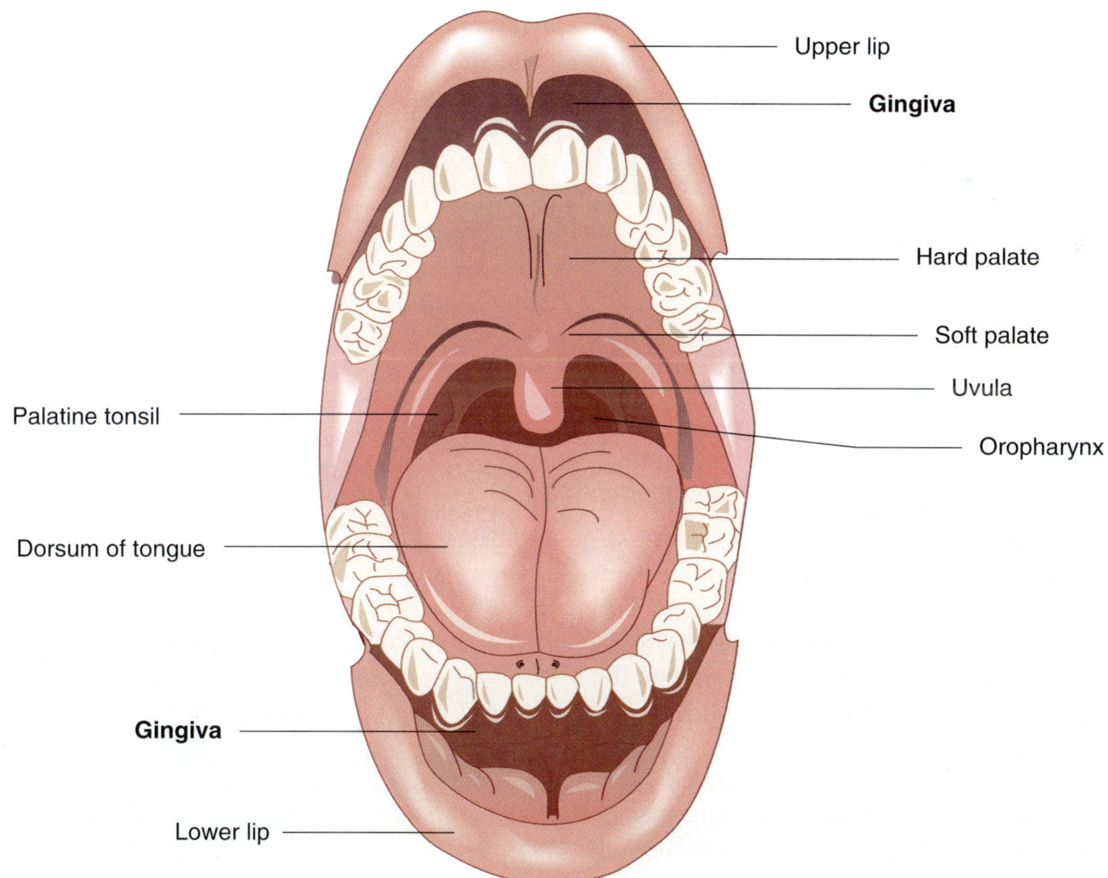

Figure 13–4 Gingivitis (inflamed gingiva).

tonsillitis the tonsils form crypts of pus, which give the tonsils a whitish appearance.

An acute type of pharyngitis is called **strep throat**. Strep throat is caused by a **virulent** (VIR-u-lent; infectious, difficult to kill) bacteria, streptococcus. This bacteria may spread into the bloodstream and produce other diseases such as scarlet fever, rheumatic fever, glomerulonephritis, and endocarditis. Diagnosis is made by examination and throat culture. Treatment of strep throat includes identification of the organism through laboratory cultures, followed by antibiotic treatment and follow-up culture to check effectiveness of antibiotic treatment. Antibiotic treatment is quite effective if taken as prescribed.

Peritonsillar and Retropharyngeal Abscesses. A peritonsillar abscess is an abscess that forms around the tonsil, and may occur up to several weeks after a severe infection. **Peritonsillar abscesses** occur most commonly in teenagers and young adults. The typical presentation includes fever, sore throat, increased salivation, and muffled voice. Examination generally reveals a single enlarged and firm tonsil. As the abscess grows, the patient may not be able to swallow or will have pain with swallowing. A **retropharyngeal abscess** is an abscess that forms in the soft tissue posterior, or behind the pharynx, in between the oral cavity and the spine. This is more common in young children and toddlers, but can also occur in adults secondary to trauma or a foreign body. In addition to the signs and symptoms listed above for peritonsillar abscess, the patient may also have neck swelling, limited or painful motion, drooling, and stridor, in young children. Airway compromise is possible in both cases, either through direct occlusion of the airway by the abscess or the inability to clear the excess saliva. Patients are generally treated aggressively with suction and airway adjuncts to prevent airway compromise. These abscesses may require surgical drainage to prevent airway compromise in addition to intravenous antibiotics.

Reflux Esophagitis. Reflux esophagitis is an inflammation of tissue at the lower end of the esophagus. This inflammation is caused by a reflux (backflow) of stomach acids through the cardiac sphincter upward into the esophagus. The most common symptom of reflux esophagitis is known as heartburn, a burning sensation in the mid-chest or epigastric (epi = above, gastric = stomach) area. The pain caused by reflux esophagitis may be similar to the pain caused by a myocardial infarction. Long-term reflux can lead to bleeding, ulceration, and scarring of the esophagus. This scarring may cause stricture and, thus, difficulty swallowing. Treatment is directed at reducing reflux and may include recommendations to avoid large meals, spicy foods, caffeine, and tight clothing. Medications such as stool softeners, laxatives, antacids and those that tighten the gastroesophageal sphincter may be helpful. Activities that increase abdominal pressure may be restricted. Sleeping with the head of the bed elevated is often helpful. Surgery on the incompetent sphincter is usually not recommended and thus only considered in extreme cases.

Hiatal Hernia. Hiatal hernia is a sliding of part of the stomach into the chest cavity. The stomach slides upward through the natural hole in the diaphragm where the esophagus passes through to the stomach (Figure 13–5). This herniation may increase in frequency related to age and the weakening of the cardiac sphincter. Many hiatal hernias are **asymptomatic** (a = without, symptomatic = symptoms), but those that do cause discomfort are usually related to esophageal reflux and are thus treated in the same manner as reflux esophagitis.

Esophageal Varices. Unusually high pressure in the veins of the esophagus causes them to enlarge and become tortuous resulting in esophageal varices. This increased pressure is caused by blockage or reduced venous blood flow through the liver known as portal hypertension. Venous blood finds an alternate pathway to return to the heart via the esophageal venous plexus located within the

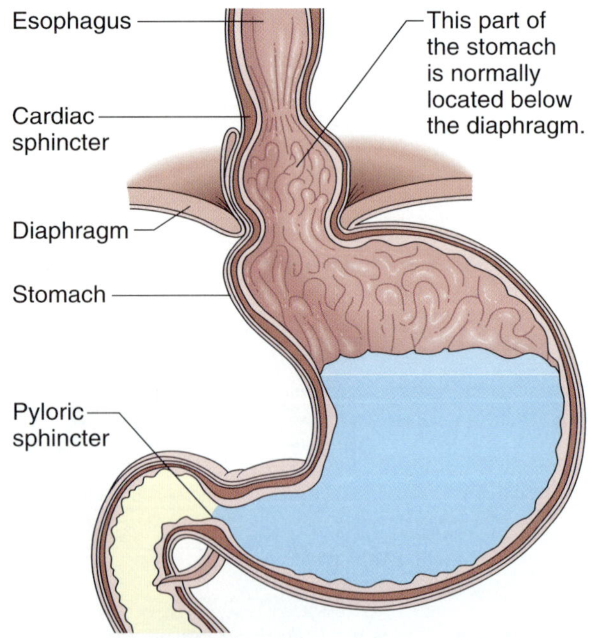

Figure 13–5 Hiatal hernia.

esophageal wall. This added blood flow through the esophageal plexus causes it to swell and bulge out into the lumen of the esophagus. These varices can rupture, causing a severe and life-threatening hemorrhage.

Any condition that leads to venous congestion in the liver may lead to esophageal varices. Usually esophageal varices are related to cirrhosis of the liver. The most common cause of cirrhosis is excessive alcohol consumption.

The goal of treatment is to decrease venous pressure by methods such as portal vein bypass surgery and medication to lower blood pressure. Other treatments include limiting the diet to soft, non-irritating foods and the use of stool softeners to prevent straining, which increases esophageal venous pressure. Chronic bleeding of the vessels may be treated with a sclerosing agent that hardens or destroys the vessel. Acute bleeding treatments include instillation of cold saline washings and/or the application of pressure to the site through a nasogastric tube.

Diseases of the Stomach

Diseases of the stomach are common problems in the digestive system. Complaints of stomach pain, especially after eating, are common. This problem increases with age because of the age-related changes in the system that are also complicated by other chronic diseases. Disorders of the stomach range from mild acute gastritis to more serious diseases such as cancer of the stomach.

Gastritis. Inflammation in the stomach is known as gastritis. Common symptoms are epigastric pain, bloating, and nausea. Acute forms of gastritis are caused by irritating agents such as aspirin, alcohol, coffee, tobacco, or bacterial-laden foods. Acute gastritis usually heals rapidly and requires no treatment.

Chronic gastritis may be identified as two separate forms, fundal gastritis and *Helicobacter* gastritis. Fundal gastritis affects the proximal area of the stomach where gastric acid-producing cells are located. As people age, there is a decrease in the number of acid-producing cells thus leading to atrophic gastritis, **achlorhydria** (AH-klor-**HIGH**-dree-ah; no hydrochloric acid), and loss of intrinsic factor (a protein produced by the gastric mucosa). Loss of this intrinsic factor leads to pernicious anemia. (See Chapter 16 for more information on anemia.) Since fundal gastritis is age related there is no specific treatment, although avoidance of irritating agents may be beneficial. The use of antacids may also be recommended.

Helicobacter gastritis is caused by small bacteria commonly found in the stomach lining. The presence of the bacteria does not cause symptoms in the majority of people. Those persons affected may experience chronic gastritis. The incidence of chronic *Helicobacter* gastritis increases with age. *Helicobacter* gastritis is now thought to be a major factor in gastric ulcer formation. Diagnosis is confirmed by biopsy. A combination of medications is utilized to reduce or eliminate *Helicobacter* bacteria and thus reduce gastritis and ulcer formation.

Peptic Ulcer. An ulcer is an area of tissue that has eroded, leaving a crater-like appearance (Figure 13–6). Peptic ulcers are those ulcers found in the stomach and duodenum that are caused in part by the action of pepsin. The stomach lining is normally protected by a thick mucous membrane lining. Pepsin is an enzyme secreted in the stomach that breaks down protein. This same enzyme, to some degree, breaks down the stomach's lining, causing ulcers. Ulcer pain is caused by the hydrochloric acid in the stomach irritating the raw ulcerated area.

Peptic ulcers found in the stomach are called gastric ulcers, while those located in the duodenum are called duodenal ulcers. Complications of peptic ulcers are massive bleeding, perforation, and obstruction. Development of peptic ulcers is unclear but it is thought that contributing factors include severe stress, heavy intake of drugs (such as aspirin, steroids and alcohol), smoking, and the presence of *Helicobacter* bacteria.

Treatment is aimed at reducing the gastric acidity and thus allowing for healing of the stomach lining. Treatment includes reduction or elimination of contributory factors. Antacids to neutralize gastric acids and other gastric medications, such as Tagamet, Pepcid, and Zantac may be helpful. Antibiotics are also used to treat ulcers caused

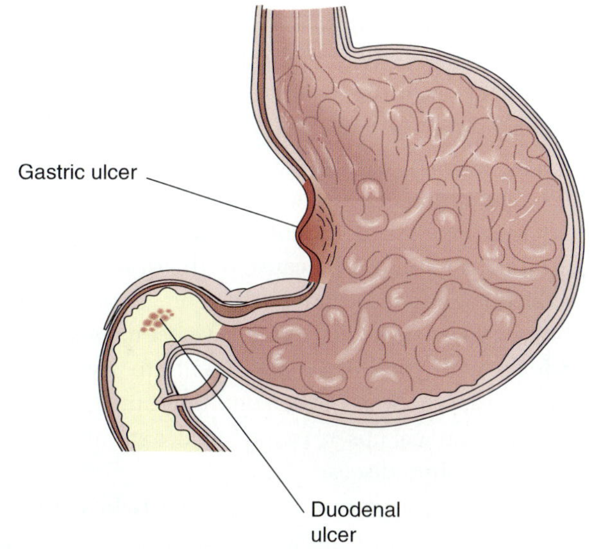

Figure 13–6 Peptic ulcers.

by *Helicobacter* bacteria. Surgery is warranted in severe cases that may lead to hemorrhage, perforation, obstruction, or extreme pain.

Diseases of the Small Intestine

The small intestine, consisting of the duodenum, jejunum, and ileum, secretes enzymes and absorbs nutrients for cellular functions. Disorders of the small intestine frequently manifest themselves in pain radiating across the abdomen. This symptom alone is not enough to diagnose the specific disease process. Additional evaluation is needed such as X-ray or CT scan. The disorders of the small intestine may range from mild intestinal upset to more severe chronic problems, such as ulcers or regional enteritis.

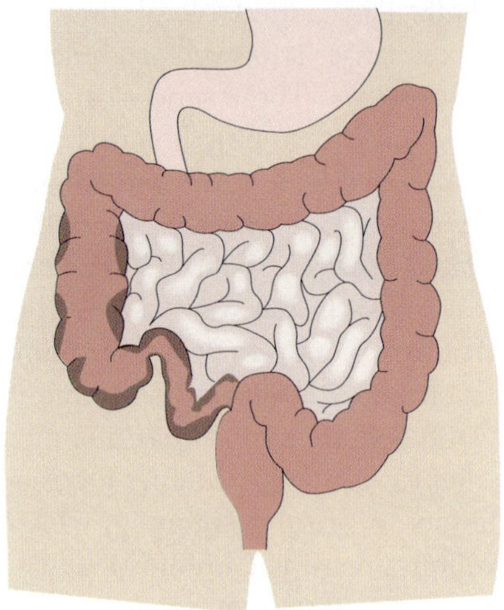

Figure 13–7 Crohn's disease.

Malabsorption Syndrome. The primary purpose of the small intestine is to absorb nutrients. When the small intestine is unable to accomplish this function, malabsorption syndrome may be diagnosed. Persons with malabsorption syndrome may be unable to absorb nutrients (especially fat) and minerals. Other organ diseases such as liver disease, gallbladder obstruction, diabetes mellitus, pancreatic deficiencies, and cardiovascular disease may lead to malabsorption syndrome. Most treatments include diet therapy for control. One of the complications of the disorder is a bleeding tendency caused by the lack of vitamin K absorption.

Crohn's Disease. Crohn's disease is a chronic inflammatory disease most commonly affecting the small intestine, but it may also affect any part of the gastrointestinal tract from mouth to anus. It is characterized by bouts of **remission** (slowing or stopping of symptoms) and **exacerbation** (x-AS-er-**BAY**-shun; flaring up of symptoms) (Figure 13–7). Crohn's is commonly classified as inflammatory bowel disease (IBD) until complete diagnosis is made. As Crohn's progresses, the intestinal wall becomes thickened resulting in a narrowing of the lumen. Symptoms include anorexia, flatulence, abdominal pain, diarrhea, and constipation. The cause of the disease has not yet been determined, although genetic, immunologic, infectious, and psychologic factors have been considered. Individuals with Crohn's disease tend to experience relapse or exacerbations of the condition during periods of stress or emotional upset. Young females are most often affected by Crohn's disease.

Treatment is supportive, but not likely to be curative. Approaches may involve a low-residue diet and medications to control diarrhea, inflammation, infection, and depression. Surgical resection is not curative and is performed to treat complications such as perforation and obstruction. Experimental treatments focusing on an immune etiology for Crohn's disease are currently undergoing research.

Gastroenteritis. Gastroenteritis (gastro = stomach, entero = intestines, itis = inflammation), as its name suggests, is inflammation of both the stomach and intestines (Figure 13–8). Causes may include bacterial, viral, or parasitic invasion, ingestion of tainted food, lactose intolerance, and allergic reaction to food or drugs. Gastroenteritis may also be caused by an enterotoxin produced by bacteria. The enterotoxin produces a change in the lining of the intestine that results in diarrhea, passage of mucus, and, sometimes, bleeding. Gastroenteritis may have an acute and violent onset with nausea, vomiting, abdominal cramping, and diarrhea leading to rapid fluid and electrolyte loss. Or, symptoms may be less violent with stomach rumbling, **malaise** (ma-LAZ; general ill feeling), nausea, and mild diarrhea. Treatment focuses on symptoms and may include anti-nausea medication, anti-diarrhea medication, antibiotics, fluids, and nutritional support. Prognosis is generally good. Prevention of gastroenteritis includes hand washing prior to food preparation, proper refrigeration of food, and avoidance of contaminated food and water.

Inguinal Hernia. An inguinal hernia is an out-pouching of the small intestine and the peritoneum (abdominal cavity lining) into the groin area (Figure 13–9). Inguinal hernias are more common in males. This may be because

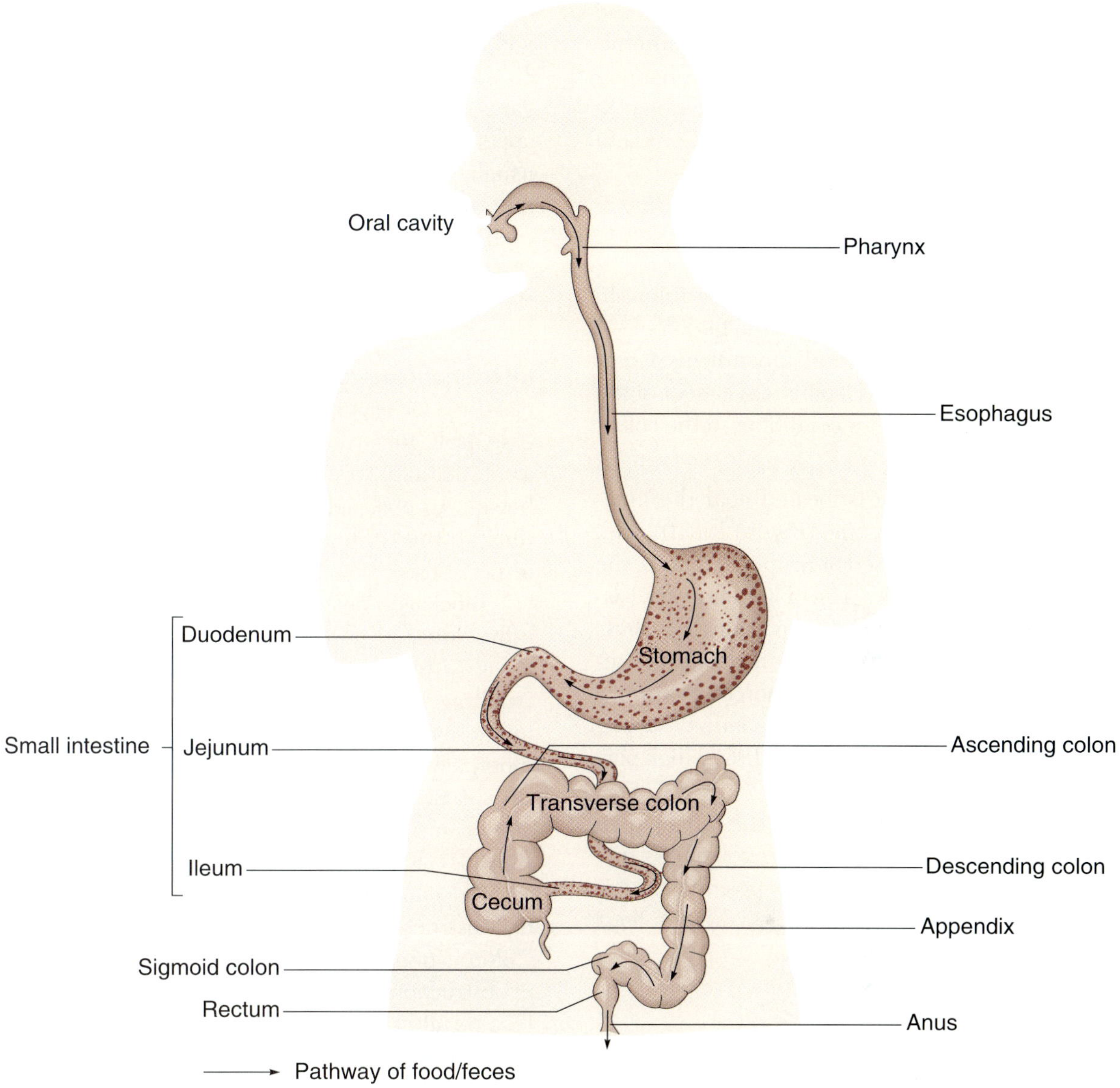

Oral cavity
Pharynx
Esophagus
Duodenum
Stomach
Small intestine
Jejunum
Ascending colon
Transverse colon
Ileum
Descending colon
Cecum
Appendix
Sigmoid colon
Rectum
Anus
Pathway of food/feces

Figure 13–8 Gastroenteritis.

of a congenital defect that developed as the testes descended from the abdomen into the scrotum, thus pulling part of the peritoneum into the inguinal area. Inguinal hernias also develop in both sexes from a weakness in the abdominal wall.

The portions of the intestine that herniate may become caught and twisted, thus cutting off blood supply to the organ. If this occurs, it is called a **strangulated hernia**. A strangulated hernia may be life-threatening and need immediate surgical intervention. Fortunately inguinal hernias can be repaired surgically in order to prevent this potentially life-threatening situation.

Portions of the small intestine may also herniate through other openings in the body such as the femoral

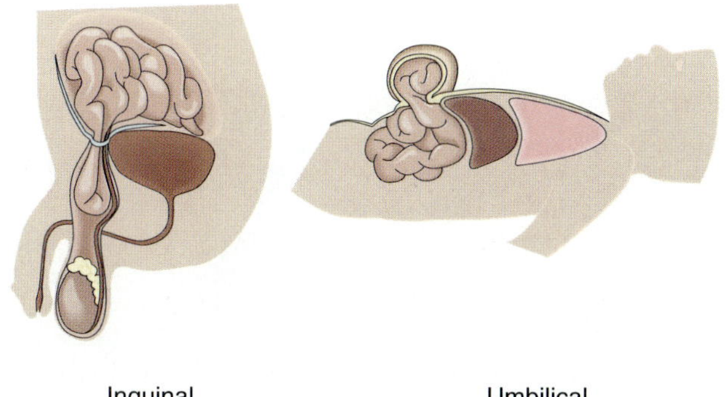

Figure 13–9 Hernias: inguinal and umbilical.

canal or the umbilicus. The femoral hernia, like the inguinal hernia, is more common in males. The umbilical hernia is most common in infants , but can happen after abdominal surgery through the surgical incision (see Figure 13–9). Like the inguinal hernia, both are corrected surgically to prevent complications.

Diseases of the Colon

Diseases of the colon or large intestine are common to all ages but are found most frequently in the middle-aged and older adult, with the exception of appendicitis. Common problems such as ulcerative colitis and cancer of the colon are two of the more serious conditions of the colon.

Appendicitis. The appendix is located near the junction of the small and large intestine (Figure 13–10), and, although it is primarily composed of lymphoid tissues, the exact function is unknown. The pain of appendicitis classically begins with generalized abdominal pain that shifts to the lower right quadrant. Other symptoms include nausea, vomiting, and fever. This combination of symptoms mimics other abdominal diseases, such as kidney stones, pelvic inflammatory disease, and pancreatitis, which may lead to an incorrect diagnosis.

Appendicitis is the inflammation of the **vermiform** (VER-my-form; worm-like) appendix. Infection or obstruction usually causes appendicitis. The position of the appendix near the colon allows for bacterial-laden fecal contents to drop into the appendix causing obstruction and infection. The inflamed appendix swells (see Figure 13–10), decreasing circulation and potentially leading to gangrene. As appendicitis progresses, the wall of the appendix thins and may rupture. Rupture of the appendix usually relieves the pain for a short time, but leads to a more severe complication of peritonitis. Prior to the development of antibiotics, peritonitis was usually fatal. Treatment for appendicitis requires surgical removal of the appendix, preferably before rupture occurs.

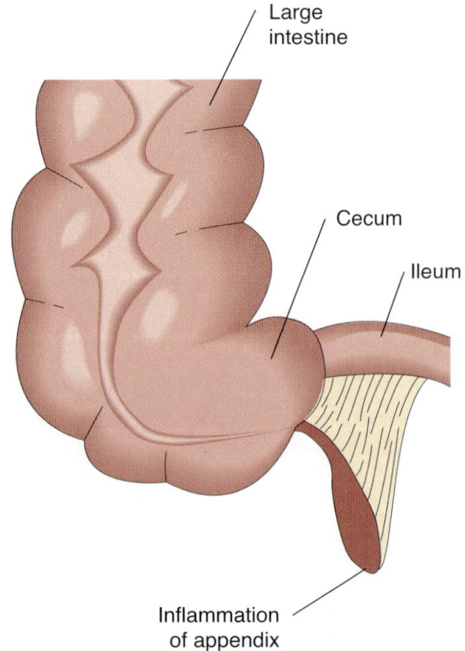

Figure 13–10 Appendix.

Intestinal Obstruction. Intestinal obstruction may be classified as a symptom of a disease process or as a disease itself. Regardless of the classification, it is identified as an inability to move intestinal contents through the bowel. An obstruction may be caused by a blockage of the intestine, or to a disease, or **ileus** (ILL-ee-us; absence of peristalsis).

Blockage may occur because of tumors, hernias, or **adhesions** (ad-He-zhuns) (Figure 13–11). Adhesions are areas within the colon that abnormally link together, resulting from a previous abdominal surgery or from inflammation. If the colon telescopes on itself, the condition may lead to a blockage called **intussusception** (IN-tus-sus-**SEP**-shun) (see Figure 13–12A). Blockage may also occur if the colon becomes twisted (**volvulus**; VOL-view-lus) (Figure 13–12B).

A decrease or absence of peristalsis that causes intestinal obstruction is classified as a **paralytic obstruction**. Colon action is paralyzed or unable to move. This type of obstruction may be a postoperative complication or may be a result of peritonitis. Symptoms depend on the type and severity of the obstruction. The individual may experience mild to severe abdominal pain and distention, nausea, and vomiting. Intestinal obstruction may be relieved by nasogastric suctioning, but more commonly surgery is required.

Ulcerative Colitis. Ulcerative colitis is a chronic inflammation of the colon (Figure 13–13). Ulcerative colitis, like Crohn's disease, is commonly called inflammatory bowel disease until diagnosis is confirmed. The colon and rectum develop multiple ulcerations which lead to lower abdominal pain, blood in the stools, anemia, and diarrhea. The cause of ulcerative colitis is unknown. Causative theories include heredity, autoimmune, and dietary factors. Patients with ulcerative colitis are at a high risk for developing colon cancer.

Treatment may include dietary limitations, stress reduction, mild sedatives, and anti-inflammatory medications. Surgery is usually considered only if conservative

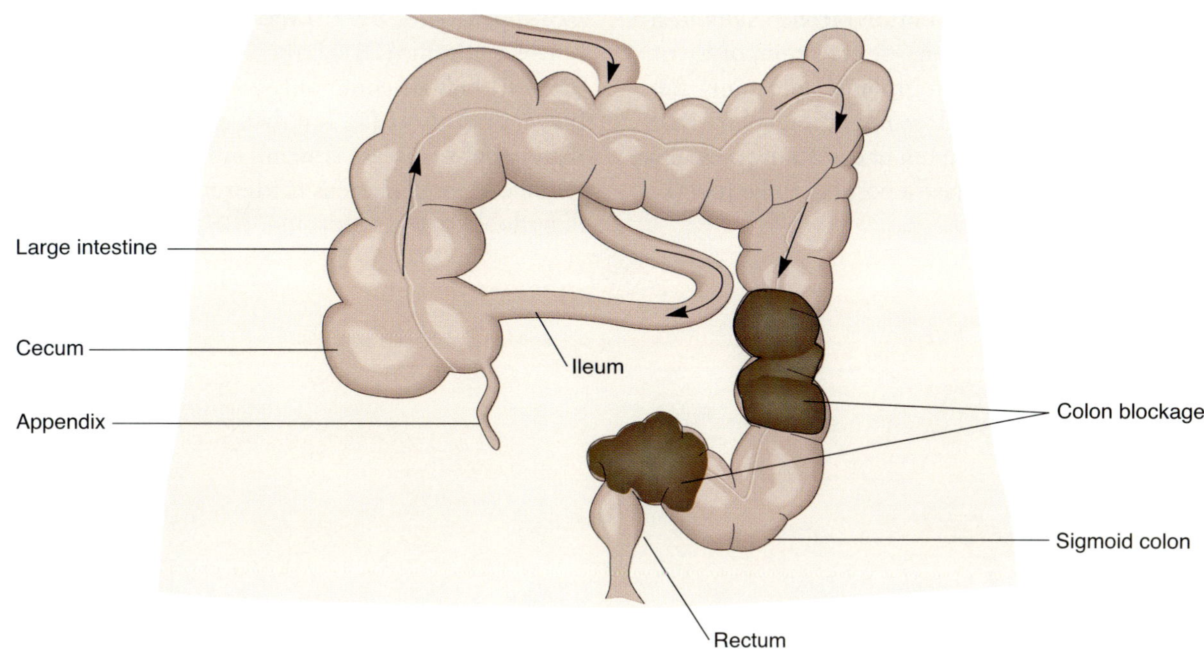

Figure 13–11 Colon blockage.

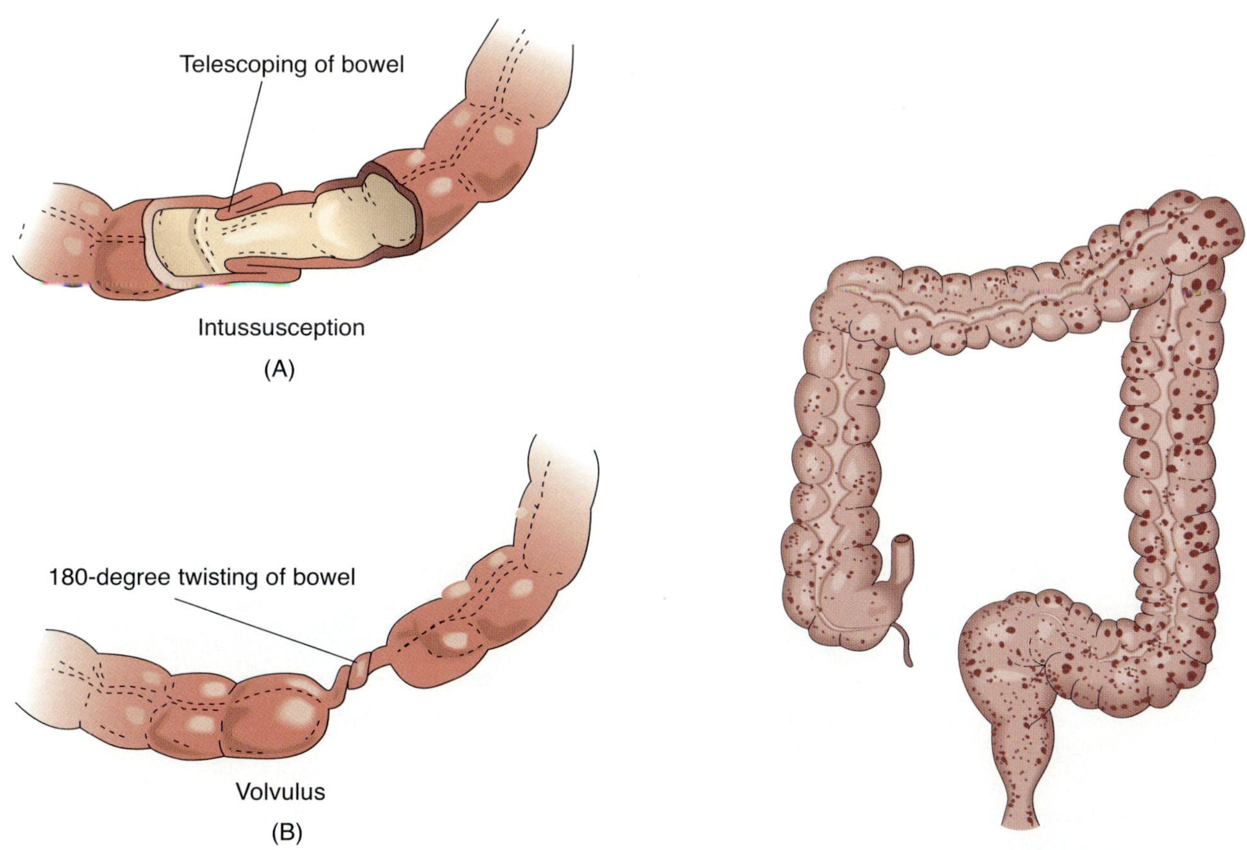

Figure 13–12 Volvulus and intussusception.

Figure 13–13 Ulcerative colitis.

treatment fails. Surgical intervention often results in a colostomy (opening in the colon)—either temporary or permanent (Figure 13–14). A temporary colostomy can be reconnected to the distal segment of colon that remained after surgery. A permanent colostomy typically cannot undergo revision because a portion of the rectum and anus have been removed.

Irritable Bowel Syndrome (Spastic Colon). Irritable bowel syndrome (IBS) is the most common intestinal disorder. It may be commonly confused with inflammatory bowel disease (IBD), but they are not the same. Inflammatory bowel disease is an inflammation of the bowel with chronic lesions. There is neither inflammation nor lesions in irritable bowel syndrome. IBS is a functional disorder

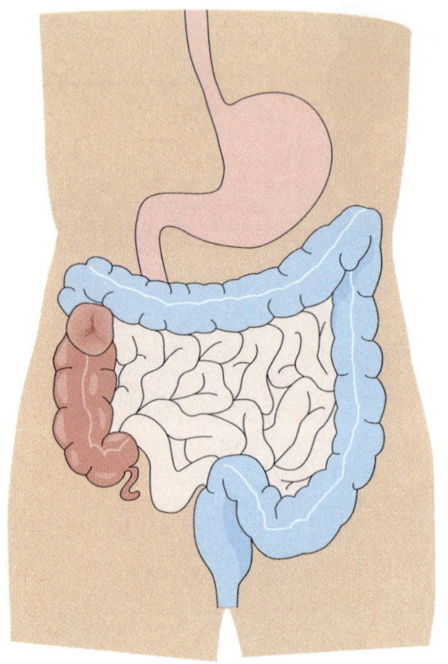

Ascending colostomy

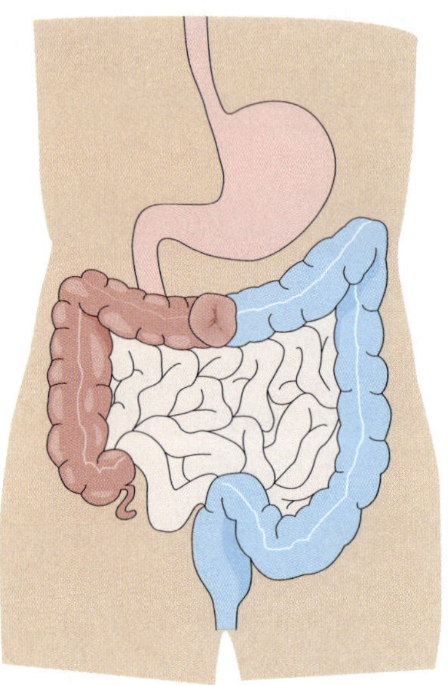

Transverse colostomy

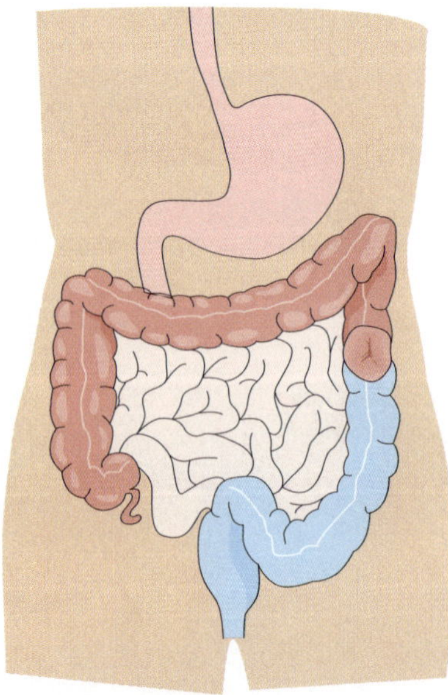

Descending colostomy

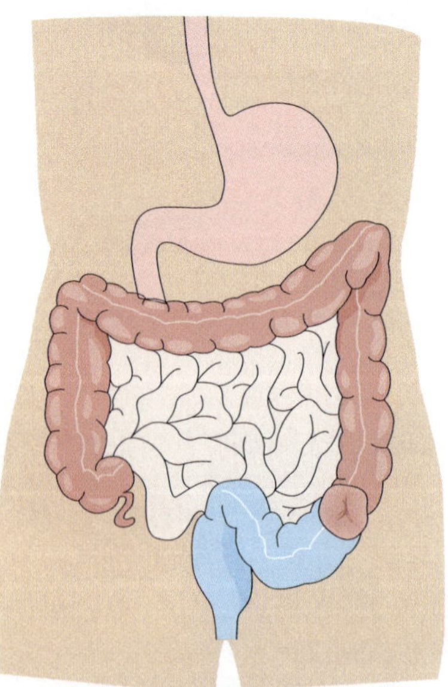

Sigmoid colostomy

Figure 13–14 Colostomy locations (blue section may be surgically removed if colostomy is permanent).

of motility and may cause a group of symptoms including abdominal pain and altered motility. Typically an individual suffering from IBS has bouts of diarrhea or constipation or both. The cause of IBS is unknown but a strong psychogenic factor has been considered. IBS is chronic and onset usually occurs in the young adult. Frequent re-occurrence over the years is very frustrating to the affected individual and the physician.

Spicy foods, caffeine, alcohol, and seasonings can irritate the colon and bring about symptoms of IBS. Stress also has an adverse effect and often causes alterations in intestinal motility. Avoidance of causative factors and stress reduction techniques often allow the colon to return to its normal functional state. Medications may be helpful in normalizing bowel motility.

Dysentery. Dysentery is an acute inflammation of the colon or colitis. The main symptom is massive diarrhea containing blood, pus, and mucus accompanied by severe abdominal pain. Dysentery is the disease and should not be confused with diarrhea the symptom. Dysentery is caused by invasion of microorganisms into the lining of the colon. This disease is usually a result of ingestion of contaminated food and/or water caused by poor sanitary conditions. Treatment is dependent on the cause of the disease. Patients will require fluid and electrolyte replacement. Antibiotics may be helpful if dysentery is caused by an infection, but not if it is caused by an enterotoxin.

Diverticulosis/Diverticulitis. Diverticulosis is a condition of having diverticula or little outpouches in the colon (Figure 13–15), especially the sigmoid colon. It may be asymptomatic (without symptoms) until the pouches become packed with fecal material and become irritated and inflamed. Once inflamed the condition is called diverticulitis. Signs and symptoms of diverticulitis include low abdominal pain, cramping, and fever. Diverticulitis increases in incidence with age, and has been associated with poor dietary habits, lack of physical activity, and poor bowel habits. As this inflammatory disease progresses, it may lead to hemorrhage, perforation, or narrowing of the lumen of the colon and thus obstruction. Treatment with antibiotics and dietary modification is usually quite effective. In severe cases or cases that do not respond to treatment, a portion of the bowel may be surgically removed.

Diseases of the Rectum

The rectum is the terminal or end part of the digestive system. The most common rectal problem is hemorrhoids.

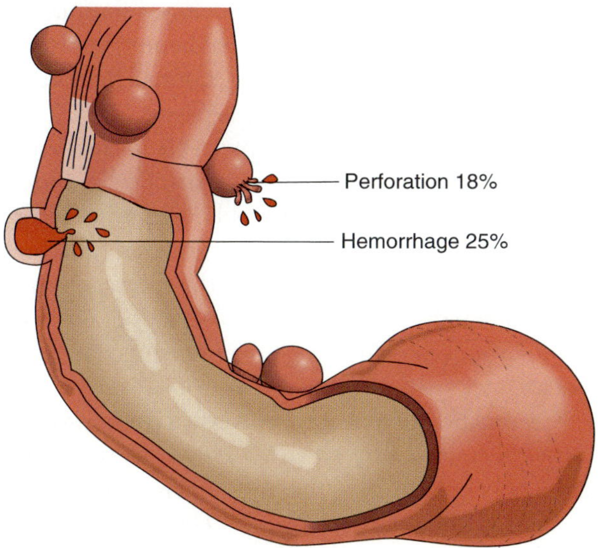

Figure 13–15 Diverticulosis.

Rectal fissures and other minor problems can also occur, but cancer of the rectum is one of the most serious diseases of the rectum to be diagnosed. It is more commonly diagnosed in the older adult than at any other age.

Hemorrhoids. Hemorrhoids are varicose veins in the rectum (Figure 13–16). Hemorrhoids can be internal or external. Internal hemorrhoids can be examined by a

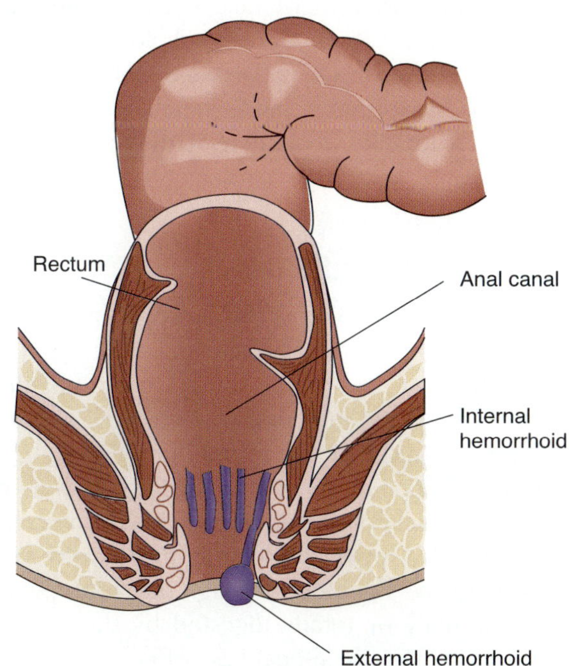

Figure 13–16 Hemorrhoids: internal and external.

physician using a proctoscope (procto = recutm, scope = instrument used to view). Internal hemorrhoids occur in the internal rectal venous plexus. External hemorrhoids occur in the external rectal venous plexus.

The internal rectal venous plexus is normally filled with venous blood. When this plexus swells, the surrounding tissue also swells and is known as an internal hemorrhoid. This hemorrhoid can grow into the bowel lumen and become compressed by the sphincter. Internal hemorrhoids are generally not painful until they become incarcerated or infected and tissue death begins to occur.

External hemorrhoids occur when a clot forms in the external rectal venous plexus. This causes a painful enlargement of the plexus that is generally visible to visual inspection without a proctoscope. These external hemorrhoids may cause bright red bleeding with bowel movements, particularly if the patient had to strain or was constipated.

Factors that increase the risk of developing hemorrhoids include any activity that increases pressure in the anal area such as straining to have a bowel movement, frequent bouts of constipation, prolonged standing, prolonged sitting, pregnancy, and childbirth. Other causes may be related to portal hypertension, heredity, and loss of muscle tone.

Preventive measures are focused at softening the stool, which will decrease constipation and straining with bowel movements. These measures include good bowel habits (defecating when reflexes are strong), adequate fluid intake, increased fiber intake, exercise, and avoiding laxative use. Treatment of hemorrhoids may include medications and warm sitz baths to ease the pain. Manual reduction, cryosurgery, and hemorrhoidectomy may be optional treatments, depending on the severity of the disease.

Gastrointestinal Bleeding

Gastrointestinal bleeding may be caused by a variety of conditions. Except in the case of an acute bleed, it can be very difficult to assess the source of the bleeding. Chronic GI bleeding may first present itself as a syncopal episode and not be found until later in the evaluation. The common sources of GI bleeding, the stomach, the small bowel, and large bowel, have already been discussed. Upper GI bleeding may involve vomiting blood or passing blood through the stool. As this blood is partially or totally digested by the stomach enzymes, it commonly appears as coffee grounds and can be very black. Acute bleeding can also manifest as frank, bright red blood, as in the case of ruptured esophageal varicies. Lower GI bleeding can also be acute or chronic. Dark black stools is an indication of GI blood loss, as the iron in the blood causes the stool to turn dark black. It can be difficult to assess the source, as both chronic upper and lower GI bleeding can cause darkened stool, though it is more commonly caused by lower GI bleeding. Frank bright red blood may be observed on the stool or in the toilet. Tumors, small bowel obstruction, and hemorrhoids can all cause lower GI bleeding. Field treatment includes assessing the patient's respiratory and hemodynamic status, and treating for shock as necessary.

Diseases of the Liver

Liver diseases can range from mild inflammation to those that destroy the liver and result in liver failure. Any disease of the liver may have serious consequences by interfering with the many functions of the liver.

Hepatitis. Hepatitis is inflammation of the liver and may be caused by the chemical action of drugs or toxic substances. Chronic alcoholism often leads to hepatitis prior to the functional changes seen with cirrhosis. The most common cause of hepatitis is a group of viruses. This form of hepatitis is often called viral hepatitis and is the form most commonly thought of when one considers hepatitis.

Viral hepatitis is the most prevalent liver disease in the world. It is often asymptomatic. When symptoms do occur they may be so vague that the disease is misdiagnosed. This explains why approximately forty percent of Americans have antibodies to hepatitis A and ten percent have antibodies to hepatitis B, yet these individuals do not recall ever having hepatitis.

Jaundice is often the first symptom that signals a liver problem, although not all individuals become yellow. Interestingly, those who become more jaundiced are more likely to have a good recovery than those who are less jaundiced. Individuals with mild jaundice are more likely to develop chronic hepatitis. Other symptoms include malaise, anorexia, myalgia (myo = muscle, algia = pain), fever, and abdominal pain. Physical examination may reveal **hepatomegaly** (HEP-ah-toh-**MEG**-ah-lee; hepato = liver, megaly = enlargement). Dark-colored urine and clay- or light-colored stools are related to the inability of the liver to form normal bile.

Treatment for viral hepatitis is symptomatic. Adequate rest and good nutrition are essential. Approximately eighty-five percent of affected individuals recover in six weeks. The most serious complications with hepatitis are development of chronic hepatitis and **fulminant** (FULL-ma-nant; to occur suddenly and with great intensity) hepatitis. Chronic hepatitis develops in one out of four cases and often leads to cirrhosis of the liver. Fulminant hepatitis is an acute hepatitis that causes extensive necrosis of liver tissue. Symptoms include a high fever, hemorrhages from the skin and mucous membranes, confusion, and stupor. Coma often develops and leads to death. Even with prompt and supportive care, fulminant hepatitis is ninety percent fatal.

Prevention of hepatitis involves good hygiene and special care when handling needles and body secretions. Vaccines are available for some types of viral hepatitis.

Viral hepatitis occurs in five basic types. A different virus causes each type. The types of hepatitis are A, B, C, D, and E.

1. Hepatitis A—the most benign or harmless form of hepatitis. Total recovery occurs ninety-eight percent of the time. This virus is spread by fecal-oral route. It commonly affects children and young adults, especially in areas where there is poor sanitation and overcrowding. Symptoms are usually very vague and similar to "flu," often leading to misdiagnosis. The virus is shed in the feces and the affected individual does not become a carrier of the disease. Hepatitis A never leads to chronic hepatitis or cirrhosis. There is a vaccine available. The vaccine is recommended for those traveling or living in a high-risk area.
2. Hepatitis B—a serious form of hepatitis formerly called "serum hepatitis." It was once thought that hepatitis B was only spread by contact with blood, as occurs with blood transfusions and contaminated needles. But it is now known that saliva, urine, feces, and semen may spread the virus, which also qualifies Hepatitis B as a sexually transmitted disease. Hepatitis B may also be spread transplacentally (across the placenta from mother to unborn infant). This virus is a major health problem as individuals may become carriers of the virus. Approximately 125,000 new infections occur every year in the United States. This virus may be carried for years or even a lifetime. Carriers are not only a threat to others but are also at high risk for developing chronic hepatitis and cirrhosis. About one out of every 250 persons is a carrier of hepatitis B. Those at high risk for hepatitis B are drug addicts, homosexuals, blood recipients, and health care workers. A vaccine is available and is ninety-five percent effective in prevention of the disease.
3. Hepatitis C—similar to hepatitis B as it also is spread by blood or sexual contact. Hepatitis C differs from B in that it attacks the RNA of a cell while hepatitis B attacks the DNA. Once hepatitis C was distinguished from hepatitis B, it was found to be the cause of most cases of hepatitis following blood transfusion (post-transfusion hepatitis). Hepatitis C is more likely to become chronic hepatitis than form B. Approximately fifty percent of those affected with hepatitis C will develop chronic hepatitis and cirrhosis. Over 12,000 individuals die each year from hepatitis C.
4. Hepatitis D—also called the "delta virus." It requires the presence of hepatitis B in order to replicate. Infection with both B and D may cause more prominent symptoms and a greater risk of developing chronic and fulminant hepatitis.
5. Hepatitis E—similar to hepatitis A in that it is spread through fecal-oral route. It is commonly caused by water contamination. Chronic hepatitis does not develop with hepatitis E, but this virus in pregnant women may be fatal.

Cirrhosis. **Cirrhosis** (sir-ROH-sis) of the liver is a chronic, irreversible, degenerative disease of the liver. Cirrhosis is characterized by the replacement of normal liver cells with non-functioning fibrous scar tissue known as "hobnail liver." This change in structure and function of the liver cells leads to impaired blood flow and altered function of the liver.

The most common cause of cirrhosis is chronic alcoholism. Cirrhosis is more common in males than females. It may also be idiopathic or it may be the end result of other diseases such as chronic hepatitis and congestive heart failure. The development of the disease often takes years. There are usually no symptoms until serious structural and functional changes in the liver tissue have occurred. If symptoms occur they are usually mild and non-specific. Symptoms may include loss of appetite, nausea, indigestion, weakness, and weight loss.

As the disease progresses, the abnormal scar tissue alters blood flow through the liver and leads to a variety of complications. Altered blood flow through the liver results in blood backing up in the hepatic portal vein. The relationship of the liver, hepatic portal system, and digestive system is as follows:

- The purpose of the hepatic portal system is to carry venous blood from the spleen and digestive organs (stomach and intestines) to the liver (Figure 13–17). The liver plays a major role in the digestive

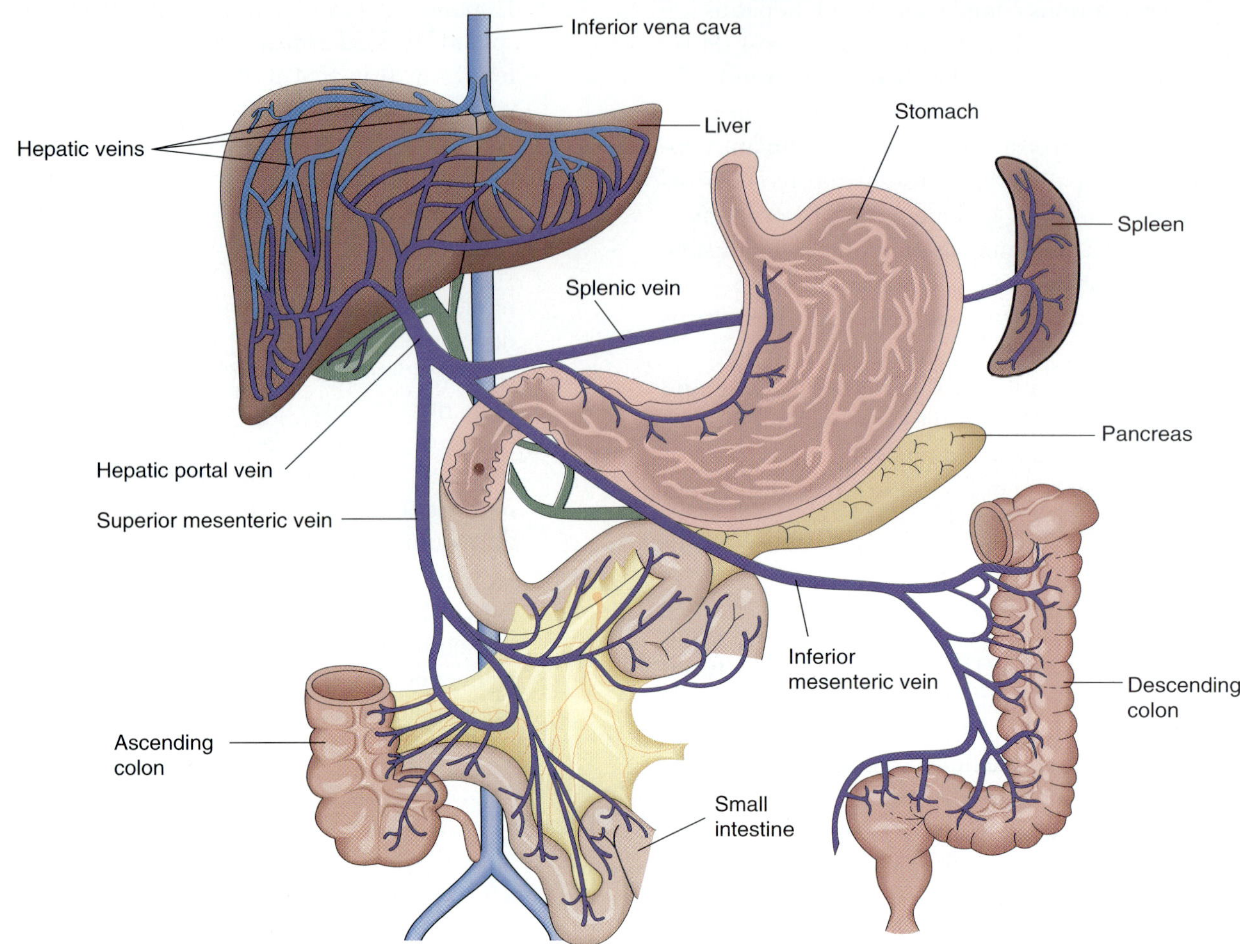

Figure 13–17 Hepatic portal system.

system by detoxifying and metabolizing nutrients before releasing them into the systemic blood in the inferior vena cava. For example, if an individual consumes a meal with an alcoholic beverage, these nutrients are absorbed into venous blood in the small intestine and transported to the liver to be filtered, detoxified, and stored. The liver's responsibility, in part, is to keep blood glucose levels from soaring when an individual eats a high carbohydrate meal. Nutrients are filtered, metabolized, stored, and released as needed into the systemic circulation by the liver. Toxins such as alcohol are detoxified. If alcohol consumption is too great or outpaces the liver's ability to detoxify the blood, the blood alcohol level will rise.

- If the liver is obstructed for any reason, blood will back up in this portal system. As blood backs up, pressure increases in the portal vein and is called **portal hypertension**.

Complications of severe cirrhosis may include:

1. Varicosities—portal hypertension causes varicosities (varicose veins) of the veins of the digestive system organs. Varicosities are commonly located in the esophagus (**esophageal varices**) (Figure 13–18). Esophageal varices (**VER**-ah-SEEZ) are prone to rupture leading to massive hemorrhage, shock, and death. Other sites of varicosities include the rectum (hemorrhoids) and anterior abdominal wall. Varicosities across the front of the abdomen are often quite tortuous and unsightly. This condition is called **caput medusae** (Medusa's head). Medusa, in Greek mythology, was a woman who had snakes on her head in place of hair.
2. Splenomegaly—portal hypertension also causes increased pressure on the organs that are connected or drained by the portal system. Often this passive congestion in the spleen leads to **splenomegaly** (SPLEE-no-**MEG**-ah-lee; spleno = spleen, megaly = enlarged). Splenomegaly often causes increased blood cell destruction leading to

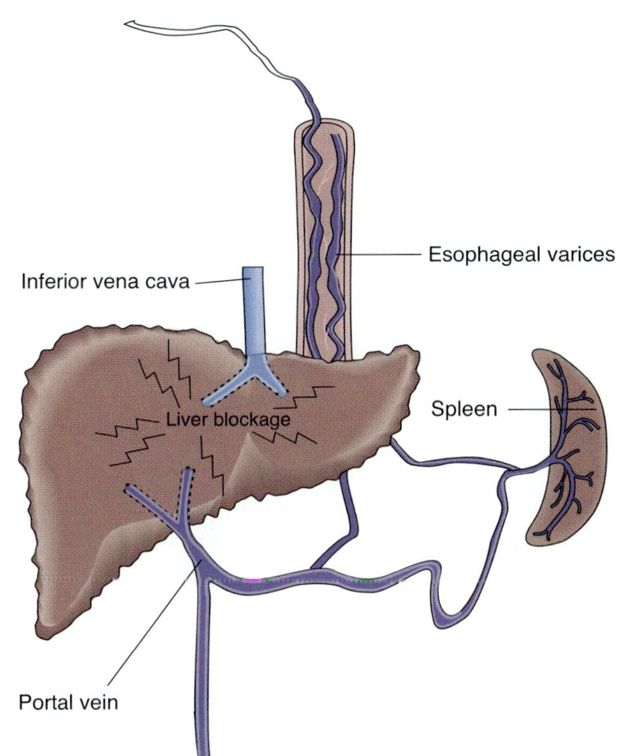

Figure 13–18 Esophageal varices.

anemia, leukopenia, and thrombocytopenia. Thrombocytopenia (thrombo = clot, cyto = cell, penia = decrease) increases the risk of bleeding.

3. Gastrointestinal hemorrhage—caused by thrombocytopenia and inability of the liver to secrete blood proteins essential for clotting. Hematemesis (HEM-ah-TEM-eh-sis; hemat = blood, emesis = vomiting) is often the first symptom of severe cirrhosis.
4. **Ascites** (ah-SIGH-teez)—is an accumulation of fluid in the abdominal cavity. This condition develops as a result of liver failure and portal hypertension. The increased pressure on the veins of the portal system causes leaking of serum into the abdomen. Often this fluid enlarges the abdomen to the point of causing difficult breathing. Excessive abdominal fluid may be drained by piercing the abdominal wall with a large bore needle. This procedure is called an **abdominocentesis** (ab-DOM-ih-no-sen-**TEE**-sis; abdomino = abdomen, centesis = puncture).
5. Edema—often develops in the ankles and feet as a result of liver failure. The normal liver produces a blood protein called **albumin** (AL-byou-men). Albumin is responsible for the osmotic pressure of blood. Osmotic pressure deals with the movement of fluid from the blood through the capillaries to the tissues and back into the blood. Without osmotic pressure, blood fluid tends to leak into the tissues and remain there. A decrease in albumin allows this to occur, leading to edema in the feet and ankles.
6. Jaundice—usually results from the obstruction of the bile ducts. This obstruction usually occurs as normal tissue is replaced by fibrous scar tissue characteristic of cirrhosis.
7. Altered sex hormone metabolism—the normal liver inactivates small amounts of estrogen secreted by the adrenal glands of both the male and female. As a result of normal liver activity, estrogen is inactivated and has no effect on the male. The cirrhotic liver is not capable of inactivating estrogen and thus the male exhibits feminizing effects. These feminizing effects are evidenced by:
   - **Gynecomastia** (GUY-neh-koh-**MAS**-tee-ah)—an enlargement of the breasts
   - **Palmar erythema**—palms of the hands become reddened in color
   - **Spider angiomas**—small dilated blood vessels on the face and chest
   - Female hair distribution—absent or reduced chest and pubic hair
   - Testicular atrophy—decrease in testicle size
8. Hepatic encephalopathy—the liver is often unable to detoxify the blood of nitrogenous waste products such as ammonia. This waste product circulates in the blood and may affect the brain, causing mental confusion, stupor, and a characteristic shaking or tremor. This shaking combined with hallucinations is called **delirium tremens** (dee-LIR-ee-um TREE-mens) or DTs. Further depression of the nervous system may lead to hepatic coma and ultimately death. The clinical features of cirrhosis of the liver in the male are shown in Figure 13–19.

Cirrhosis has an unfavorable prognosis with most individuals surviving only ten to fifteen years after diagnosis. The appearance of ascites is a prognostic indicator as a majority of individuals with cirrhosis die within five years after the onset of ascites. Individuals die of massive bleeding from esophageal varices, hepatic encephalopathy, and other metabolic disorders.

Treatment of cirrhosis is directed at the cause in order to attempt to prevent further liver damage. Alcohol is strictly prohibited no matter the cause of the cirrhosis.

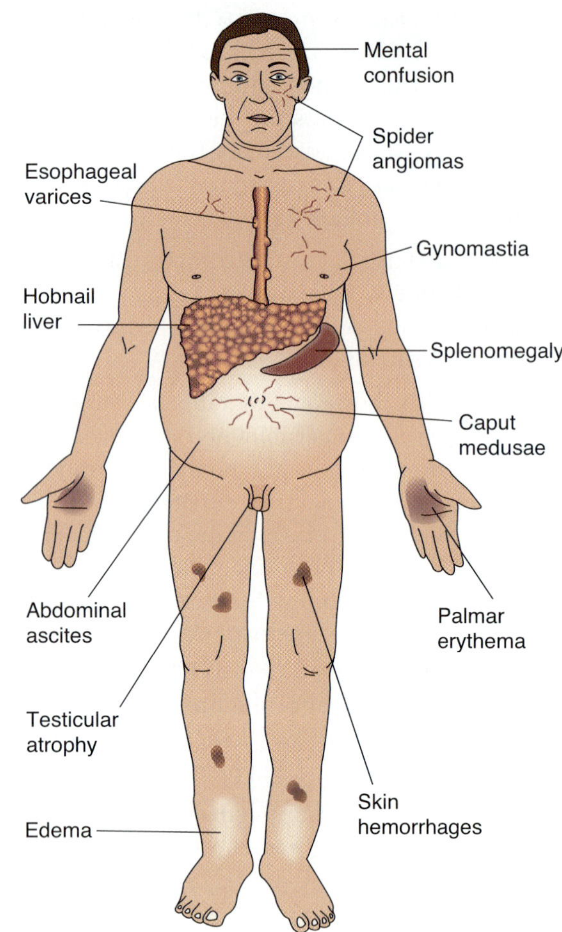

Figure 13–19 Clinical features of cirrhosis of the liver in the male.

Adequate nutrition and rest are necessary. Vitamins, minerals, and diet supplements may be needed to prevent malnutrition. Diuretics may be needed to reduce edema and ascites.

Diseases of the Gallbladder

Gallbladder disorders usually cause symptoms related to indigestion when eating fatty foods. Nausea, pain, and excessive gas are the most common symptoms. Nutritional changes and a variety of surgical procedures may be used to treat the disease.

Cholecystitis. Cholecystitis (KOH-lee-sis-**TYE**-tis; chole = bile or gall, cyst = bladder, itis = inflammation) or inflammation of the gallbladder is usually caused by obstruction of bile flow caused by a gallstone. When bile flow is obstructed, bile in the gallbladder becomes overly concentrated and irritates the lining of the gallbladder, leading to inflammation. When a fatty meal is eaten, fat in the duodenum stimulates the gallbladder to contract and release bile. This contraction of the inflamed gallbladder causes mild to severe pain in the right upper quadrant of the abdomen. This pain combined with a history of nausea and vomiting after meals is indicative of cholecystitis. Ultrasound and cholecystogram confirm diagnosis of cholecystitis. Cholecystogram involves swallowing a dye that is absorbed by the liver and excreted into the bile. Radiographic pictures are made to confirm the presence of stones.

Complications of cholecystitis include rupture of the gallbladder, leading to peritonitis. Chronic cholecystitis may cause bile to back up into the liver leading to liver damage and cirrhosis. Treatment for cholecystitis is aimed at the cause. Gallstones often obstruct the gallbladder or one of its ducts. Treatment of choice for cholecystitis caused by stones is surgical removal by a procedure called **cholecystectomy** (KOH-lee-sis-**TECK**-toh-me; chole = bile or gall, cyst = bladder, ectomy=removal). Cholecystectomy may be performed using an abdominal incision or it may be removed using a laparoscope (laparo = abdomen, scope = scope). Removal of the gallbladder using a laparoscope is called laparoscopic cholecystectomy (LAP-ah-**ROW**-skop-ic KOH-lee-sis-**TECK**-toh-me). Laparoscopic cholecystectomy is performed through several small abdominal incisions. This type of procedure drastically reduces discomfort and the length of hospital stay as compared to the larger abdominal incision.

After a cholecystectomy, the bile continues to be excreted by the liver into the common bile duct and simply drips into the duodenum as it is produced. As long as the individual does not take in an excessive amount of fatty foods, the amount of bile will be sufficient to break down the consumed fat and normal digestion will occur.

Cholelithiasis. Cholelithiasis (KOH-lee-lih-**THIGH**-ah-sis; chole = bile or gall, lith = stone, iasis = condition) is the presence of gallstones in the gallbladder or bile ducts (Figure 13–20). Over one million people in the United States are diagnosed each year with gallstones and approximately 500,000 undergo surgery for removal of the stones (American Liver Foundation, 1997). Gallstones are often asymptomatic. If symptoms do occur they are usually related to blocking the outflow of the gallbladder or of its ducts. Symptoms include nausea, vomiting, and right upper quadrant pain following meals with fat. A cholecystogram and ultrasound along with a positive history will confirm the diagnosis.

Gallstones form from bile salts and cholesterol. The stones may vary in size, shape, number, color, and composition. The reason for stone development is not under-

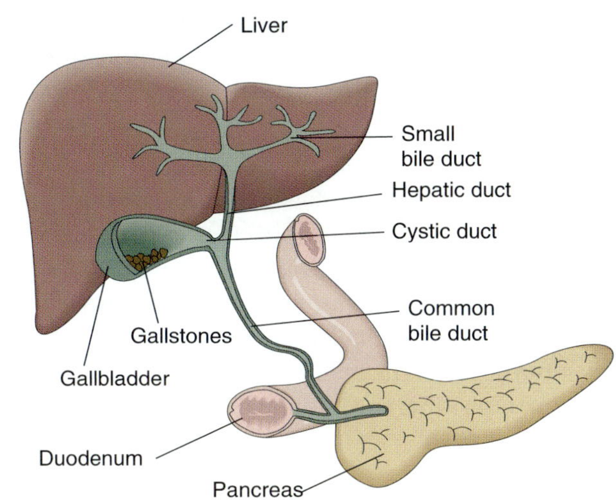

Figure 13–20 Cholelithiasis.

stood, but females develop stones more commonly than males. The three most important risk factors for developing gallstones include excessive body weight, increasing age, and being female. In general, individuals developing cholelithiasis have several factors in common called the five Fs of cholelithiasis. They include 1. **F**emale 2. **F**air complexion 3. **F**at or obese 4. **F**ertile or has had children 5. **F**orty years in age or older.

Complications of cholelithiasis include cholecystitis and jaundice. Extracorporeal shockwave lithotripsy (litho = stone, tripsy = destruction) ESWL may be performed in an effort to break up the stones so they can be passed. If this procedure is not effective or is not recommended, cholecystectomy is performed.

Diseases of the Pancreas

Diseases of the pancreas are often quite advanced by the time symptoms appear. Some pancreatic disorders are associated with alcoholism. Replacement or supplements of pancreatic enzymes and insulin may be necessary when the pancreas is not functioning properly or is surgically removed.

Pancreatitis. Pancreatitis is an inflammation of the pancreas that may range from mild to fatal. With pancreatitis, the pancreas becomes inflamed, edematous, hemorrhagic, and necrotic. This disease is similar to cirrhosis of the liver in that most cases of severe pancreatitis are caused by alcoholism. Pancreatitis differs from inflammation of other organs because of the powerful digestive enzymes that are produced by the pancreas. As this organ becomes diseased these enzymes often escape the pancreatic cells and ducts causing digestion of the pancreas (**autodigestion**) and the surrounding tissues. If this destruction extends into blood vessels, hemorrhage occurs, leading to severe pain and shock. Acute hemorrhagic pancreatitis usually follows an alcohol-drinking spree and is often fatal in spite of emergency medical attention.

An acute attack of pancreatitis causes sudden, severe abdominal pain that often radiates to the back. The individual may find some relief by drawing the knees up toward the abdomen. Other symptoms exhibited during an acute attack are nausea, vomiting, diaphoresis (sweating), and tachycardia. Individuals with chronic pancreatitis may complain of constant back pain and frequent bouts of mild symptoms similar to those of an acute attack. As the disease progresses, the pancreatic tissue is replaced with fibrous tissue and function is lost. As endocrine function is lost the individual has symptoms of diabetes mellitus. Digestive disorders including malabsorption occur when exocrine function is impaired.

Pancreatitis may also be caused by blockage of pancreatic ducts by gallstones, also known as gallstone pancreatitis. Many cases of pancreatitis are idiopathic (of unknown cause). Diagnosis of pancreatitis is often made based on the individual's history and is confirmed by blood testing. A high blood **amylase** (pancreatic enzyme) is indicative of pancreatitis. Treatment and prognosis of pancreatitis depends on the cause. Pancreatitis caused by gallstones is treated successfully by removing the gallbladder and the involved stones. Treatment for idiopathic and alcohol-related pancreatitis is palliative as there is no cure. Individuals must stop drinking alcohol and are treated with analgesics and nutritional support. Prognosis for these types of pancreatitis is poor.

TRAUMA

Trauma to the GI system varies depending upon the cause (i.e., blunt or penetrating trauma) and the specific organ involved. The abdominal organs, most of which are components of the GI system, can be divided into solid organs and hollow organs

Solid Organ Trauma

The solid organs of the gastrointestinal system include the liver, spleen, and pancreas. The kidneys (renal system) are also classified as solid organs. As their name implies, they are solid compared to the other organs in the abdominal cavity and have a rich blood supply. These organs, if lacerated, can bleed profusely. The trauma surgeon may not be able to halt the flow of blood from these organs, and part of or the entire organ many need to be removed. In some cases, the organ capsule, which is made up of several layers of peritoneum surrounding the organ, may remain intact and limit bleeding by the increase in pressure caused by bleeding into a confined space. Solid organs may be damaged by both blunt trauma and penetrating trauma.

Hollow Organ Trauma

In contrast, hollow organs have a thin wall and a lumen, and can generally withstand blunt impact to the abdomen. The rest of the digestive tract, the urinary bladder, and female reproductive organs are considered hollow organs of the abdomen. The esophagus may be damaged as a result of blunt trauma because it lies in a relatively fixed position, connected to the pharynx, adhered to the heart and aorta in the chest, and passing through the diaphragm. Rupture of the esophagus can cause bacteria and stomach acid to leak into the chest cavity directly damaging the heart and lungs. Blunt trauma may cause a full urinary bladder to rupture, potentially spilling irritating urine into the abdominal and pelvic cavities. Penetrating trauma to the abdomen may cause perforation of the hollow organs of the gastrointestinal system, allowing bacteria normally present in the digestive tract access to the peritoneal cavity.

EVALUATION OF ABDOMINAL PAIN

One of the most challenging aspects of patient care to EMS providers is evaluating a patient who is complaining of abdominal pain. **Visceral pain** is pain that originates from the organs, for example, stomach or spleen. **Somatic pain** is pain that originates from the soft tissue or muscles in the body. **Referred pain** is pain that is located in one area but caused by a disease process located in another area. Palpation to the area of referred pain does not cause pain, however palpation over the organ responsible for the referred pain may cause both direct or referred pain. When assessing a patient complaining of abdominal pain, it is important to determine if peritonitis is present. Blood, byproducts of infection or inflammation, and other fluids that are irritating to the peritoneal lining can cause peritonitis. Peritoneal signs may indicate a surgical emergency, as in the example of a ruptured appendix. Rebound tenderness and an increase in pain with movements such as walking or driving over a bumpy road are indicative of peritonitis.

The abdomen can be divided into quadrants to help in describing symptoms and assessing signs in the patient (Figure 13–21). Table 13–1 correlates the quadrants with the abdominal organs that are located within the quadrants.

Pain originating from abdominal organs tends to not only cause localized pain, but referred pain. These pain referral patterns are well documented and can be used to narrow down the list of organs causing the pain (Figure 13–22). Some patients will present with complaints of pain limited to the pain referral pattern, providing an additional diagnostic challenge. Knowledge of the common referral patterns will assist you in evaluating the patient complaining of abdominal pain.

DEVELOPMENTAL AND GENETIC DISORDERS

Digestive system disorders, both genetic and developmental, range from mild to severe. Many are diagnosed at birth, especially if the disorder interferes with ingestion, digestion, or elimination. Some of them are incompatible with life and must be corrected immediately or the infant would not survive.

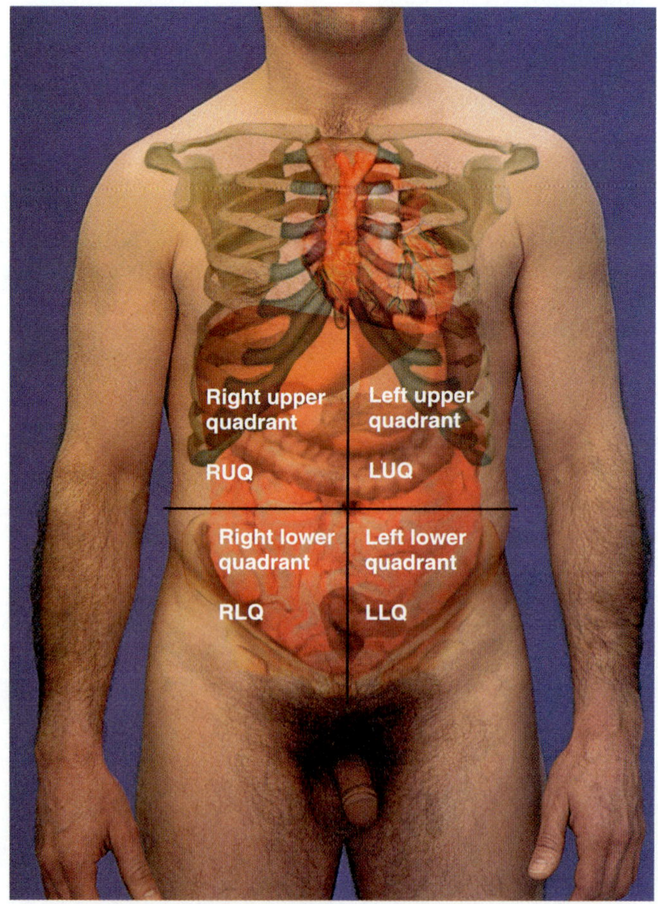

Figure 13–21 The four quadrants of the abdomen.

TABLE 13-1 Contents of the Abdominal Quadrants

Right Upper Quadrant	Left Upper Quadrant
Liver	Liver
Gallbladder	Spleen
Stomach (pyloric part)	Stomach
Duodenum	Jejunum and first part of ileum
Right kidney	Left kidney
Ascending colon (upper half)	Descending colon (upper half)
Transverse colon (right half)	Transverse colon (left half)
	Pancreas
Right Lower Quadrant	**Left Lower Quadrant**
Ascending colon (lower half)	Descending colon (lower half)
Appendix	Sigmoid colon
Most of ileum	Left ureter
Right ureter	Left ovary and tube (female)
Right ovary and tube (female)	Uterus (if enlarged)
Uterus (if enlarged)	Urinary bladder (if very full)
Urinary bladder (if very full)	

Developmental Malformations

Several developmental malformations occur in the digestive system. Surgical correction is the treatment of choice for these malformations. A few of the more common malformations are briefly discussed here.

- Meckel's diverticulum is an outpouching or diverticulum of the ileum (Figure 13–23A). During fetal life the intestine is connected to the yolk sack by a duct. Failure of the duct to disappear leads to formation of this diverticulum. Meckel's diverticulum

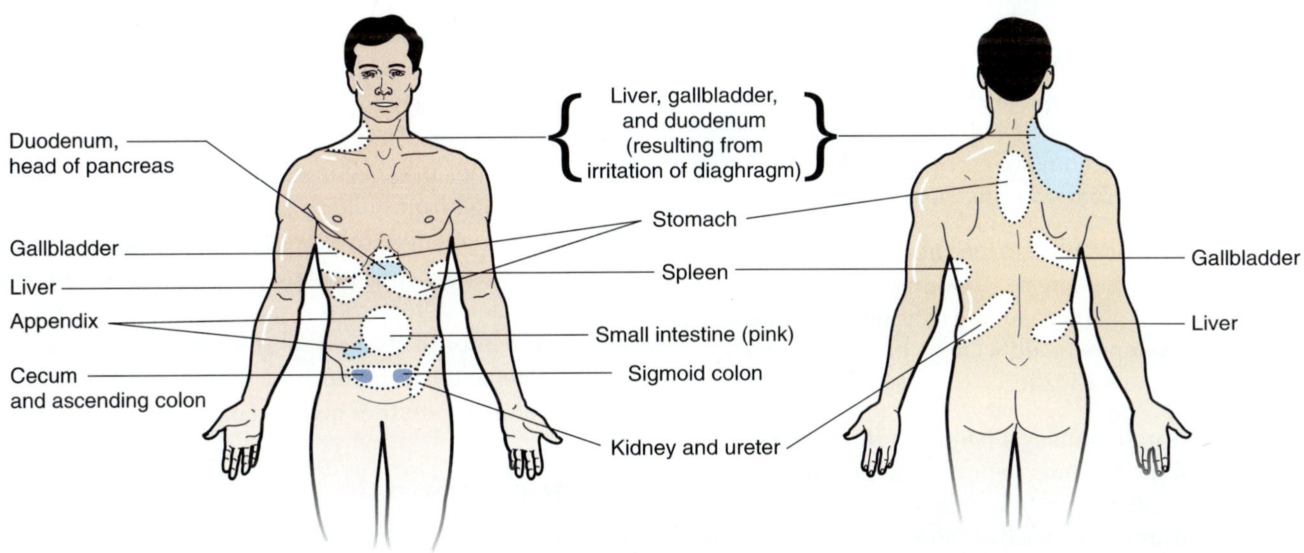

Figure 13–22 Pain referral patterns of abdominal organs.

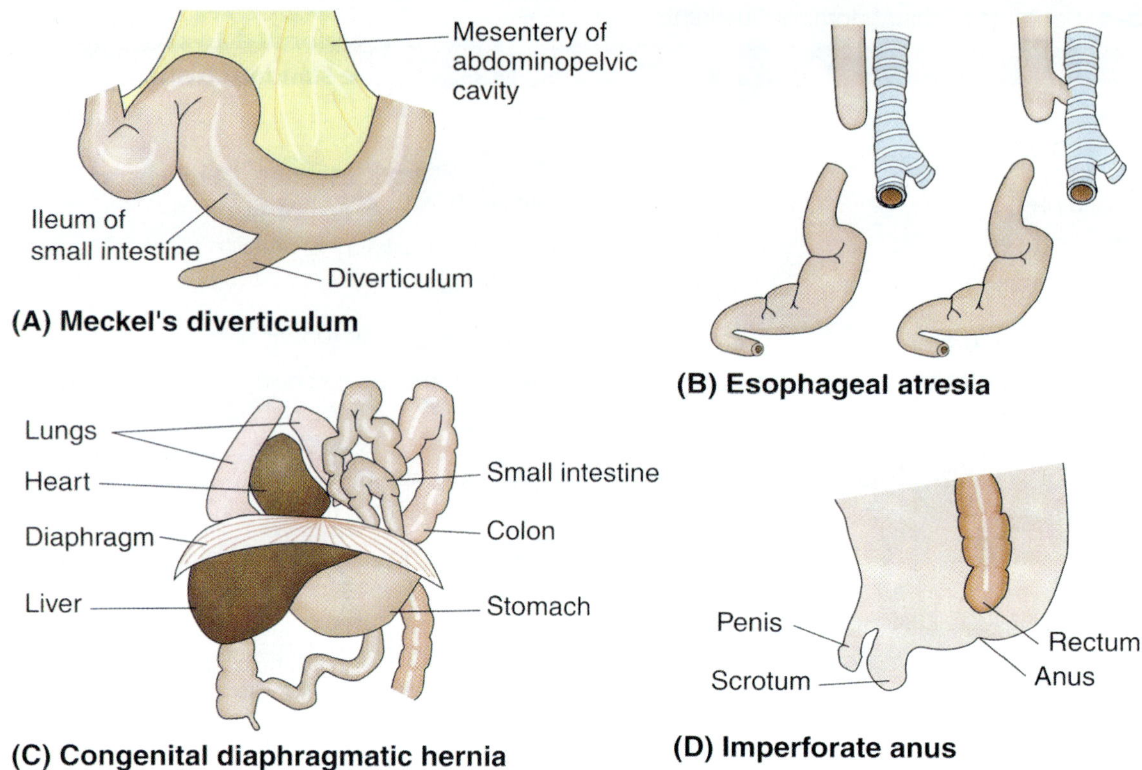

Figure 13–23 Developmental malformations.

is the most common malformation of the gastrointestinal system, occurring in approximately two percent of the population. The diverticulum may be asymptomatic the entire life of the individual and found only on autopsy. If symptoms do occur, it is usually during infancy. The most common symptom is painless bloody stools.

- Esophageal atresia is the absence of part of, or abnormal closure of, the esophagus. An **atresia** (ah-TREE-ze-ah) is the congenital absence or closure of a normal opening or lumen in the body and may occur in a variety of areas. Esophageal atresia is often accompanied by a fistula connecting the trachea to the esophagus (Figure 13–23B).
- Congenital diaphragmatic hernia is a congenital hole in the diaphragm. Abdominal organs may herniate through this opening causing problems with lung development, difficulty in breathing and chest pain (Figure 13–23C).
- Imperforate anus is a failure of the anus to connect to the rectum (Figure 13–23D). Infants with imperforate anus commonly have other developmental anomalies such as those affecting the heart, kidneys, esophagus and spine.

Cleft Lip and Palate

Cleft (a split) lip, formerly commonly called a harelip, consists of one or more abnormal splits in the upper lip (Figure 13–24A). This is a common anomaly occurring in approximately one in 1,000 births. The defect occurs more frequently in boys and may vary from slight to severe. A cleft palate involves the palate or roof of the mouth (see Figure 13–24B). A cleft palate is more serious than a cleft lip as it forms an opening between the nasopharynx and the nose. This anomaly not only leads to difficulty with feeding but also increases the risk of respiratory and middle ear infections. Cleft palate is more common in girls. Both conditions may occur separately or in combination and may range from mild to severe. The cause of clefts appears to be related to a hereditary factor coupled with an alteration in intrauterine environment. Surgical repair for cleft deformities is usually performed as soon as possible after birth. Several surgeries may be needed in order to achieve the desired results. Special feeding devices and speech therapy are common needs.

Pyloric Stenosis

Pyloric stenosis is a narrowing (stenosis) of the outlet of the lower end of the stomach, the pylorus (Figure 13–25).

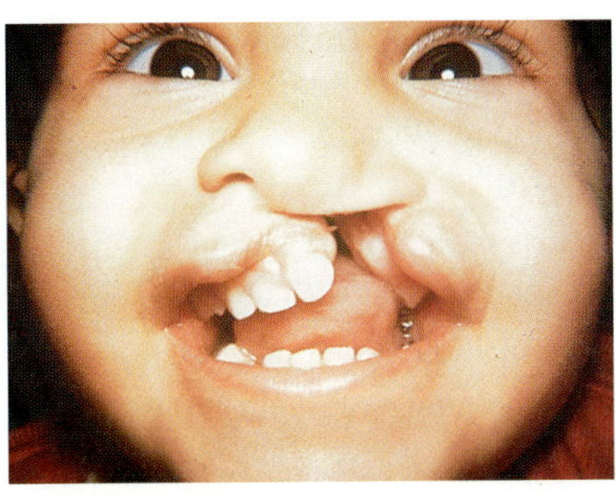

(A)

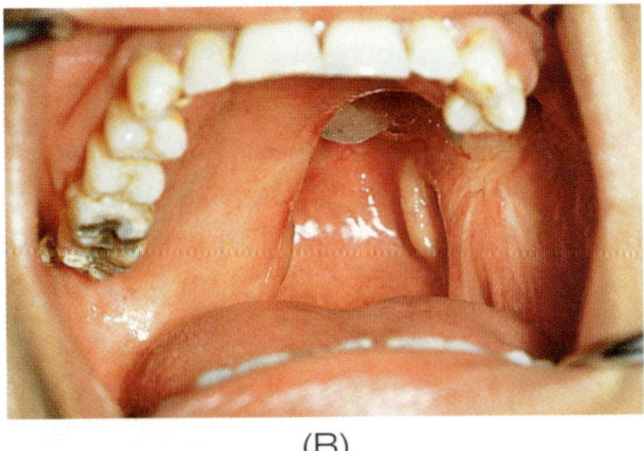

(B)

Figure 13–24 (A) Cleft lip. (B) Palate. (Courtesy of Dr. Joseph Konzelman, School of Dentistry, Medical College of Georgia.)

This condition is one of the most common developmental abnormalities of the digestive tract. It is caused by a hypertrophy or thickening of the pyloric sphincter. This sphincter controls the flow of contents out of the stomach or pyloric area. The hypertrophy of the pyloric sphincter slows the flow of stomach contents resulting in a backup of contents. The most common symptom of pyloric stenosis is projectile or forceful vomiting. Symptoms of pyloric stenosis usually begin at two to four weeks of age. This condition occurs almost exclusively in boys. A simple operation, called a **pyloromyotomy** (pyloro = pyloric, myo = muscle, otomy = cut into), which involves incising and suturing the pyloric sphincter muscle, can be performed to correct the problem. This surgery is the standard treatment and is usually very effective.

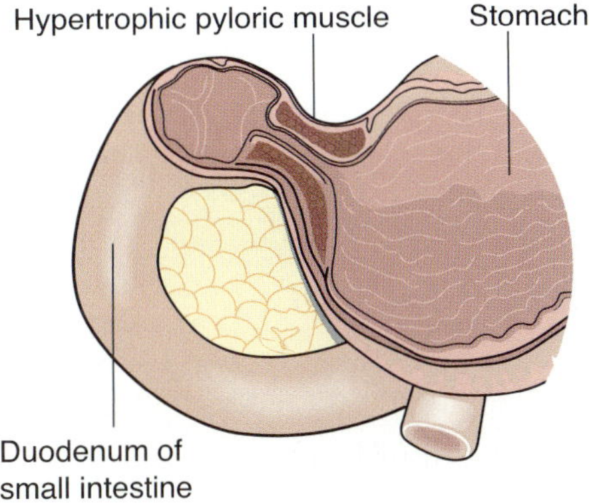

Figure 13–25 Pyloric stenosis.

Hirschsprung's Disease

Hirschsprung's disease is caused by an absence of nerves (ganglion) in a segment of the colon, usually the sigmoid colon. Without normal ganglion, the affected segment of colon lacks peristalsis, causing massive distention of the colon with feces (Figure 13–26). Common symptoms include chronic constipation and abdominal distention. Hirschsprung's disease is seen more often in boys and those affected with Down syndrome. It has a familial tendency and occurs in approximately one in 5,000 births. Diagnosis is made on the basis of a biopsy to determine the absence of ganglion cells. Treatment is surgical removal of the affected segment. A temporary colostomy may be necessary to allow adequate healing of the colon.

EFFECTS OF AGING ON THE SYSTEM

Disorders of the digestive system are common in the aging population. The incidence of problems increases with age. Some of the problems occurring in the system with age are caused by changes in the cardiovascular or neurologic system, which cause disruptions in the functioning of the digestive system. In the upper digestive system, the most common problem with aging is related to loss of teeth.

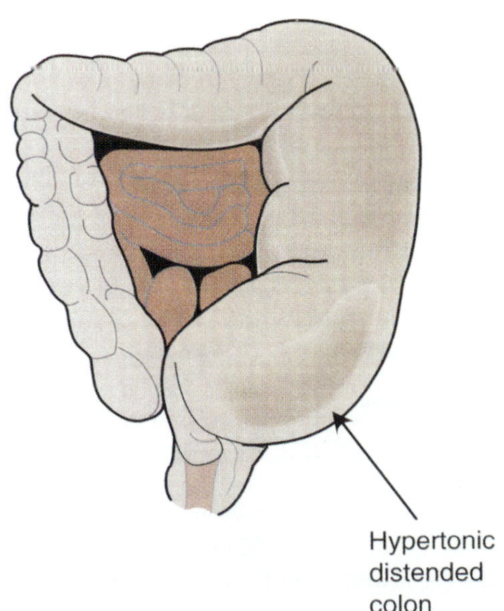

Figure 13–26 Hirschsprung's disease.

Preventive dentistry has lessened teeth and gum problems in recent years, but it is still a significant factor in the older adult. The sense of taste becomes less sensitive. The motility in the esophagus decreases and may cause some distress, but it is generally asymptomatic.

Changes in the lining of the stomach and decreased secretion of hydrochloric acid increase the likelihood of digestive disorders in the older adult. Decreased circulation to the stomach increases the incidence of ulcer disease.

Lower digestive disorders are common in the older adult. The lower intestinal lining is affected much like the stomach lining. There is a decreased absorption of some nutrients, such as vitamin B_{12} and fats. Decreased circulation to the intestines may cause ischemia and pain in the abdomen. Decreased motility may contribute to constipation problems. The development of inflammatory disease and hemorrhoids is common to the aging process, but may also be caused by earlier problems or other predisposing factors.

The older adult who develops hepatitis usually undergoes a more severe infection than a younger person does with the same disease. The mortality rate for hepatitis increases with age. The elderly may be at an increased risk for developing hepatitis if any of the following factors are present:

- a depressed immune system
- increased contact with a variety of caregivers
- poor nutrition
- increased intake of medications
- poor hygiene
- multiple blood transfusions

Cirrhosis in the elderly may be of unknown etiology or caused by chronic alcohol intake. It is usually progressive, severe, and the prognosis is poor. Bile stones are also seen more frequently in the older adult. Surgery is usually the treatment of choice but may not be an option because of the age of the individual and other complicating disorders. Pancreatic disease is also common in the older adult population. Replacement of pancreatic enzymes may be needed if the pancreas is not producing adequate amounts.

SUMMARY

The gastrointestinal system consists of a long hollow tube that extends from mouth to anus and several accessory organs. The purpose of this system is the ingestion, digestion, and absorption of fluids and nutrients, and elimination of waste products. Diseases of the esophagus, stomach, and small and large intestine include infections, inflammatory processes, and cancers. The liver has several additional functions that can affect the circulatory system, reproductive system, and hematological system when it is diseased. Hepatitis is the most common liver disorder and is usually caused by a virus. Cirrhosis of the liver is most commonly related to long-term alcoholism and leads to portal hypertension. Gallbladder disease affects thousands of individuals annually. Pancreatic disorders are often not diagnosed until late in the disease process because early symptoms are often not apparent. Supplementation of pancreatic enzymes may be required if they are deficient. Trauma to the solid organs may involve profuse hemorrhage. Trauma to the hollow organs may cause rupture or perforation. Knowledge of anatomy and pain referral patterns are helpful in assessing a patient complaining of abdominal pain. Developmental disorders of the gastrointestinal system are not common but often require surgical correction. Physiologic and lifestyle changes in older adults put them at higher risk for diseases of the digestive system.

REVIEW QUESTIONS

Short Answer

1. What are the functions of the digestive system, including liver, gallbladder, and pancreas?

2. Which signs and symptoms are associated with common digestive system disorders?

3. Which signs and symptoms are associated with common liver, gallbladder, and pancreas disorders?

4. Which diagnostic tests are most commonly used to determine type and/or cause of the digestive system disorders?

5. Which diagnostic tests are more commonly used to determine type and/or cause of the liver, gallbladder, or pancreas disorder?

Matching

6. Match the disorders listed in the left column with the correct region of the digestive system in the right column:

_____ Pharyngitis	a. disease of the small intestine
_____ Gastritis	b. disease of the mouth
_____ Hemorrhoids	c. disease of the colon
_____ Periodontal disease	d. disease of the throat or esophagus
_____ Regional enteritis	e. disease of the rectum
_____ Irritable bowel syndrome	f. disease of the stomach

Multiple Choice

7. Which of the following behaviors may contribute to digestive system problems?
   a. Eating four to six small meals per day
   b. Improperly cooking food
   c. Failure to wash hands after toileting
   d. Poor dietary habits
   e. Straining with bowel movements
   f. Drinking plenty of fluids daily
   g. Frequent use of laxatives and enemas

8. Which of the following is the cause of jaundice?
   a. Increased levels of amylase in the blood
   b. Decreased levels of pancreatase in the blood
   c. Increased levels of bilirubin in the blood
   d. Decreased levels of lipase in the blood

9. Impaired liver function leads to an elevation in which of the following tests?
   a. Bilirubin and alkaline phosphatase
   b. Albumin and bilirubin
   c. Alkaline phosphatase and amylase
   d. Amylase and albumin

10. Diseases of the liver, gallbladder, or pancreas generally have an adverse effect on which of the following?
    a. The immune system
    b. Digestion and metabolism
    c. The inflammatory process
    d. The endocrine system

11. Which of the following types of hepatitis is the most common?
    a. Hepatitis A
    b. Hepatitis B
    c. Hepatitis C
    d. Hepatitis D

12. Individuals at high risk for developing hepatitis B include which of the following?
    a. Drug addicts
    b. Blood recipients
    c. Health care workers
    d. All of the above

13. Which of the following is the best definition of cirrhosis?
    a. A chronic, degenerative disease of the pancreas
    b. An acute irreversible disease of the liver
    c. An abnormality of the liver caused by alcoholism
    d. A chronic, degenerative, irreversible disease of the liver

14. Ascites is an accumulation of fluid in the abdominal cavity usually caused by which of the following conditions?
    a. Pancreatic cancer
    b. Liver failure and portal hypertension
    c. Cholelithiasis
    d. Cirrhosis

True or False

15. T F The alimentary canal is a continuous tube from the mouth to the anus.
16. T F Strep throat should always be treated since it may lead to rheumatic heart disease.
17. T F The main function of the large intestine (colon) is the digestion of food.
18. T F The *Helicobacter* bacteria are thought to be a contributing factor for the development of peptic ulcers.
19. T F The effects of aging put the older adult at an increased risk for digestive system problems.
20. T F Gallbladder disorders usually cause symptoms related to indigestion when eating high fat foods.
21. T F A cholecystogram is a radiographic exam used to diagnose cholecystitis.
22. T F Gallstones are most commonly found in obese middle-aged men.
23. T F A high serum amylase is usually diagnostic for pancreatitis.
24. T F The older adult who develops hepatitis usually experiences a much milder episode of the disease than a young person.

CASE STUDY

You are called to the home of Adelide Fisher, a 68-year-old retired female who is complaining of right upper quadrant pain and right shoulder pain. She states that this has happened before and often occurs after fatty meals. She ate two slices of pepperoni pizza for lunch and states that this is the worst pain she has ever experienced. What organs are located in the right upper quadrant? What pain referral pattern explains Ms. Fisher's symptoms? What is the pathophysiology associated with the organ causing Ms. Fisher's symptoms?

BIBLIOGRAPHY

American Liver Foundation. (1997). *http://gi.ucsf.edu/alf.html* 1425 Pompton Avenue, Cedar Grove, NJ 07009 1-800-465-4837.

Corish, C. (1997). Nutrition and liver disease. *Nutrition Reviews, 55*(1), 17–20.

Evans, R. W. (1997). Liver transplants and the decline in deaths from liver disease. *American Journal of Public Health, 87*(5),868–869.

Hahn, R. G. (1995). Pelvic pain from cholelithiasis with kyphoscoliosis. *American Family Physician 51*(3), 750.

Isselbacher, K. J., Epstein, A. (1998). Chapter 288: Diverticular, vascular, and other disorders of the intestine and peritoneum. Harrison (Ed.). *Internal Medicine* (14th Ed.). McGraw-Hill Company.

Kalman, D. R. (1996). Nutrition status predicts survival in cirrhosis. *Nutrition Reviews, 54*(7), 217–219.

Moore, K. I., Dalley, A. F. (1999). Chapter 2: The Abdomen, and Chapter 3: Pelvis and Perineum. *Clinically oriented anatomy.* Lippincott, Williams & Wilkins.

Outcome of pancreatic or liver resection in elderly persons. (1996). *American Family Physician,* 53(3), 1401.

Reid, C. D. (1996). Probing the pancreas. *FDA Consumer, 30*(10), 27–28.

Rinaldo, P. (January 30, 1997). Liver disease in pregnancy. *The New England Journal of Medicine, 336*, 377–379.

Russell, R. M. (1997). The impact of disease states as a modifying factor for nutrition toxicity. *Nutrition Reviews, 55*(2), 50–53.

Sriramachari, S. (March 30, 1996). Excess zinc and progressive cholestastis: A new disease? *Lancet, 347*, 845–846.

Thiel, D. H. V. (1996). Liver transplantation for alcoholics with terminal liver disease. *Alcohol Health and Research World, 20*(4), 261–265.

Tintinalli, J. E. (1999). Chapter 202: Otolaryngologic emergencies, and Chapter 205: General dental emergencies. *Emergency medicine: A comprehensive study guide* (5th Ed.). American College of Emergency Physicians.

Travis, J. (January 20, 1996). New pancreatic cancer gene identified. *Science News, 149*, 39.

CHAPTER 14

Renal and Urologic Diseases and Disorders

CONTENT OUTLINE

- Anatomy and Physiology
- Common Signs and Symptoms
- Diagnostic Tests
- Common Diseases of the Renal and Urologic System
  - Urinary Tract Infection (UTI)
  - Diseases of the Kidney
  - Diseases of the Bladder
- Trauma
  - Straddle Injuries
  - Neurogenic Bladder
- Effects of Aging on the System

KEY TERMS

Albuminuria
Anuria
Blood urea nitrogen (BUN)
Catheterization
Clean catch
Colicky pain
Costovertebral angle tenderness
Creatinine
Creatinine clearance test
Cystogram
Cystoscopy
Dysuria
Frequency
Hematuria
Intravenous pyelogram (IVP)
Kidneys-ureter-bladder (KUB)
Lithotripsy
Nephrectomy
Nocturia
Oliguria
Polyuria
Proteinuria
Pruritis
Pyuria
Radical cystectomy
Transurethral resection (TUR)
Urea
Uremia
Urgency
Urinalysis
Urine culture and sensitivity (C & S)

LEARNING OBJECTIVES

Upon completion of the chapter, the student should be able to:

1. Define the terminology common to renal and urologic disorders.
2. Identify common disorders of the renal and urologic system.
3. Discuss the basic anatomy and physiology of the renal and urologic system.
4. Identify the important signs and symptoms associated with common renal and urologic system disorders.
5. Describe the common diagnostic tests used to determine type and/or cause of the renal and urologic disorders.
6. Describe the typical course and management of the common renal and urologic disorders.
7. Describe the effects of aging upon the renal and urologic system and the common disorders of the system.

OVERVIEW

The renal and urologic system maintains homeostasis in the body by excreting and reabsorbing important electrolytes, compounds, and water. It also excretes wastes from the body in the form of urine. Disturbances in other systems, such as the circulatory or nervous systems, can adversely affect the functioning of the renal and urologic system. Renal and urologic disorders range from mild infections to very serious diseases such as cancer of the bladder or kidneys.

ANATOMY AND PHYSIOLOGY

The renal and urologic system includes the kidneys, ureters, bladder, and urethra (Figure 14–1). The kidneys are located behind the intestines at the mid-back level. Each kidney is about the size of a man's fist and weighs about 150 grams. The kidneys are responsible for removing waste products from the bloodstream. Every minute, about one quarter of the blood circulating in the body passes through the kidneys. Toxic wastes and unused nutrients are filtered and pass out of the body as urine. The kidneys also regulate fluid and electrolyte balance, acid-base balance, assist in the metabolism of calcium, and help regulate blood pressure. The kidneys are composed of nephrons that act as filters, selectively filtering, excreting, or reabsorbing what is needed by the body to maintain homeostasis. They monitor the amount of salts and other chemicals needed for proper body functioning. The kidneys also produce an active form of vitamin D necessary for strong bones.

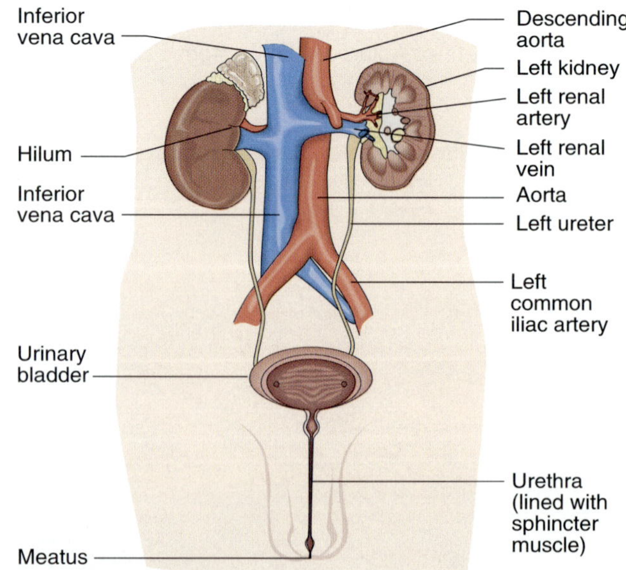

Figure 14–1 The urinary system.

The ureters are tubules that run from the kidney to the bladder (see Figure 14–1). They transport the urine from the renal pelvis to the bladder, where it is stored until emptied, usually a conscious effort by the individual. The bladder, a muscular organ that holds urine, can usually store about 350–500 ml. This amount varies some from individual to individual and is affected by many other factors, especially bladder tone, neurologic disease, and urologic disorders. Micturition is the process of voiding or emptying the bladder. This usually occurs in response to stimuli to the pelvic nerves.

The urethra is a hollow tube running from the bladder to the external opening (the meatus) for excretion (see Figure 14–1). The urethra is significantly longer in males than in females. The urethra serves as the passageway for urine in the female, and for both urine and semen ejaculation in the male.

Urine is normally clear, slightly yellow to gold in color, and free of sediments. Some drugs can change the color of urine. Urine has its own distinct odor but is not foul smelling unless disease is present. There are some foods that will change the odor of urine as their byproducts are excreted, such as asparagus. Urine has a normal specific gravity of 1.005–1.030, and a pH of about 6. Changes in these values may indicate disease.

COMMON SIGNS AND SYMPTOMS

Common signs and symptoms of urinary tract diseases include any abnormality in urine or in the ability to urinate. Some of these include:

- **hematuria** (hem-ah-TOO-ree-ah; hema = blood, uria = urine) or blood in the urine
- **pyuria** (pye-YOU-ree-ah; py = pus, uria = urine) or pus in the urine
- **proteinuria** or protein in the urine. If a specific protein, albumin, is present in the urine, then the term **albuminuria** is used.
- **dysuria** (dis-YOU-ree-ah; dys = difficult or painful, uria = urine) or difficulty or pain with urination
- **nocturia** (nock-TOO-ree-ah; noc = night, uria = urine) or increased voiding at night
- **oliguria** (OL-ih-**GOO**-ree-ah; olig = scanty or few, uria = urine) or a decrease in urine output
- **anuria** (ah-NEW-ree-ah; an = without, uria = urine) or no urine output
- **polyuria** or a great increase in the amount and frequency of urination
- **frequency** or urinating frequently
- **urgency** or the need to urinate immediately

Pain from the renal system causes typically begins with flank or mid-back pain and may radiate down to the groin or to the mid-back around the lower thoracic/upper lumbar vertebrae (see Chapter 10). The pain is typically described as sharp and stabbing or dull and achy like a toothache. The pain is often described as **colicky pain** or pain that comes and goes in waves. This pain is a visceral pain, meaning the origin of the pain is the abdominal organ and the pain is more diffuse. Pain from the kidneys can refer to the lower thorax and to the groin. Pain from the lower urinary tract, the bladder and the urethra, can refer to the pubic symphasis or to the sacral area. One test that the EMS provider may perform that may differentiate kidney pain from other origins is to percuss the patient's back at the costovertebral angle, or the area of the lower ribs almost out at the patient's flank. Tenderness to percussion at this location is called **costovertebral angle** (CVA) **tenderness** and indicates the kidneys are the most likely source of the pain.

Other signs and symptoms associated with renal system disorders include nausea, vomiting, and fever as in the case of an infection. Malaise, fatigue, mental status changes, and intense itching, or **pruritis** can occur in renal failure. Kidney disorders can also affect the cardiovascular system and respiratory system, leading to hypertension, fluid overload, peripheral and pulmonary edema, and shortness of breath.

DIAGNOSTIC TESTS

A **urinalysis** (YOU-rih-**NAL**-ih-sis; urine analysis) is the most common test performed by the emergency department to diagnose urinary system diseases. This test is important because the results can confirm the presence of many different urinary tract disorders. A urinalysis uses a urine sample to test for pH, specific gravity, presence of protein, glucose or sugar, and blood. It also includes a microscopic examination to determine the presence of bacteria, blood, and other materials.

A **urine culture and sensitivity (C&S)** may be performed in the laboratory if the urinalysis shows an abnormal number of white cells or bacteria in the urine. A culture helps determine the type of bacteria present while a sensitivity helps determine the most effective antibiotic to prescribe for treatment. A urine specimen collected for a culture may be obtained by the clean catch method or sterile technique. The **clean catch** method involves cleaning the urethral meatus, voiding a moderate amount of urine to flush out the urethra, then catching a urine specimen in a sterile container. A sterile technique involves placing a sterile urinary catheter into the bladder to obtain a sterile urine specimen.

Blood tests may be performed to determine if waste products are being filtered out adequately by the glomerulus, thus checking kidney function. The two most common nitrogenous waste products that are normally filtered from the blood are **urea** and **creatinine**. A **blood urea nitrogen** (**BUN**) test will determine the levels of urea nitrogen or waste product in the blood. A **creatinine clearance test** is a blood test to determine the ability of the renal glomeruli to filter creatinine out of the blood after creatinine is ingested by the subject. High levels of waste products in the blood is called **uremia** (you-REE-me-ah; ur = urine, emia = blood). Uremia is a toxic condition of the blood.

Radiologic examination of the urinary system include **kidneys-ureter-bladder (KUB)**, **intravenous pyelogram (IVP)**, and **cystogram**. A KUB is a common X-ray of the structures of the urinary tract to determine abnormalities. An IVP is an X-ray taken after injecting dye into the individual's bloodstream. The dye accumulates in the urinary tract improving the ability to visualize and identify obstructions, tumors, and deformities. A cystogram (cysto = bladder, gram = picture) is an X-ray taken of the bladder after a radiopaque dye is instilled into the bladder using a urinary catheter. A cystogram helps determine shape and function of the bladder and is used in trauma patients to assess for a bladder rupture. If a rupture is present, the dye will leak out of the bladder, and will be seen on the X-ray. If a pelvic fracture is suspected, a retrograde urethrogram will be performed by infusing contrast dye into the urethra and taking an X-ray. This test is performed to ensure the urethra is not damaged before a foley catheter is inserted into the patient.

Cystoscopy (sis-TOS-koh-pee; cysto = bladder, scopy = procedure to look) is an invasive procedure to directly visualize the urethra and bladder using a lighted scope. Additional instruments may be used to allow the physician to biopsy tissue or crush bladder stones.

Biopsies of the kidney and bladder are often performed to determine the presence of disease. Bladder biopsies are often obtained by using a cystoscope. Renal biopsies are often obtained by using X-ray technique to guide a fine needle through the flank to remove a core of renal tissue.

Catheterization of the urinary bladder is a sterile procedure of passing a soft catheter through the urethra and into the bladder for the purpose of (1) instilling or pouring fluids or medication into the bladder or (2) removing urine. Sterile technique must be maintained to prevent urinary tract infections. Urinary catheterization to remove urine may be done to (1) relieve urinary retention (2) empty the bladder prior to a procedure (3) obtain a sterile urine specimen for testing or (4) as a treatment for incontinence.

COMMON DISEASES OF THE RENAL AND UROLOGIC SYSTEM

Diseases of the urinary system can affect either gender at any age. Approximately twenty million Americans are affected by disorders of the renal system each year. Approximately 50,000 deaths per year are attributed to renal disorders, with 260,000 Americans in need of dialysis and 35,000 awaiting kidney transplant. Renal and urinary system disorders are also responsible for twenty-seven million physician visits, and six million hospitalizations per year, a major cause of time lost from work. Diabetes and hypertension are the two most common causes of chronic renal failure, responsible for thirty-five percent and thirty percent, respectively, of the new cases of chronic renal failure diagnosed each year. Many of the diseases of the urinary system have similar symptoms in their early stages of development, such as dysuria, oliguria, and frequency of urination.

Urinary Tract Infection (UTI)

Urinary tract infection is a broad diagnosis covering any infection of the urinary tract including the urethra, bladder, and kidneys (Figure 14–2). UTIs may be caused by virus and fungus, but by far the most common infection is due to bacteria.

Bacteria may reach the urinary tract through the blood (hematogenous infection) or by entering the tract through the urethra (ascending infection). Hematogenous infection is less common and is usually the result of septicemia. In this case the urinary tract is a site of secondary infection. Primary infection may begin in the respiratory or gastrointestinal tract and be carried to the urinary tract through the blood.

Ascending infection is by far the most common route of infection. With ascending infection, bacteria enter the urethra and climb or ascend upward toward the kidneys infecting the various organs as they progress. Approximately eighty percent of the time the bacteria causing ascending infection is *Escherichia coli (E. coli)*. This bacterium is a normal flora of the intestine and is commonly found in large numbers around the anal and perineal area. Sexual intercourse, bladder catheterization, and surgical procedures increase the risk of ascending infection.

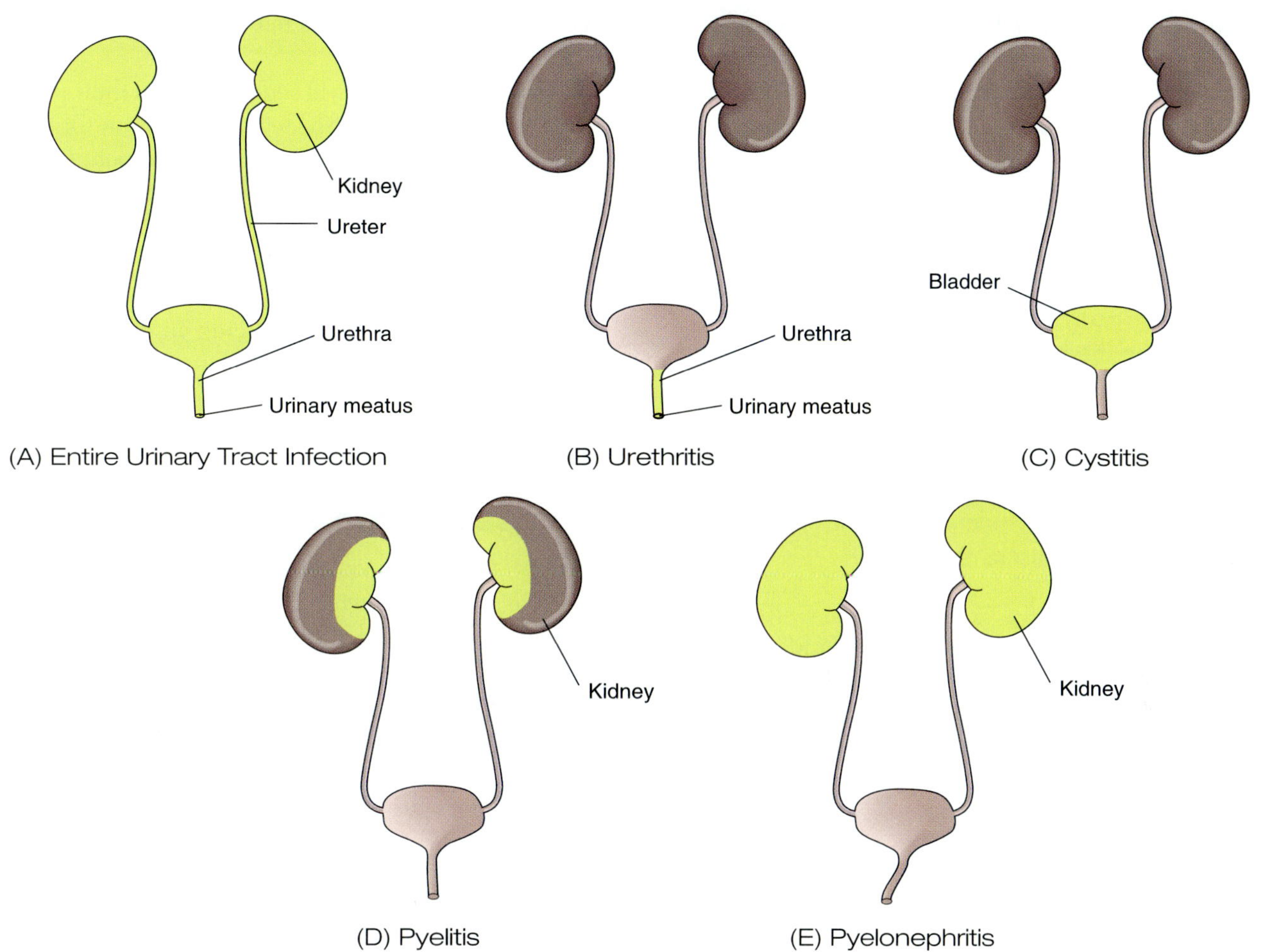

Figure 14–2 Sites of urinary tract infections.

UTIs in males are quite rare and are usually related to obstruction of the tract by an enlarged prostate or a sexually transmitted disease. Ascending UTIs are far more common in females than in males for the following reasons:

- Anatomically the female urethra is shorter than the male urethra, allowing bacteria to ascend more easily.
- Anatomically the female urethral opening is closer to the rectal area than the male, allowing migration of bacteria from the rectal area to the urethra.
- Improper female toileting habits or wiping improperly from the back (rectal area) toward the front (vulva area) pulls rectal bacteria toward and into the urethral opening. This is especially true for female toddlers who are potty training.
- Vaginal secretions may harbor bacteria and contaminate the urethral area.
- Sexual intercourse may cause trauma to the urethra and bladder, leading to inflammation and potential infection.
- Pregnant females are more susceptible to infection because of the pressure of the heavy uterus on the urinary tract and the fact that pregnancy hormones tend to relax the organs of the urinary tract allowing easier entry by bacteria.
- Male prostatic secretions have an antibacterial effect reducing the risk of UTI.

UTIs are commonly diagnosed utilizing a urinalysis and culture of a urine specimen. Bacterial counts of 100,000 bacteria or greater per milliliter of urine confirm UTI. Antibiotic treatment is usually effective. A bacterial sensitivity test helps in the selection of the most effective antibiotic for treatment. Signs and symptoms may include dysuria, flank pain, urinary frequency and urgency, hematuria, and low back pain.

As previously discussed, UTI includes infection of any of the organs of the urinary tract. Types of urinary tract infection include urethritis, cystitis, ureteritis, pyelitis, and pyelonephritis. A brief discussion of each follows.

Urethritis. Urethritis (YOU-reh-**THRIGH**-tis; urethri = urethra, itis = inflammation) is more common in males than females and is often a symptom of gonorrhea (Figure 14–2B), a sexually transmitted disease. In females, urethritis may be the result of irritation caused by tight clothing, application of soaps or powders to the genital area, and sexual intercourse. Urethritis commonly occurs in conjunction with cystitis. In males and females it may be a symptom of herpes genitalis or chlamydia. Symptoms of urethritis may include swelling of the urethra, dysuria, and a urethral discharge.

Cystitis. Cystitis (sis-TYE-tis; cyst = bladder, itis = inflammation) is commonly called "bladder infection" (Figure 14–2C). Antibiotic treatment is usually effective. Antispasmodic medications, such as Pyridium, may be prescribed in addition to antibiotics to decrease the discomfort of bladder spasms. The pain associated with bladder spasms is typically on the midline just above the pubic bone and can worsen with urination.

Pyelitis. Pyelitis (PYE-eh-**LYE**-tis; pyelo = pelvis of kidney, itis = inflammation) is a fairly common disease among young female children (Figure 14–2D). Pyelitis is usually the result of an ascending infection from the bladder (cystitis) but it may also be spread by blood (hematogenous infection). Rapid diagnosis and treatment must be initiated to prevent the spread of infection to adjacent tissue, which can cause pyelonephritis.

Pyelonephritis. Pyelonephritis (PYE-eh-loh-neh-**FRY**-tis; pyelo = pelvis of kidney, nephr = kidney, itis = inflammation) may be caused by an ascending or a hematogenous infection and may affect one or both kidneys (Figure 14–2E). Obstruction or blocking of urine flow in the urinary tract caused by pregnancy, prostate enlargement, stones, or tumors increases the risk of pyelonephritis. Commonly, abscesses form in the kidney and rupture, filling the kidney pelvis with pus and leading to pyuria (pyo = pus, uria = urine). Other symptoms include a sudden onset of fever and chills with flank pain and hematuria. Pyelonephritis is usually treated effectively with antibiotics, but repeated bouts of acute pyelonephritis or chronic pyelonephritis lead to scarring of the kidney. Chronic pyelonephritis may eventually lead to uremia and kidney failure.

In general, patients will seek care from their primary care provider or obtain private transportation for simple urinary tract infection symptoms unless the patient is otherwise disabled. Urinary tract infections are common in patients who are repeatedly catheterized and is often found as the source of infection in this population of patients. In contrast, patients with pyelonephritis can become septic from the advancing infection. These patients may require airway protection if they become obtunded and may require fluid resuscitation if severely dehydrated or in shock.

Diseases of the Kidney

Diseases of the kidney affect the filtering system of the body. This, in turn, affects the homeostatic balance of fluids and electrolytes. If left untreated, kidney diseases can affect all other body systems, interrupting their functioning. Symptoms of kidney disease may first appear in an affected system rather than in the urinary system. An example of this is an elevated blood pressure caused by inappropriate reabsorption of sodium and water.

Glomerulonephritis (Acute). Acute glomerulonephritis is an inflammation of the glomerulus or filtering unit of the kidney. It is the most common disease of the kidney. This disease usually affects children and young adults within one to four weeks following a strep throat infection. Other streptococcus infections such as scarlet fever and rheumatic fever may also be the cause of this problem. Glomerulonephritis with this etiology may also be called acute post streptococcal glomerulonephritis. In addition to streptococcus bacterial infections, virus, other bacteria, and parasites may also lead to this disease.

Glomerulonephritis is nonsuppurative, or not associated with bacterial infection and pus formation. Inflammation in this case is the result of tissue destruction caused by the individual's immune system. Glomerulonephritis is a type of allergic or immune disease caused by an antigen-antibody reaction. The causative agent (bacteria, virus, parasites) produce antigens that stimulate the individual's immune system to produce antibodies. These antibodies stick to the antigen thus producing large antigen-antibody complexes. These large complexes circulate in the bloodstream until they become trapped in the tiny capillaries of the glomerulus. The trapping of these complexes blocks the glomerulus, leading to increased pressure, irritation, and the inflammatory response.

The outpouring of neutrophils and serum as a part of the inflammatory response increases pressure and decreases blood flow to the glomerulus. Ultimately the glomerulus weakens and becomes permeable, allowing red blood cells and blood plasma proteins to leak into Bowman's capsule and appear in the urine.

Signs and symptoms of glomerulonephritis are flank pain, fever, loss of appetite, and malaise (general ill feeling). The eyes and ankles may appear edematous (swollen). Oliguria and hematuria are frequent signs of glomerulonephritis. A urinalysis may show albuminuria (albumin = a blood protein, uria = urine) and casts (proteins that mold to the shape of the kidney tubules).

Treatment is usually supportive. Antipyretic (anti = against, pyretic = fever) and diuretic (increase urine output) medications may be prescribed. Dietary management may include restrictions on salt and protein foods, and increased fluids. If a secondary bacterial infection occurs, antibiotics may be prescribed. Prevention is aimed at proper antibiotic treatment for streptococcal infections. Proper treatment of strep throat in children and young adults decreases the number of antigen-antibody complexes, thus reducing the risk of developing glomerulonephritis.

Prognosis for glomerulonephritis is generally good. Children usually recover at a slightly better rate than adults. Those who do not recover may progress into chronic glomerulonephritis.

Glomerulonephritis (Chronic). Repeated bouts of acute glomerulonephritis may lead to a chronic condition. This chronic condition may extend over several years with periods of remission and exacerbation. During this time a number of the glomeruli are destroyed, leading to an inability of the kidney to produce urine. This decrease in urine output leads to an increase in fluid volume in the blood, retention of salt, edema, and ultimately hypertension.

Symptoms of chronic glomerulonephritis include those mentioned in the acute disease plus hypertension. Uremia (you-REE-me-ah; ur = urine, emia = blood or urine waste in the blood) and kidney failure may occur during late stages of the disease. Prevention of chronic glomerulonephritis is prompt treatment of the acute form. Treatment for symptoms of uremia and renal failure may include peritoneal or hemodialysis.

Hydronephrosis. Hydronephrosis (HIGH-droh-neh-**FROH**-sis; hydro = water, nephro = kidney, osis = condition of) is a collection of urine in the renal pelvis caused by some type of obstruction. This accumulation of urine leads to dilation and distention of the kidney pelvis. Causes of obstruction include congenital defects in urinary tract structure, kidney stones, tumors, enlarged prostate, and urinary tract infections. If the obstruction is unrelieved, permanent damage may occur and the kidney pelvis becomes non-functioning. One or both kidneys may be affected depending on the position of the obstruction (Figure 14–3). If one kidney is affected the disease may go undetected as the other kidney continues to function adequately. If both kidneys are involved, anuria and uremia may develop. Diagnosis is confirmed by pyelogram. Treatment involves immediate draining of the kidney pelvis by surgical intervention, or immediate relief of the obstruction.

Renal Calculi. Renal calculi are commonly called "kidney stones." Approximately 500,000 Americans suffer from kidney stones each year. These stones are often composed of calcium salts and other substances. Size, location, and number of stones may vary (Figure 14–4). Staghorn calculi are one of the more common types of stones. These calculi form in the pelvis of the kidney and may become so large that they fill the entire kidney pelvis. Calculi commonly form in the kidney, but they may also form in the urinary bladder. Bladder stones cause difficulty with emptying the bladder, often leading to frequent or chronic bladder infections. Individuals may frequently form small kidney stones that easily pass through the

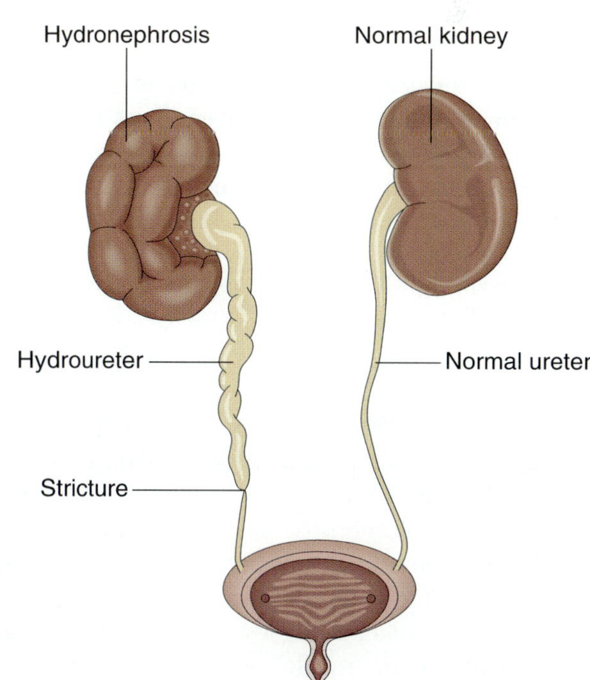

Figure 14–3 Hydronephrosis.

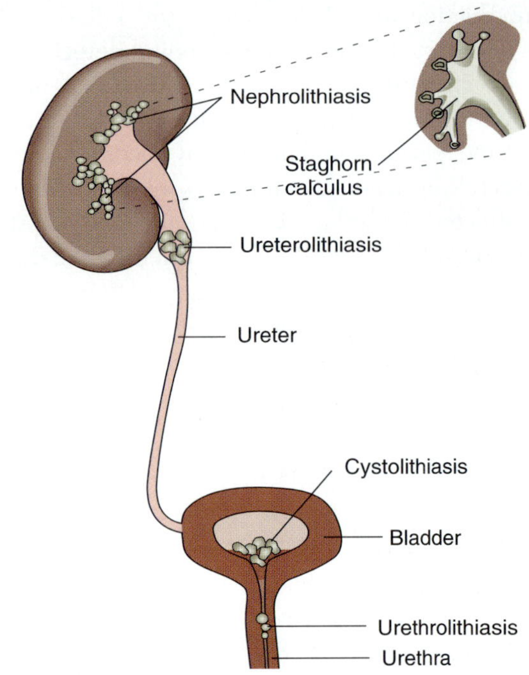

Figure 14–4 Types and locations of renal calculi.

urinary tract unnoticed. Stones may be present in the kidney yet cause no problems. It is only when stones become caught in the ureters or obstruct the urinary tract that problems and symptoms arise. Typical symptoms of kidney stones are hematuria and renal or urinary colic. Urinary colic is an extreme, spasmodic flank pain often described as "the worst pain I've had in my entire life." This pain is caused by the spasmodic contraction of an obstructed ureter.

Urinary stones are more common in males than females and commonly occur between ages thirty and fifty. Cause of stone formation is unknown in most cases but some precipitating factors include dehydration, chronic urinary tract infection, and immobility or prolonged bed rest leading to release of calcium from the bones. Less commonly stones are the result of metabolic disorders such as hyperparathyroidism, severe bone disease, cancer, and gout. Diagnosis is commonly confirmed by utilizing an IVP. A KUB and renal ultrasound may also be beneficial for diagnosis. Treatment during an acute attack of kidney stones includes pain medication and increasing fluid intake with the hope that the stone will pass in the urine. Urine is often strained through a filtering device in an effort to catch the stone for identification. Even though stones feel like they should be quite large to the individual passing a stone, the ones that are voided and filtered are usually quite small ranging in size from a grain of salt to a small piece of rice.

If the urinary tract is totally obstructed, emergency surgery must be performed to prevent hydronephrosis and kidney damage. The stone may be removed either by inserting an instrument into the urinary tract or by using a specialized ultrasound probe to break the stone into smaller pieces. This breaking of the stone is called a **lithotripsy** (litho = stone, tripsy = breaking).

Field treatment of suspected renal calculi includes assessing and treating shock and providing adequate pain management. Shock can result from internal bleeding that occasionally accompanies calculi. More often the presence of shock indicates another etiology is present. Intravenous or intramuscular NSAIDs, for example ketorolac, are commonly used in the emergency department and work well for renal colic. Narcotic analgesics can also be used to provide adequate pain relief while still allowing proper examination of the abdomen.

Prevention of further stone development may include medications, correcting any causative metabolic conditions, and increasing water intake.

Renal Failure. Renal failure is the failure of the kidneys to perform the function of cleansing the blood of waste products. The primary method of cleansing the body of waste involves the liver forming urea and the kidneys filtering this product out of the blood to be excreted in urine. Blood urea nitrogen and creatinine are nitrogenous wastes, an end product of protein metabolism. The amount of urea in the blood can be measured with a blood test called a BUN, blood urea nitrogen. Creatinine levels can also be measured in the blood. BUN and creatinine levels are utilized to measure kidney function. A high urea level in the blood is called uremia. Urea that is not excreted by the kidneys is eventually converted to ammonia, leading to toxicity and related symptoms in all systems of the body (Figure 14–5).

Renal failure may occur suddenly (acute renal failure) or progress over a longer period of time (chronic renal failure). Acute renal failure is usually related to decreased blood flow to the kidneys caused by conditions such as hemorrhagic or surgical shock, embolism, congestive heart failure, and dehydration. Blockage of urine flow, caused by tumors, stones, or enlarged prostate, may also lead to acute failure. Reversal of acute renal failure, which involves treating the cause of the failure, is usually quite successful. Dialysis may be needed temporarily to remove toxic wastes from the individual's blood until kidney function is restored. Individuals in acute renal failure are placed on a limited diet to allow the kidneys to rest and regenerate function.

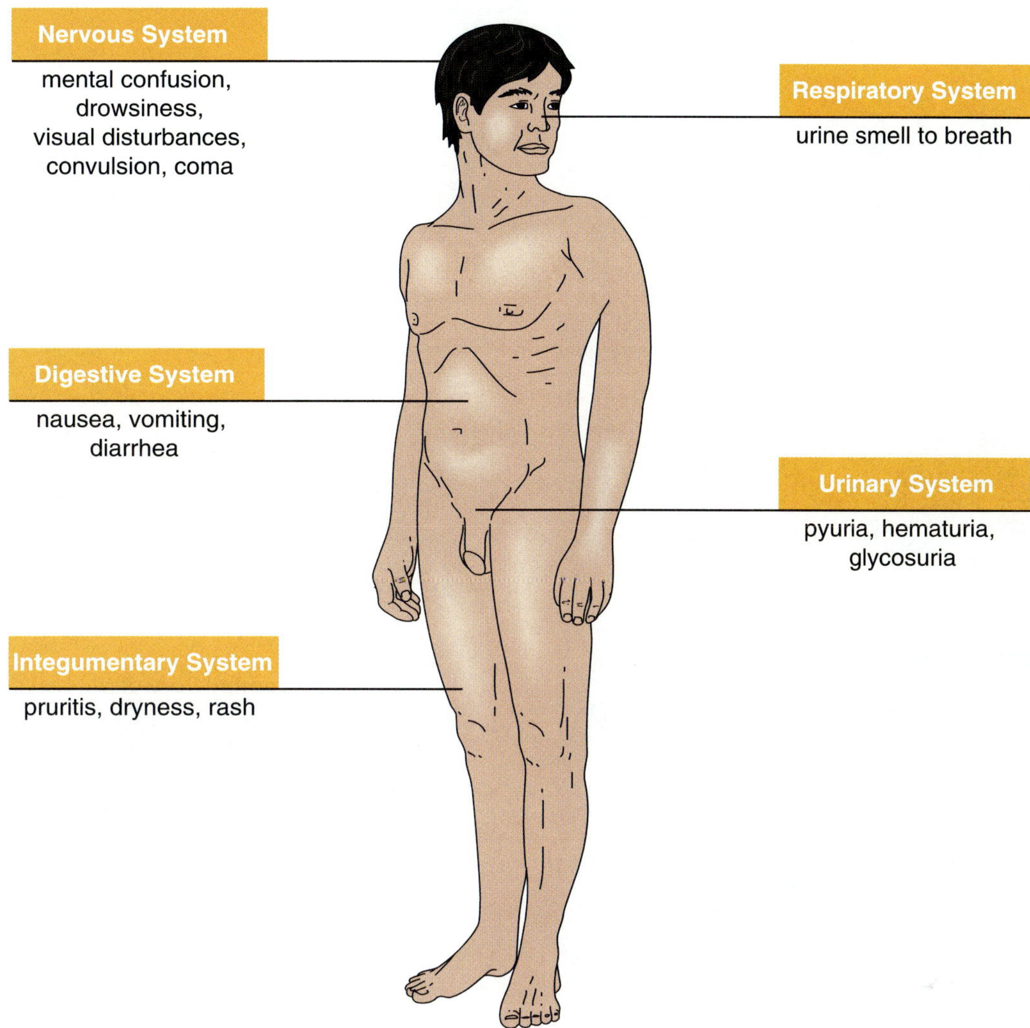

Figure 14–5 Areas of the body affected by toxic levels of circulating ammonia.

Chronic renal failure occurs slowly and isusually the result of chronic kidney disease such as glomerulonephritis, pyelonephritis, renal hypertension, and other genetic diseases. Long-term substance abuse, alcoholism, and diabetes may also cause chronic renal failure. Symptoms of renal failure are not significant until approximately seventy-five percent of kidney function has been destroyed. Symptoms may include those of acute failure, plus problems of infertility, impotence, and bone weakness leading to pain and fractures. Treatment includes management of the related cause of the failure, limiting protein and sodium in the diet, and monitoring intake and output. Medications may include antihypertensives, diuretics, and antibiotics as needed. Dialysis and kidney transplantation may be options for long-term treatment.

Dialysis is a procedure that cleanses the blood of waste products when the kidneys have failed or are failing to perform this function. There are two types of dialysis. Both of the types of dialysis require the same components—the patient's blood, a semi-permeable membrane, and a washing or dialyzing solution. In both types of dialysis, the waste products in the individual's blood pass through the semi-permeable membrane by diffusion to enter the dialyzing solution thus cleansing the blood.

The most common type of dialysis is hemodialysis (Figure 14–6). During hemodialysis, the individual's blood is routed out of an artery (usually the brachial or radial artery) and through a hemodialyzer, which mechanically cleans the blood. This machine is filled with semi-permeable cellophane-like material and dialyzing solution.

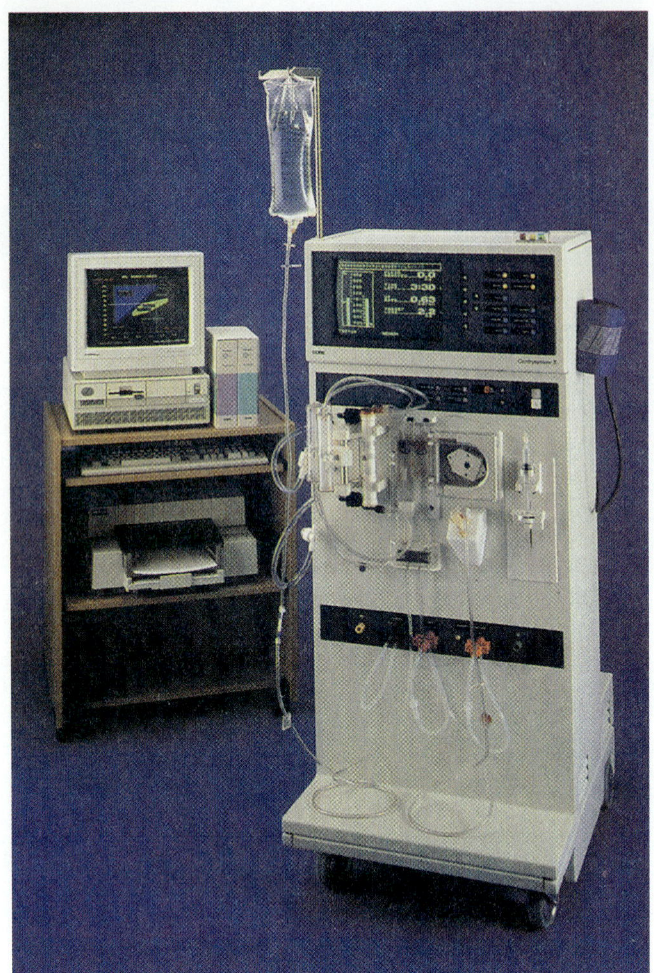

Figure 14–6 Hemodialysis unit.

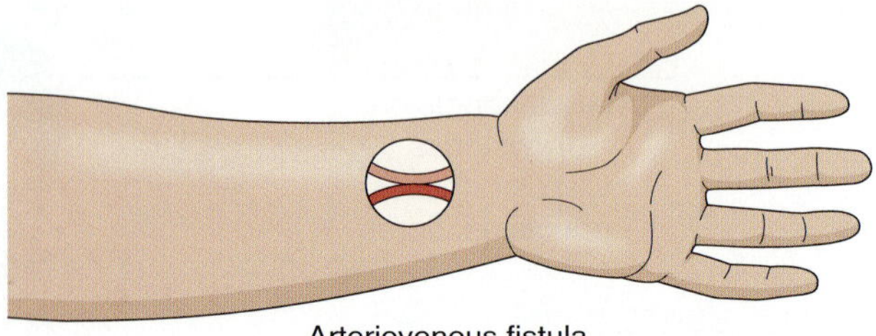

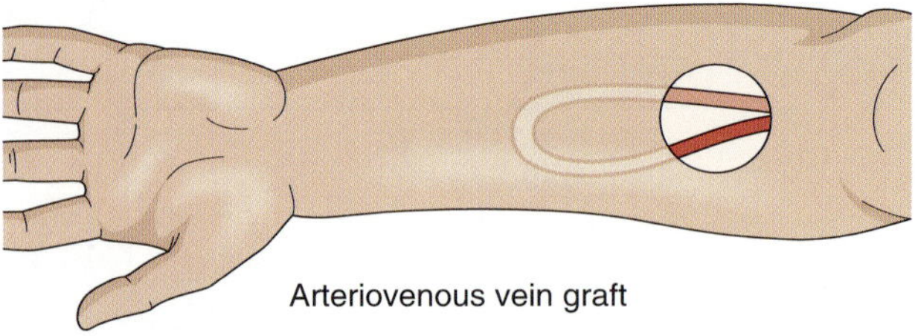

Figure 14–7 Hemodialysis sites: AV shunts.

As blood passes through the machine, the waste products diffuse through the membrane into the dialyzing solution to cleanse the blood. The clean blood re-enters the patient through a venous access. One common problem with hemodialysis is maintaining vascular access. Commonly an arteriovenous (AV) shunt is created by placing catheters in the needed artery and vein (Figure 14–7). These vessels are connected (shunted) with silicone rubber tubing. Common complications of AV shunts include infection and clotting.

The other type of dialysis is peritoneal dialysis. This procedure involves performing a paracentesis to instill dialyzing solution into the peritoneal cavity. This type of dialysis utilizes the membrane that lines the peritoneal cavity to act as the semi-permeable membrane. The dialyzing solution is allowed to stay in the abdomen for varying amounts of time (dwell time). During this time, waste products diffuse out of the peritoneal capillaries and into the dialyzing solution. Solution is then drained and disposed. Peritoneal dialysis may be performed by several methods.

- Continuous ambulatory peritoneal dialysis (CAPD) is a self-dialysis that does not utilize a machine. Solution drains by gravity into and out of the peritoneal cavity by way of a permanently connected catheter. The waste solution drains into a bag worn around the individual's waist. CAPD is performed several times a day and usually once at night (Figure 14–8).
- Continuous cycling peritoneal dialysis (CCPD) uses a cycling machine and takes place while the individual sleeps.
- Intermittent peritoneal dialysis (IPD) is performed several times a week usually in a medical clinic.

Hemodialysis is a much faster and more efficient process than peritoneal, but it is also much more expensive and more time consuming. Also, access to a hemodializer may be limited in rural areas.

Renal transplantation is a procedure to transplant a kidney of a donor into an individual recipient. This surgical procedure is performed on individuals with chronic renal failure commonly caused by diabetes, hypertension, and glomerulonephritis. Best results from kidney transplants are obtained when the donor and recipient are close human leukocyte antigen (HLA) matches or are histocompatible. An identical twin provides the greatest probability of match, with a fraternal twin, sibling, parent, and child the next best matches in that descending order. The greatest problems with renal transplant are obtaining a kidney that is compatible with the recipient, postoperative organ rejection, and complications with life-long administration of immunosuppressant medications.

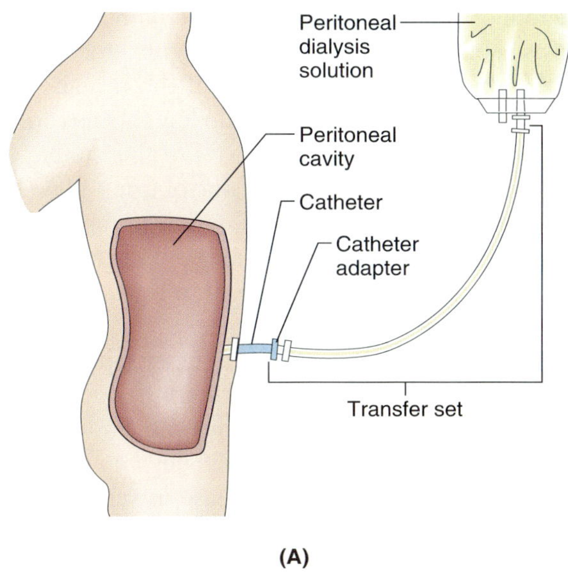

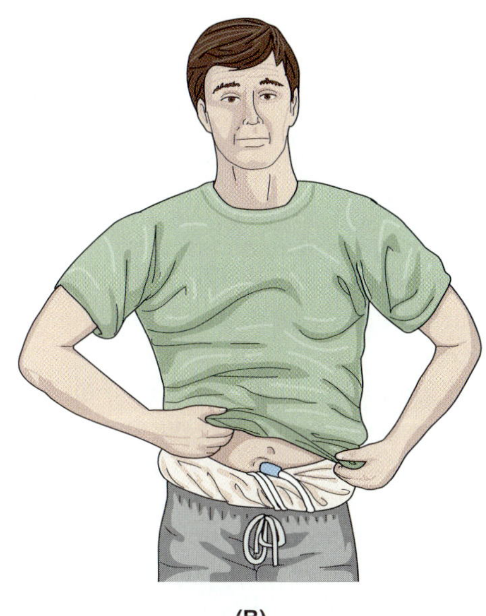

Figure 14–8 Continuous ambulatory peritoneal dialysis.

The different causes of renal failure may be difficult to assess and treat in the field. Much of the diagnosis is dependent upon blood and urine analysis that is not available in the field. Managing the airway, maintaining adequate ventilations, and treating shock are important. Aggressive infusion of fluid is generally avoided in patients who cannot produce urine, as the patient will be unable to remove excess fluid and pulmonary edema will result. Diuretics may be helpful in patients who are still able to produce urine or who are in acute renal failure to help encourage urine production. Consultation with medical control where appropriate can assist the EMS provider in determining proper treatment for the specific situation.

Adenocarcinoma of the Kidney. Cancer of the kidney is relatively uncommon. The cause of this tumor is unknown although cigarette smoking is considered to be a risk factor. Adenocarcinoma of the kidney frequently metastasizes to the liver, brain, and bone before symptoms appear. The most common initial symptom is painless hematuria. Later, as the tumor increases in size, the individual experiences flank pain and fever. A KUB, IVP, computerized tomography (CT), and biopsy of the kidney may be utilized to confirm the diagnosis. Treatment, whether metastasis has occurred or not, is **nephrectomy** (neh-FRECK-toh-me; nephr = kidney, ectomy = excision or removal). If metastasis has occurred, chemotherapy and radiation may also be utilized. Prognosis varies with the extent of spread. Cure may be possible if no metastasis has occurred, but with metastasis prognosis is poor.

Diseases of the Bladder

Cystitis. This condition was discussed earlier under urinary tract infection.

Transitional Cell Carcinoma of the Bladder. Bladder cancer is the most common neoplasm of the urinary tract. It usually occurs in males after age sixty and is three times more common in males than females. Transitional carcinoma arises from the lining of the bladder. Bladder cancer commonly metastasizes before symptoms appear, making it highly malignant. The cause of these tumors is unknown, but the most important risk factor is cigarette smoking, which increases the chance of cancer proportionate to the number of cigarettes smoked during the life of the affected individual. Other predisposing factors include exposure to industrial chemicals and chronic cystitis. Symptoms include hematuria, dysuria, and nocturia, but as previously mentioned these symptoms do not usually appear until late in the course of the disease. Diagnosis may be confirmed by cystoscopy and biopsy. Treatment depends on the stage of the tumor. **Transurethral resection (TUR)** (trans = through, urethral = urethra; resection = partial excision) may be performed to remove the tumor, or more frequently, a **radical** (radical = a treatment that seeks to cure, aggressive, not pallative or conservative) **cystectomy** (sis-TECT-toh-me, cyst = bladder, ectomy = excision or removal) is performed. If metastasis has occurred, radiation and chemotherapy may also be utilized. Prognosis depends on the stage of the tumor when discovered. Usually discovery is late in the course of the disease and thus prognosis is poor.

TRAUMA

Trauma to the genitourinary system is relatively uncommon, estimated at approximately two percent of injury, and typically occurs with blunt mechanisms of injury. Much of the system is well protected, either by the ribs, pelvis, or surrounding musculature. However, when injury is present to the genitourinary system, the EMS provider should carefully assess for significant trauma to the pelvis, lower thorax, and abdomen.

Straddle Injuries

Straddle injuries commonly cause injury to the urethra. This type of injury occurs when an individual accidentally falls in a straddling position. Straddle injuries are more common in males. Instances when straddle injuries may occur include walking a fence or roof beam, or in some cases, riding a horse or motorcycle. Treatment varies depending on the severity of the injury.

Neurogenic Bladder

Neurogenic bladder is dysfunction of the bladder caused by some type of injury to the nervous system supplying the urinary tract or bladder. A common trauma that causes neurogenic bladder is a spinal cord injury such as those sustained in motor vehicle accidents or diving accidents. Other traumatic causes include cerebrovascular accidents, strokes, tumors, and herniated lumbar disks. Diabetes, dementia, and Parkinson's disease are metabolic disorders that often lead to neurogenic bladder.

Symptoms of neurogenic bladder vary depending on the nerves involved. Individuals may have no feeling of the need to void, or they may feel like they need to void all the time. Other symptoms are mild to severe urinary incontinence, difficulty or inability to empty the bladder, and bladder spasms. Treatment goals are aimed at prevention of urinary tract infections and controlling incontinence. Indwelling urinary catheters may be utilized to control incontinence. Intermittent self-catheterization may be taught to individuals unable to empty the bladder to prevent hydronephrosis and possible renal failure.

EFFECTS OF AGING ON THE SYSTEM

The most common problem of the urinary system in the older adult is urinary incontinence, affecting an estimated three million older Americans. It is frequently caused by changes in other body systems in the aging process rather than the urinary system. Because of the urinary elimination process is primarily controlled by the nervous system, changes with aging or diseases of this system may affect the individual's ability to control urine flow. Individuals with Alzheimer's disease, brain tumor, or other disorders of the nervous system may not be aware of the urge to urinate or be able to communicate the need to urinate.

In older males, benign prostatic hypertrophy is a common disorder that often causes urinary frequency, dribbling, pain or burning with urination, and difficulty starting the urine flow. In older females, the changes in estrogen levels may cause a decrease in vaginal muscle tone, and along with the changes in structure, may cause increased frequency and some urine incontinence. Changes in lower abdomen muscle tone, usually the result of multiple pregnancies or obesity, also contribute to some urinary incontinence in the older adult female. (See Chapter 21 for more information on changes in the female and male reproductive systems.)

Older individuals with other common system disorders such as stroke or severe circulatory impairment may not feel the urge to urinate and thus have urinary incontinence. Chronic urinary tract infections may also affect bladder function so that the result over time is urinary incontinence.

Urinary problems in the older adult may not be caused by the aging process at all, but to many other events occurring in the individual's life. Fecal impactions that are common in the institutionalized elderly individual can also cause urinary incontinence.

Some medications can cause changes in the ability of the bladder to empty thoroughly, causing overflow incontinence. Many older adults take medications such as antidepressants, narcotic pain relievers, or cardiac drugs that may cause some urinary retention, eventually resulting in incontinence.

Older adults who have mobility problems frequently have urinary incontinence. Individuals who have some difficulty rising from a chair or bed and walk slowly often have periods of incontinence just because they cannot get to the restroom in time. Lack of mobility causes the individual to be dependent upon others for toileting and this frequently leads to urinary incontinence problems. This is extremely common in the institutionalized older adult.

SUMMARY

The urinary system includes the kidneys, ureters, bladder, and urethra. It maintains homeostasis in the body by excreting and reabsorbing important electrolytes, compounds, and water. Urinary disorders range from infections to cancer. The most common signs and symptoms of urinary dysfunction include an abnormality in the urine or in the individual's ability to urinate. The most common disorder of the urinary system by EMS providers is renal calculi. In the older adult, urinary incontinence is the most frequent problem of the system. Urinary disorders may be the result of urinary system pathology or the result of disease or malfunction of other body systems.

REVIEW QUESTIONS

Short Answer

1. What are the functions of the urinary system?

2. Which signs and symptoms are associated with common urinary system disorders?

3. Which diagnostic tests are most commonly used to determine type and/or cause of the urinary system disorder?

4. What is the most common urinary problem in the older adult population?

Matching

5. Match the disorders listed in the left column with the correct definition in the right column:

_____ Urethritis
_____ Pyuria
_____ Oliguria
_____ Anuria
_____ Nocturia
_____ Cystectomy
_____ Dysuria
_____ Nephrectomy
_____ Urinalysis
_____ Pyelonephritis
_____ Glomerulonephritis

a. most commonly used diagnostic test for urinary system disorders
b. pus in the urine
c. an inflammation of the filtering components of the kidney
d. difficulty urinating
e. excision of the kidney
f. inflammation of the urethra
g. frequent urination at night
h. surgical removal of the bladder
i. scanty urine output
j. absence of urine output
k. inflammation of the kidney pelvis

CASE STUDY

You respond to an office building in the business district for a female patient in her early fifties who is complaining of abdominal pain. When you arrive, you find Julie Hayden, a secretary, sitting at her chair writhing in pain. She states the left side of her mid-back began hurting suddenly and the pain came and went. The pain quickly moved toward her groin and is the worst pain she ever felt in her life. She states, "This is worse than childbirth!" She jumps when you percuss her left flank. What is that sign called? What do you think is the source of her pain? How will you and the emergency department treat this patient?

BIBLIOGRAPHY

A new approach to female urethral syndrome. (1996). *American Family Physician, 54*(10), 1704.

Atkins, M. B. (March 13, 1997). Renal-cell carcinoma. *The New England Journal of Medicine, 336*, 809–811.

Feinfeld, D. A. (1995). Sequential changes in renal function tests in the old: Results from the Bronx Longitudinal Aging Study. *Journal of the American Geriatrics Society, 43*(4), 412–414.

Gray, R. (1995). Lower urinary tract dysfunction in Parkinson's disease: Changes related to age not disease. *Age and Ageing, 24*(11), 499–504.

Grieder, K. (1997). You and your bladder. *Harper's Bazaar, 4*, 116+.

Kidney stones? (1997). *Flying, 124*(1), 50.

Levallois, P. (1995). Assessing exposure to carcinogens in drinking water. *American Journal of Public Health, 85*(9), 1298–1300.

Li, D. (1996). Maternal smoking during pregnancy and the risk of congenital urinary tract anomalies. *American Journal of Public Health, 86*(2), 249–253.

Linnenbach, A. J. (February 3, 1994). Urothelial carcinogens. *Nature, 367*, 419–420.

Lloyd, S.E. (February 1, 1996). A common molecular basis for three inherited kidney stone diseases. *Nature, 379*, 445–449.

McConnell, E. A. (1995). Assessing flank pain. *Nursing 95, 25*(11), 74–75.

Mylonakis, E. (1997). Periurethral abscess: Complication of UTI. *Geriatrics, 52*(8), 86–88.

National Kidney Foundation website: http://www.kidney.org

Rodman, J. S. (1997). Stop kidney stones cold. *Prevention, 49*(5), 106–109.

Sadovsky, R. (1997). Urinary tract infections in young febrile children. *American Family Physician, 55*(4), 1933–1934.

Save your bones, lose those stones. (1996). *Prevention, 48*(7), 57.

Seeds of hope. (1996). *Prevention, 48*(2), 48+.

Service, R. F. (April 25, 1997). New vaccines may ward off urinary tract infections. *Science, 276*, 533.

Stamler, J. (February 15, 1997). Dietary salt and renal stone disease. *Lancet, 349*, 506–507.

Stranded in midstream. (1997). *Esquire, 128*(9), 134–135.

Winterling, C. A. (January 30, 1997). Urinary tract infections in young women. *The New England Journal of Medicine, 336*, 381–382.

CHAPTER 15

Toxicologic Emergencies

CONTENT OUTLINE

- Routes of Entry
  - Ingestion
  - Inhalation
  - Injection
- Absorption
- General Management of Toxicologic Emergencies
- Toxidromes
  - Cholinergic Toxidrome
  - Anticholinergic Toxidrome
  - Opioid Toxidrome
  - Hallucinogenic Toxidrome
  - Sympathomimetic Toxidrome
- Substances of Abuse
  - Alcohol
  - Cocaine
  - Narcotics
  - Marijuana
  - Mushrooms
- Chemical Agents
  - Caustic Agents
  - Common Household Chemicals
  - Carbon Monoxide
  - Hydrocarbons
  - Alcohols
  - Organophosphates
  - Metals
- Medications
  - Cardiovascular Medications
  - Psychiatric Medications
  - Sedatives and Hypnotics
  - Analgesics
  - Xanthines
- Food Poisoning
- Insect and Snakebites

KEY TERMS

Absorption

Alkalemia

Analgesia

Anticholinergic toxidrome

Cholinergic toxidrome

Delirium tremens

Hallucinogen

Hallucinosis

Hydrocarbons

Ingestion

Inhalation

Injection

Neuromuscular junction

Organophosphates

Serotonin syndrome

Sympathomimetic toxidrome

Therapeutic range

Tinnitus

Toxidrome

LEARNING OBJECTIVES

Upon completion of this chapter, the student should be able to:

1. Describe the four routes of entry for toxins and list at least two examples of toxins that use each route of entry.
2. Describe the four steps in the general management of toxicologic emergencies
3. Describe the pathophysiology, signs, and management of the five toxidromes presented in this chapter.
4. Describe the pathophysiology, signs, and management of poisoning with substances of abuse.
5. Describe the pathophysiology, signs, and management of poisoning with chemical substances.
6. Describe the pathophysiology, signs, and management of poisoning with cardiac medications.
7. Describe the pathophysiology, signs, and management of poisoning with psychiatric medications.
8. Describe the pathophysiology, signs, and management of poisoning with analgesics.
9. Describe the pathophysiology, signs, and management of poisoning with xanthines.
10. Describe the pathophysiology, signs, and management of food poisoning.
11. Describe the pathophysiology, signs, and management associated with insect and snakebites.

OVERVIEW

The American Association of Poison Control Centers (AAPCC) estimates that approximately 4 million poisonings occur each year in the United States with poison control centers assisting in roughly half of these poisonings. Toxicologic emergencies vary across the spectrum from an ingestion of a household chemical by a young child to a drug overdose in a young adult, and an accidental overdose of prescribed medication by an elderly individual. The EMS provider who responds to the scene of a patient who is unconscious or has an alteration of their mental status needs to keep an open mind and look for evidence of poisoning. While field treatment for the majority of these emergencies is focused on managing the ABCs, clues extracted from the scene assist in definitive care of the poisoned patient. In this chapter, we discuss the routes by which toxic substances enter the body, general management of toxicologic emergencies, common toxidromes, and the pathophysiology and treatment of specific substances.

ROUTES OF ENTRY

In order for a toxic substance to act on the body, it must gain entry through the protective barrier that separates the cells from the outside environment. Once access to the body has been achieved, the toxins act in a way to alter the cellular processes that occur in the body and allow us to function properly. There are four ways poisons bypass this protective barrier: ingestion, inhalation, injection, and absorption. Most toxins can actually enter the body through more than one route of entry; however, the major route of entry is typically what is used in discussing the poison.

Ingestion

Ingestion is a route of entry by which the poison is taken in by mouth and enters the blood stream by crossing the mucous membranes in the upper GI tract or by transport across the intestinal walls in the small intestine (Figure 15–1). Examples of poisons that enter the body by ingestion include medications, caustic substances, and bacteria or endotoxins that cause food poisoning. Toxins that enter through the route of ingestion can act quickly, as in the case of a caustic substance that produces physical damage to the GI tract, or act more slowly, as in the case of a medication overdose that must be broken down by the digestive system and absorbed into the blood stream. With ingested poisons, there may be time to block the GI absorption of the toxin.

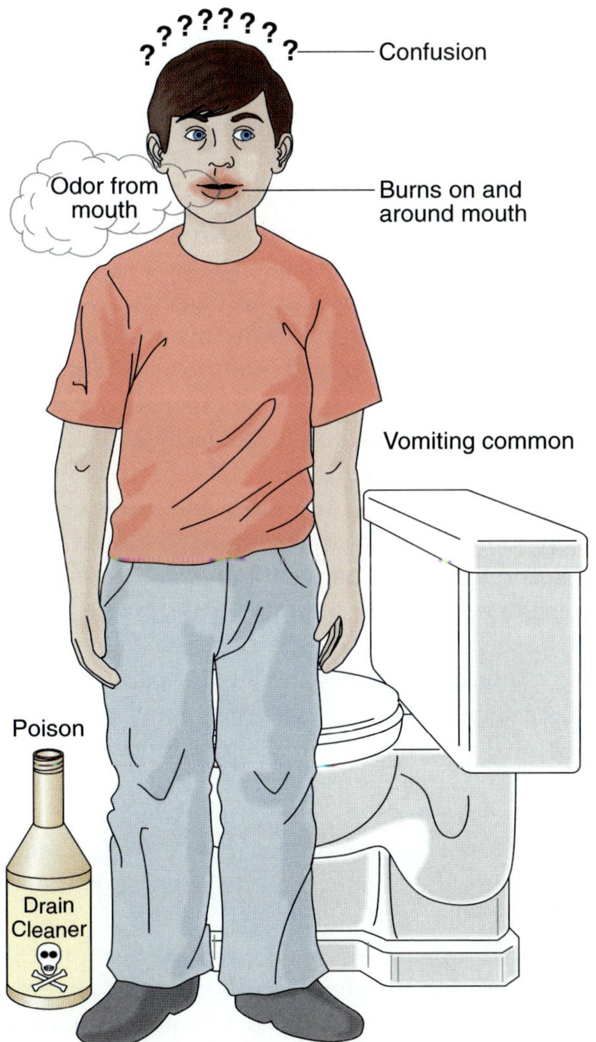

Figure 15–1 Ingested poisons can cause injury to the mouth and throat and will absorb into the stomach vessels and be distributed throughout the body.

Inhalation

Inhalation occurs when the poison is in a vapor form and is taken into the lungs during inhalation. The poison crosses the thin barrier between the alveoli and pulmonary capillary bed, gaining access to the bloodstream (Figure 15–2). Examples of poisons that enter through the inhalation route include carbon monoxide and some cholinergic nerve agents (e.g., sarin gas). Inhalation allows the toxin almost immediate access to the central circulation and rapid distribution throughout the body. This explains the rapid onset of signs in patients exposed to nerve gas agents. The speed of onset is limited only by the exact mechanism of action of the toxin, as the toxin will cross the thin alveolar wall rapidly.

Injection

Injection is the route of entry where the toxin is carried directly across the skin and into the blood or subcutaneous tissues (Figure 15–3). This route of entry involves an object that is either contaminated with the toxin or carries the toxin and pierces the skin. Examples of toxins

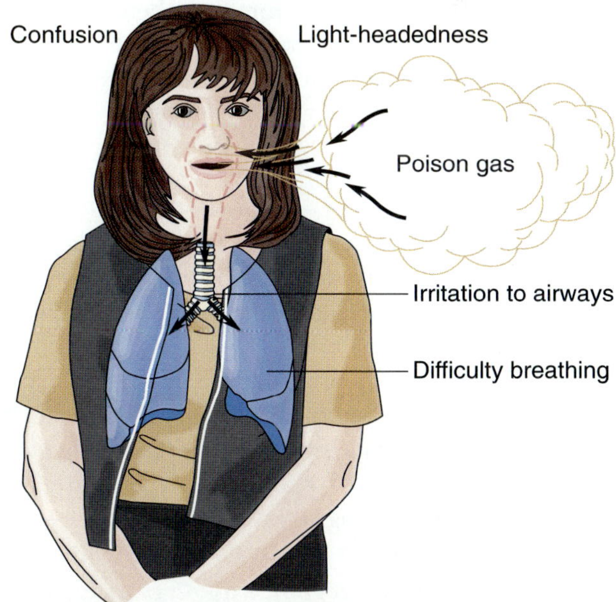

Figure 15–2 Inhaled poisons can cause irritation and injury to the upper and lower airways and may impede effective oxygenation.

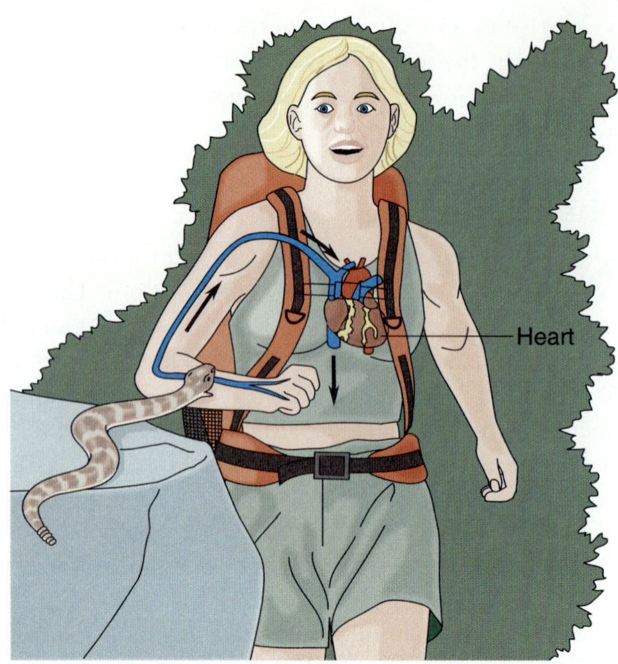

Figure 15–3 An injected poison will directly enter the bloodstream and be distributed around the body. Local blood vessel irritation is often seen.

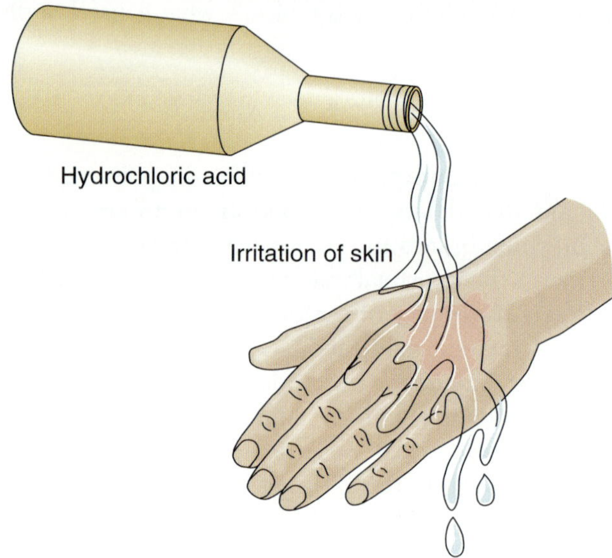

Figure 15–4 Some substances can be absorbed directly through the skin into the surface blood vessels; others cause injury to the skin itself.

that utilize injection include IV narcotics and insect stings. Toxins that utilize this route of entry are generally able to act fairly quickly, especially if direct access to the circulatory system is available, as in the case of injecting heroin into a vein. Even in the case of a toxin deposited in the subcutaneous tissue, onset can be relatively rapid as the toxin is either absorbed from the subcutaneous tissue into the bloodstream or carried by lymphatic drainage from the site of the injection to the central circulation.

Absorption

Absorption is the route of entry that utilizes the largest organ in the body, the skin, to gain access into the body (Figure 15–4). Examples of toxins that utilize absorption include some organophosphate compounds and chemical compounds. Absorption through the skin can be enhanced if the skin is not completely intact, as can occur in dry or cold climates. The speed of onset is greatly dependent upon the specific substance, with some toxins being readily absorbable and other requiring repeated or extended exposure before producing signs and symptoms.

GENERAL MANAGEMENT OF TOXICOLOGIC EMERGENCIES

Assessment and management of the poisoned patient can be a challenge. Information gathering about the specific substance or substances involved can be hampered by patient condition, witnesses who are unwilling to provide information regarding the patient, or lack of witnesses to the event. The EMS provider must quickly assess the situation and the patient in order to maintain safety, support the patient, and provide information required for definitive treatment in the emergency department. Overall care of the poisoned patient includes the following steps: scene safety, securing the ABCs, decontaminating the patient, eliminating the toxin, and providing a specific antidote as appropriate (Figure 15–5).

Scene safety is paramount in field emergency care, especially when dealing with toxicologic emergencies. Specific scene hazards will vary with the situation but can include threats of violence from individuals at the scene, toxic substances that remain on the ground or in the air, or confined spaces filled with toxic gas or low oxygen levels. The scene must be assessed and the EMS crew must make the decision of either entering the scene or calling for response of appropriate backup in the form of law enforcement, fire department, or Hazardous Materials team.

Once the scene is safe for the EMS team to enter, securing the ABCs is the first priority. The Hazardous Materials team may perform these tasks if it is not safe for the EMS team to come in contact with the patient prior to decontamination. The patient's airway, ventilatory status, and circulatory status should be rapidly assessed. Supplemental oxygen should be provided and

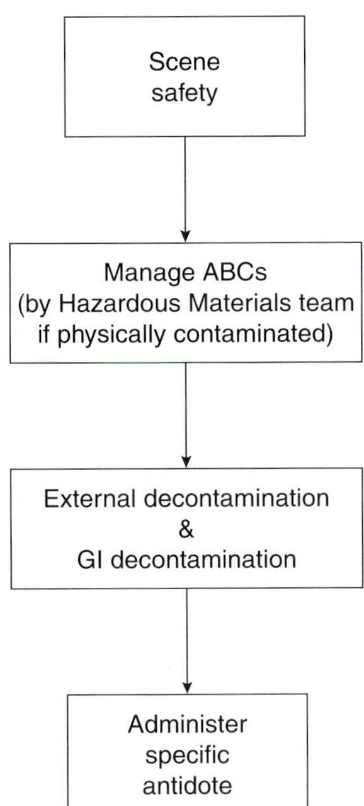

Figure 15-5 General management of toxicologic emergencies.

ventilations assisted as appropriate. Endotracheal intubation should be considered for patients who are obtunded or cannot maintain an open airway. IV access should be initiated and IV fluids infused as needed for hypotension. If additional responders are available, EMS providers should obtain as complete a history as possible and look for evidence of the toxic agent involved. Assessing blood glucose level is appropriate to rule out hypoglycemia as a cause for the decreased mental status, and 50% dextrose administered IV if indicated. If chronic alcohol abuse is suspected, 100 mg thiamin should be administered prior to dextrose. Administration of a narcotic antagonist (e.g., naloxone 0.4–2 mg, IV or IM) may be appropriate if there is a possibility of narcotic overdose; it can be titrated to respiratory effort.

Decontamination and elimination of the toxin can involve either an external decontamination or internal decontamination. External decontamination involves removing the patient from the toxic environment and physically removing the toxic agent from the patient. The specific decontamination procedure is performed by the Hazardous Materials team and is beyond the scope of this text. Internal decontamination is used to remove the toxin from the GI tract and depends upon the length of time from ingestion to treatment. In the emergency department, gastric lavage with copious amounts of water is performed until clear fluid returns from the orogastric tube. Activated charcoal (1 g/kg) can be administered to bind to and slow absorption of the toxin. Cathartic compounds, for example sorbitol or magnesium citrate, may be administered to help speed the toxin through the GI tract, limiting the amount of time the toxin is in contact with the intestinal wall and decreasing the amount of toxin absorbed. Syrup of ipecac, commonly used to induce vomiting, is a treatment that has limited value in gastric decontamination unless it can be administered within the first few minutes after the ingestion and before the substance has had time to begin absorption. In that case, syrup of ipecac should be used only on certain substances. When in doubt, medical control or the poison control center should be contacted for guidance.

If the specific toxin or toxins involved are known, a specific antidote can be administered to the patient to counteract the effects of the toxin. The elimination of some toxins can be facilitated by an IV infusion of sodium bicarbonate. The sodium bicarbonate infusion is titrated to produce an **alkalemia**, or blood that is alkalotic. The alkalemia improves filtering and elimination of the toxin by the kidneys. Some toxins may require dialysis in order to completely remove the toxin from the blood.

Consultation early in the encounter with either medical control or the regional poison control center may be beneficial in patient management, especially when the specific toxin is known or suspected. Contact with the receiving facility early in transport is essential in transporting a partially decontaminated patient so appropriate measures can be taken at the emergency department, including isolation, proper personal protective equipment, and decontamination facilities.

TOXIDROMES

A **toxidrome**, short for *toxic syndrome*, is a collection of signs and symptoms that are associated with groups of similar toxic agents. Grouping similar agents into toxidromes is helpful in remembering signs, symptoms, and treatment, as similar treatments are used to treat the agents in the toxidrome. Toxidrome groupings can be helpful for cases where the toxin is unknown by directing treatment until the substance can be confirmed by witness or laboratory screening. The five major toxidromes that are discussed include cholinergic, anticholinergic, opioid, hallucinogenic, and sympathomimetic toxidromes. These toxidromes are summarized in Table 15–1.

TABLE 15-1 Common Toxidromes, Associated Signs, and Treatment

Toxidrome	Signs	Treatment
Cholinergic	SLUDGE signs (salivation, lacrimation, urination, defecation, GI upset, emesis); headache; dizziness; muscle weakness, tremors or fasciculations; bradycardia; wheezing; diaphoresis; myosis; coma; seizures	Atropine. Pralidoxime chloride (2-PAM). Diazepam or midazolam for seizures.
Anticholinergic	Hot as Hades (hyperthermia); Blind as a Bat (mydriasis); Dry as a Bone (dry skin); Red as a Beet (red rash); Mad as a Hatter (delirium); hypertension; tachycardia; urinary retention; absent bowel sounds; dysrhythmias; cardiovascular collapse; seizures	Supportive using traditional therapies to treat findings. Physostigmine use is controversial and reserved for hospital use.
Opioid	Altered mental status; respiratory depression; miosis (pinpoint pupils); bradycardia; hypotension; hallucinations; decreased GI movement (constipation)	Naloxone IV or IM
Hallucinogenic	Distortion of reality; euphoria; intense colors & sounds; sensory misrepresentations (e.g., hear colors); distorted body/object image	Supportive. Provide reassurance. Diazepam or midazolam for a "bad trip" or increased sympathetic effects.
Sympathomimetic	CNS excitation; seizures; tachycardia; tachypnea; hypertension; hyperthermia	Diazepam/midazolam. β-blockers contraindicated unless used in conjunction with an α-blocker. Nitrates for MI symptoms or hypertension.

Cholinergic Toxidrome

The **cholinergic toxidrome** involves agents that alter the action of acetylcholine, a neurotransmitter that is used in the autonomic nervous system and at the neuromuscular junction, where the motor neurons interface with the muscle. Common agents that cause these effects include insecticides (Figure 15–6), for example organophosphates and carbamates, and nerve agents, for example sarin and Soman.

The neurotransmitter acetylcholine normally binds to a specific receptor to either produce muscle contraction or autonomic nervous system changes. This neurotransmitter is broken down and removed from the receptor site by acetylcholinesterase after a set period of time. If additional muscle contraction is required, then more acetylcholine is released from the nerve terminal and reactivates the muscle. If the acetylcholine is not removed from the receptor site, the receptor will be continuously activated, leading to muscle paralysis and enhanced autonomic nervous system effects. The cholinergic agents listed above bind to acetylcholinesterase, disabling it and impairing its ability to remove acetylcholine from its receptor. As acetylcholine is involved in both the parasympathetic and sympathetic nervous systems, both systems are activated by continuous stimulation. Insecticides tend to cause symptoms over a period of days as they are absorbed slowly and the exposure tends to be smaller. Nerve agents, on the other hand,

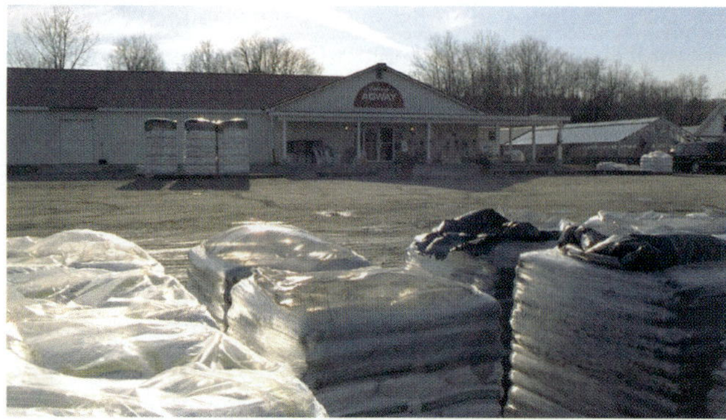

Figure 15-6 Agricultural supply stores have a large quantity of hazardous materials, including pesticides, herbicides, and fertilizers.

tend to be very powerful and can cause immediate signs and death within several minutes of exposure.

The signs associated with the cholinergic toxidrome include headache, dizziness, weakness, abdominal cramps, nausea, and vomiting in mild exposures. As the exposure increases, additional signs of salivation, lacrimation, urination, defecation or diarrhea, GI upset, and emesis (some providers use the mnemonic SLUDGE to recall the signs of cholinergic toxidrome) are seen, along with increased confusion and anxiety, muscle tremors or fasciculations, and miosis (constricted pupils) leading to blurred vision. The patient may have trouble protecting the airway because of the increased oral and respiratory secretions. In severe exposures, the patient is unable to breathe adequately, and bradycardia, wheezing, diaphoresis, and seizures develop.

Specific management of cholinergic toxidrome includes administering atropine until secretions have cleared and pralidoxime chloride (2-PAM) until signs resolve. Atropine is used to selectively block acetylcholine in the parasympathetic nervous system, thus reducing secretions and treating bradycardia. Atropine is initially administered at a dose of 2–4 mg IV and repeated every 10 minutes until secretions resolve. Doses of atropine required for organophosphate poisoning can easily exceed what is normally carried on board an advanced life support unit, as upwards of hundreds of milligrams of atropine may be required for severe poisonings. 2-PAM acts to replenish the levels of acetylcholinesterase, dislodging the acetylcholine from its receptor and eventually restoring normal action. Diazepam or midazolam may be administered IV or IM to treat seizures that can accompany severe poisonings. For mild exposures, the only treatment required may be to remove the patient from the offending substance.

Anticholinergic Toxidrome

The **anticholinergic toxidrome**, like the cholinergic toxidrome, also involves agents that have action at acetylcholine receptors; however, these agents bind to the acetylcholine receptor and block the action of acetylcholine in the autonomic nervous system. There are many agents that have anticholinergic effects to differing degrees, with atropine and scopolamine, both derived from the belladonna plant, as the prototypic agents. Many antihistamines, medications used to treat Parkinson's disease and diarrhea, certain antidepressants, skeletal muscle relaxants, and some plants have anticholinergic effects.

Signs of the anticholinergic toxidrome include a very witty memory aid: hyperthermia (Hot as Hades), mydriasis (dilated pupils—Blind as a Bat), dry skin (Dry as a Bone), red rash (Red as a Beet), and delirium (Mad as a Hatter). Other signs of anticholinergic overdose include hypertension, tachycardia, urinary retention, absent bowel sounds, cardiovascular collapse, and seizures. Sinus tachycardia is the most common dysrhythmia that presents with anticholinergic overdose, however AV conduction blocks, bundle branch blocks, and atrial or ventricular tachycardias can develop.

Specific management of the anticholinergic toxidrome is generally supportive and findings can be treated using the standard medications and treatment therapies (e.g., antiarrhythmics for arrhythmias). The ECG should be continually monitored for dysrhythmias. As anticholinergic activity tends to slow down transport through the GI system, charcoal, gastric lavage, or cathartics may be employed to decontaminate the GI tract. Mild and moderate forms of the anticholinergic toxidrome will typically resolve with supportive measures; however, severe cases may require physostigmine, a medication that inhibits acetylcholinesterae, to reverse the anticholinergic action. This is an area of toxicology that is controversial and the use of physostigmine should be used with extreme care as it may precipitate a cholinergic syndrome caused by the decreased action of acetylcholinesterase.

Opioid Toxidrome

The class of drugs derived from opium is appropriately named opioids. Opium is produced from the poppy seed and was a popular drug of abuse in China in the 19th Century. Morphine and codeine are natural derivatives of opium and other drugs, for example, heroin, oxycodone, meperidine (Demerol), and methadone are synthetic or semisynthetic derivatives of opium. Heroin, a commonly abused drug in the late 1960s and 1970s has found new life as a relatively inexpensive and potent drug of abuse in the late 1990s and early 21st century (Figure 15–7).

Opioids act on the naturally occurring opioid receptors located in the spinal cord and brain. The body produces natural opioid chemicals that include endorphins, enkephalins, and dynorphins that serve as natural analgesics and euphorics. These receptors are responsible for the effects of natural and synthetic opioid substances, including **analgesia**, euphoria, sedation, respiratory depression, decreased movement of materials through the GI system, hallucinations, and dysphoria. Bradycardia, hypotension, coma, and non-reactive miosis (pinpoint pupils) also occur with varying degrees of opioid usage. The decreased movement of materials through the GI system can produce constipation. Dependence occurs in patients who take opioids because, with repeated usage, the body creates an increased number of opioid receptors,

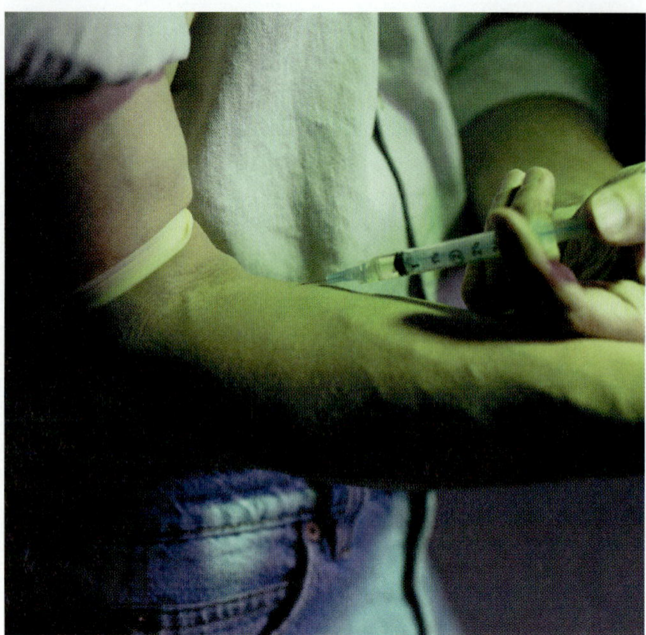

Figure 15-7 Heroin is once again a popular drug which is often abused. (Courtesy of PhotoDisc)

and additional drug is required to achieve the same effect. Patients who abuse opioids can run into danger as respiratory depression and mental status changes can occur at doses that are less than the dose required for an euphoric effect in the chronic abuser. Many patients who present to EMS with an opioid overdose have a significantly altered mental status, and may require ventilatory and circulatory assistance. It is important to note that opioid overdoses are possible with prescription pain medications if taken in sufficient amounts over short periods of time.

Scene safety should be a primary concern when responding to the scene of a drug overdose and sufficient law enforcement manpower should be available to control the scene. Management of patients who have an opioid overdose focuses on ensuring a patent airway, adequate ventilation, and adequate circulatory system status. Supplemental oxygen and ventilation should be employed as appropriate. IV access should be attempted, but can be difficult in patients with a history of IV drug abuse as the veins become scarred and sclerosed with repeated injections and infections. An opioid antagonist, for example naloxone, can be administered either IV or IM to counteract the action of the opioid. This presents an interesting dilemma to the EMS provider in the field, as significant management of the airway may be necessary before the naloxone becomes effective; however, once it begins to work, endotracheal intubation may not be necessary. The half-life of naloxone is also much shorter than the half-life of the opioid so there is a good chance that repeated doses will be required, otherwise respiratory depression and altered mental status will recur. Another dilemma in the management of the patient with an opioid overdose involves the quick resolution of the "high" the patient was experiencing with the opioid. Most patients who are abusing opioids will not appreciate the loss of the high and will plunge into withdrawal precipitated by naloxone administration. These patients can become highly combative and easily overcome available scene resources. If IV access is available, the dose of naloxone may be initially titrated to treat the respiratory depression but not produce significant withdrawal symptoms until the patient is in a more controlled environment. Once naloxone is determined to be effective, the emergency department may elect to initiate a naloxone infusion. Gastric lavage and charcoal may be employed in the emergency department for cases of oral opioid ingestion as the opioid slows movement through the GI tract and lavage and charcoal may limit absorption.

Hallucinogenic Toxidrome

Hallucinogens are substances that produce a distortion of reality to the extent that the person who ingested the substance believes the hallucination is real. Many people report distortion of shapes, greater intensity to colors and sounds, a heightened awareness, and hallucinations. Some also report a misrepresentation of sensory data, for example, they "hear" colors or "see" sounds. **Hallucinosis** is a state of constant hallucinations. Treatment is generally supportive as long as the individual is having a "good trip." In a "bad trip," the patient can become highly agitated and signs of sympathetic overdrive may be apparent. In this situation, reassurance and diazepam or midazolam in addition to supportive measures can be helpful in decreasing the effects of a bad trip.

Sympathomimetic Toxidrome

The **sympathomimetic toxidrome** occurs when there is heightened stimulation of the sympathetic nervous system. This can occur with medications such as aminophylline and ephedrine, found in many over-the-counter cold remedies and appetite suppressants, caffeine, and illicit substances such as cocaine and amphetamines. These agents either act directly on the α–adrenergic and β–adrenergic receptors in the sympathetic nervous system or they work to prolong the action of neurotransmitters at these receptors. The signs and symptoms of sympathomimetic action include tachycardia, tachypnea, hypertension, central nervous system excitation, and possibly seizures. Cocaine induced MI has increased in prevalence among younger individuals and cardiotoxicity from appetite suppressant overdose has also been reported.

Treatment includes supporting the ABCs. β–blockers should be avoided to prevent significant hypertension associated with unopposed α–adrenergic effects, however a benzodiazepime, for example diazepam, may be used to diminish the effects of a sympathomimetic until arriving at the emergency department. Nitrates can be used to treat MI symptoms or hypertension.

SUBSTANCES OF ABUSE

According to the 1999 National Household Survey performed by the U.S. Substance Abuse and Mental Health Services Administration, there were an estimated 14.8 million Americans currently using an illicit substance, which has decreased from the 1979 high of 25 million Americans. In the year 2000, the Drug Abuse Warning Network reported over 600,000 drug related emergency department episodes and over 1.8 million drug mentions in the United States. The drugs most frequently mentioned in order of most to least frequent were alcohol, cocaine, heroin/morphine, and marijuana/hashish. Of these emergency department visits, the two most cited reasons for drug use were dependence and suicide.

Alcohol

Alcohol is one of the most widely abused substances in the United States and was responsible for over 700,000 hospital admissions for substance abuse in 1998. Alcohol consumed for abuse is ethanol; methanol, ethylene glycol, and isopropyl alcohol are covered later in this chapter. Ethanol is also found in many over-the-counter preparations and food flavorings. Ethanol is easily distributed throughout all body tissues and is metabolized at a constant rate by the liver. The central nervous system effects are the primary result of ethanol ingestion; however hypoglycemia, liver damage, GI tract damage, and a predisposition to hypothermia and trauma are also associated with ethanol abuse.

Signs of ethanol intoxication include slurred speech, ataxia, incoordination, and euphoria. With more severe intoxication, stupor, respiratory depression, and aspiration can occur. Chronic ethanol abuse can lead to cirrhosis or hepatitis, gastric irritation and rupture of esophageal varices, cardiac dysrhythmias associated with electrolyte imbalance, and sensory neuropathy and encephalopathy. Withdrawal from chronic ethanol abuse includes anxiety, tachycardia, headache, palpitations, and tremors. These symptoms can progress to **delirium tremens**, a syndrome consisting of seizures, tachycardia, hyperthermia, and delirium which can be life-threatening. Delirium tremens usually manifests itself between 48 and 72 hours after cessation of ethanol intake; however, it may present earlier.

EMS treatment of acute ethanol ingestion includes maintaining a patent airway and supporting ventilation and circulation. If the patient is hypoglycemic, as many chronic abusers are, EMS providers should administer 100 mg thiamin prior to administering glucose to avoid encephalopathy. Seizures can often be controlled with diazepam, and it can be given prophylactically if the patient is beginning to show early signs of delirium tremens. Activated charcoal does not bind ethanol and is not indicated unless another substance was ingested along with ethanol. There is no specific antidote and most patients will easily metabolize the alcohol to freedom.

Cocaine

Cocaine is a naturally occurring alkaloid found in the *Erythroxylon coca* plant in Central America and Indonesia. It was and is still used by native populations in religious ceremonies. Cocaine can be used by snorting, smoking, or IV injection. Crack or free-based cocaine is a super-concentrated compound with greater purity that can be easily smoked.

Cocaine is a powerful sympathomimetic in addition to potentiating the action of several neurotransmitters in the brain. At the peripheral receptor level, cocaine enhances the effects of epinephrine and norepinephrine by decreasing removal of these neurotransmitters from the receptors, providing longer and more intense stimulation of the receptor. In the central nervous system, the mechanism of action is not well understood, but it appears that cocaine also interferes with the removal of several neurotransmitters from their receptors. When applied locally, cocaine acts as an effective anesthetic because it interrupts nerve transmission. Cocaine was used locally after surgery involving the mucous membranes of the nose or mouth to decrease the amount of bleeding, taking advantage of its vasoconstrictive properties.

Signs and symptoms of cocaine use depend upon the amount of the substance ingested. The central nervous system is first stimulated producing restlessness and agitation. Seizures are produced by increased stimulation of the motor system. Cocaine will initially increase respiratory rate by stimulating the respiratory centers in the brain stem, and cause respiratory depression with increased doses. As discussed above, cocaine's effects on the circulatory system stem from its sympathomimetic effects: tachycardia from increased sympathetic action on the heart and hypertension from vasoconstriction. It is interesting to note that cocaine will initially produce a bradycardia by stimulating the vagus nerve; however, this is a transient condition that will revert to the tachycardia that is seen by the time the patient receives medical attention. The pupils become dilated from the increased sympathetic activity. Vomiting occurs from stimulation of the vomiting center in the brain and hyperthermia occurs from either stimulation of the thermoregulatory center in the brain, an increase in metabolism, or severe vasoconstriction. Cocaine induced myocardial infarctions and strokes can also occur and should be suspected in any young patient presenting with signs and symptoms of an infarction or stroke.

Management of a patient with a cocaine overdose includes managing the ABCs, and performing interventions as appropriate. IV access should be initiated and blood glucose level checked if the patient is exhibiting signs of altered mental status. Diazepam or lorazepam can be used to treat seizures or anxiety, and may indirectly treat the sympathomimetic effects of tachycardia and hypertension. Suspected cocaine induced MI can be treated using normal methods, including nitroglycerin and aspirin, with the nitroglycerin potentially alleviating coronary artery spasm that sometimes accompanies cocaine overdose. Hypertension that does not respond to diazepam should be treated with nitrates as β–blockers can produce additional coronary artery spasm. The use of β–blockers in a patient who has taken cocaine can also lead to unopposed α–adrenergic stimulation, producing severe hypertention and tachycardia. Dysrhythmias should be treated following normal advanced cardiac life support algorithms.

Narcotics

Both prescription and non-prescription narcotics are abused. Heroin has regained its popularity in the late 1990s as a non-prescription narcotic that is abused. Prescription narcotics have always been the subject of abuse, with some unscrupulous individuals obtaining prescriptions to sell to others or obtaining several prescriptions from different providers or altering prescriptions to support their own addiction. The specific prescription narcotic or combination analgesics that are abused vary with time and between communities. Local law enforcement is a good resource to find out what is the "drug of choice" for abuse in a specific community.

Please refer to the discussion on the mechanism of action and management of narcotic overdose in the opioid toxidrome section above.

Marijuana

Marijuana is the most commonly abused substance among 18- to 25-year-old Americans and was the primary substance of abuse that prompted hospital admission in over 200,000 admissions in 1998 (Figure 15–8). Marijuana is made from the leaves and flowering portions of the *Cannabis sativa* plant. It is most commonly smoked or added to food. Hashish is formed from drying and compressing resin that is made from the plant. The primary psychoactive ingredient is THC, although several other compounds are likely to contribute to the psychoactive effects of marijuana. THC binds to receptors in the brain that can produce stimulation, sedation, or hallucination depending upon the dose. THC can stimulate catecholamine release and simultaneously inhibit sympathetic

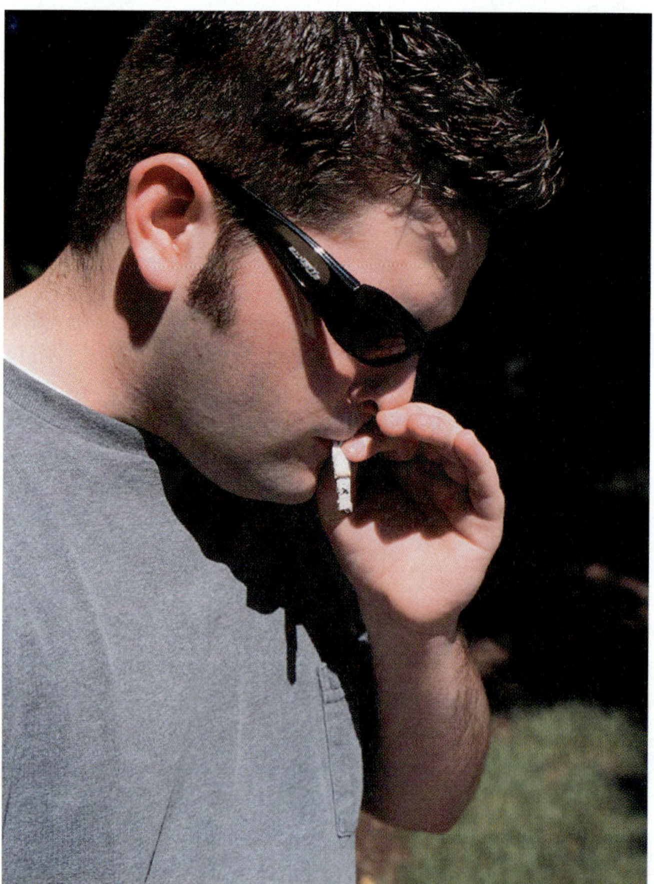

Figure 15–8 Adolescents may suffer from poisoning from marijuana use because of experimentation.

reflexes, for example, the postural reflex that prevents orthostatic hypotension. THC has been synthesized into pill form and is prescribed as an appetite stimulant for patients with AIDS and cancer. The medical use of marijuana in the United States is currently a very controversial topic, with several states having passed legislation allowing the use of marijuana for medicinal purposes under certain conditions. So far, the United States federal government does not support this movement.

Symptoms of marijuana use include palpitations, euphoria, increased sensory awareness, and sedation. At higher doses, marijuana can impair short-term memory and produce visual hallucinations and paranoid psychosis. Signs of marijuana use include tachycardia, orthostatic hypotension, slurred speech, injection of the conjunctiva surrounding the eyes, a loss of coordination, or even ataxia. Intravenous use of the hashish oil can produce dyspnea, abdominal pain, shock, disseminated intravascular coagulation, acute renal failure, and death.

Treatment of marijuana overdose is primarily supportive, providing reassurance. Anxiety may respond to a sedative, for example, diazepam or midazolam and orthostatic hypotension generally responds to IV fluids. Syrup of ipecac may be helpful if given within a few minutes of ingestion, and charcoal can help decrease the absorption of oral marijuana.

Mushrooms

The *Psilocybe* genus of mushrooms is a commonly used hallucinogenic mushroom. These mushrooms grow wild in the United States and are available through illegal drug markets. Psilocybin, the active compound in the mushroom, acts on the serotonin system in the brain and can produce sympathomimetic symptoms in addition to euphoria and anxiety. In rare cases, mushroom ingestion can produce seizures and hyperthermia. EMS treatment of mushroom ingestion is largely supportive, as respiratory depression does not usually occur unless other substances are ingested along with the mushroom. Diazepam or midazolam can be effective at treating seizures and anxiety. Patients should be transported with minimal stimulation.

CHEMICAL AGENTS

Chemical agents are found everywhere in our environment, from the large factories that produce chemicals to the household cleaners under the kitchen sink. Some chemical agents are produced during manufacturing operations and other toxic chemicals are produced by mixing the cleaners in the home. According to the 1999 annual report of the American Association of Poison Control Center TESS database, cleaning substances were the most frequently involved substance in human toxic exposure and the second most common exposure for children under six years old. This section covers caustic agents, common household chemicals, carbon monoxide, hydrocarbons, alcohols, organophosphates, and metals.

Caustic Agents

Many forms of caustic agents are available, both at home and at work, with a variety of mechanisms. All of them share a common result of damage to the skin, damage to the GI tract if ingested, and permanent scarring. Corrosives can be inhaled, ingested, or contacted. Inhaled corrosives produce airway obstruction, stridor, wheezing, hoarseness, and pulmonary edema. Ingestion will cause pain, difficulty swallowing, and drooling, and perforated stomach or intestine can occur producing chest or abdominal pain. Contact irritation to the mucous membranes causes pain, redness, and blistering. Swallowed button batteries can produce extensive tissue destruction through their corrosive effects and possibly by discharge of electrical current into the local tissues. Button batteries lodged in the esophagus can erode into the aorta, producing a severe hemorrhage.

EMS treatment includes removal from the environment, appropriate decontamination with copious amounts of water or saline, and attention to the ABCs. EMS providers should administer milk or water orally to help buffer the caustic substance. Drinking vinegar or other buffers is not recommended.

Common Household Chemicals

There are numerous products around the typical household which are non-toxic or produce minimal symptoms if ingested or contact mucous membranes (Figure 15–9). The manufacturer's label will often describe the contents or the local poison control center or emergency department will have a database available that describes the specific toxicity, signs and symptoms, and recommended treatment for the substance. Most household products will cause mild gastrointestinal discomfort if ingested and minor skin or mucous membrane irritation if contacted. Household cleaners pose a unique risk as the combination of cleaners can produce deadly gasses and should be avoided.

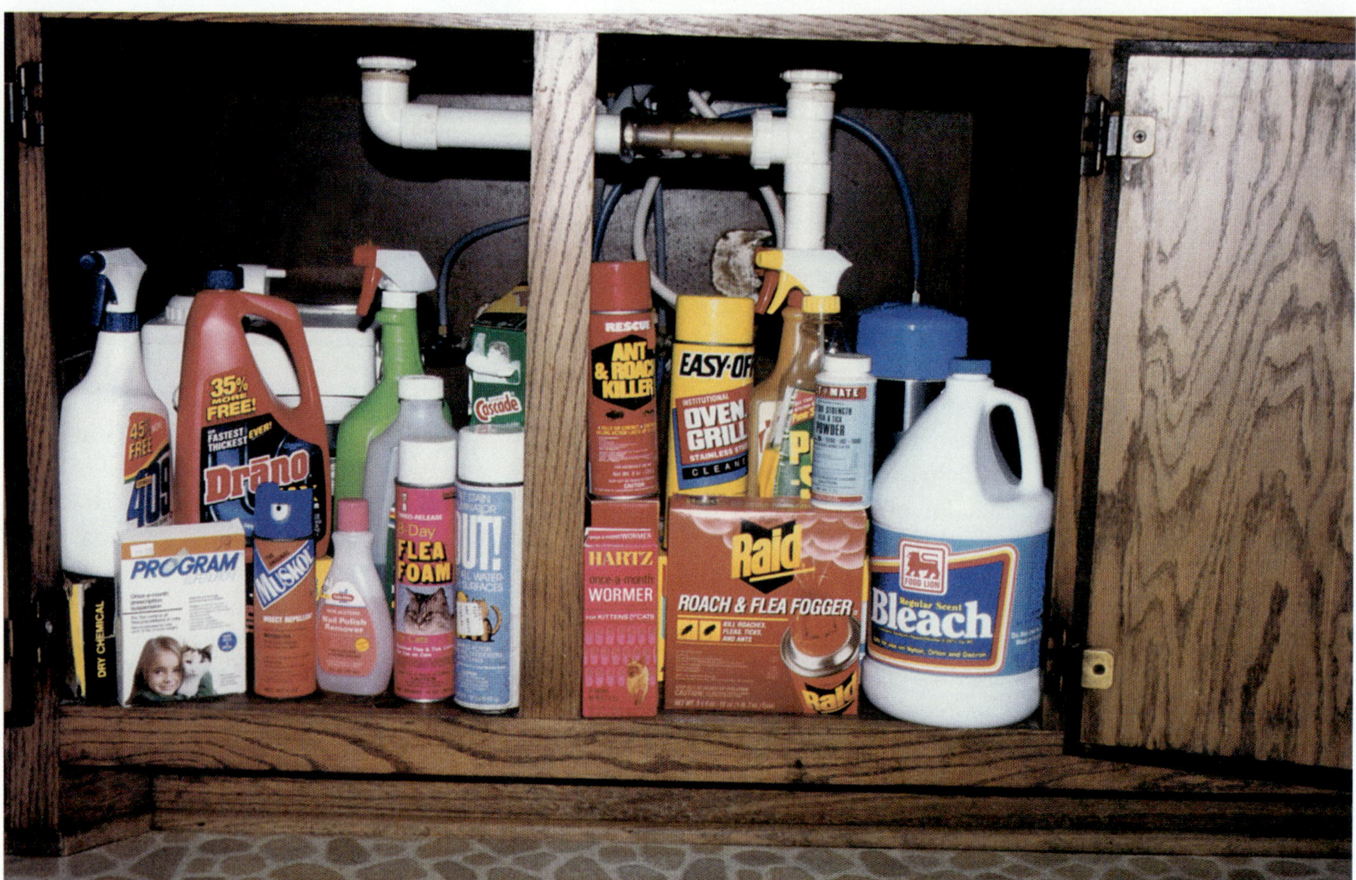

Figure 15-9 A look under the kitchen sink yields a number of poisonous items. (Courtesy of Mark Zeringue)

EMS treatment follows the general principles outlined above. EMS providers should remove the patient from the environment ensuring adequate personal protection for rescuers. Secure the airway, assist respiration with supplemental oxygen or mechanical ventilation, and support circulation with IV fluids if needed. Flush skin or mucous membranes with copious amounts of water or saline to help dilute the substance and contact the local poison control hotline or emergency department for advice on specific treatment.

Carbon Monoxide

Carbon monoxide is a colorless and odorless gas produced as a byproduct of incomplete combustion. Exposure typically occurs in a poorly ventilated area exposed to exhaust fumes from a variety of fossil fuel powered equipment, including garages, coal stoves, or kerosene heaters. Carbon monoxide directly binds to hemoglobin approximately 200 times better than oxygen does, thus displacing oxygen from hemoglobin and causing a decrease in tissue oxygen perfusion. The brain is most susceptible to the lack of oxygen caused by carbon monoxide poisoning. Carbon monoxide may also be directly toxic to the myocardium. Signs and symptoms of carbon monoxide exposure include headache, irritability, somnolence, nausea, and dizziness. Some patients may also complain of anginal symptoms or present with an MI and dysrhythmias. Syncope, seizures, coma, and death can also result from sustained exposure. In significant exposure, the patient's skin may become the classic "cherry red" color associated with carbon monoxide exposure. Pulse oximetry machines are considered unreliable to measure oxygen saturation because the carbon monoxide bound to the oxygen sites on hemoglobin produces the same molecular change as does oxygen and this change is what is measured to determine oxygen saturation.

EMS treatment includes removing the patient from the environment using appropriate breathing apparatus, securing the airway, assisting ventilation, and maintaining circulation. 100% oxygen should be administered, as it will help to displace the carbon monoxide from the hemoglobin binding sites quicker than room air. Elimination of carbon monoxide can be enhanced by hyperbaric oxygen and can be useful in patients who do not respond to initial oxygenation or are severely intoxicated.

Hyperbaric oxygen treatment remains a controversial area in medicine, even in the treatment of carbon monoxide poisoning.

Hydrocarbons

Hydrocarbons consist of products manufactured from petroleum products, including gasoline, pesticides, solvents, and degreasers. These substances produce direct tissue damage from contact with the respiratory system, gastrointestinal tract, and skin. Signs of systemic toxicity may present after any route of entry. Inhalation will typically produce immediate coughing, gasping, and wheezing, and chemical pneumonitis can develop to the point where death ensues. Ingestion will typically produce nausea, vomiting, and bloody vomitus or bloody diarrhea. Systemic signs, which also occur with ingestion because of absorption of the hydrocarbon from the GI tract, include confusion, headache, ataxia, dysrhythmias, syncope, liver or renal failure, and respiratory arrest. Skin contact typically only produces localized irritation; however, some hydrocarbons are absorbed through the skin.

EMS treatment involves removal from source and thorough decontamination with copious amounts of water or saline, and attention to the ABCs. Activated charcoal can be administered on the advice of poison control or medical command if the substance is one that will likely cause systemic toxicity. At this time there are no specific antidotes for hydrocarbon toxicity, although specific antidotes may be available in the future.

Alcohols

There are several alcohols that are used in everyday chemicals and solvents. Ethanol, the alcohol that is commonly consumed, was discussed previously. The other alcohols are isopropyl alcohol, methanol, and ethylene glycol.

Isopropyl alcohol is commonly found in rubbing alcohol, solvents, hair care products, paint thinners, and antifreeze. It acts in a similar fashion to ethanol, but with a much longer duration of action. Signs and symptoms of a severe overdose include respiratory depression, coma, hypotension, and bloody vomitus. EMS treatment is generally supportive, managing the airway, assisting breathing, and administering IV fluids for hypotension. Activated charcoal does not bind alcohols and is not indicated. Patients who have ingested isopropyl alcohol may require emergent dialysis for definitive treatment.

Methanol and ethylene glycol are commonly found in solvent, paint thinners, windshield wiper fluid, antifreeze, coolant, and as a preservative in nail polishes and detergents. Methanol and ethylene glycol are metabolized by the same pathways as ethanol; however, formaldehyde and formic acid are the very toxic byproducts formed from that process. Signs and symptoms of poisoning may not be evident for up to eighteen hours after ingestion and include CNS depression, visual disturbances (looking through a snowstorm), abdominal pain, nausea, vomiting, and other signs of GI irritation. Within the first 12–24 hours, the patient may develop tachycardia, hypertension, and increased respiratory rate, putting the patient at risk for developing CHR, pulmonary edema, and ARDS. After 24 hours kidney irritation occurs and the patient develops flank pain and hypertension.

EMS treatment of methanol and ethylene glycol ingestion include managing the airway, ensuring adequate respiration, and supporting circulation. As with the other alcohols, activated charcoal is contraindicated if the airway is not protected and if only an alcohol was ingested. In the emergency department, the patient may receive sodium bicarbonate if acidotic. Fomepazole is an agent that decreases alcohol metabolism and reduces the amount of formaldehyde produced during the process. If fomepazole is not available, then an ethanol drip is used to treat methanol and ethylene glycol intoxication because ethanol will be preferentially metabolized. Emergent dialysis may also be required.

Organophosphates

Organophosphates are commonly used as insecticide agents and can be present in the home or in the industrial (e.g., farm, greenhouse) setting. Organophosphates, as discussed above in the cholinergic toxidrome section, inhibit acethylcholinesterase, producing prolonged contact between acetylcholine at the **neuromuscular junction**, which is the interface between the nerve and muscle, and throughout the autonomic nervous system. The effect of organophosphate exposure typically presents after prolonged exposure to the insecticide of up to a week in duration unless the patient is exposed to a massive amount of the insecticide. Please refer to the discussion in the cholinergic toxidrome section for signs, symptoms, and management of organophosphate poisoning.

Metals

Humans come into contact with metals every day. Certain types of free metals can be dangerous when ingested or the powder inhaled because of the alteration of the normal biochemical processes that occurs in the body. Three common metals that can be dangerous are iron, lead, and mercury.

Iron Iron is a commonly found element that is used in the treatment of iron deficiency anemia and is also found in iron fortified baby formula. Iron is an important substrate for the synthesis of hemoglobin, the oxygen carrying compound found in red blood cells. The toxic effects of iron can easily occur because of its affects on the GI lining and cellular dysfunction. Iron is corrosive on GI tract mucosa, producing ulcerations, hemorrhage, and hypovolemia from blood loss. On a cellular level, iron toxicity can interrupt metabolism, producing lactic acidosis and cellular necrosis, or cell death. The signs and symptoms of iron toxicity are divided into four stages; however, the signs and symptoms can overlap and death can occur at any stage.

- Stage I: In the first few hours after ingestion, symptoms of GI irritation predominate, including abdominal pain, vomiting, diarrhea, and blood in the vomitus (hematemesis). If there are no symptoms within six hours after reported ingestion, then a significant iron overdose can be excluded.
- Stage II: Up to 24 hours later, the GI symptoms will resolve and the patient may not have any specific complaints but appears ill with abnormal vital signs and evidence of poor tissue perfusion.
- Stage III: This stage can present early or after Stage II and consists of shock and a metabolic acidosis. Bleeding and hypovolemia will worsen caused by changes in coagulation produced by the excess iron. Liver, heart, and kidney failure can also occur.
- Stage IV: In two to five days after ingestion, the patient may develop liver failure.
- Stage V: Within four to six weeks after ingestion, the corrosive effects of iron may produce an obstruction of the GI tract where the stomach empties into the duodenum.

Treatment of iron overdose includes managing the airway, ventilation, and circulation, including providing supplemental oxygen, initiating intravenous access and monitoring the ECG. Activated charcoal is not effective against iron overdose. Fluid resuscitation may be required as the patient is hypovolemic. Gastric lavage may be performed in the emergency department if ingestion occurred less than six hours before presentation. Whole bowel irrigation, Vitamin K, fresh frozen plasma transfusion, or chelation therapy may be considered by the emergency department. Whole bowel irrigation will limit the time that the iron is in contact with the GI mucosa and may reduce absorption and irritation. Vitamin K and fresh frozen plasma are used to counteract the coagulation deficiencies produced by liver toxicity. Chelation therapy can be used on many heavy metal ingestions and utilizes an agent that directly binds to the metal, inactivating it. This compound is then excreted from the body.

Lead. Lead is the most common cause of heavy metal poisoning in children. It can produce toxicity by ingestion or by the inhalation of lead particles. Lead paint was commonly used in older houses, and inquisitive toddlers can easily ingest paint chips. If the house was renovated, lead dust may be present in the soil surrounding the house in sufficient levels to produce toxicity in children and adults. Lead is irritating to the GI tract and interferes with hemoglobin production. Lead also interacts with calcium and zinc producing nervous system and musculoskeletal effects. The American Association of Pediatrics recommends lead testing for all toddlers between the ages of 9 months and 12 months of age, and then again at 24 months in higher risk groups.

Acute lead toxicity can produce altered mental status and colicky abdominal pain. Chronic exposure can produce painful joints, anemia, GI distress, weight loss, and a peripheral motor weakness that tends to affect the upper extremities. Childhood encephalopathy from lead exposure can produce long lasting behavioral effects, delirium, ataxia, and coma. Developmental effects of lead exposure include decreased intelligence, stunted growth, and impaired development. Lead poisoning may be difficult to detect because many of the symptoms are not specific and developmental delays can take a long time to be discovered.

Treatment includes maintaining the airway, breathing, and circulation, assessing and treating seizures as usual, and using syrup of ipecac if ingestion was within a few minutes of arrival. Fluids may be beneficial; however, overhydration can worsen the cerebral edema that commonly occurs with lead overdose. Charcoal can help delay absorption in acute ingestion and gastric lavage and cathartics may be employed at the emergency department to decontaminate the GI tract. As with iron overdose, chelation may be considered in the hospital.

Mercury. Mercury is another common compound that is used in industry for a variety of chemical processes. Mercury also is present in home thermometers and fillings used in cavities, although the use of mercury outside industry has decreased. Mercury alters CNS cell membranes and inhibits many enzymes. Mercury salts are very corrosive to the mucous membranes, skin, and eyes, and are toxic to the kidneys. Mercury exposure can occur by contact, ingestion or inhalation.

Acute inhalation of mercury vapor may produce pulmonary edema or a chemical pneumonitis, an inflammation of the lungs caused by chemical irritation of lung tissue. Chronic inhalation may produce a tremor, ataxia, and behavioral changes, including memory loss, severe mood swings, and depression. Acute ingestion of mercury may produce a GI hemorrhage and abdominal pain that can produce shock, renal failure, necrosis of the GI lining, or death. Chronic lead exposure typically presents with CNS disturbances rather than GI disturbances.

Treatment of mercury toxicity includes ensuring a patent airway, and adequate ventilation and circulation. EMS providers should administer supplemental oxygen and treat pulmonary edema in the usual manner. If mercury salts were ingested and the airway is patent, activated charcoal should be administered. The patient may require dialysis or chelation agents for definitive treatment.

MEDICATIONS

Every medication prescribed comes with side effects and untoward reactions. Medications are intended to act within the **therapeutic range**, or the blood level of the medication that has been found to be beneficial to most patients. Some patients may metabolize medications slightly faster than others, and require additional medication to reach the therapeutic range. Other patients with liver or kidney damage or who are taking other medications may process certain medications at a slower rate, and thus require less medication to reach the therapeutic range. Many medication dosages are adjusted for individuals over age 70 as the metabolism and excretion of the medication tend to occur more slowly as the individual ages.

Every medication has the ability to become toxic or lethal. Typically the lethal dosage level is significantly greater than the dosage required to achieve a blood level in the therapeutic range; however, the therapeutic dose for some medications is close to the toxic or lethal dose. In this section, five types of medications are examined for features and treatment of toxicity.

Cardiovascular Medications

Cardiovascular medications are commonly prescribed for conditions such as heart failure, dysrhythmias, and hypertension. When used within their therapeutic ranges, they can be quite safe and effective. However, when dosages outside the therapeutic range are taken, toxicity can occur. Three classes of cardiovascular medications that are particularly troublesome in toxic doses are the cardiac glycosides, β–blockers and calcium channel blockers.

Cardiac Glycosides. Cardiac glycoside medications include digoxin and digitoxin and are prescribed for congestive heart failure as well as atrial dysrhythmias. This class of medication is derived from the foxglove plant. Digoxin and digitoxin increase the heart's strength of contraction by providing additional calcium for the cardiac muscle to use for contraction. These medications also increase the parasympathetic tone and decrease the sympathetic tone which results in a decrease in rate and slower electrical conduction through the heart's conduction system, making these medications useful as antiarrhythmic medications.

The clinical features of acute toxicity include nausea, vomiting, diarrhea, headache, confusion, and potentially coma. Cardiovascular manifestations of acute toxicity include supraventricular tachycardia, AV node blocks, or severe bradycardia. These dysrhythmias may develop because of the high levels of potassium (hyperkalemia) that can occur during acute toxicity. The features of chronic toxicity include symptoms of an upper respiratory infection and generally do not include dysrhythmias.

Treatment of acute cardiac glycoside toxicity includes activated charcoal to slow absorption of the medication, atropine or cardiac pacing for symptomatic bradycardias, and lidocaine or magnesium sulfate for ventricular dysrhythmias. Cardioversion should be avoided unless absolutely necessary as it may precipitate a ventricular dysrhythmia that is resistant to treatment. In the emergency department, a digoxin specific antibody can be administered to directly bind and inactivate the digoxin for patients who have ventricular dysrhythmias, symptomatic bradycardia, or a significantly elevated potassium level.

ß–adrenergic Blockers. ß–blockers are first line agents used to treat hypertension. Two types of ß receptors are involved in the sympathetic nervous system, the $ß_1$ receptors located in the heart which affect heart rate, electrical conduction, and decrease hypertension and the $ß_2$ receptors located in the lungs which affect bronchial smooth muscle to create bronchodilation. Some ß–blocker medications are selective for the $ß_1$ receptor and affect only heart rate and blood pressure while others are less selective and can affect bronchodilation. At toxic doses, ß–blockers lose their selectivity and may precipitate bronchospasm. Other signs of ß–blocker overdose include hypotension, bradycardia, AV blocks, cardiogenic shock, and even asystole. CNS effects of ß–blocker overdose can produce seizures, coma, and respiratory arrest. Hypoglycemia and hyperkalemia can also result as insulin release is affected.

Treatment of ß–blocker overdose includes maintaining a patent airway and adequate ventilation. Bradycardia can be treated with atropine or transcutaneous pacing and bronchodilators, for example, albuterol, can be used to treat wheezing from bronchospasm. If the airway is patent, activated charcoal should be administered. Glucagon 5–10 mg can be administered IV or an epinephrine infusion may be required to treat hypotension that is resistant to basic therapies. Wide complex dysrhythmias, indicative of ventricular conduction delay, may respond to a soduim bicarbonate infusion of 1–2 mEq/kg. Polymorphic ventricular tachycardia, or Torsades, may respond to magnesium sulfate or overdrive pacing.

Calcium Channel Blockers. Calcium channel blockers are used for a variety of cardiac illnesses, including atrial arrhythmias, and to treat hypertension. These medications bind to the calcium channel which is located in the cardiac conduction system, myocardium, and coronary artery and peripheral artery smooth muscle. Calcium channel blockers act as negative chronotropes by decreasing SA node automaticity and AV conduction, and negative inotropes by decreasing myocardial force of contraction. These actions work to control the ventricular response to atrial arrhythmias, specifically atrial fibrillation and atrial flutter, improve oxygenation of the myocardium, and decrease blood pressure.

Signs and symptoms of a calcium channel overdose include hypotension and bradycardia. Additional cardiovascular manifestations include AV blocks, sinus arrest with a junctional rhythm, and prolonged PR and QT intervals. Noncardiac manifestations of calcium channel overdose include hyperglycemia, nausea, vomiting, confusion, and altered mental status.

As with ß –blocker overdose, airway and ventilation are the first management priorities. If the airway is patent, charcoal can be administered. Transcutaneous pacing for bradycardia should be considered. Either calcium chloride 10% (0.1–0.2 ml/kg) or calcium gluconate 10% (0.3–0.4 ml/kg) can be administered intravenously every five to ten minutes as needed as a specific antidote. The patient may also respond to glucagon or an epinephrine infusion.

Psychiatric Medications

Psychiatric medications used to treat a variety of psychiatric disorders can be very helpful to the patient in alleviating or controlling symptoms. However, these medications can become deadly when taken in toxic dosages. These medications work by altering the levels of one or more of the neurotransmitters serotonin, norepinephrine, and dopamine in the brain. The main categories of psychiatric medications that are commonly involved in toxic dosages are the tricyclic antidepressants (TCAs), lithium, and monoamine oxidase inhibitors. Another condition, called serotonin syndrome, is also discussed.

Tricyclic Antidepressants. Up until the introduction of the safer selective serotonin reuptake inhibitors (SSRIs—Prozac as an example), tricyclic antidepressants (TCAs) were commonly prescribed as a means of treating major depression and obsessive compulsive disorder. TCAs are still prescribed for these conditions as well as for chronic pain issues and to assist with insomnia. TCAs increase the amount of serotonin and norepinephrine available in the brain. TCAs also bind to the sodium channel on myocardial cells, producing the cardiovascular effects seen with TCA overdose.

Serious toxicity can occur within 6 hours of ingestion. Cardiovascular effects include hypotension, cardiac conduction delays, and dysrhythmias. Common dysrhythmias include sinus tachycardia and prolonged PR, QRS, and QT intervals. CNS effects include a decrease in mental status, respiratory depression, seizures, and coma. Complications of TCA overdose include aspiration pneumonia, pulmonary edema, hyperthermia, and rhabdomyolysis.

Treatment of TCA overdose includes rapidly securing the ABCs and aggressively treating hypotension with fluid boluses. As pulmonary edema is a complication of TCA overdose, the patient should be assessed regularly for both pulmonary and peripheral edema. Dysrhythmias and refractory hypotension tend to respond to administration of sodium bicarbonate. Hypotension that is refractory to fluids may require vasopressor support. Seizures should be managed with benzodiazepines, for example lorazepam or diazepam, to help control the seizure.

Serotonin Syndrome. **Serotonin syndrome** is a rare and life-threatening complication of antidepressant use. Both TCAs and SSRIs act to increase the level of serotonin in the brain to assist with depression. In serotonin syndrome, there is a significant increase in serotonin levels in the brain that causes cognitive impairment, autonomic nervous system dysfunction, and neuromuscular dysfunction. This dramatic increase in serotonin is generally caused by an interaction between medications that produce effects on the serotonin system, with the monoamine oxidase inhibitors (MAOIs) and SSRI combination often used as an example. The added medication does not even have to be another antidepressant.

Serotonin syndrome can be produced by administering meperidine (Demerol), dextromethorphan, or codeine to patients who are on MAOIs or SSRIs because of the increase in serotonin that can occur with those medications. Fortunately, morphine, fentanyl, NSAIDs, and Tylenol are generally safe for these patients.

Signs and symptoms of serotonin syndrome can be divided into CNS, autonomic nervous system, and neuromuscular effects. CNS effects include confusion, agitation, hallucinations, lethargy, coma, and seizures. Autonomic nervous system effects include hyperthermia, tachycardia, hypo- or hypertension, tachypnea, mydriasis, diaphoresis, flushed skin, and diarrhea. The neuromuscular effects in serotonin syndrome include myoclonus or hyperreflexia, tremor, muscle spasms especially in the lower extremities, ataxia, and nystagmus.

Treatment for serotonin syndrome includes maintaining a patent airway, and supporting ventilation and circulation. Benzodiazepines may be helpful for treating muscle rigidity, and other medications are under investigation for treating serotonin syndrome at the receptor level.

Lithium. Lithium is an ion that is used in the treatment of bipolar and other psychiatric disorders. In the nerve cell, it substitutes for sodium and potassium, acting to stabilize the nerve cell membrane and decrease its excitability. In toxic doses, this inhibition is amplified and both nerve conduction and transmission between neurons at the synapse are significantly reduced. As there is a lag between blood lithium level and central nervous system lithium level, the onset of symptoms can lag for hours behind ingestion. Dehydration can also produce lithium toxicity as the body decreases elimination of the ion in the same way it decreases elimination of sodium in an attempt to decrease fluid loss.

Signs of mild to moderate lithium overdose include weakness, slurred speech, lethargy, tremor, myoclonus, and ataxia (see Chapter 9, Nervous System Diseases and Disorders). Severe lithium toxicity can produce agitation, delirium, seizures, coma, and hyperthermia. ECG changes that commonly occur with lithium overdose include inverted T waves, and, less commonly, bradycardia or sinus arrest. Acute ingestions can include nausea and vomiting from gastric irritation while toxicity from chronic ingestion present with more CNS signs and symptoms.

Treatment of lithium toxicity includes managing the airway, breathing, and circulation. Seizures and unresponsiveness should be managed with usual treatment. If the patient is dehydrated, fluid replacement with up to two liters of normal saline may assist in reducing lithium level; however, replacing with more than two liters of normal saline may produce hypernatremia, or high serum sodium concentration, and should be avoided. Activated charcoal does not bind lithium and therefore does not affect toxicity unless other substances are involved. Syrup of ipecac may be useful to induce vomiting if used within a few minutes after an acute ingestion, as in the case of a small child who accidentally ingests their parent's lithium. Diuresis to excrete lithium is not recommended unless the patient has decreased urinary output. There is no specific antidote, and in severe cases of lithium toxicity dialysis may be required.

MAO Inhibitors. Monoamine oxidase inhibitors (MAOIs) are powerful antidepressants that were popular before the advent of SSRIs. This medication inhibits the enzyme monoamine oxidase, increasing the level of catecholamine in the brain and providing effects similar to α–adrenergic stimulation. St. John's wort, a commonly used nutriceutical, is believed to act as a mild MAO inhibitor. While effective at treating depression, MAOIs interact with numerous medications and foods, producing symptoms of toxicity or precipitating serotonin syndrome. Symptoms can be delayed for up to 24 hours after ingestion as the signs and symptoms are produced by an increase in central catecholamines.

Mild toxicity can produce anxiety, flushing, headache, tremor, restlessness, myoclonus, and hyperreflexia (increased reflexes). Sweating, shivering, hypertension, tachycardia, and tachypnea can also accompany mild MAOI toxicity. Severe toxicity can produce significant hypertension, hyperthermia, delirium, and multi-organ system failure.

Treatment of MAOI toxicity includes ensuring adequate airway, ventilation, and circulation. Hypotension may respond to fluid challenge and labetalol, a nonselective ß –blocker. If the airway is patent, charcoal should be administered. As with lithium overdose, syrup of ipecac administered at the scene within several minutes from an acute ingestion may help evacuate the tablets from the stomach.

Sedatives and Hypnotics

Sedatives and hypnotics are medications that are widely prescribed for the treatment of anxiety and insomnia. They act centrally to depress the CNS, providing relaxation or sleep. The major complications of sedative or hypnotic toxicity are CNS depression, respiratory depression, aspiration, and death. There are four subgroups of sedatives and hypnotics that are discussed, barbiturates, benzodiazepines, gamma-hydroxybutyrate (GHB), and chloral hydrate.

Barbiturates act to depress nerve and muscle cell function and also have been used for seizure control. The signs and symptoms mimic ethanol intoxication in mild to moderate doses including confusion, slurred speech, and ataxia. In severe ingestions, the patient may present with coma, complete neurologic unresponsiveness, hypotension, respiratory depression, and noncardiogenic pulmonary edema. Death commonly occurs as a result of respiratory arrest. EMS treatment includes managing the ABCs, initiating an IV of normal saline and administering activated charcoal. Forced diuresis with furosemide and saline or a sodium bicarbonate infusion may assist the body in excreting the barbiturate.

Benzodiazepines also produce CNS depression in the form of drowsiness, confusion, slurred speech, and cognitive impairment. Headache, nausea and vomiting, diarrhea, and joint aches may also occur. Benzodiazapines commonly present in multi-substance overdose. Supportive care is recommended, paying attention to the airway and breathing. Flumazenil is a benzodiazepine antidote that acts much in the same way naloxone works on opioids; however, its use is not recommended as it can cause seizures from interaction in multiple drug overdoses. Diuresis and alkalinazation of the blood and urine with sodium bicarbonate are also not recommended as treatment for benzodiazepine overdose.

Gamma-hydroxybutyrate (GHB) is an illegal drug commonly used among partyers as a date rape drug, because of the rapid onset of unconsciousness that is produced by the drug. It has also been touted as a drug to enhance sexual potency. GHB is structurally similar to GABA, a naturally occurring neurotransmitter that acts to decrease nerve impulse transmission. In acute GHB ingestion, there is a sudden loss of consciousness and loss of protective airway reflexes, with bradycardia, myoclonus, and seizure. In milder intoxication, GHB produces a euphoric state. EMS treatment includes protecting the airway, and supporting ventilation and circulation. If GHB is ingested alone, the patient will usually regain consciousness in two to four hours; however, this is prolonged if other substances, for example, alcohol, were ingested along with GHB. Activated charcoal may be useful in acute ingestions within a short period of time after ingestion, but the use of syrup of ipecac is not recommended.

Chloral hydrate is another sedative/hypnotic drug that produces effects similar to that described above. One of the metabolites of chloral hydrate is also toxic to the central nervous system and can produce ventricular dysrhythmias caused by increased sensitivity to catecholamines. EMS treatment includes protecting the airway, ensuring adequate ventilation and circulation, and treating tachycardias and ventricular dysrhythmias.

Analgesics

Analgesia is defined in *Dorland's Medical Dictionary* as the absence of pain sensation. Analgesic medications act in a way to reduce or eliminate the sensation of pain. According to the 1999 annual report of the American Association of Poison Control Center TESS database, toxic exposure to analgesics was the category with the largest number of deaths. The four main classifications of analgesics include narcotic or opioid analgesics, non-steroidal anti-inflammatory analgesics (NSAIDs), salicylates, and acetaminophen. Each of these medications acts in a different way. Their overuse can produce toxicity.

Narcotic Analgesics. Narcotic analgesics are prescription opioid medications that are prescribed for pain relief in a variety of conditions. Opioids vary in strength and dosing frequency. Some opioids are formulated as a combination medication containing either acetaminophen (e.g., vicodin, a brand name for hydrocodone/acetaminophen) or, less commonly, ibuprofen (e.g., vicoprofen, a brand name for hydrocodone/ibuprofen). The pathophysiology and management of opioid overdose has been discussed under the heading of substance abuse. One additional danger that patients may run into is taking a combination medication such as vicodin and additional over-the-counter acetaminophen. Patients who have been prescribed one of these combination opioid/non-opioid analgesics should be warned by their physician against taking additional over-the-counter analgesics with the combination medication. The pathophysiology and management of ibuprofen and acetaminophen toxicity are discussed below.

NSAIDs. Non-steroidal anti-inflammatory drugs (NSAIDs) are widely available analgesics that can be purchased over-the-counter. They are effective at both analgesia and in stopping the inflammatory cascade. Overuse of NSAIDs often produces only mild GI upset, although significant gastrointestinal bleeds have been reported related to NSAID use. NSAIDs work to decrease prostaglandin production, which is a key element in the inflammatory cascade. Prostaglandins are known to maintain the lining of the GI system and control blood flow through the kidney, so NSAID overdose directly affects these organs. The role of prostaglandins in the liver, lung, and central nervous system is not as well known, although these systems can be involved in NSAID overdose. Finally, NSAIDs also decrease the collection ability of platelets, predisposing the patient to easy bruising or extended bleeding.

Most patients with an NSAID overdose are asymptomatic or present with signs and symptoms of gastric irritation. Other signs present in more significant overdoses include drowsiness, nystagmus, lethargy, ataxia, disorientation, and **tinnitus**, or ringing in the ears. Patients who ingest a massive amount of ibuprofen can present with renal failure, coma, metabolic acidosis, liver failure, and cardiac arrest.

Treatment of an NSAID overdose includes securing the airway, ensuring adequate ventilation with supplemental oxygen or assisted ventilation, and maintaining circulation. Seizures and hypotension can be treated in the usual manner. If the airway is patent, EMS providers should administer charcoal or, if the ingestion occurred within minutes before arrival, induce vomiting with syrup of ipecac. There is no specific antidote for NSAID overdose.

Salicylates. Salicylates are another common, over-the-counter form of analgesia. Many cold formulas and sports creams contain salicylates. Aspirin overdose was the leading cause of death in children before the advent of child-proof caps on medication bottles. On a positive note, aspirin is one very inexpensive medication that has been shown to help reduce mortality and morbidity immediately after an MI and stroke. Another source of salicylates that many people do not consider is in wintergreen flavoring, as many college chemistry students know aspirin is produced from oil of wintergreen.

Salicylate toxicity can produce several different effects. Salicylates stimulate the central respiratory center and produce hyperventilation, and respiratory alkalosis. Within the cells, salicylates interrupt and disconnect the mechanism used to produce energy, producing hyperthermia and acidosis. Cerebral and pulmonary edema are caused by an unknown mechanism. As with NSAIDs, salicylates interfere with platelet aggregation and can prolong bleeding. The signs and symptoms associated with mild salicylate overdose include nausea, vomiting, and GI irritation. Moderate salicylate overdose can also produce hyperventilation, diaphoresis, and tinnitus. Severe salicylate overdose is associated with fever, renal failure, pulmonary edema, adult respiratory distress syndrome, and altered mental status. Rare complications include rhabdomyolysis and gastric perforation.

EMS treatment includes maintaining a patent airway, adequate ventilation, and preventing circulatory collapse. EMS providers should use care in administering IV fluids to avoid pulmonary edema. Activated charcoal should be administered if the airway is patent and inducing vomiting with syrup of ipecac in the first thirty minutes of ingestion may be helpful. Sodium bicarbonate may be administered to help treat acidemia as well as to assist in renal elimination of the salicylate. Hyperthermia can be treated with cooling. There is no specific antidote for salicylate overdose.

Acetaminophen. Tylenol is another common analgesic that is easily available over-the-counter and is a component of several commonly prescribed narcotic–Tylenol combination medications, for example vicodin or lortab. Acetaminophen toxicity predominantly affects the liver, where Tylenol is broken down into a toxic byproduct that is quickly neutralized by a tripeptide, glutathione. The amount of the toxic byproduct released in an overdose exhausts the liver's supply of glutathione, allowing the toxic compounds to build up. Acute ingestions of up to 150–200 mg/kg is potentially dangerous. A nomogram was developed to assist in determining the risk for liver damage using the time from ingestion and the blood level drawn at that time to determine the risk of damage (Figure 15–10). The nomogram begins at four hours from the time of acute ingestion, so accurate determination of the time of ingestion is essential for predicting the likelihood of liver damage and guiding hospital treatment. This nomogram is not helpful in guiding treatment of chronic acetaminophen ingestion.

In an acute ingestion, early symptoms are relatively benign: nausea, vomiting, malaise, and loss of appetite. If untreated, by day two, the patient's nausea and vomiting typically disappear; however, patients develop right upper quadrant pain and tenderness that indicate hepatic toxicity. This may progress to complete liver failure after three or four days if untreated. If the patient survives the liver failure, then there will usually be complete resolution over the course of several weeks.

EMS treatment of acetaminophen overdose includes securing the airway, breathing, and circulation. The EMS provider may need to treat the patient for narcotic overdose if one of the prescription narcotic–acetaminophen tablets was ingested by administering enough naloxone so the patient can maintain an adequate respiratory rate, but not enough to precipitate complete withdrawal. Vomiting can be treated with an antiemetic, and activated charcoal should be administered if less than four hours has passed since the ingestion, except in cases where extended-release acetaminophen was ingested. The specific antidote administered in the hospital is N-acetylcysteine (NAC), a compound that replenishes the

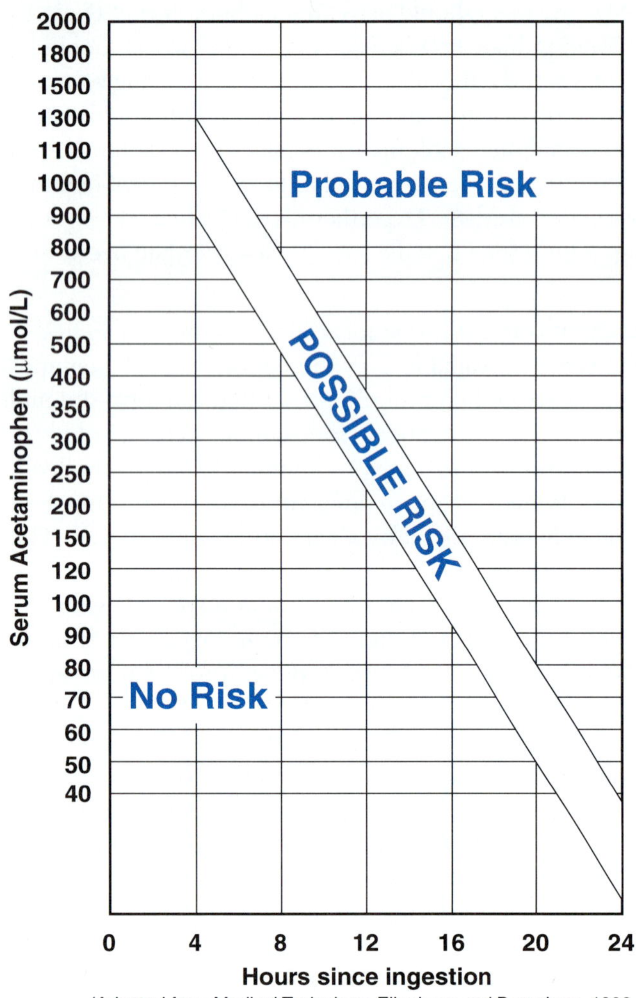

Figure 15-10 Acetaminophen toxicity nomogram in acute overdose. This nomogram should not be used in overdose from chronic ingestion or sustained release preparations. (Reproduced with permission from *Pediatrics*, Vol. 55, Page 971, Figure 1, Copyright 1975.)

liver's supply of glutathione. NAC should be started within eight to ten hours of the time of ingestion. NAC is used to treat all patients who fall above the top line on the nomogram and patients at high risk who fall between the two lines. NAC is not used if the blood acetaminophen level falls below the lower line. This treatment continues for 36 to 72 hours after ingestion. NAC is sometimes used to treat chronic ingestions, for example, a patient who has exceeded the prescribed dosage of acetaminophen over a period of a day or more, if they appear to be at high risk for liver failure.

Xanthines

Theophylline is a methylxanthine used to treat chronic obstructive pulmonary disease, and is believed to act by blocking the adenosine receptor, although the exact mechanism of toxicity is not well established. Caffeine is another commonly used methylxanthine; however, the toxic effects of caffeine are usually not as severe as theophylline. Theophylline has a very small therapeutic window and levels can be artificially raised by interaction with many other medications.

Signs and symptoms of an acute xanthine overdose include tremor, anxiety, vomiting, tachycardia, and electrolyte disturbances. At higher doses, hypotension, status seizures, and ventricular arrhythmias can occur. In chronic overdose, vomiting, electrolyte imbalances, and hypotension are not as common; however, tachycardia is very common and seizures can occur at lower blood levels. EMS treatment of xanthine overdose includes ensuring a patent airway, providing for adequate ventilation, and maintaining the circulatory status. Seizures should be treated in the usual fashion; however, they may be resistant to antiseizure medications. EMS providers should monitor the ECG and treat dysrhythmias according to standard protocols, and administer activated charcoal if the airway is patent in the setting of acute ingestion. As discussed before, syrup of ipecac may be beneficial in the setting of an acute overdose within the first few minutes after the ingestion. Patients with significant elevation of theophylline may require dialysis to clear the medication.

FOOD POISONING

Food poisoning is caused by food-borne bacteria and results from improper preparation of food. In most cases, the toxin is a substance that is produced by the bacteria and is not the direct result of a bacterial infection. The majority of the time, the symptoms include nausea, vomiting, and diarrhea, which begin between two hours and three days after ingestion and usually resolve within twenty-four hours of onset of symptoms. Food poisoning associated with salmonella, shigella, botulism, and some strains of *E. coli* can be deadly, especially for the elderly and children. Signs and symptoms associated with bacterial food poisoning include nausea, vomiting, diarrhea, and abdominal cramps. Profuse vomiting or diarrhea may produce electrolyte imbalances. More severe bacterial food poisoning can present with bloody stools and profuse diarrhea. *E. coli* and shigella can produce significant bloody diarrhea and renal failure with a high mortality rate in children.

Certain fish and shellfish also contain toxins that can produce a variety of signs and symptoms in humans. These toxins are often heat-stable, meaning that cooking the food does not destroy the toxin. Certain toxins are neurotoxic, and can produce numbness, paralysis, and respiratory arrest. Other toxins can produce excitation, headache, and seizures, and produce other GI symptoms.

EMS treatment of food poisoning includes maintaining a patent airway and adequate ventilation, and treating hypotension or dehydration. If the ingested substance is a fish or shellfish and the airway is patent, activated charcoal should be administered. Activated charcoal is not beneficial in bacterial food poisoning. EMS providers should treat anaphylaxis if present. There are no specific antidotes for bacterial food poisoning and fish and shellfish poisoning.

INSECT AND SNAKE BITES

Insects that sting are classified in the order *Hymenoptera* and consist of four families of insects: honeybees; bumblebees; ants; and wasps, hornets, and yellow jackets. Wasps, hornets, and yellow jackets can sting without provocation, while the other insects will sting only if in danger or if the nest is disturbed. Bumblebee stingers will stay in the victim after injection, causing death to the bee. Wasps, hornets, and yellow jackets can sting multiple times, as the stinger is not released from the insect's body. Ants can either sting or deposit their venom into wounds created by biting the host. For most people, stings cause a local inflammatory reaction with redness, swelling, blisters, pain, and occasionally nausea and vomiting. For those allergic to insect stings or in severe stings, respiratory distress, airway or throat edema, hypotension, coagulation disturbances, and rhabdomyolysis can present within fifteen minutes of the sting and become life-threatening. EMS treatment includes assessing and managing the airway, ventilation, and circulation, treating anaphylaxis and hypotension, and if an isolated sting, applying ice to the stinger site to control local inflammation.

There are only five families of poisonous snakes of the fourteen families of snakes that inhabit the United States. Of the few thousand reported snakebites per year, there are only a handful of deaths with the rattlesnake as the most common offender. Snake venom is a mixture of several substances that allow the snake to immobilize, kill, and then digest its prey. Local signs and symptoms of snakebites include fang marks, redness, swelling, and hemorrhagic blisters and a stinging, burning pain (Figure 15–11). Limb swelling, compartment syndrome, and hypovolemic shock can occur within a few hours. Systemic signs and symptoms include nausea, vomiting, weakness, diaphoresis, muscle spasm, tingling around the eyes and mouth, metallic taste, and coagulation changes. In some cases, pulmonary edema and cardiac arrest can occur. EMS treatment includes maintaining a patent airway and adequate ventilation, treating shock with fluid replacement, applying ice to the area of the bite, and removing constricting clothing or jewelry. If possible, EMS providers should wash the bite with soap and water. Making an incision across the fang marks and mouth suction is not recommended. Suction applied to the site within fifteen minutes of the bite may reduce the amount of venom absorbed. EMS providers should immobilize the extremity at the level of the heart. Specific antivenoms are available; however, it is important, if possible, to identify the offending snake so the proper antidote can be administered. EMS providers should not try to capture the snake; but should allow an animal control officer to safely capture or identify it.

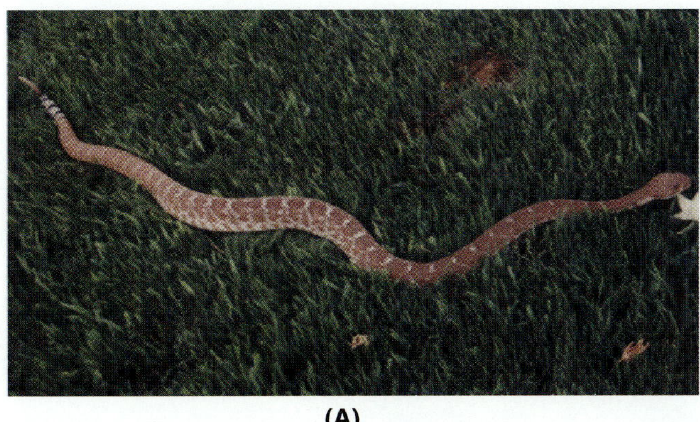

(A)

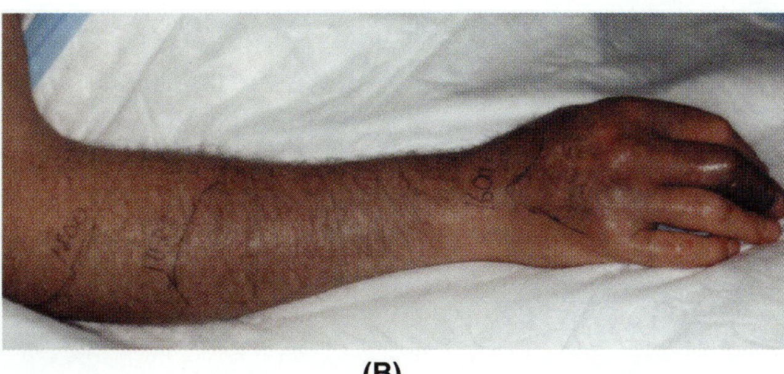

(B)

Figure 15–11 (A) A pit viper can be recognized by the sunken pit in front of each eye. (B) The bite produces local pain and swelling. (Courtesy of Dr. Sean Bush, Loma Linda University Medical Center, Loma Linda CA)

SUMMARY

The field of toxicology involves assessment and management of a wide variety of toxic materials. These materials can involve chemical agents, substances of abuse, medications, food, insect stings, and snakebites. Several toxidromes, or collection of symptoms and signs that occur with a particular class of poison, were presented to assist the reader in assessing and treating similar agents. The assessment and treatment of specific substances were also discussed. General management principles involve scene safety for responders, managing the ABCs, physical decontamination and GI decontamination, and administration of the specific antidote. Guidance for EMS providers managing toxicologic emergencies can be obtained by contacting the regional poison control center or local medical control.

REVIEW QUESTIONS

1. Which of the following toxins utilize injection as the route of entry?
   a. Hymenoptera
   b. Organophosphates
   c. Acetaminophen
   d. Cocaine
2. What is the first priority during a call involving a toxicologic emergency?
   a. Establishing a patent airway.
   b. Initiating intravenous access.
   c. Patient decontamination.
   d. Assessing the scene for safety and utilizing proper personal protective equipment.
3. In order, the four steps in the general management of toxicological emergencies are:
   a. Manage ABCs; External/GI decontamination; Administer specific antidote; Scene safety.
   b. Scene safety; External/GI decontamination; Manage ABCs; Administer specific antidote.
   c. Scene safety; Administer specific antidote; External/GI decontamination; Manage ABCs.
   d. Scene safety; Manage ABCs; External/GI decontamination; Administer specific antidote.
4. Administration of which medication can assist the kidney in eliminating many toxins or toxic byproducts?
   a. Dopamine
   b. Sodium bicarbonate
   c. Atropine
   d. Calcium carbonate
5. Which of the following toxidromes is associated with the SLUDGE signs and symptoms (Salivation, Lacrimation, Urination, Defecation, GI upset, Emesis)?
   a. Sympathomimetic toxidrome
   b. Opioid toxidrome
   c. Cholinergic toxidrome
   d. Anticholinergic toxidrome
6. Which of the following toxidromes is associated with the following memory aid for signs and symptoms: Hot as Hades, Blind as a Bat, Dry as a Bone, Red as a Beet, Mad as a Hatter?
   a. Sympathomimetic toxidrome
   b. Opioid toxidrome
   c. Cholinergic toxidrome
   d. Anticholinergic toxidrome

7. Which of the following medications is the specific antidote for opioid toxicity?
   a. Atropine 2–4 mg IV, repeated as necessary to relieve symptoms.
   b. Naloxone 2 mg IV regardless of respiratory status.
   c. Ethanol drip.
   d. Naloxone 0.4–2 mg IV, titrated to maintain adequate respirations.
8. The state of constant hallucination is called:
   a. Continuous hallucinations
   b. Hallucinosis
   c. Status hallucinosis
   d. Myers' hallucination syndrome
9. Which medication is contraindicated in the setting of cocaine induced myocardial infarction?
   a. Sublingual nitroglycerine
   b. β–blocker
   c. Diazepam
   d. Diltiazem
10. Delirium tremens consists of:
    a. Tachycardia, seizures, and hyperthermia.
    b. Seizures, hyperthermia, and bradycardia.
    c. Tachycardia, seizures, and hypothermia.
    d. Stupor, tachycardia, and hyperthermia.
11. On average, untreated withdrawal from chronic ethanol abuse will progress to delirium tremens between:
    a. 6 and 12 hours after withdrawal.
    b. 18 and 24 hours after withdrawal.
    c. 48 and 72 hours after withdrawal.
    d. 84 and 96 hours after withdrawal.
12. Your patient is stuporous and is suspected of overdosing her prescription pain reliever, Lortab. What other compound do you need to be concerned with toxicity?
    a. Aspirin
    b. Ibuprofen
    c. Salicylate
    d. Acetaminophen
13. Your patient is reported to have accidentally ingested acid from a used car battery. You should administer large quantities of:
    a. Syrup of ipecac.
    b. Activated charcoal.
    c. Vinegar.
    d. Milk.
14. Which assessment modality may produce an incorrect value in the setting of a carbon monoxide poisoning?
    a. Sphygmomanometer
    b. Pulse oximeter
    c. ECG monitor
    d. Pressure readings on the portable ventilator
15. Carbon monoxide binds to hemoglobin:
    a. 200 times better than oxygen.
    b. 20 times better than oxygen.
    c. 20 times less than oxygen.
    d. 200 times less than oxygen.

16. Organophosphates prolong the action of acetylcholine at the:
    a. Presynaptic sympathetic neuron.
    b. Postsynaptic sympathetic neuron.
    c. Neuromuscular junction.
    d. Presynaptic parasympathetic neuron.
17. Chronic lead exposure in children is responsible for:
    a. Decreased intelligence.
    b. Stunted growth.
    c. Impaired development.
    d. All the above.
18. ECG signs of tricyclic antidepressant overdose include:
    a. Widened QRS.
    b. ST segment depression.
    c. Prolonged QT interval.
    d. Both a and c are correct.
19. You are treating a patient who is exhibiting confusion, agitation, and hallucinations, tachycardia, and skin that is very warm to the touch. You find he has been taking phenelzine, a MAO inhibitor, for depression for a long time and dextromethorphan, which he began recently for a cough. You suspect this patient may have:
    a. Serotonin syndrome.
    b. Recently used marijuana.
    c. Recently used cocaine.
    d. Malignant hyperthermia.
20. Acute acetaminophen ingestion above which of the following ranges may be toxic to the liver?
    a. 50–100 mg/kg
    b. 100–150 mg/kg
    c. 150–200 mg/kg
    d. 200–250 mg/kg

CASE STUDY

You respond for a 34-year-old male found unresponsive by family. You note the patient is breathing at a rate of approximately 4 breaths per minute, vomitus on the floor, and several empty beer and liquor bottles in the room. The patient's sister also hands you an empty pill bottle that was for 30 vicodin tablets that was filled yesterday. The patient's brother also states that the patient was "feeling down" the last few days because his chronic back pain was acting up. What are your priorities in assessment and management of this patient? What specific treatments should you consider for this patient?

BIBLIOGRAPHY

Bureau of Justice Statistics. *Drug use*. United States Department of Justice. Available on-line at *http://www.ojp.usdoj.gov/bjs/dcf/du.htm*.

Bureau of Justice Statistics. *Drug use and crime*. United States Department of Justice. Available on-line at *http://www.ojp.usdoj.gov/bjs/dcf/duc.htm*.

Committee on Environmental Health. *Screening for elevated blood lead levels: Policy statement* (RE9815). American Association of Pediatrics, 1998. Available on-line at *http://www.aap.org/policy/re9815.html*.

Cline, D. M., (Ed.) (2000). *Emergency medicine companion handbook* (5th ed.). New York: McGraw Hill.

Goldfrank, L. R., (Ed.) (1994). *Toxicologic emergencies* (5th ed.). Norwalk, CT: Appleton & Lange.

Litovitz, T. L., Klein-Schwarta, W., White, S., Cobaugh, D. J., Youniss, J., Drab, A., & Benson, B. (2000)/1999. Annual report of the American Association of Poison Control Centers toxic exposure surveillance system. *American Journal of Emergency Medicine*, *18*(5), 517–574.

Office of Applied Studies. Summary of findings from 1999 national household survey on drug abuse. U.S. Substance Abuse and Mental Health Services Administration. Available on-line at *http://www.samhsa.gov/oas/oas.html*.

Olson, K. R. (Ed.) (1999). *Poisoning and drug overdose*. Stamford, CT: Appleton & Lange.

Rothrock, S. G. (1999). *Adult emergency pocketbook*. Loma Linda, CA: Tarascon Publishing.

Tintinalli, J. E., (Ed.) (1996). *Emergency medicine: A comprehensive study guide* (4th ed.). New York: McGraw Hill.

CHAPTER 16

Hematologic System Diseases and Disorders

CONTENT OUTLINE

- Anatomy and Physiology
- Common Signs and Symptoms
- Diagnostic Tests
- Common Diseases of the Hematologic System
  - Disorders of Red Blood Cells
  - Disorders of White Blood Cells
  - Disorders of Platelets
- Trauma
- Developmental and Genetic Disorders
- Effects of Aging on the System

KEY TERMS

Anemia
Bence Jones protein
Bleeding time
Complete blood count (CBC)
Differential
Dyspnea
Ecchymosis
Epistaxis
Erythrocytopenia
Erythrocytosis
Extrinsic pathway
Fibrinolysis
Hemarthrosis
Hematemesis
Hematocrit
Hematuria
Hemoglobin
Hemolyzed
Hypovolemia
Intrinsic pathway
Leukemia
Leukocytopenia
Leukocytosis
Lymphopenia
Neutropenia
Pallor
Pancytopenia
Petechiae
Purpura
Reed-Sternberg cell
Syncope
Tachycardia
Tachypnea
Thrombocytopenia
Thrombocytosis

LEARNING OBJECTIVES

Upon completion of the chapter, the student should be able to:

1. Define the terminology common to the hematologic system and the disorders of the hematologic system.
2. Identify the common disorders of the hematologic system.
3. Discuss the basic anatomy and physiology of the hematologic system.
4. Identify the important signs and symptoms associated with common hematologic system disorders.
5. Describe the common diagnostic tests used to determine type and/or cause of the hematologic system disorders.
6. Describe the typical course and management of the common hematologic system disorders.
7. Describe the effects of aging upon the hematologic system and the common disorders of hematologic system.

OVERVIEW

The hematologic system consists of the blood and the organs that produce and filter the blood.The blood is the body's life fluid. It is responsible for transporting nutrients to cells and removing wastes. The hematologic system organs are the lymph nodes, bone marrow, spleen, and liver. Disorders of the system may have severe effects on other systems because of the responsibilities of the blood and these organs. Altered nutrition, medications, and diseases of other systems, in turn, can greatly affect the functioning of the hematologic system.

ANATOMY AND PHYSIOLOGY

The major function of the blood is to transport necessary oxygen and nutrients to the cells and to aid in the removal of wastes. The blood also transports hormones secreted by the endocrine system. In addition, the white blood cells (leukocytes) are important in infection prevention. The blood is composed of a variety of substances. The plasma portion of the blood is a straw-colored liquid and makes up about fifty-five percent of the total. The formed elements constitute the other forty-five percent of the total. They include the erythrocytes (red blood cells or RBCs), leukocytes (white blood cells or WBCs), and platelets (clotting fragments) (Figure 16–1).

Descriptive properties of the blood include its color, volume, viscosity, and pH. Blood is bright red in the arteries because of its oxygen content. Blood in the veins is a dark red (often pictured as blue) because of the loss of oxygen. The average adult has about seventy-five ml/kg of body weight of circulating blood (five to six liters or approximately one and a half gallons). The viscosity or density of blood is about three or more times greater than water. Blood is slightly alkaline (pH 7.35–7.45).

The erythrocytes transport oxygen from the lungs to the tissues. The normal erythrocyte count is 4.2 to 6.3 million and their life span is only about 120 days. Erythrocytes formed in the bone marrow do not contain a cell nucleus, and do not reproduce. Erythrocyte production increases when oxygen demand increases. During their life span, the red cells become worn and often ragged from bumping and bouncing into the vessel walls of the circulatory system. The worn RBCs are filtered out of circulation by the spleen and liver. These organs are responsible for breaking down the RBC and

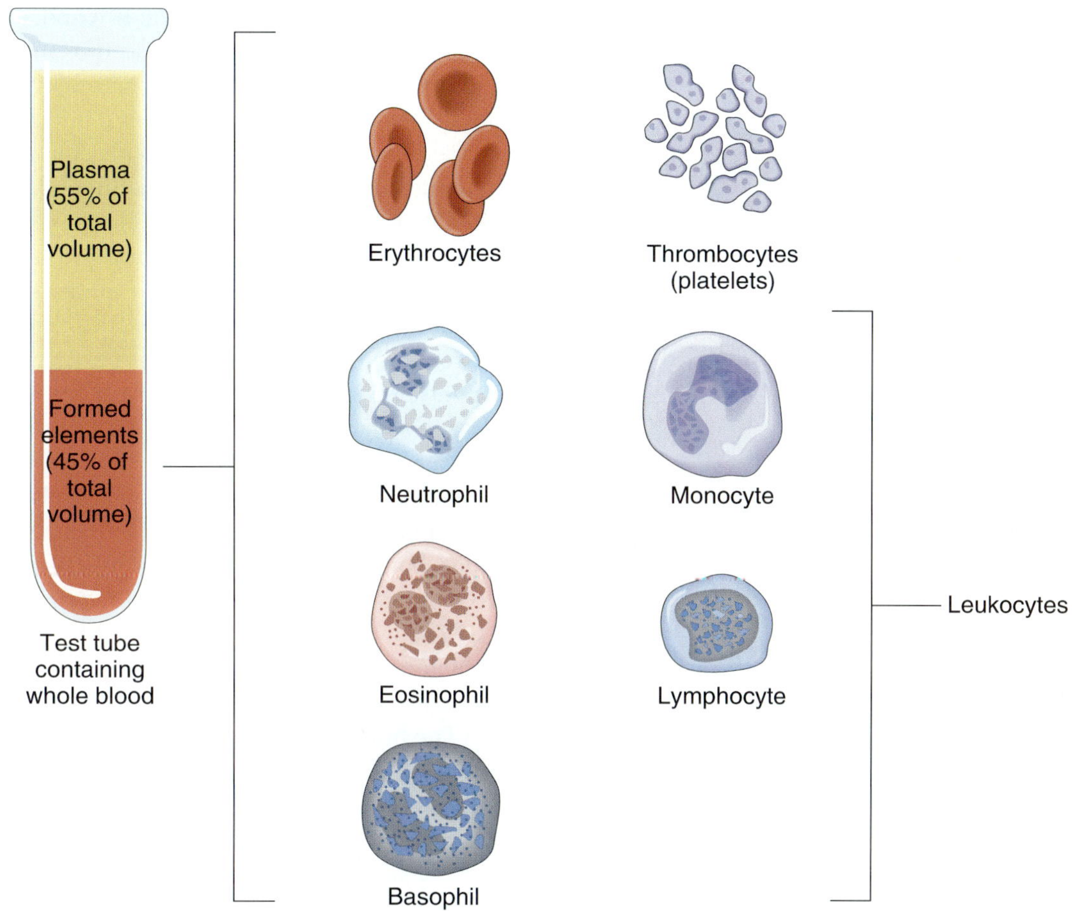

Figure 16–1 Blood components.

saving the iron component for reuse in the development of new RBCs.

Hemoglobin, a component of the red blood cell, is important in the transport of oxygen. A low level of hemoglobin in the blood reduces the level of circulating oxygen. The normal level of hemoglobin for an adult male is 13.5–18g/100 ml and 12–16g/100 ml for an adult female.

Leukocytes are concerned with protecting the individual from infections. The functions of the five types of leukocytes, neutrophils, eosinophils, basophils, monocytes, and lymphocytes (Figure 16–1), are discussed in Chapter 12. The average white blood cell count for an adult is 4,500–11,000 mm^3. A count higher than 11,000 usually indicates the presence of an infection. See Chapters 4 and 12 for more information about leukocytes.

Platelets (also called thrombocytes) produce the thrombokinase used in the clotting process. The average number of platelets in adults is 150,000– 350,000/mm^3 of blood. Platelets also participate in tissue repair and release proteins that promote coagulation.

The plasma portion of blood is composed of ninety-one percent water and nine percent plasma proteins. The plasma proteins include (1) albumin, responsible for maintaining osmotic pressure; (2) globulin, responsible for infection fighting; (3) fibrinogen, responsible for a part of the clotting process; and (4) prothrombin, also responsible for a part of the clotting process.

Coagulation, or the formation of blood clots, is a process that occurs continuously. At the same time, the body is continuously breaking down clots that have formed and are no longer needed. These two mechanisms operate in a balance to allow the body to repair itself and prevent it from producing too many clots. Tipping this balance in either direction can have serious consequences.

The coagulation system operates as a cascade of events that results in the formation of fibrin clots. This system has two pathways to activate clots, an **intrinsic pathway** and an **extrinsic pathway** (Figure 16–2). Each pathway is composed of different clotting factors and feeds into the common pathway to producing fibrin. These clotting factors are proteins that will undergo a

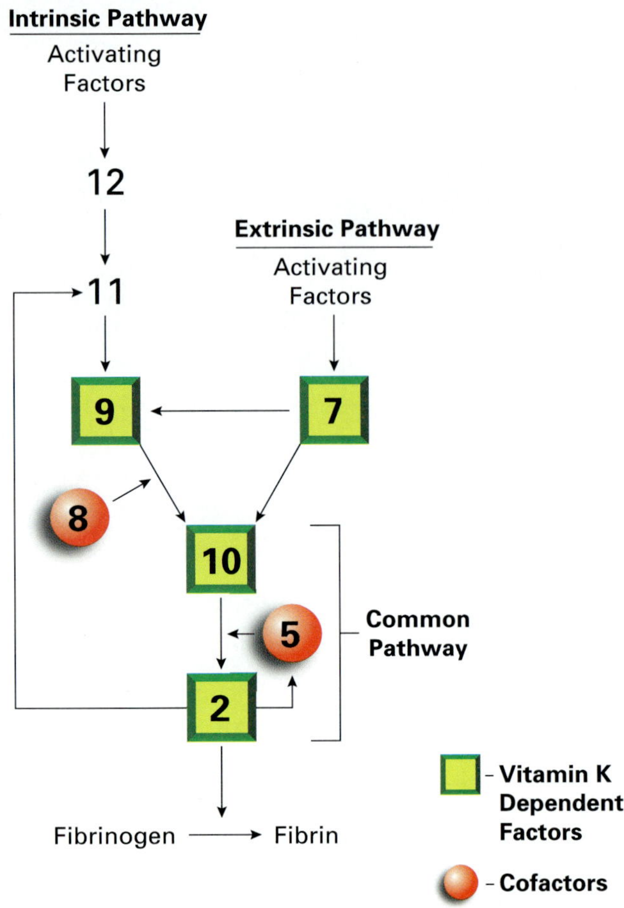

Figure 16–2 Coagulation pathways. The vitamin K dependent factors are shown in green. Factors 5 and 8 are cofactors necessary to carry out the next step in the pathway. Factor 2 (thrombin), when activated, also activates factors 5 and 11 promoting additional coagulation.

change when activated that will in turn activate the next factor in the pathway. Several of these factors require Vitamin K, a vitamin found in green vegetables, to work properly; all factors are produced in the liver. Therefore, a deficiency in Vitamin K or liver disease will affect a patient's ability to clot. Calcium is also required for these clotting factors to work properly.

When the wall of a blood vessel is damaged, even on a microscopic level, it releases several factors that promote clotting. Healthy tissue will release proteins that serve as the body's natural anticoagulants to prevent formation of unnecessary clots that could become lodged in blood vessels. These proteins also dissolve old clot after the tissue heals. This process is called **fibrinolysis**. Calcium is required for this system to work properly.

Blood is classified by the antigens in the red blood cells and the antibodies in the plasma. The antigens are A and B and the antibodies are anti-A and anti-B. In addition, a factor called Rh is also used in the classification system (see Chapter 12 under erythroblastosis fetalis and blood transfusion reaction for more information). Blood is typed as A, B, AB, and O. Type A blood has A antigens and anti-B antibodies, type B blood has B antigens and anti-A antibodies, type AB blood has A and B antigens and does not have anti-A or anti-B antibodies, and type O blood has neither A nor B antigens but has both anti-A and anti-B antibodies. The Rh designation is based on twelve different antigens. Rh positive blood has this antigen present while Rh negative does not. Because of these designations and blood properties, blood transfusion recipients must have a type and crossmatch of blood to be certain a reaction will not occur (Table 16–1).

The hematologic system organs include the lymph nodes, bone marrow, spleen, and liver. The lymph nodes are found throughout the body along the lymphatic vessels. The lymph system is important for protection from pathogens. The nodes filter the lymph and produce lymphocytes and antibodies.

The bone marrow is found in the center part of long bones and in the spongy part of other bones. The bone marrow is the major blood cell producing organ in the body.

The spleen is found in the upper left quadrant of the abdomen. It produces lymphocytes, plasma cells, and antibodies, and filters microorganisms from the blood. It also removes old blood cells from the body.

The liver is a large organ found in the right upper quadrant of the abdomen. It has multiple responsibilities for many body systems. The liver functions as a blood-forming organ in intrauterine life and is active the rest of the individual's life as a producer of prothrombin and fibrinogen for blood clotting.

COMMON SIGNS AND SYMPTOMS

Signs and symptoms of this system include those related to increases and decreases in the number of blood cells. Diseases affecting the blood-forming organs (primarily spleen, bone marrow, and lymph nodes) may lead to decreased or increased production of cells. Diseases that hemolyze, destroy, or use up the cells, will also lead to a decrease in cell number and volume.

Erythrocytopenia (erythro = red, cyte = cell, penia = decrease) leads to **anemia** (an = without, emia = blood). Anemia does not mean without any blood, it means a low number of red blood cells or decreased blood volume. Anemia may be asymptomatic to life-threatening depend-

TABLE 16–1 Blood Donor and Recipient Chart

		Recipients			
	Blood Types	**O**	**A**	**B**	**AB**
Donors	O	YES	YES	YES	YES
	A	NO	YES	NO	YES
	B	NO	NO	YES	YES
	AB	NO	NO	NO	YES

YES = This type (row) can donate blood and this type (column) can receive the blood.

NO = This type (row) cannot donate blood and this type (column) cannot receive the blood without a transfusion reaction.

ing on cause. Common signs and symptoms include a low erythrocyte count, headache, fatigue, **pallor**, and shortness of breath.

Erythrocytosis (erythrocyte = red cell, osis = condition) is a condition of increased red blood cells. Common signs and symptoms include a high red blood cell count, reddened skin tones, blood shot eyes, increased blood volume and pressure, and an increase in the workload of the heart.

Leukocytopenia (leuko = white, cyte = cell, penia = decrease) is a decrease in white cell count. Leukocytopenia weakens the immune system as these cells are primary players in our defense system. **Neutropenia** (neutrophil decrease) and **lymphopenia** (lymphocyte decrease) may be associated with chronic infection as the cells are "used up" during a long-term battle. Signs and symptoms are related to the particular type of infection.

Leukocytosis (leukocyto = white cell, osis = condition of) is an increase in white cell count. This condition is a normal response to acute infection. If leukocytosis is related to a tumor these numbers may be extreme, as in the case of **leukemia** (leuk = white, emia = blood).

Thrombocytopenia (THROM-boh-SIGH-toh-**PEE**-nee-ah; thrombocyte = platelet, penia = decrease) is a decrease in platelets, resulting in a coagulation problem. Signs and symptoms include small hemorrhages in the skin called **petechiae** (pee-TEE-kee-ee), large areas of bruising or hemorrhage called **ecchymoses** (ECH-ih-**MOH**-ses), and **epistaxis** (EP-ih-**STACK**-sis; nosebleeds). Bleeding lesions in the mouth, gums, and mucous membranes are also common.

Thrombocytosis (THROM-boh-sigh-**TOE**-sis; thrombocyte = platelet, osis = condition of) is an increase in platelets. This condition is uncommon and usually has no serious side effects (Table 16–2).

TABLE 16–2 Blood Cell Abnormalities and Associated Symptoms

RED BLOOD CELLS
INCREASED—Erythrocytosis–reddened skin, increased blood pressure, increased workload on the heart
DECREASED—Erythrocytopenia–anemia
WHITE BLOOD CELLS
INCREASED—Leukocytosis–increased white cell count
DECREASED—Leukocytopenia–weakened immune system
THROMBOCYTES (PLATELETS)
INCREASED—Thrombocytosis–increased clotting
DECREASED—Thrombocytopenia–increased bleeding

DIAGNOSTIC TESTS

Diagnostic tests for blood and blood-forming organ disorders include complete blood count (CBC) with differential and indices. Biopsy of the blood-forming organs may also be helpful in diagnosing disorders of the spleen, lymph nodes, and bone marrow.

A **complete blood count** (CBC) identifies the number of red blood cells (RBCs), white blood cells (WBCs), and platelets per cubic millimeter (Table 16–3). A CBC may be utilized in the determination of most blood diseases. Red blood cell count and indices can assist in the determination of the different anemias, polycythemia, and erythrocytosis. A **differential** is a more detailed count identifying the number of each type of leukocyte. A white

TABLE 16-3 Complete Blood Count (CBC) Normal Values

Cells	Values
Erythrocytes	**Males**
	4.6–6.3 million/mm^3
	Females
	4.2–5.4 million/mm^3
Hematocrit	**Males**
	40–54%
	Females
	38–47%
Hemoglobin	**Males**
	13.5–18 g/dl
	Females
	12–16 g/dl
Red Blood Cell Indices	
MCV	80–96 um^3
MCH	27–31 pg
MCHC	32–36%
Leukocytes	4500–11,000 million/mm^3
Differential	
Myelocytes	0 /mm^3
Band neutrophils	1500–3000 /mm^3
Segmented neutrophils	300–500 /mm^3
Lymphocytes	50–250 /mm^3
Monocytes	15–50 /mm^3
Eosinophils	15–50 /mm^3
Basophils	15–50 /mm^3
Platelets	150,000–350,000 /mm^3
Reticulocytes	25,000–75,000 /mm^3

Key:
mm^3 = cubic millimeter
g/dl = grams per deciliter
pg = picograms

blood cell count and differential may assist in determination of the cause of inflammation and infection or white cell tumors. **Hematocrit** (Hct) reflects the amount of red cell mass as a proportion of whole blood. The red cell mass depends upon both the number and size of the red blood cells. If the number of red cells increases or the size of the red cells increases, then the hematocrit will increase. Conversely, if the number or size of the red blood cells decreases, then the hematocrit will decrease. The hematocrit will also change based on the amount of plasma in the blood because the value is computed as a percent of the whole blood. If the patient is dehydrated, his hematocrit will increase because the total amount of red blood cell mass has not changed, but the total volume of whole blood has decreased. In the early stage of bleeding, the patient is losing the same proportion of plasma and red blood cells, therefore the hematocrit will initially remain constant. The body will then compensate for the loss of blood by drawing fluid into the blood vessels; however, the patient is unable to increase red cell production to equal the rate of red blood cell loss. In this case, the hematocrit will decrease because the net loss of fluid is less than the loss of red blood cells. If a patient is not producing red blood cells fast enough to replace the ones that die, then his hematocrit will also decrease.

Hemoglobin (Hgb) reflects the amount of hemoglobin or oxygen carrying potential available in the blood. Special measurements of red cells are called indices and include:

- MCV—mean corpuscular volume, reflects average size of the red cell
- MCH—mean corpuscular hemoglobin or average hemoglobin content
- MCHC—mean corpuscular hemoglobin concentration, or average hemoglobin concentration.

The morphology, or shape, of each of the cells and platelets may be observed by performing a blood smear. A blood smear is performed by placing a drop of blood on a glass slide, smearing it to spread the cells to a thin layer, and staining and examining it microscopically for abnormal cell morphology or shape. Adding a staining solution to the slide helps in the identification of the different types of WBCs. A blood smear may be helpful in determination of the cause of anemia, especially sickle cell disease.

A **bleeding time** test may assist in determination of platelet disorders such as hemophilia, thrombocytopenia, and disseminated intravascular coagulation (DIC). A bleeding time test is performed by pricking the earlobe of the involved individual and measuring the amount of time it takes for the area to clot or stop bleeding. Prothrombin time (PT) and partial thromboplastin time (PTT) are both blood tests measuring the ability of the blood to clot related to clotting factors. The PT measures the extrinsic clotting pathway and the PTT measures the intrinsic clotting pathway.

Biopsy of blood-forming organs may be helpful in diagnosing diseases and disorders. A bone marrow biopsy is performed by boring a needle into the bone of the iliac crest of the hip to obtain tissue. This tissue is prepared and microscopically examined. Lymph node biopsy may be performed to determine proper functioning of the marrow, detect anemias, and diagnose neoplasms.

COMMON DISEASES OF THE HEMATOLOGIC SYSTEM

The most common problem related to this system is anemia. Anemia is a decrease in red blood cell mass which may be caused by a number of different disease processes. Anemia is generally a symptom of a disease, but is commonly used as a diagnosis until the cause is discovered. Anemia may be serious if the cause is not determined or cannot be corrected.

Disorders of white blood cells are usually secondary to other diseases rather than a primary disease. Infections demand an increased need for WBCs, as they are used up while fighting the invader. This may lead to leukocytopenia or a decrease in white blood cell number.

Any disorders of the organs (spleen, bone marrow, and lymph nodes) may lead to secondary disorders of this system. Leukemias, lymphomas, and myelomas are the primary tumors affecting the system.

Disorders of Red Blood Cells

Any increase or decrease in number or size of red blood cells will affect the mass or volume. Red cell mass is important as it directly affects the amount of hemoglobin available and thus oxygen-carrying potential. Commonly the problem is not enough red cell mass leading to anemia. Too much red cell mass is called erythrocytosis. The most common type of erythrocytosis is a condition called polycythemia.

Anemia. Anemia is any decrease in oxygen-carrying ability of the red blood cell. This is commonly caused by a low number of RBCs, or a decrease in hemoglobin in RBCs. Acute hemorrhage or chronic bleeding may lead to a low number of circulating RBCs, and thus anemia.

Any disease of the liver, spleen, or bone marrow may also lead to anemia. If the cells are broken down (**hemolyzed**) too soon this may lead to a decrease in cell number. If cells are not formed quickly enough to replace the worn cells, the number of circulating cells will be low. If cells are formed abnormally, their ability to carry oxygen may be impaired. In this case the number of cells may be adequate, but oxygen-carrying ability is not adequate. Dietary deficiencies may lead to an inadequate supply of needed nutrients to make RBCs.

Despite the cause, the symptoms of anemia are fairly common. The individual suffering from anemia commonly is pale or has a condition of **pallor**. Facial paleness may be difficult to determine, but further examination of the mucous membranes of the mouth and conjunctiva of the eyes will reveal definite paleness. The nail beds may also be noticeably pale in color.

Anemic individuals are weak and suffer with fatigue caused by poor oxygenation of muscle tissue. Shortness of breath, **dyspnea** (DISP-nee-ah; dys = difficult, pnea = breathing), **tachycardia** (TACH-ee-**KAR**-dee-ah; tachy = fast, cardia = heart), and **tachypnea** (TACK-ihp-**NEE**-ah; tachy = fast, pnea = breathing) are common as the heart and lungs attempt to meet the body's oxygen need. Headache, irritability, and **syncope** (SIN-koh-pee; fainting) are also common symptoms.

Determining the cause of anemia is very important as treatment is directed at the cause. Complete blood counts will often indicate low cell number, and low hemoglobin and hematocrit. Treatment for anemia varies depending on cause or type of anemia. Some anemias may be cured with treatment, while others, like sickle cell anemia, are not curable.

Iron Deficiency Anemia. Iron deficiency anemia may be caused by a loss of iron or an inadequate intake of iron. Chronic blood loss may lead to loss of iron and thus this type of deficiency anemia. Chronic blood loss may be caused by bleeding hemorrhoids, gastrointestinal bleeding, and heavy or prolonged menstrual flow. Low dietary intake of iron may also lead to this type of anemia. Iron deficiency anemia is commonly seen in females during times of increased iron demand. Increased iron is needed during pregnancy and with breastfeeding. During menstrual years, females often have the combination of iron loss with menstruation and inadequate dietary intake of iron. Treatment is aimed at the cause and may include increasing dietary intake of iron.

Folic Acid Deficiency Anemia. Folic acid is a B complex vitamin that is needed for the maturation of red blood cells. Deficiency of folic acid may be related to poor diet, overcooking vegetables, or as a consequence of alcoholism. The deficiency may occur during times of high folic acid need like those associated with infancy and pregnancy. Treatment is aimed at increasing dietary intake of folic acid by eating green and yellow vegetables.

Pernicious Anemia. Pernicious anemia has an unusual cause. The mucosa or lining of the stomach secretes a protein called intrinsic factor. This factor is needed for vitamin B_{12} to be absorbed in the small intestine. Vitamin B_{12} is essential for red blood cell formation. Pernicious anemia is caused by a lack of intrinsic factor leading to inadequate absorption of vitamin B_{12} and thus anemia. Increasing the dietary intake of vitamin B_{12} will not alleviate the problem. Treatment is a monthly injection of vitamin B_{12} for the life of the individual. Pernicious anemia usually affects older individuals and is thought to be related to an autoimmune disorder.

Hemolytic Anemia. Hemolytic anemia is characterized by increased destruction of red blood cells. It may be related to an antigen-antibody reaction as with Rh factor in blood transfusion reaction or erythroblastosis fetalis (see Chapter 12 for detailed information). Hemolytic anemia may also occur from a disorder of the immune system leading to destruction of one's own erythrocytes. This type of anemia may be severe and lead to the death of the individual. Hemolytic anemia may be brought on by exposure to chemicals such as benzene, medications, including aspirin and penicillin, and bacterial toxins. Treatment may include prompt exchange transfusion (removal of the individual's blood and replacement by donor blood). A splenectomy (removal of the spleen) may also be required for some patients.

Sickle Cell Anemia. Sickle cell anemia is a hereditary anemia found in the black race that causes an abnormal sickle shape of the erythrocyte. The sickle cell has abnormal hemoglobin that causes it to elongate when deoxygenated or as it loses the oxygen load. The cell regains its normal shape once it is re-oxygenated or picks up an oxygen load (Figure 16–3). The sickle shape causes a problem in that it does not allow the cell to travel smoothly through small blood vessels. Sickle cells tend to stick and clump together in small vessels leading to occlusion of the vessel, ischemia, and infarction. This occlusion may occur in any vessel causing multiple thrombi (clots) and emboli (traveling clots) formations that may lead to infarctions throughout the body, including the vital organs.

Symptoms of the disease may vary from mild to severe. Individuals suffering severe symptoms often die in infancy or childhood. Few severely affected individuals live beyond age twenty. Even mildly affected individuals usually die before age fifty.

There is no cure for sickle cell disease. Treatment is symptomatic. An increase in fluid intake to two times the normal amount may be beneficial. Additional fluids increase blood volume and improve sickle cell movement. Analgesia is also administered to treat the severe pain that accompanies attacks.

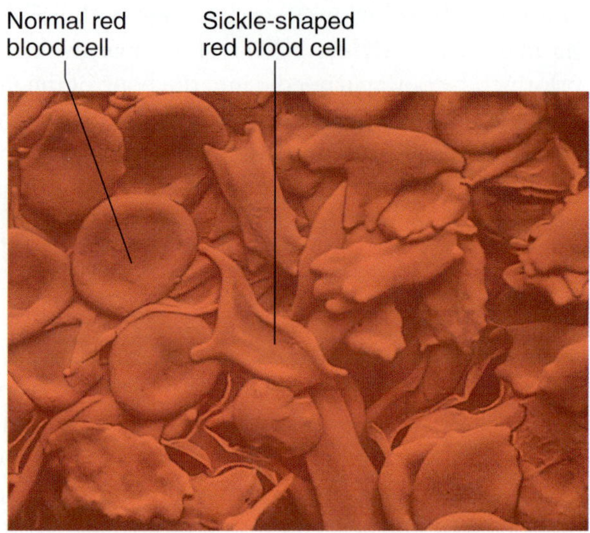

Figure 16–3 Sickled erythrocytes. (Courtesy of Philips Electronic Instrument Company.)

Hemorrhagic Anemia. Acute loss of large amounts of blood leads to hemorrhagic anemia. This may lead to **hypovolemia** or low blood volume. Severe hypovolemia may lead to life-threatening shock (low blood pressure). If the loss is not severe, blood fluid will be replaced within a few hours, decreasing the risk of shock. The decreased number of circulating erythrocytes will stimulate the bone marrow to step up production of erythrocytes. Bone marrow has the potential to replace large amounts of blood cells thus correcting this type of anemia. If the individual is symptomatic, blood transfusions may be the treatment of choice.

Aplastic Anemia. Aplastic anemia is characterized by failure of the bone marrow to produce blood components. A severe decrease or total absence of erythrocytes, leukocytes, and thrombocytes, called **pancytopenia** (pan = all, cyto = cell, penia = decrease), is commonly seen. This decrease in blood cells leads to anemia, infection, and hemorrhage respectively. This anemia is caused by injury or destruction of the blood-forming area of the bone marrow. Causes include chemotherapy, radiation, viruses, and chemical toxins. Severe cases of aplastic anemia have a poor prognosis with fifty percent fatality. Treatment includes discontinuing or avoiding the causative agent. Other treatment may include bone marrow transplantation and blood transfusions.

Polycythemia. Polycythemia is also called primary polycythemia or polycythemia vera. It is a condition of too many blood cells. This condition is caused by hyperplasia (hyper = excessive, plasia = growth) of the cell-forming tissues of the bone marrow leading to an increase in the production of erythocytes, leukocytes, and thrombocytes. This disease has an unknown etiology. The increase in erythrocytes leads to an increase in blood volume. Increased blood volume raises blood pressure and causes an increase in the workload of the heart. The spleen, an organ of blood cell storage, is enlarged. The mucous membranes are reddened in color and the eyes often appear bloodshot. The palms of the hands are noticeably a deeper red color. Treatment is to reduce the red cell count and thus blood volume. Radiation of the bone marrow may be effective in reducing red cell count. Phlebotomy or donating blood at regular intervals will reduce the volume.

Another type of polycythemia is called secondary polycythemia or erythrocytosis (erythocyte = red cell, osis = condition of). Secondary polycythemia differs from primary polycythemia in that only red cell numbers are increased. Erythrocytosis is a protective mechanism of the body to meet the need for extra oxygen. This is a normal compensatory mechanism for people in high altitudes, where oxygen content of air is low. Also highly trained athletes may have erythrocytosis in order to meet the high oxygen demands of the body's muscle tissue. Certain respiratory and circulatory conditions cause a decrease in oxygen supply to the tissues and thus stimulate erythrocytosis. When the condition for extra oxygen is returned to normal, the erythrocytosis disappears. For example, if people living in high altitudes move to a lower altitude, the red cell count will return to a normal level.

Disorders of White Blood Cells

Disorders of white blood cells are common problems of the hematologic system, especially among certain age groups. The common symptom of white blood cell disorders is a compromised immune response leaving the individual susceptible to infections.

Mononucleosis. Mononucleosis is a viral infection that affects primarily children and young adults. It is somewhat contagious and is commonly called "kissing disease." Symptoms include fatigue, sore throat, and swollen lymph glands. Diagnosis is confirmed by a white blood cell count showing a marked elevation in monocytes. Treatment is symptomatic, including rest, analgesics, and throat gargles.

Leukemia. Leukemia is a malignant neoplasm of the blood-forming organs (bone marrow, lymph nodes, and spleen). It is characterized by an abnormally high production of leukocytes that are immature and function abnormally. This increase of white cells in the blood-forming organs causes a decrease in the production of erythrocytes and platelets.

Leukemia may be classified as acute or chronic. Acute forms commonly affect children, progress rapidly, and may be fatal. Chronic forms occur more commonly in older adults, are often asymptomatic, and may not be the cause of death. Leukemia is also classified as myelogenous (affecting the bone marrow) and lymphocytic (affecting the lymph nodes). The cause of leukemia is unknown. It is usually diagnosed by clinical history and blood studies. A bone marrow biopsy is the most definitive test confirming the diagnosis.

Symptoms of leukemia include fatigue, headache, sore throat, dyspnea, bleeding of the mucous membranes of the mouth and gastrointestinal system, bone and joint pain, and enlargement of lymph nodes, liver, and spleen. Infections are common as white cells are not functioning properly. Bleeding disorders and anemia are caused by erythrocytopenia and thrombocytopenia, respectively.

Treatment includes aggressive chemotherapy utilizing several neoplastic agents. Once in remission, a bone marrow transplant to replace the neoplastic tissue with normal tissue may be performed. Pain from enlargement of lymph nodes, spleen, and liver may be treated with analgesics. Complete remission occurs approximately fifty percent of the time depending on the type of leukemia and the individual's tolerance of the treatment.

Lymphoma. Lymphoma refers to several types of neoplasms that affect lymphoid tissue (lymph nodes, tonsils, spleen, and lymph fluid). There are many types of lymphoma, but all affect normal lymphocyte production leading to an impaired immunity.

Hodgkin's Disease. Hodgkin's disease is the most common lymphoma. It is characterized by painless enlargement of the lymph nodes in the neck, weight loss, and fever. Hodgkin's primarily affects young adults with the average age of thirty-five years. Men are affected with Hodgkin's at a slightly higher rate than women. Diagnosis is made by the presence of a large cell called **Reed-Sternberg cell** in lymphatic tissue. The diagnosis may be confirmed by lymph node and bone marrow biopsy. Treatment with radiation and chemotherapy is usually effective to bring about remission. If the disease is kept in remission for five years or longer, complete cure may be possible. Mortality rate is approximately twenty percent.

Non-Hodgkin's Lymphoma (NHL). Non-Hodgkin's lymphoma (NHL) is a group of lymphomas not containing the Reed-Sternberg cell characteristic of Hodgkin's. NHL initially is more widespread than Hodgkin's. Usually there is painless enlargement of lymph nodes in the neck, axilla, and inguinal areas. Other symptoms include fever, night sweats, and weight loss. NHL affects older adults with the average age of fifty years. Men are affected one and a half times more often than women. The cause of NHL is unknown, but individuals receiving or who have received immunosuppressive medications have more than 100 times greater chance of developing NHL. Treatment and prognosis depends on the type of NHL, but some combination of radiation and chemotherapy is usually of benefit.

Multiple Myeloma. Multiple myeloma is a malignant neoplasm of plasma cells or B lymphocytes. The plasma cells multiply abnormally in the bone marrow causing weakness in the bone leading to pathologic fractures and bone pain (Figure 16–4). Multiple myeloma occurs increasingly with age, peaking in the seventies, and is more common in men. It is one of the most common neoplasms affecting the bone.

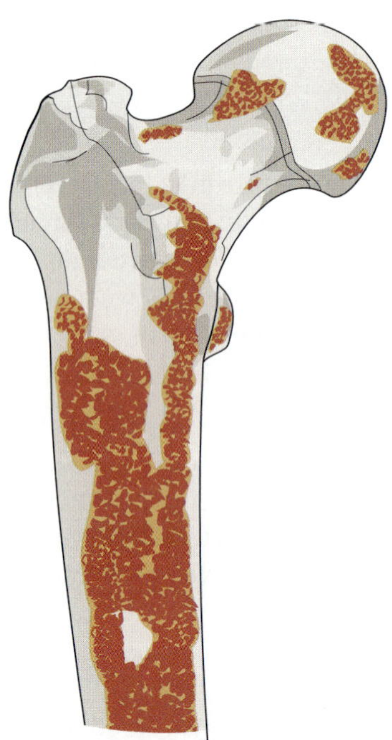

Figure 16–4 Multiple myeloma—Extensive bone destruction caused by disease.

Overgrowth of plasma cells leads to a decrease in other blood components causing anemia, leukocytopenia, and thrombocytopenia. The breakdown of bone leads to hypercalcemia (hyper = excessive, calc = calcium, emia = blood) or excessive blood calcium levels. Antibodies secreted by the plasma cells attach to kidney tubules (see Chapter 14) causing tissue damage leading to kidney failure.

Diagnosis is confirmed by:

- X-ray exhibiting a honeycombed bone pattern caused by tumor involvement
- Hypercalcemia caused by the tumor breaking down bone
- A special protein called **Bence Jones**, found in the blood and urine
- A bone marrow biopsy confirming the presence of an excessive number of plasma cells

Prognosis is poor for multiple myeloma. Chemotherapy and radiation are not very effective and death is usually within two to three years as the result of infection and kidney failure.

Disorders of Platelets

Platelet disorders are varied in terms of cause, severity, treatment, and prognosis. However, they all share the common symptom of bleeding. The bleeding may be mild or severe depending on the particular condition. Many disorders of platelets are inherited diseases.

Hemophilia. Hemophilia (hemo = blood, philia = lover) is an X-linked hereditary bleeding disorder. The characteristic inability to clot blood makes hemophiliacs "love blood" or require transfusions. There are several types of hemophilia but the most common is Type A. Hemophilia commonly occurs in male children and is passed to these children often by their mother who is usually asymptomatic and unaffected. Hemophiliacs lack a blood protein that plays a part in clot formation. Symptoms of frequent epistaxis (nosebleeds), bruising, and prolonged bleeding in a male child may be indicative of hemophilia. Diagnosis is confirmed by blood testing and clinical history of the involved individual.

This condition may vary from mild to severe. A hemophiliac may experience severe and prolonged bleeding with a minor injury. Severe hemophilia often leads to **hemarthrosis** (hem = blood, arthro = joint, osis = condition) or bleeding into joints. This is extremely painful. Recurrent episodes often lead to joint deformity. There is no cure for hemophilia. Treatment is aimed at prevention of injury and treatment of symptoms. Whole blood transfusions may be needed along with a concentrated form of the needed clotting protein.

Von Willebrand's disease. Von Willebrand's disease is a hereditary congenital bleeding disorder caused by a deficiency in clotting factor and platelet function. This disorder is also called angiohemophilia. It affects females as well as males.

Thrombocytopenia. Thrombocytopenia, also known as thrombocytopenia purpura is a decrease in platelets that leads to an inability to normally clot blood. This condition is characterized by abnormal bleeding in the skin, mucous membranes, and internal organs. The skin may exhibit small hemorrhagic spots called petechiae or larger purplish hemorrhagic spots called ecchymoses. This purple coloring of the skin leads to another descriptive term, **purpura** (PUR-pew-rah; purplish color of the skin caused by hemorrhaging). Symptoms of thrombocytopenia include gastrointestinal hemorrhages, frequent epistaxis (nosebleeds), and **hematuria** (HEM-ah-**TOO**-ree-ah; hema = blood, uria = urine, blood in the urine).

Thrombocytopenia may be caused by inadequate or abnormal platelet production or destruction. In the case of abnormal destruction, platelet life may be reduced to hours instead of days. The cause of this disorder is frequently unknown. In this case, the condition may be called idiopathic thrombocytopenia purpura.

Diagnosis is made utilizing individual clinical history along with platelet count and bleeding time. Treatment includes avoiding tissue trauma to reduce the potential for bleeding, administration of vitamin K to improve clotting, and transfusion of platelets. If the disorder persists, a splenectomy may alleviate symptoms as the spleen is the main site of platelet destruction. Splenectomy is usually the last treatment of choice but is very effective.

Disseminated Intravascular Coagulation (DIC). Disseminated intravascular coagulation is a condition of abnormal clotting followed by abnormal bleeding. DIC can occur after major surgery, burns, trauma involving major tissue destruction, septicemia, shock, some forms of cancer, eclampsia in pregnancy, and trauma caused by complicated childbirth.

Multiple microscopic clots form mostly in the capillaries causing infarctions throughout the body with resulting consequences. Clotting factors are used up during the formation of all the microthrombi. Reduced clotting factor leads to the inability to clot blood resulting in multiple hemorrhages. The individual with DIC often oozes blood, forming petechiae, ecchymosis, hematoma, and hematuria. Other symptoms include gastrointestinal bleeding causing **hematemesis** (HEM-ah-TEM-eh-sis; hema = blood, emesis = vomiting), blood in the stool, and symptoms associated with anemia.

Diagnosis is made on the basis of history and blood studies. Treatment includes heparin, an anticoagulant medication, to halt the formation of thrombi and platelet administration to stop hemorrhage or increase clotting ability. This disorder is very difficult to manage as one administers agents to clot and thin blood at alternating intervals. The condition usually is life-threatening and leads to death.

TRAUMA

Any traumatic injury to the bone marrow, spleen, or lymph nodes may lead to a decrease in the production of blood cells. Enlargement of the spleen or splenomegaly may lead to premature breakdown of blood cells. Chemotherapy and radiation treatments affecting bone marrow often lead to symptoms of anemia and infection related to decreased production of red cells and white cells respectively. Hemorrhage can be life-threatening and produce shock (Chapter 6).

DEVELOPMENTAL AND GENETIC DISORDERS

Genetic and developmental disorders of the blood are more common in certain population groups. For example, some anemias are most commonly found in black populations, while other anemias are more common in European populations. Sickle cell anemia and hemophilia were both discussed earlier in this chapter. Sickle cell anemia is a chronic hereditary form of anemia found predominately in black individuals. Hemophilia is an X-linked hereditary bleeding disorder passed from a carrier mother to a son.

EFFECTS OF AGING ON THE SYSTEM

Older adults may be more prone to developing diseases of the hematologic system because of the age-related changes occurring in other systems, such as the immune or digestive system, leaving them more susceptible to infections and nutritionally related blood disorders. However, total serum iron, total iron-binding capacity, and intestinal iron absorption all decrease with age. Aging does not change the number of lymphocytes, but their functioning decreases to some degree over time.

The most common disorder of the blood in the older adult is anemia. This is not usually caused by a defect in the system, but by poor nutrition (iron deficiency anemia) or inability to absorb the needed nutrients (pernicious anemia). Anemia often complicates other chronic diseases of the affected individual.

Some types of leukemia are more common in the older adult. Problems can arise during treatment for the condition because of decreased gastric motility and impaired circulation. These age-related changes can reduce the effectiveness of some therapies and increase the chance of experiencing side effects of the treatment.

SUMMARY

The hematologic system forms the body's life fluid, transports nutrients to cells, removes wastes, and helps prevent infection. The main components of the system include the blood, lymph nodes, bone marrow, spleen, and liver. Common signs and symptoms of diseases of the hematologic system are fatigue, shortness of breath, bleeding, lesions, pain, and increased susceptibility to infections. The most common disorder of the system is anemia. Although there are several types of anemia, they all have common symptoms. White blood cell disorders include mononucleosis, and leukemia as the most common. Disorders of platelets include the major bleeding diseases of the hematologic system such as hemophilia. The older adult may develop problems of the hematologic system, such as anemia, but it is usually caused by other problems or disorders in other systems.

REVIEW QUESTIONS

Multiple Choice

1. Which of the following are major functions of blood? (Select all that apply.)
   a. transportation of nutrients
   b. metabolism of nutrients
   c. removal of wastes
   d. protection from infection
   e. production of lymphocytes
   f. production of erythrocytes
2. Which of the following are common signs and symptoms of disorders of the hematologic system? (Select all that apply.)
   a. inflammation
   b. fatigue
   c. shortness of breath
   d. paralysis
   e. urinary frequency
   f. bleeding
   g. pain
   h. lesions
3. A patient with a history of a bleeding disorder who sustained minor trauma to his knee may develop what condition because of his bleeding disorder?
   a. fractured patella
   b. hemearthrosis
   c. osteoarthritis
   d. torn ligament

4. Treatment of a patient during a sickle cell crisis includes
   a. ice applied over achy joints
   b. IV fluids at least twice the normal daily intake
   c. analgesia
   d. both b & c are correct
5. Bone marrow biopsies are performed to:
   a. determine the presence and number of platelets.
   b. diagnose cancers, anemias, and bone marrow functional disorders.
   c. diagnose vitamin B_{12} deficiency.
   d. test for antigens to prevent antigen/antibody reactions.
6. You are transferring an unconscious male multiple trauma patient on a portable ventilator from a community hospital to a tertiary care facility. During the transfer, you notice that your patient begins to bleed from his mouth, nose, and both IV sites. You suspect this patient has developed:
   a hemophilia
   b. von Willebrand's factor deficiency
   c. disseminated intravascular coagulation
   d. eclampsia
7. In which of the following ways does primary polycythemia differ from secondary polycythemia (erythrocytosis)?
   a. The most common symptom of the primary type is shortness of breath while fatigue is the most common symptom of the secondary type.
   b. The primary type disease responds to radiation therapy while the secondary type does not.
   c. The primary form of the disease is considered to be a type of cancer while the secondary form is not.
   d. Both red and white cell numbers are increased in the primary type but just red cell numbers are increased in the secondary type.
8. Which of the following statements is true about hemophilia?
   a. It is most common in the older adult.
   b. It results in continuous minor bleeding internally.
   c. It is caused by a deficiency of clotting factor.
   d. It is found in male children of mothers who carry the defective gene.
9. Which of the following statements is true about leukemia?
   a. It is considered to be a group of disorders with a cancerous development occurring in the bone marrow.
   b. It is the most common cause of death in young children.
   c. Chemotherapy is ineffective against leukemia.
   d. There are several types of leukemias but most types are diagnosed in the young or middle-aged adult.

Short Answer

10. List some of the common tests used to diagnose disorders of the hematologic system.

11. Describe the common effects of a hemorrhagic disorder on an individual.

12. Why would an individual with Hodgkin's disease be instructed to avoid individuals with coughs, colds, and fever?

13. Why are older adults more susceptible to infections if there is a hematologic disorder present?

CASE STUDY

You are transporting Mr. Avery, a 73-year-old gentleman who was recently diagnosed with lymphoma, to his daily radiation treatment. What are some things you will need to consider for this patient during transport?

BIBLIOGRAPHY

Anemia: Knowledge for practice, Part 1. (1995). *Nursing Times, 91*(5), 1.
Anemia: Revision notes, Part 3. (1995). *Nursing Times, 91*(7), 9.
Anemia: The role of the nurse, Part 2. (1995). *Nursing Times, 91*(6), 5.
Antman, K. (1996). When are bone marrow transplants considered? *Scientific American, 275*(9), 124–125.
Blood drug is approved. (1997). *New York Times* p. C10.
Borson, R., & Loeb, V. (1994). Acute and chronic leukemias in adults. *CA—Cancer Journal for Clinicians, 44*(6), 323.
Carroll, P. A. (1995). When a Jehovah's Witness refuses a transfusion. *Nursing, 95*(8), 60.
Cook, J. D., Skikne, B. S., & Baynes, R. D. (1994). Iron deficiency: The global perspective. *Advances in Experimental Medicine and Biology, 356*, 219.
Darby, S. C. (July 25, 1996). Links in childhood leukemia. *Nature, 382*, 303–304.
Devine, S. M., & Larson, R. A. (1994). Acute leukemia in adults: Recent developments in diagnosis and treatment. *CA—A Cancer Journal for Clinicians, 44*(6), 326.
Dumas, M. A. S. (1996). What it's like to belong to the cancer club. *American Journal of Nursing, 96*(4), 40–42.
Erickson, J. M. (1994). Update on Hodgkin's Disease. *Nurse Practitioner, 19*(11), 63.
Frum, L. (1996). Barbara Frum: Canadian television journalist dies from leukemia. *Saturday Night, 111*(10), 50–52.
Goldstein, K. H. (February 15, 1996). Efficient diagnosis of thrombocytopenia. *American Family Physician, 53*, 915–920.
Graydon, J. E., Bubela, N., Irvine, D., & Vincent, L. (1995). Fatigue-reducing strategies used by patients receiving treatment for cancer. *Cancer Nursing, 18*(1), 23.
Huston, C. J. (1994). Disseminated intravascular coagulation. *American Journal of Nursing, 94*(8), 51.
Inskip, H. (April 5, 1997). Childhood leukemia near nuclear sites re-examined. *Lancet, 349*, 969-970.
Is cancer patient's anxiety overestimated? (1997). *American Journal of Nursing, 97*(2), 10.
Kajs-Wyllie, M. (1995). Thrombotic thrombocytopenic purpura: Pathophysiology, treatment, and related nursing care. *Critical Care Nurse, 15*(6), 44.
Kolata, G. (July 3, 1997). Big study sees no evidence power lines cause leukemia. *New York Times*, A1.
Kurtz, A. (1993). Disseminated intravascular coagulation with leukemia patients. *Cancer Nursing, 16*(6), 456.
Lee, L. S. (1997). Managing chronic cancer pain. *Nursing, 97* 27(4), 74.
Leukemia studies continue to draw a blank. (1996). *Science, 272*, 358.
Lundquist, D. M., & Stewart, F. M. (1994). An update on non-Hodgkin's lymphoma. *Nurse Practitioner, 19*(10), 41.
Lusher, J. M. (June 19, 1996). Hematology. *Journal of the American Medical Association, 275*, 1814-1815.
McCance, K. L., & Huether, S. E. (1994). *Pathophysiology: The biological basis for disease in adults and children.* (2nd ed.). St. Louis: Mosby-Year Book.
McKinney, B. (1996). When this rare cancer strikes. *RN, 59*(12), 36–41.
Messinezy, M., & Pearson, T. (1995). Polycythemias. *The Practitioner, 237*, 355.
Miller, C. (1994). The role of transfusion therapy in the treatment of sickle cell disease. *Journal of Intravenous Nursing, 17*(2), 70.
Purandare, L. (1995). Caring for patients with chronic leukemia. *Nursing Times, 91*(31), 27.
Schneider, A. S., & Szanto, P. A. (1993). *Pathology Board Review Series.* (pp 32–36). Baltimore: Williams & Wilkins.

Sickle Cell Disease Guideline Panel. (1993). Sickle Cell Disease: Screening, Diagnosis, Management, and Counseling in Newborns and Infants. *Clinical Practice Guidelines No. 6*. AHCPR Pub. No. 93-0562. Rockville, MD: Agency for Health Care Policy and Research, Public Health Service, U.S. Dept. of Health and Human Services.

Tierney, L. M., McPhee, S. J., & Papadakis, M. A. (1996). *Current medical diagnosis and treatment,* (35th ed.). Stamford, CT: Appleton & Lange.

Warmkessel, J. H. (1997). Caring for patient's with non-Hodgkin's lymphoma. *Nursing, 97 27*(6), 48–49.

Warne, I. (1994). Chemotherapy for acute monoblastic leukemia. *Nursing Times, 90*(17), 43.

Waters, J. (1995). Pain from sickle-cell crises. *Nursing Times, 91*(16), 29.

Young, N. S., & Barnett, A. J. (1995). The treatment of severe acquired aplastic anemia. *Blood, 85*(12), 3367.

CHAPTER

17 Integumentary Diseases and Disorders

CONTENT OUTLINE

- Anatomy and Physiology
- Common Signs and Symptoms
- Diagnostic Tests
- Common Diseases of the Integumentary System
  - Infectious Diseases
- Trauma
  - Mechanical Skin Injury
  - Thermal Skin Injury
  - Electrical Injury
  - Radiation Injury
  - Pressure Injury
- Effects of Aging on the System

KEY TERMS

Abrasion
Alopecia
Avulsion
Blunt trauma
Contusion
Erythema
Exacerbation
Hirsutism
Incision
Keratin
Laceration
Lesion
Paronychia
Pilonidal cyst
Pruritus
Pustule
Sebum
Ulcer
Vesicles
Wheals
Xerosis

LEARNING OBJECTIVES

Upon completion of the chapter, the student should be able to:

1. Define the terminology common to the integumentary system and the disorders of the system.
2. Identify common disorders of the integumentary system.
3. Discuss the basic anatomy and physiology of the integumentary system.
4. Identify the important signs and symptoms associated with common integumentary system disorders.
5. Describe the common diagnostic tests used to determine type and/or cause of the integumentary system disorder.
6. Describe the typical course and management of the common integumentary system disorders.
7. Describe the effects of aging upon the integumentary system and the common disorders of the system.

OVERVIEW

The integumentary system is composed of all the skin and its layers. The skin is known as the largest organ of the body. It makes up about fifteen percent of the total body weight. The skin is the first line of defense against disease. Many diseases of the integumentary system are the result of other body or system disorders. For instance, measles is a viral disease of the respiratory system but it is characterized by the maculopapular rash seen on the skin. Skin disorders such as psoriasis are traumatic to the individual because of the obvious lesions and the effect it has on body image. Skin disorders range from mild to severe, and acute to chronic.

ANATOMY AND PHYSIOLOGY

The skin is the largest organ of the body. It is a large durable and pliable organ and is the first line of protection for the body against invading organisms. The skin also provides a sense of touch, heat, cold, and pain, and helps stabilize temperature, and fluid and electrolyte balance. The skin is composed of three layers: the epidermis, dermis, and subcutaneous level (Figure 17–1).

The epidermis or outer layer is composed of five layers: the stratum corneum, stratum lucidum, stratum granulosum, stratum spinosum, and stratum basale. The cells of the epidermis are called stratified squamous epithelial cells. Most of these are keratinocytes and the others are melanocytes that produce melanin, the pigment that darkens the skin and gives it color. The dermis is the middle layer, consisting of connective tissue and a variety of cell types. Blood vessels transverse the dermal layer to provide nutrients and oxygen, regulate heat, and remove waste products. Nerves also form a network in the dermis. They provide the sensations of heat, cold, pain, and touch.

The subcutaneous layer is composed of connective tissue containing fat cells and blood vessels. The amount of fat varies considerably with the individual. This layer protects the body against cold.

Imbedded in the dermis and extending to the epidermis are the sebaceous, apocrine, and eccrine sweat glands. The sebaceous glands produce oil called **sebum**. The apocrine sweat glands are located in the underarms (axillae), around the nipples of the breasts, and around the umbilicus, anus, and genital areas. These glands are inactive until puberty and initiate their function with hormonal changes at that time. Their secretions are odorless, but bacteria that accumulate in these areas cause the

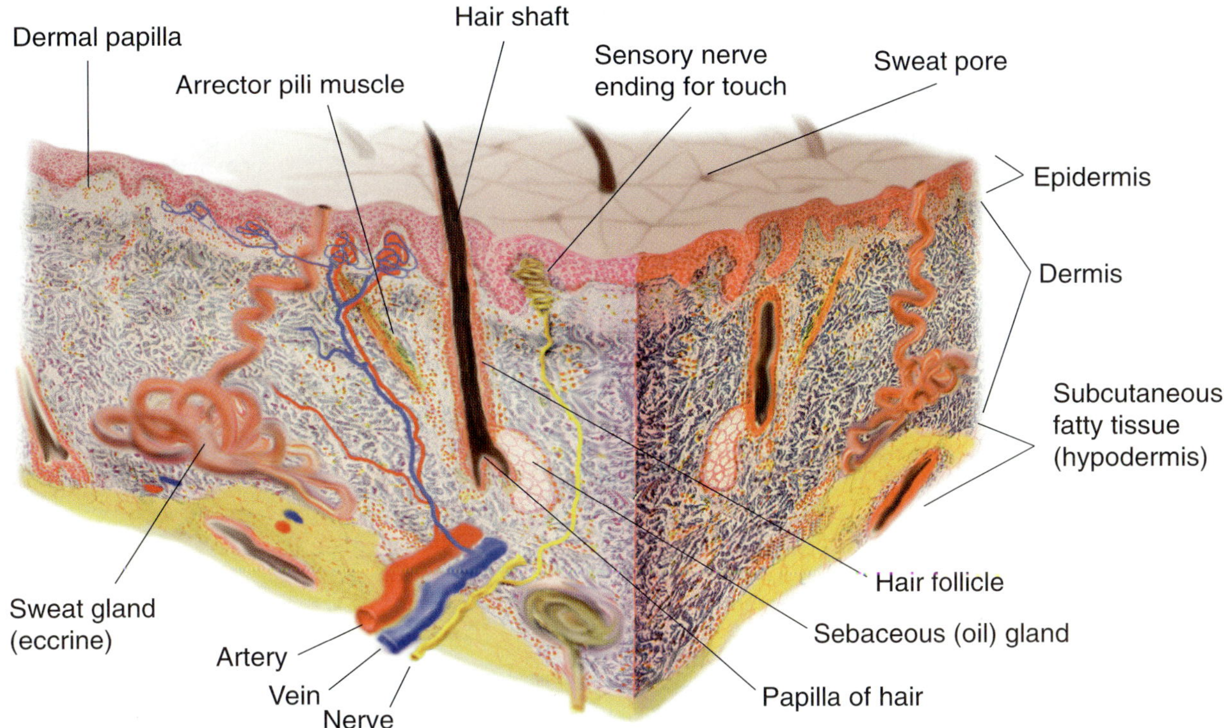

Figure 17–1 The structures of the skin.

smell referred to as body odor. Both the sebaceous glands and the apocrine glands secrete through the hair follicles. The eccrine sweat glands are found throughout the body surfaces. They secrete through the skin pores to help the body regulate heat. Some electrolytes are also lost through these sweat glands.

The hair follicles are found in the dermal layer and extend through the epidermis. The hair follicles grow in cycles, which vary with the individual, with an average growth of about 1 cm per month. Hair loss occurs continually but is not usually obvious until a large amount is lost and not replaced. The male hormone testosterone influences hair growth, especially at puberty when hair begins to appear in the axillae and groin. It also causes the male's level of baldness later in life. Generally soft tiny hairs cover most of the body and terminal hairs (stiffer, longer, and often darker) are found on the scalp, axillae, groin, eyebrows, and eyelashes of both sexes, and the face and trunk of males.

The nails are composed of **keratin** (epidermal cells in a tight web). Fingernails grow more rapidly than toenails but they are composed of the same material. The thickness and growth rate of the nail varies with the individual. Health status, nutrition, and other factors may influence nail strength and growth.

COMMON SIGNS AND SYMPTOMS

Common signs and symptoms of integumentary diseases include:

- Skin **lesion** (LEE-zhun). A lesion is a very broad term meaning any discontinuity or abnormality of tissue. Lesions may be hard, soft, flat, raised, large, small, reddened, crusted, fluid filled, or pus filled to name only a few characteristics (Figure 17–2).
- Pain
- **Pruritus** (proo-RYE-tus) or itching
- Edema (swelling)
- **Erythema** (ER-oh-**THEE**-mah) or skin redness
- Inflammation

DIAGNOSTIC TESTS

There are numerous skin diseases. Several have very characteristic lesions leading to an easy diagnosis. But many exhibit the same or similar types of lesions and symptoms making diagnosis difficult. Biopsy may be used in diagnosing nodules and chronic lesions. Culture and sensitivity are effective in determining the presence of bacterial

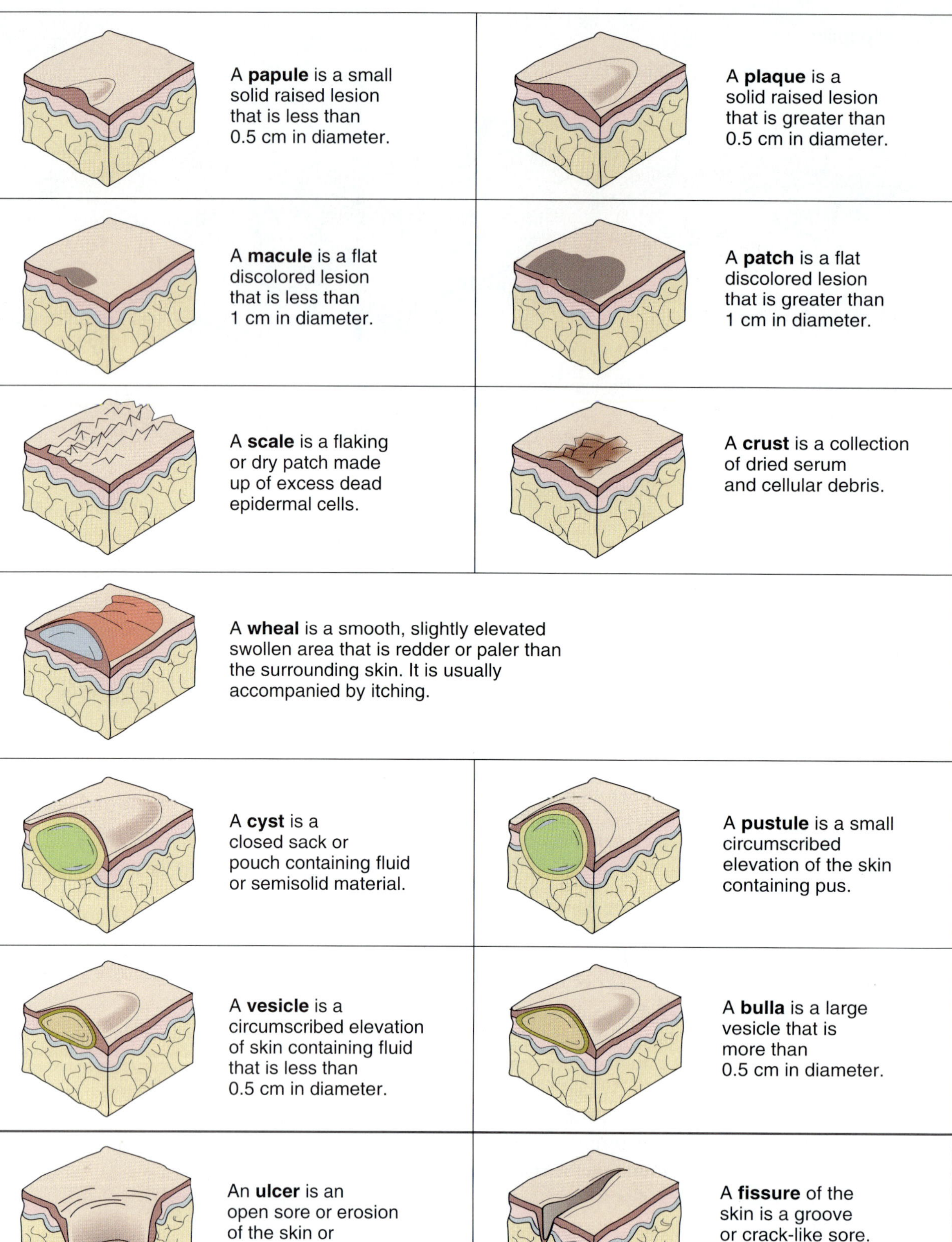

Figure 17-2 Skin lesions.

infections. Blood tests are helpful especially if there is concern about a systemic infection or metabolic disorder. Diagnosis and identification of fungal and parasitic infections may be determined by utilizing cultures and microscopic smear examinations.

COMMON DISEASES OF THE INTEGUMENTARY SYSTEM

There are numerous diseases and disorders of the integumentary system. Diagnosis of skin disorders is often very difficult because several diseases may be characterized by the same type or similar types of lesions. Common diseases may be categorized as to cause and include: infections, metabolic, hypersensitivity, idiopathic, and tumors.

Infectious Diseases

Skin infections are quite common and usually contagious. Care must be taken to prevent spread from one area of the body to another and from one person to another. Most infections are not serious unless systemic involvement occurs. Infections of the skin may be caused by virus, bacteria, fungus, and parasites.

Viral Diseases. Viral skin diseases may be acute or chronic. Acute viral diseases commonly affect children and usually resolve spontaneously. Many viral infections become lifelong with periods of remission and **exacerbation** (flaring up).

Herpes. Herpes is a large family of viruses characterized by inflammation of the skin and clusters of fluid-filled **vesicles** (VES-ih-kul). The virus is not treatable and remains in the affected individual's body for life. Some type of balance between the host and the virus exists, with periods of viral remission and exacerbation. The virus exacerbates or flares up often during times of decreased immunity as occurs with stress. Common types of herpes virus are:

- Herpes simplex type I—commonly called "fever blisters" and "cold sores" as febrile conditions and the common cold often bring about an exacerbation. The vesicles commonly appear around the lips and nose (Figure 17–3). Lesions appearing around the lips may be further identified as *herpes labialis* (labia = lip) and those occurring in conjunction with a fever may be further identified as *herpes febrilis*.

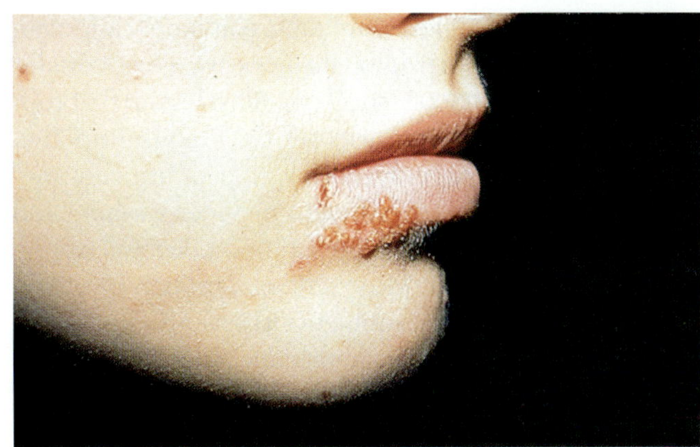

Figure 17–3 Herpes simplex virus I.

- Herpes genitalis, herpes simplex type II—commonly called genital herpes. This is a highly contagious disease and is spread by direct contact. Genital herpes may be a sexually transmitted disease but transmission is not limited to sexual contact. Autoinoculation with the hands is also possible by touching the lips then the genitals and vice versa. Genital herpes type II and herpes simplex type I cause the same type of lesions and clinically cannot be separated. (See Chapter 21 for more information.)
- Herpes Varicella—commonly called chickenpox is an acute, highly contagious childhood disease. Varicella is discussed in detail in Chapter 23.
- Herpes zoster—commonly called shingles. The virus that causes chickenpox in children causes zoster in adults. Shingles is characterized by painful lesions that follow the course of a spinal nerve. (More detailed information may be found in Chapter 9.)

Measles. Measles is a highly contagious childhood disease. This viral disease causes a characteristic maculopapular skin rash. (For more information on measles, see Chapter 23.)

Bacterial Diseases. Bacterial skin infections are often highly contagious and affect individuals who are immunosuppressed or practice poor personal hygiene. These skin infections are generally caused by normal flora bacteria and are treated effectively with antibiotics.

Impetigo. Impetigo is a highly contagious skin disease caused by *Streptococcus* and *Staphylococcus* bacteria. The face and hands of children are most commonly affected. Impetigo is characterized by the appearance of vesicles and **pustules** (PUS-tyouls; small pus-filled lesion) that rupture producing a yellow crust over the lesions. Impetigo occurs more readily in individuals with poor hygiene, anemia, and malnutrition. Treatment includes washing and drying the affected area several times a day and applying antibiotic ointment. More serious conditions may also require the use of oral antibiotics. Prevention is aimed at correcting anemia and malnutrition, and following good personal hygiene guidelines.

Abscess, Furuncle, Carbuncle. Abscess, furuncle, and carbuncle are all characterized by inflammation, infection, and the formation of a capsule to wall off and prevent the spread of infection. These lesions are commonly caused by the pyogenic, normal flora bacteria *Staphylococcus*. All these encapsulated lesions are extremely painful, usually develop a soft spot or "come to a head," and need to be opened or surgically drained. Antibiotic treatment is generally effective. Predisposing factors for these lesions include a lowered immunity caused by the presence of other diseases and poor personal hygiene. There are some differences in these lesions. An abscess is a localized collection of pus occurring in any tissue of the body including the skin. Abscesses commonly occur around sites of trauma, embedded foreign material such as splinters, and hair follicles. A small abscess occurring in the tissues of the skin is a furuncle, commonly called a boil. Furuncles generally occur around a hair follicle and may develop during an acute case of folliculitis. Boils may develop in any hairy area of the body, with common sites including the skin of the neck, back, and buttocks. Carbuncles are larger abscesses and involve several interconnected furuncles. These lesions arise in a cluster of hair follicles and have multiple drainage sites. Needless to say, carbuncles are much larger than furuncles and are less common.

Cellulitis and Erysipelas. Cellulitis is a diffuse or spreading inflammation of the skin and subcutaneous tissue. The cause of cellulitis is usually the bacterium *Staphylococcus*. Cellulitis may be the extension of a wound, **ulcer**, or other skin infection. The involved area is swollen, red, and painful. Cellulitis is generally treated successfully with oral antibiotics. Any cellulitis involving the face may be dangerous as this has the potential of spreading into the sinuses of the skull. Erysipelas is a form of cellulitis commonly involving the skin of the face. This infection is caused by the bacterium *Streptococcus* and may be transferred from the respiratory system to the face. Fever, chills, headache, vomiting, and red, painful, edematous skin are characteristic symptoms. Complications include endocarditis and septicemia. Affected individuals are often hospitalized and treated with intravenous antibiotics.

Lyme Disease. Lyme disease is a multisystem infection caused by bacteria transmitted to humans by the bite of a deer tick. The bacteria may affect any organ causing a variety of symptoms and possibly delaying diagnosis. Symptoms may include flu-like symptoms, arthritis, malaise, chills, and fever. A characteristic "bull's eye" skin rash is a common symptom. The bull's eye is a reddened circle with a lighter center and may appear days to weeks after the infected bite. Positive blood testing for antibodies confirms the diagnosis. Antibiotic treatment is necessary, as untreated the disease may cause arthritis and various neurologic and cardiovascular complications. Lyme disease is more prevalent in the northeast and was first discovered in 1975 in Lyme, Connecticut, hence the name. Prevention of lyme disease is aimed at preventing tick bites by using insect repellant, wearing long-sleeved shirts, pants and socks, and tucking the pants into the socks and boots when hiking or camping in grassy or wooded areas. Showering and inspecting the skin immediately after outside activities may also aid in prevention of bites. In May, 1998 the Food and Drug Administration approved the lyme vaccine LYMErix® for use in individuals over fifteen years of age. It is still being tested for use in children.

Fungal Diseases. Fungal infections are very common and usually affect the nails and hair. Pathogenic fungi are called dermatophytes and tend to live in dead tissue. Dermatophytes often cause the skin to itch and crack, leaving it open to bacterial infections. Fungal infections are difficult to eradicate and may cause life-long symptoms.

Candidiasis. Candidiasis (KAN-dih-**DYE**-ah-sis) is a fungal infection caused by the fungus *candida*. This infection commonly affects individuals with chronic diseases such as diabetes mellitus, those who are on immunosuppressive medications or antibiotics, and those dealing with long-term water immersion, such as dishwashers, bartenders, and waitresses. Candidiasis infection may produce patches of red, itchy skin with blisters and pustules. This infection commonly affects the fingernails, interdigital space or area between the fingers, mouth, and vagina. Candidiasis of the mouth is commonly called thrush. The inner cheeks and tongue are often covered with white patches of infection. Thrush is common in infants and immunosuppressed adults. Candidiasis of the vagina causes vaginitis and is discussed in detail in Chapter 21. Antifungal medications are useful in treatment, but, again, fungal infections are often difficult to eradicate and may become chronic in some cases.

Parasitic Diseases. Parasites are organisms that feed upon a host, that host sometimes being a human. Human parasites affecting the skin are easily spread and cause intense itching. Parasites commonly occur in crowded living conditions with inadequate bathing facilities. The two most common skin parasites are pediculosis (lice) and scabies.

Pediculosis. Pediculosis is infestation with lice. Lice are easily spread by direct contact with an infected individual or may be carried by sharing of combs, brushes, towels, clothing, or bed linens. Lice are not partial to any of the socioeconomic classes, and thus affect anyone coming in contact with them. Treatment generally includes bathing and shampooing with medicated shampoo (for example, Kwell). There are three types of lice commonly affecting humans.

1. Head lice—commonly spread among school-aged children and their families. (Figure 17–4) (See Chapter 23 for more information.)
2. Body lice—often occur in individuals with poor hygiene practices, such as transients and homeless. Body lice can spread disease and were responsible for the spread of typhus during war times.
3. Pubic lice—are spread by sexual contact with an affected individual and are commonly called "crabs." Pubic lice infect males and females and cause intense itching in the genital area. These lice may also spread to the eyelashes and eyebrows. Treatment includes bathing in medicated shampoo, and treating clothing and bed linens. Petroleum jelly may be applied to the eyelashes to kill lice.

Scabies. Scabies is a condition caused by a tiny mite. The condition is commonly called the "seven year itch." Mites are transferred from one infected individual to another by direct contact. Scabies commonly affect the folds of the skin, such as areas beneath the breasts, under the arms, in the groin area, wrists, and between the fingers and toes (Figure 17–5). The pregnant female mite burrows into the skin and lays her eggs in a short tunnel near the surface of the skin. These burrows often appear as slightly elevated greyish white lines. Intense itching, vesicles, and pustules develop from hypersensitivity to the bite, the mite's feces, and the presence of the ova. The eggs hatch in three to five days; the mite matures on the surface of the skin in two to three weeks, then mates, and the cycle begins again. Diagnosis is made on the basis of microscopic skin examination often revealing the presence of mites. Female mites may be viewed at the end of the burrowed tunnel and appear as tiny black dots. Treatment includes application of lindane cream to the entire body, leaving the cream on for eight to fourteen hours before showering or bathing. All infected individuals must be treated to prevent reinfection. Itching may persist for three to four weeks after successful treatment.

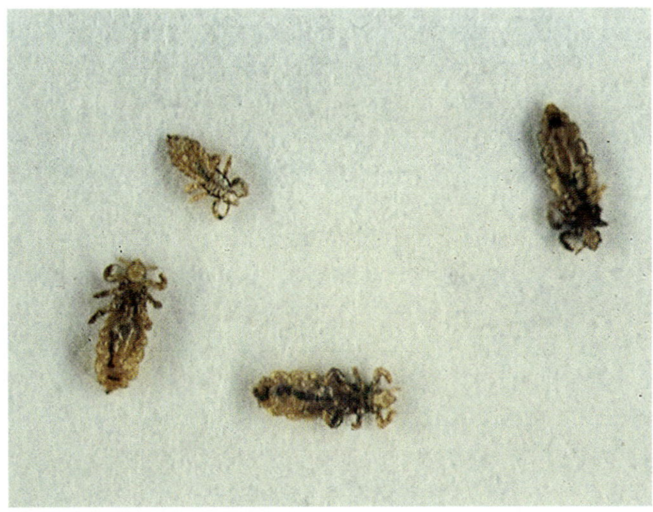

Figure 17–4 Head lice.

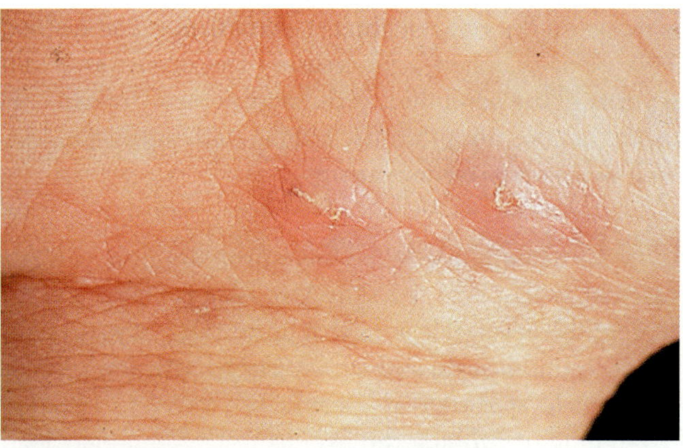

Figure 17–5 Scabies. (Courtesy of Robert A. Silverman, MD, Clinical Associate Professor, Department of Pediatrics, Georgetown University.)

Metabolic Diseases. Hyperactivity of the sebaceous gland is the cause of several different skin diseases. Inflammation and infection may also play a role in these diseases although the primary cause is metabolic.

Sebaceous Cyst. A sebaceous (seh-BAY-shus) cyst develops when a sebaceous gland becomes blocked and the sebum collects under the skin. This cyst can form anywhere on the body except in the palms of the hands and soles of the feet. Sebaceous cysts commonly develop in the scalp, neck, and groin area. A special type of sebaceous cyst is a **pilonidal cyst**. This cyst develops around a hair in the sacrococcygeal area. Treatment of sebaceous cyst includes incising and draining the cyst although it tends to recur. Permanent treatment is surgical removal.

Hypersensitivity or Immune Diseases. Hypersensitivity diseases are those that are caused by an immune reaction within the body. Frequently the cause is unknown and treatment is symptomatic.

Eczema. Eczema (ECK-zeh-mah) is an inflammation of the skin or type of dermatitis characterized by itching, redness, vesicles, pustules, scales, and crust appearing alone or in combination (Figure 17–6). It is also called atopic dermatitis, as it tends to occur in atopic individuals or those with a genetic predisposition to allergies. Eczema is a common allergic reaction in children often beginning in infancy. It is believed to be caused by allergies to milk, orange juice, or some other foods. Eczema in infants often disappears when the offending food is discontinued. In adults eczema often produces dry leathery skin lesions. Stress, humidity, and severe changes in temperature are a few of the identified factors causing an exacerbation or flare-up of the condition. Diagnosis is made on the basis of clinical examination and history. Treatment is aimed at decreasing the occurrence and severity of the condition, as there is no cure. Topical cortisone creams are often used along with antihistamines and sedatives to treat pruritus.

Urticaria. Commonly called hives or nettle rash, this is a vascular reaction of the skin. Urticaria is characterized by slightly elevated lesions that are redder or paler than the surrounding skin and are associated with severe itching. The elevated areas are called **wheals** (WEEL)s or hives. Scratching or rubbing the hypersensitive area may lead to formation of larger or additional wheals. This condition is caused by contact with an external irritant such as insect bites, pollen, or plants. Urticaria may also be caused by internal irritants such as food, drugs, and contrast dye.

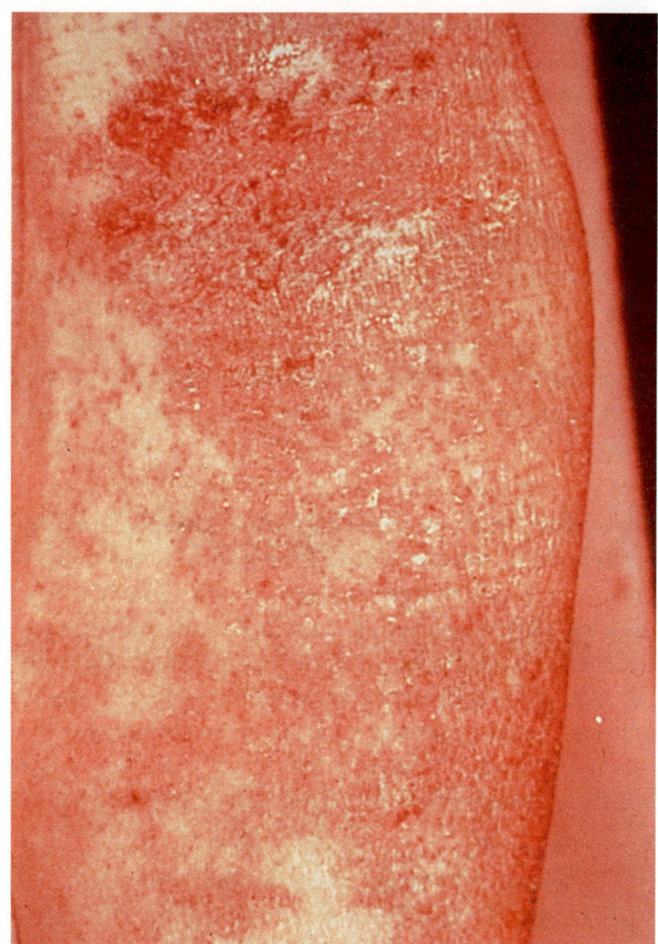

Figure 17–6 Eczema. (Courtesy of the Centers for Disease Control and Prevention.)

Treatment includes antihistamines and avoidance of the allergen. (See Chapter 12 for more information.)

Contact Dermatitis. Contact dermatitis is an acute or chronic allergic reaction affecting the skin. Often the allergen is some type of cosmetic, laundry product, plant, jewelry, paint, drug, plastic, or a variety of other agents. Often it is difficult to determine the causative agent and once found complete avoidance may not be possible. Allergic lesions may range from small red localized lesions to vesicular lesions that cover the entire body. A common example of a contact dermatitis is poison ivy. (See Chapter 12 for more information.)

Skin Cancer. Skin cancer is the most common type of cancer in humans and, in most cases, is caused by exposure to sun. Skin cancers generally occur in multiples and appear on the face, arms, and hands of middle-aged and older individuals. The most common skin cancer is basal cell carcinoma, but the most deadly is malignant melanoma. Diagnosis is made on the basis of clinical examination and positively confirmed by biopsy. Prevention for all forms of skin cancer is aimed at avoiding overexposure to the sun and life-long use of sunscreen with a high sun protection factor (SPF).

Basal Cell Carcinoma. Basal cell carcinoma is the most common type of skin cancer. It is most common in fair-skinned, blonde hair and blue or gray eyed individuals. Basal cell carcinoma is a slow growing, locally invading tumor that does not metastasize. This is not to say that left untreated it is not dangerous. Tumors near the eyes and mouth may invade these spaces and cause much concern. Tumors on the nose, lip, and ear may lead to the loss of these tissues. There is variability in the appearance of this tumor. It may appear as a raised nodule with a depressed or dented center, a smooth shiny bump that is pink to pearly white in color, or a non-healing lesion that bleeds easily (Figure 17–7). Treatment of basal cell carcinoma is surgical removal.

Squamous Cell Carcinoma. Squamous cell carcinoma is less common than basal cell carcinoma but it tends to grow more rapidly and become metastatic. This tumor, like basal cell, tends to occur on sun-exposed skin. As a general rule, basal cell carcinoma occurs on the face above the lip line while squamous cell occurs below the lip line. This tumor is often preceded by another skin lesion, such as actinic keratosis, chronic ulcers, sinus tracts, or scars. Squamous cell carcinoma may appear as a firm, red nodule with crusts or a slightly elevated plaque (Figure 17–8). Treatment is wide surgical excision with radiation treatments and follow-up for at least five years for signs of recurrence.

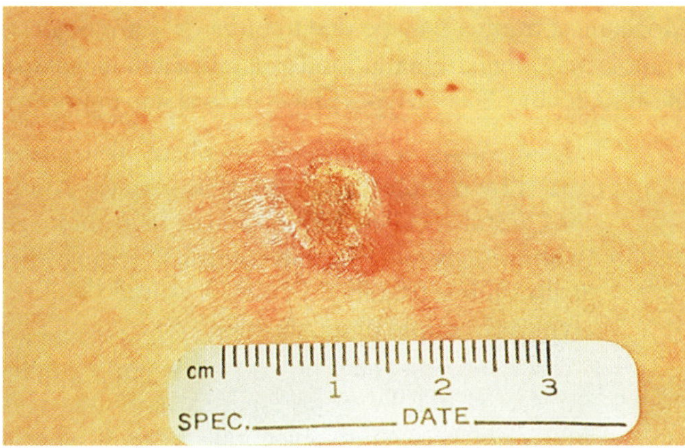

Figure 17–7 Basal cell carcinoma. (Courtesy of Robert A. Silverman, MD, Clinical Associate Professor, Department of Pediatrics, Georgetown University.)

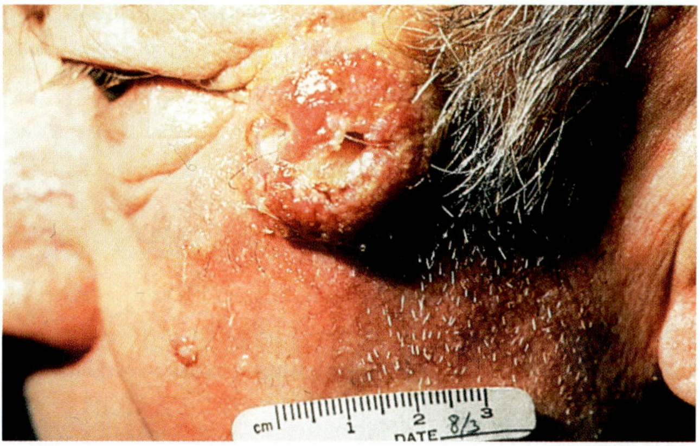

Figure 17–8 Squamous cell carcinoma. (Courtesy of Robert A. Silverman, MD, Clinical Associate Professor, Department of Pediatrics, Georgetown University.)

Malignant Melanoma. Malignant melanoma (melan = black, oma = tumor) is the most serious type of skin cancer. This tumor arises from melanocytes or skin-coloring cells and is usually tan, brown, or dark brown in color (Figure 17–9). Often this tumor arises in a mole and causes a change in size and color of the mole. Malignant melanoma rarely occurs before the age of twenty and may be related to a severe childhood sunburn. Malignant melanoma metastasizes quickly and is highly malignant. This tumor spreads into the lymph nodes and may metastasize to all organs of the body. Treatment depends on

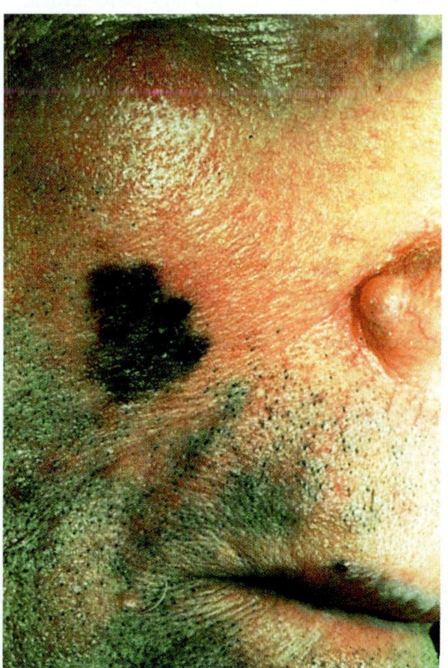

Figure 17–9 Lentigo malignant melanoma. (Courtesy of the American Academy of Dermatology.)

the degree of spread and may include wide surgical excision, radiation, chemotherapy, and immunotherapy. Prognosis depends on the degree of spread when discovered, but approximately twenty percent of those diagnosed with this tumor die from effects of metastasis.

Kaposi's Sarcoma. Kaposi's sarcoma (KAP-oh-seez sar-KOH-mah) is a malignant vascular skin tumor characterized by bluish-red cutaneous nodules. These tumors generally develop on the toes, feet, and legs, often increasing in number and size and spreading upward. Previous to the discovery of AIDS, Kaposi's sarcoma was relatively rare, but with the recent epidemic of AIDS the development of this neoplasm has increased drastically. The relationship between Kaposi's sarcoma and AIDS is not fully understood. This tumor usually is not highly malignant except in the case of AIDS, where it tends to be widespread and is often the cause of death in these individuals. There is no adequate treatment for this sarcoma.

Abnormal Pigmented Lesions. The epidermis of normal skin contains melanocytes that produce melanin or the coloring pigment of skin. Skin color varies from light to dark depending on the number of melanocytes present. Pigment or coloring protects the skin from burning. This explains why individuals with a fair or pale complexion burn more easily than individuals with a darker complexion. An individual's skin may contain several variations or abnormal lesions associated with pigment. These abnormal pigmented lesions include ephilis, lentigo, nevus, albinism, vitiligo, and melasma. These conditions may be unsightly but are usually harmless and easily diagnosed by a physician. Moles may cause increased concern if they undergo a change in size and shape, which are possible indicators of cancer. Lesions may be biopsied if cancer is suspected.

Diseases of the Nails. Nails act as coverings for the toes and fingers and may be considered an extension of the skin. Diseases of the nail may cause abnormal shape, thickening, and color changes. Fungal and bacterial infections are the most common cause of nail disease. Bacterial infection of the nails is **paronychia** (PAR-oh-**NICK**-ee-ah), an infection of the skin around the nail. This condition is commonly seen in individuals whose hands are in water for long periods of time, such as dishwashers, for example. This infection may cause the nail to lift away from the bed causing acute pain. Antibiotics are usually an effective treatment. In addition to antibiotics, severe cases may require incision and drainage of the paronychia. Fungal infections frequently affect the feet, are often chronic in nature, and commonly cause permanent nail deformity. Tinea pedis (athlete's foot) is a common cause of fungal nail infections of the feet. Fungal infections are difficult to treat and recurrence is common.

Diseases of the Hair. Hair color, texture, and distribution are genetically determined and influenced by hormones. **Hirsutism** (HER-soot-izm; in Latin meaning shaggy) is excessive growth of hair. Men typically have facial and chest hair caused by stimulation by male sex hormones. Hair growth in these areas in females is quite distressing and is usually caused by hormone abnormalities caused by such disorders as adrenal tumors, ovarian tumors, and polycystic ovaries. **Alopecia** (AL-oh-**PEE**-shee-ah; in Greek meaning fox mange, which caused hair loss) is partial or complete hair loss, usually from the head Alopecia may be caused by a number of factors including aging, heredity, thyroid disease, iron deficiency, chemotherapy, radiation, and dermatitis. Alopecia may occur suddenly or over a period of time and may be temporary or permanent. One of the most common causes of sudden, temporary alopecia is related to chemotherapy and radiation treatment. Hair growth normally returns when treatments are stopped.

TRAUMA

The skin is the outermost organ of the human body and the body's first line of defense. The position of the skin allows it to be at high risk for receiving frequent trauma. Trauma may be the result of mechanical, thermal, electrical, radiation, or pressure injury.

Mechanical Skin Injury

Skin is exposed to mechanical trauma in a variety of ways. Mechanical trauma may be due to blunt or sharp objects. Trauma may range from mild and insignificant to major and life-threatening. Several types of mechanical skin injury are:

- **Abrasion**—is a common mechanical trauma caused by scraping away the skin surface. Abrasions are also called friction burns or rug burns. An abrasion is red, raw, and painful. Bleeding with an abrasion is usually minimal. A skinned knee is a typical example of an abrasion.
- **Blunt trauma**—may be caused when an individual is struck by items such as hammers and clubs, or is thrown into objects like steering wheels and walls. Falls may also be the cause of blunt trauma. Blunt trauma often causes a large bruise

called a **contusion** (kon-TOO-zhun). A contusion is an accumulation of blood in the tissue without breaking the skin. The bleeding comes from injured or disrupted blood vessels.

- **Avulsion**—occurs when a portion of skin or appendage is pulled or torn away. Avulsion injuries usually occur when tissue is caught up in some type of machinery. If an appendage is completely torn away it is termed an amputation.
- Crush trauma—occurs when tissue is caught between two hard surfaces. Crush injuries commonly involve fingers, hands, feet, and toes. The hands and fingers may be caught in doors or between objects. Crush trauma also occurs when heavy items are dropped on the fingers, hands, feet, and toes.
- Puncture injury—occurs when a sharp object such as a knife, nail, or splinter of glass or metal is forced into the tissue. Bleeding is usually minimal. A feared complication of puncture injury is tetanus, as puncture injuries set up an anaerobic condition favorable to tetanus bacteria.
- **Laceration**—is a cut in the skin caused by a sharp object such as a knife, razor, glass, or metal. The edges of the laceration may be smooth, making repair easy, or the edges may be jagged, leading to a more difficult repair. A laceration with smooth even edges is commonly called an **incision**.

Thermal Skin Injury

Thermal skin injury may be caused by excessive heat or cold. Injury may be caused by short-term or long-term exposure to varying temperatures. Skin injury may range from mild to severe. Untreated, severe skin injuries may become life-threatening. In this chapter, we will discuss burns. Other heat and cold related emergencies are discussed in Chapter 19.

Burns. Burns may be caused by fire, steam, exposure to hot liquids or items, chemicals, and electricity. The degree of tissue injury is related to the intensity of the heat and duration of exposure. Burns are classified by depth of skin injury and include first-, second- and third-degree burns.

- First-degree burns are fairly common. This burn is characterized by pain, skin redness, and swelling. First-degree burns involve only the epidermis and are often the result of sunburn. Healing generally occurs within a week, followed by peeling of the damaged epidermis.
- Second-degree burns, also called partial thickness burns, involve the epidermis and dermis. This burn is characterized by extreme pain, redness, blisters, and open wounds. Second-degree burns usually heal in two to three weeks. If the burned area becomes infected, a second-degree burn may progress into a third-degree wound.
- Third-degree burns, also called full thickness burns, involve the epidermis and entire dermis, exposing layers of fat, muscle, and bone. This burn is characterized by charred and broken tissue layers. The affected individual may exhibit signs and symptoms of shock. Tissue burned to the third degree is painless since the nerves in the dermis have been destroyed. This is not to say that individuals with third-degree burns do not have pain; there is extreme pain, but the pain is caused by the first- and second-degree burns surrounding the third degree burn. Third-degree burns do not consist exclusively of third-degree burn areas; there is a layering of degrees of burn, with first- and second-degree areas surrounding the third-degree areas. Third-degree burns often need tissue grafting in order to heal. Scarring and deformity are common with third-degree tissue damage.

The amount of body surface burned generally correlates with the chance of survival for the affected individual. Body surface may be determined by applying the "rule of nines" (Figure 17–10). Burns exceeding nine percent of the body are serious and should be treated in large medical centers with special burn units. Generally

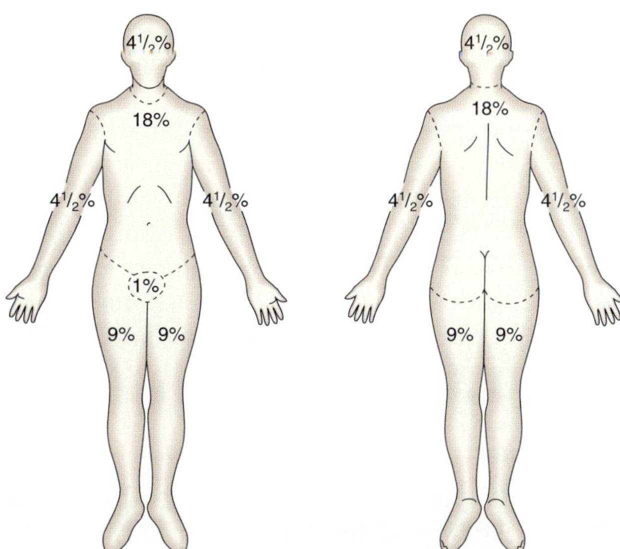

Figure 17–10 Rule of nines—used to calculate percentage of body surface burned.

speaking, body burns of twenty-five to thirty percent of the body are extremely serious, and sixty percent body burns are usually fatal. Other factors affecting the chance of survival include age, health, quality of care, and complications. The elderly and very young do not survive serious burns as well as other age groups. The main complications of burns are fluid loss and infection. Open tissue affected by second- and third-degree burns may leak pints to quarts of serous fluid per day, leading to dehydration and shock. *Pseudomonas* is the bacterium often causing infection. This bacterium is noted for its ability to spread to the blood, leading to septicemia and death.

Treatment of burns depends on the degree and type of burn. Generally treatment will include cooling the tissue with cool water to prevent further burning. Pain is treated with analgesics ranging from over-the-counter products to narcotic analgesics depending on the severity of pain. Antibiotics are given orally and intravenously to prevent or treat infection. Antibiotic ointments may also be applied directly to the burned area. Surgical débridement may be needed to remove charred and necrotic tissue or this may be accomplished by whirlpool treatments. Surgery is often necessary to graft skin, remove excessive scar tissue, and reshape deformities. Surgical treatment may be needed multiple times over a period of months or years to obtain the desired results.

Electrical Injury

Electrical tissue injury is the result of contacting unprotected or inadequately insulated electrical wiring or coming in contact with lightning. Whatever the cause of injury, electrical tissue damage has a point of entry and an exit point. The point of entry is the area coming in contact with the electrical source while the exit point is the grounded area. Electricity travels through the body from point of entry to point of exit, causing burns and often causing deep tissue injury. A common cause of death related to electrical injury is caused by respiratory and cardiac arrest. The physical jolt of electricity may cause respiratory arrest. Electrical current passing through the body may interfere with the conduction system of the heart leading to cardiac arrest.

Radiation Injury

Radiation injury may be caused by ionizing radiation, such as X-rays, and by sunlight. Of the two, sunlight injury is the most common. Exposure to sunlight for short amounts of time leads to skin redness, but prolonged exposure may cause first- and second-degree burns to the skin. Fair-skinned persons are the most easily burned because of a lower number of pigment cells in the skin. Tanning of the skin occurs as a protective mechanism. Tanned skin returns to normal color when pigmented keratocytes in the epidermis are shed. Pigmented skin cells shed approximately every thirty days. Radiation injury may also occur from exposure to sun tanning beds. Tanning of the skin occurs in the same manner as with sun exposure. Tanning of the skin is a popular activity because of the cosmetically pleasant color produced. The long-term effects of tanning are not so pleasant. Prolonged exposure to sun or tanning beds causes the skin to prematurely become dry, brittle, wrinkled, and lose elasticity. These effects cause the skin to appear much older than the natural age. Another unpleasant effect of sun exposure is the development of skin cancers, as discussed earlier in this chapter. (See Healthy Highlight 17–1.)

Pressure Injury

Pressure injury is caused when placing pressure against tissue leads to a decrease in blood flow to this area. The most common type of pressure injury is a decubitus ulcer. Corns and calluses are also the result of pressure injury.

Decubitus Ulcer. Decubitus (dee-KYOU-bih-tus) ulcer is a pressure injury commonly called a bedsore or pressure sore. Decubitus actually means the act of lying

HEALTHY HIGHLIGHT 17–1

Sunburn Prevention

Fair-skinned persons and those working in the sun, such as sailors, farmers, ranchers, road crew workers, and construction personnel, are at the greatest risk for development of sunburn and ultimately skin cancer. Prevention of sunburn includes:

- Avoiding sun exposure during the hours of 10:00 A.M. and 3:00 P.M., when sunrays are the strongest
- Using sunscreen with SPF (sun protection factor) of 15 or higher on all exposed skin
- Wearing a large brimmed hat to reduce sun exposure to the face, ears and head
- Avoiding tanning beds

down or the position of lying. Decubitus ulcers commonly affect the bony areas of the body, such as the heels, sacrum, elbows, and head of individuals who spend prolonged amounts of time in bed. Increased pressure in these areas slows blood flow thus leading to tissue ischemia and necrosis. Pressure sores can be avoided by frequent turning and repositioning to decrease tissue pressure and allow blood flow to the tissues. Massaging the affected area may also improve circulation.

EFFECTS OF AGING ON THE SYSTEM

There are numerous changes in the integumentary system during the aging process. The epidermal layer becomes thinner and retains less water. This accounts for the easy tearing and dryness of the skin common to older adults. **Xerosis** (zee-ROE-sis; dry skin) is a major problem in older adults. They may have flaky, scaly skin and pruritus. The sweat and sebaceous glands do not function as well, further contributing to the dry skin problem. The youthful elasticity of the skin is lost causing wrinkles and an aged appearance. If the individual has spent a great deal of time in the sun over the years, these problems will be exaggerated. The nails become thicker and may be difficult to trim. The hair becomes thinner and brittle. There may be extensive hair loss and graying.

Skin lesions are common in the elderly. Keratoses and skin cancers are the most common problems, especially in individuals who have been exposed to sunlight for many years without using protection. Seborrheic dermatitis and psoriasis are frequently seen disorders. Older adults with chronic disorders such as diabetes or peripheral vascular diseases are particularly prone to develop skin problems, especially pressure injuries. Older adults are also more likely to experience burn or cold injuries as they have decreased touch sensation.

SUMMARY

The skin is important in protecting the body from pathogens, in providing sensations of touch, heat, and cold, and in regulating body temperature. There are numerous skin conditions, some being manifestations of other body system diseases. Skin problems are very traumatic to the individual because they affect appearance and can cause extreme discomfort. Skin diseases range from mild to severe and from acute to chronic. Treatment for many of the skin conditions is symptomatic. Changes in the integumentary system in the older adult cause dry skin; thick, brittle nails; and graying, thinning hair. The elderly are at increased risk for secondary skin disorders related to other system diseases.

REVIEW QUESTIONS

Short Answer

1. What is the main function of the integumentary system?

2. What are the most common symptoms of integumentary system disorders?

3. Which diagnostic tests are used to diagnose integumentary system disorders?

Matching

4. Match the skin condition in the left column with its description in the right column.

____ Herpes
____ Scabies
____ Erysipelas
____ Eczema
____ Pediculosis
____ Pilonidal cyst
____ Urticaria
____ Candida
____ Paronychia

a. a form of cellulitis commonly involving the face
b. a cyst developing around the hair in the sacrococcygeal area
c. a viral disease characterized by inflammation and fluid-filled blisters
d. fungal infection commonly associated with immuno compromised patients
e. vascular reaction of the skin commonly called hives
f. a condition caused by a tiny mite that burrows into the skin
g. bacterial infection of the nail
h. an inflammation of the skin known as atopic dermatitis
i. infestation with lice

True or False

5. T F Carbuncles are most commonly caused by *Staphylococcus* bacteria.
6. T F Pediculosis is an infestation of lice.
7. T F An avulsion is a traumatic crushing injury often caused by heavy objects dropped on parts of the body, such as the fingers.
8. T F Skin cancer is the most common type of cancer diagnosed in individuals.
9. T F Radiation injury may be caused by ionizing radiation, such as X-rays, and by sunlight.
10. T F In burn injuries, the amount of body surface burned generally correlates with the chance of survival of the affected individual.
11. T F Third-degree burns, also called partial thickness burns, involve the epidermis and dermis.
12. T F Your patient suffered second-degree burns on the rear of both arms and the rear of both legs. The total body surface area burned is 27%.
13. T F Complications of severe burns include infection, dehydration, and shock.
14. T F Decubitus ulcers commonly occur over bony areas of the body, for example, the sacrum.
15. T F As one ages, the epidermal layer retains more water, accounting for easier tearing in the older adult.
16. T F In the aging process, the elasticity of the skin is lost, causing wrinkles and an aged appearance only if the individual has had constant exposure to sunlight over the years.

CASE STUDY

Mr. James is a firefighter who is pulled from a burning building that had collapsed several moments earlier. After you remove his bunker gear, you notice second and third-degree burns across his chest, abdomen, back, and the back of his right leg. How severe are Mr. James' burns? What are your priorities as the EMS provider on scene? What are some of the modalities that may be used to treat Mr. James? What complications are likely with burns?

BIBLIOGRAPHY

Albert, R. E. (1997). Allergic contact sensitizing chemicals as environmental carcinogens. *Environmental Health Perspectives, 105*(9), 940–948.

Brodin, M. B. (1997). Dermatology in Primary Care I and II. *Journal of the American Medical Association, 278*, 524.

Fisher, G. J. (1997). Pathophysiology of premature skin aging induced by ultraviolet light. *The New England Journal of Medicine, 337*, 1419.

Gordon, M. L. (1997). Care of the skin at midlife: Diagnosis of pigmented lesions. *Geriatrics, 52*(8), 56–58.

Levine, N. (1997). Pruritic lesions on extremities. *Geriatrics, 52*(9), 89.

Levine, N. (1998). Chronic irritation of the lips. *Geriatrics, 53*(2), 83.

Levine, N. (1998). Persistent rash around lip and eyes. *Geriatrics, 53*(1), 33.

Ramsey, M. L. (1997). Avoiding and treating blisters. *The Physician and Sportsmedicine, 25*(12), 91–92.

Rietschel, R. L. (1997). Occupational contact dermatitis. *Lancet, 349*, 1093–1095.

Roberts, J. R. (1997). Ascending hemorrhagic signs after a bite from a copperhead. *The New England Journal of Medicine, 336*, 1262–1263.

Strauss, R. H. (1997). Grappling with skin infections. *The Physician and Sportsmedicine, 25*(12), 3.

CHAPTER 18

Eye and Ear Diseases and Disorders

CONTENT OUTLINE

- Anatomy and Physiology
  - Eye
  - Ear
- Common Signs and Symptoms
- Diagnostic Tests of the Eye
- Diagnostic Tests of the Ear
- Common Diseases of the Eye
  - Refractive Errors
  - Inflammation and Infection
  - Cataract
  - Glaucoma
  - Nystagmus
- Common Diseases of the Ear Infection
  - Ménière's Disease
  - Labyrinthitis
- Trauma
  - Corneal Abrasion
  - Conjunctival Hemorrhage
  - Hyphema
  - Ruptured Globe
  - Orbital Fracture
  - Chemical Trauma
  - Retinal Detachment
  - Ruptured Tympanic Membrane
  - Basilar Skull Fracture
  - Separation of Ear Cartilage
- Effects of Aging on the System

KEY TERMS

Angiography
Audiometry
Cerumen
Mastoidectomy
Myringotomy
Ophthalmoscope
Otalgia
Otoscope
Photophobia
Pruritis
Purulent
Suppurative
Tinnitus
Tonometry
Topical
Tympanoplasty
Tympanostomy
Vertigo

LEARNING OBJECTIVES

Upon completion of the chapter, the student should be able to:

1. Define the terminology common to the eye and ear.
2. Identify common disorders of the eye and ear.
3. Discuss the basic anatomy and physiology of the eye and ear.
4. Identify the important signs and symptoms associated with common eye and ear disorders.
5. Describe the common diagnostic tests used to determine type and/or cause of eye and ear disorders.
6. Describe the typical traumatic injuries to the eye and ear and discuss the pathophysiology of each injury.
7. Describe the effects of aging upon the eye and ear and the common disorders of these organs.

OVERVIEW

The eyes and ears are the major sensory organs of the body. They are extremely important to most individuals to maintain the quality of life and ease of functioning. However, although sensory deficits affect many people adversely, a high quality lifestyle is still possible after sensory losses. Individuals with visual and hearing impairment learn to function extremely well in activities of daily living. Disorders of the sensory organs are frequently the result of other system problems. Early detection of vision or hearing impairment may prevent permanent loss of these senses.

ANATOMY AND PHYSIOLOGY

The eye and ear are sensory organs that perform highly complex functions in the individual. They each are unique in their structure and function.

Eye

The eye is the sensory organ of sight located in the bony orbit of the skull. It is about one inch in diameter. The eye consists of extraocular and intraocular structures (Figure 18–1). The extraocular structures include the following:

- muscles that hold the eye in place and allow movement of the eye
  - superior and inferior rectus—move eye up and down
  - medial and lateral rectus—move eye toward the nose and toward the temple
  - superior and inferior oblique—move the eye to the right and left vertically
- cranial nerves that innervate the eye and its structures
  - optic (II)—transmits visual information to the brain
  - oculomotor (III)—all muscles that move the eyes except superior oblique and lateral rectus; pupil reaction
  - trochlear (IV)—superior oblique muscle
  - trigeminal (V)—sensation (except vision)
  - abducens (VI)—lateral rectus muscle
  - facial (VII) —closes eyelid; lacrimal gland
- eyelids that cover the anterior portion of the eyeball, protect the eye, and lubricate the eye
- conjunctivae (clear transparent membranes) protect the eye from foreign objects

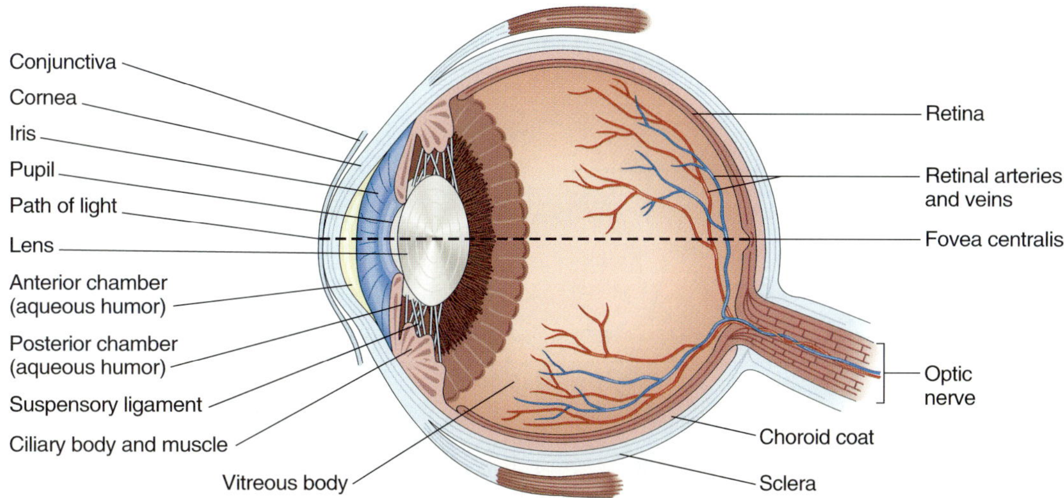

Figure 18–1 The eyeball—cross section view.

- lacrimal glands (tear glands) clean and moisten the eye

The intraocular structures consist of some parts of the eye visible externally and parts visible only through an ophthalmoscope. The intraocular structures include the following:

- sclera—white area covering the outside of the eye except over the pupil and iris
- cornea—clear tissue covering the pupil and iris that provides the majority of refraction
- iris—round disk of smooth and radial muscles giving the eye its color
- pupil—round opening in the iris that changes size as the iris reacts to light and dark
- anterior chamber—space between cornea and iris/pupil filled with clear fluid called aqueous humor
- posterior chamber—space between the iris and lens that is filled with aqueous humor
- lens—clear fibers enclosed in a membrane that refract and focus light to the retina
- posterior cavity—the space in the posterior part of the eyeball filled with a thick, gelatinous material called vitreous humor
- posterior sclera—white opaque layer covering the posterior part of the eyeball
- choroid layer—the layer between the sclera and retina containing blood vessels
- retina—the inside layer of the posterior part of the eye that receives the light rays (visual stimuli)

The mechanism of vision occurs after impulses leave the retina and travel through the optic nerves to the brain. At the optic chiasm the nerve fibers cross and continue to the thalamus. These fibers synapse with other neurons that send the impulses to the right and left visual area of the occipital lobe of the brain. The two optic tracts cross at the optic chiasm (Figure 18–2), which results in some information from the right visual fields translated into the visual area of the left occipital area, and some information from the left visual fields translated into the visual area of the right occipital lobe.

There are two parts to vision, central vision and peripheral vision. Central vision is located in the center of the retina and is responsible for the majority of what a person sees. Destruction to the portion of the retina that is responsible for central vision can significantly affect the patient's vision. Peripheral vision is the part of vision that is on the periphery or boundary of the visual field. Loss of peripheral vision will still allow the patient to function, however it will affect activities such as driving that rely on peripheral vision.

Ear

The structures of hearing and equilibrium are divided into the external ear, the middle ear, and the inner ear (Figure 18–3). The external ear includes the pinna (auricle) and the external auditory canal. The pinna is mostly cartilaginous tissue with a small amount of adipose tissue in the earlobe. The external auditory canal is about one inch in length and contains hair and wax (**cerumen**,

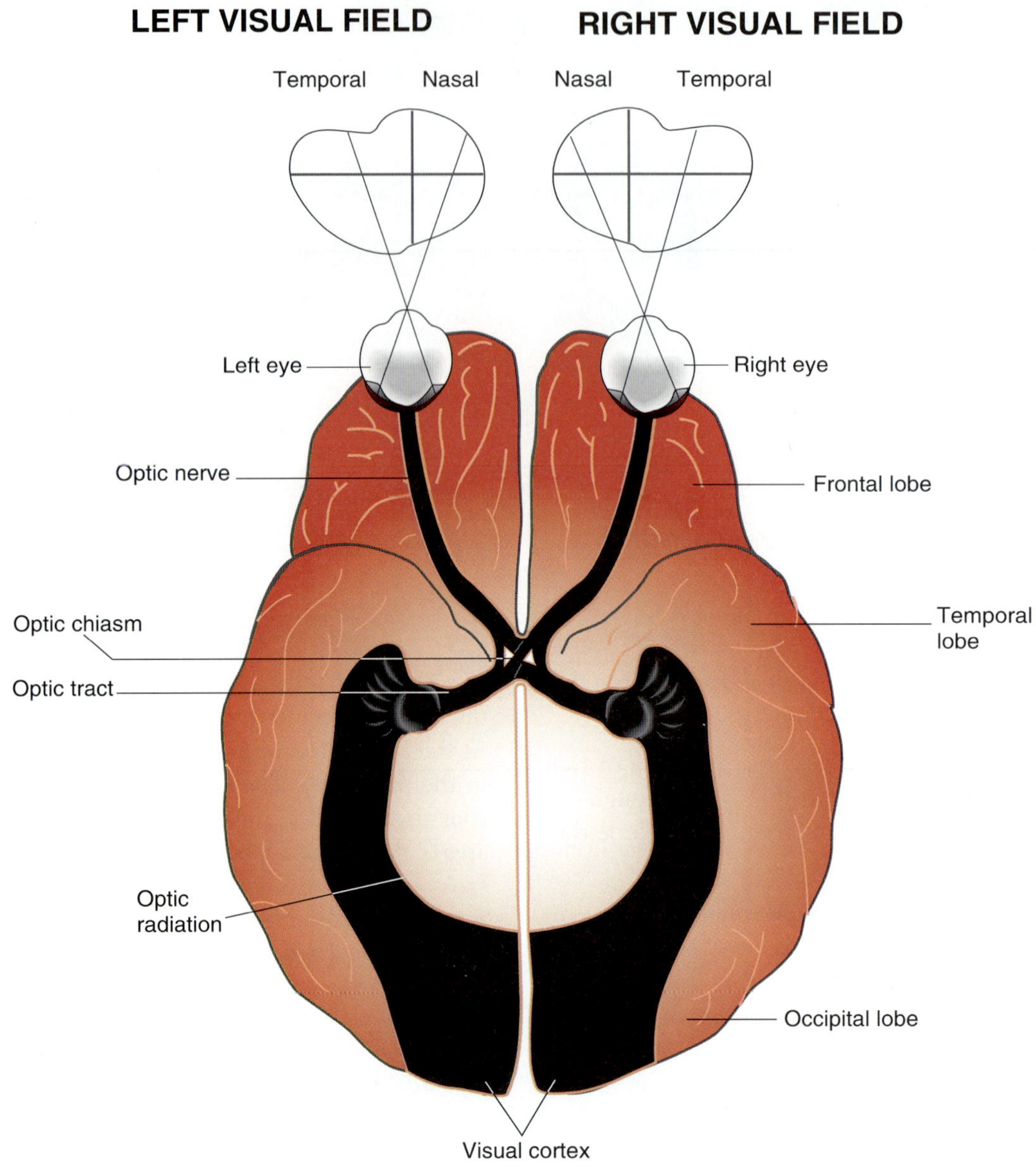

Figure 18–2 The visual pathways of the eye.

se-ROO-men) producing glands. The external ear and middle ear are separated by the tympanic membrane (eardrum).

The middle ear, also called the tympanic cavity, is a small space containing three bones, the malleus (hammer), incus (anvil), and stapes (stirrup). Next to the stapes is the oval window that leads to the inner ear.

The inner ear is the most sophisticated part of the ear. It is responsible for both hearing and equilibrium (balance). The inner ear consists of a fluid-filled space housing the vestibule, the semicircular canals, the round window, and the cochlea. The structures in the vestibule are responsible for maintaining equilibrium during movement of the head. The semicircular canals assist the body to adjust to changes in direction. Changes in the internal components of the semicircular canal or a disparity in sensation between the two sets of canals can cause the symptom of dizziness. The cochlea is the organ of hearing.

The outer ear (pinna) picks up sound waves that are funneled through the external auditory canal to the tympanic membrane. The membrane vibrates in reaction to the sound waves striking it. These vibrations pass through the three tiny middle ear bones through the oval window and into the fluid in the cochlea. Receptor cells respond and transfer the sounds into electrical impulses

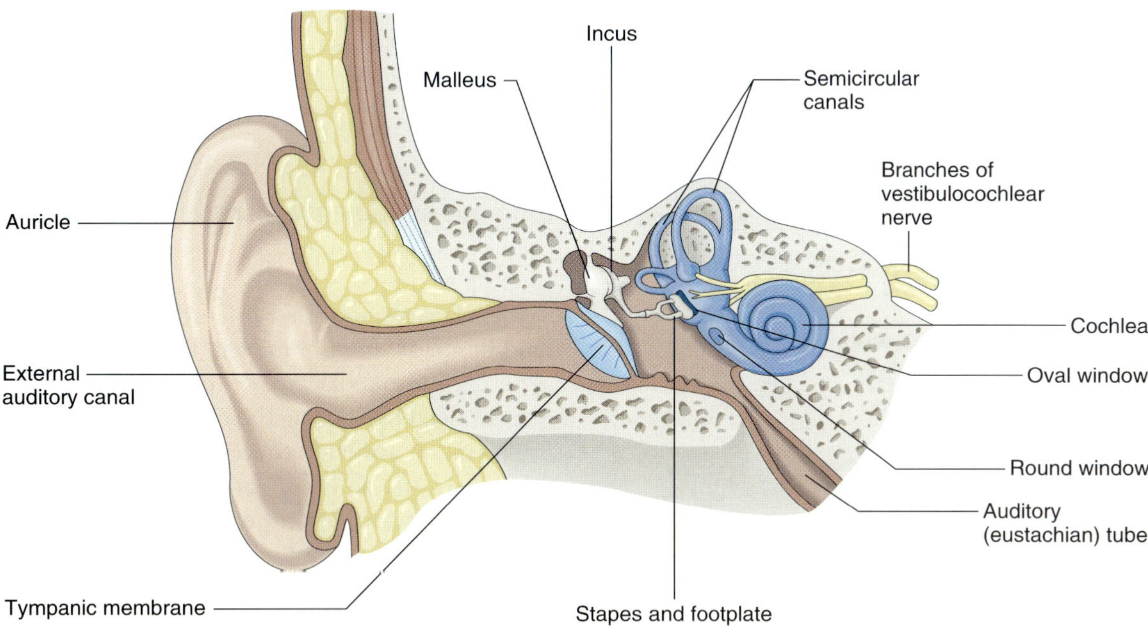

Figure 18–3 The ear.

that travel to the brain via the acoustic nerve. The receiving area of the brain for auditory impulses is in the temporal lobe.

COMMON SIGNS AND SYMPTOMS

Common signs and symptoms of eye disease that need medical attention include:

- Pain or burning in or around the eye
- Decreased visual acuity or ability to see
- Any visual disorder such as seeing flashes of light
- Eye redness

Common signs and symptoms of ear disease that need medical attention include:

- Otalgia (oh-TAL-gee-ah; oto = ear, algia = pain; ear pain)
- Deafness
- Vertigo (VER-tih-go; dizziness)
- Tinnitus (tin-EYE-tus; ringing in the ears)

DIAGNOSTIC TESTS OF THE EYE

An **ophthalmoscope** (aft-THAL-moh-skope; ophthalm = eye, scope = instrument used to look) is the instrument used for a basic examination of the eye. During an ophthalmoscopy (ophthalm = eye, oscopy = procedure to look), the fundus or interior aspect of the eye is examined. The retina, vessels, and optic disc of the eye can be easily visualized.

Visual acuity is measured by the use of a Snellen chart (Figure 18–4). The chart contains lines of letters in varying sizes with predetermined numbers at the end of each line. The predetermined numbers indicate the distance from which an individual with normal vision can see that particular line of letters. Normal vision is expressed as 20/20 and is considered normal vision for an individual viewing a particular line of the chart from 20 feet. For testing, the individual is positioned 20 feet from the chart or this distance may be simulated with the use of reflective mirrors. During the testing one eye is covered allowing measurement of each eye separately. The smallest line of letters the individual can read is noted and the predetermined numbers at the end of that line are recorded in a fraction. The first number, 20, expresses the fact that the individual is tested from 20 feet, and the second number expresses the distance an individual with normal vision could view those same images. For example 20/220 means that the tested individual can see at 20 feet what most people can see at 220 feet.

Diagnostic testing includes tonometry, slit-lamp examination, and retinal angiography. **Tonometry** (toh-NOM-eh-tree; tono = tone or pressure, metry = measurement) is a procedure to measure the pressure inside the eye. Tonometry is useful in determining the presence of glaucoma. A slit-lamp examination utilizes a microscope to magnify the surface of the eye. A beam of light, narrowed to a slit is directed at the cornea. A slit-lamp

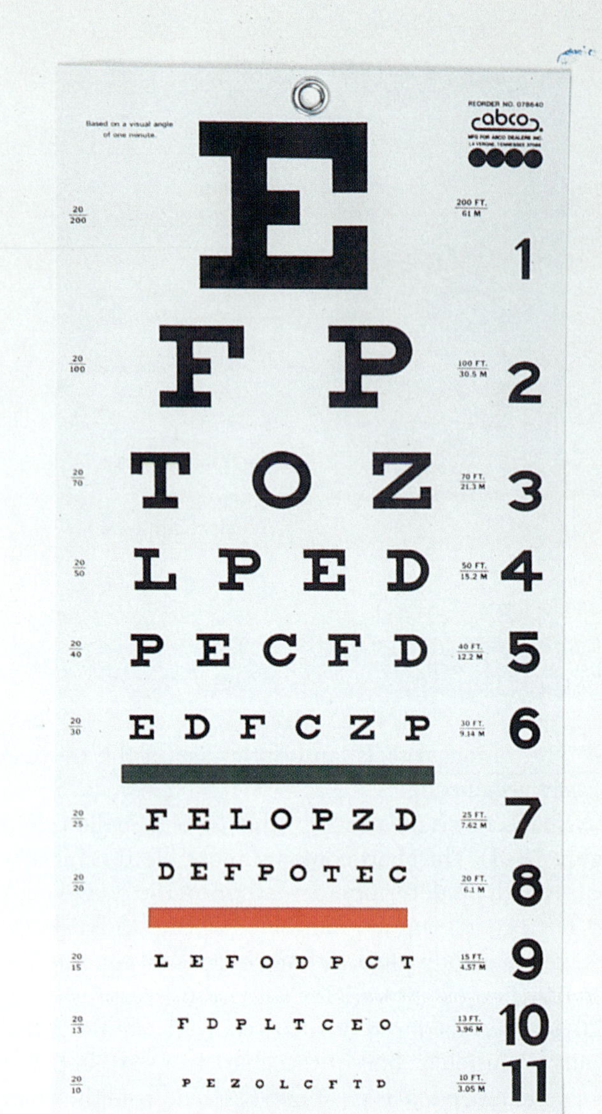

Figure 18–4 The Snellen chart.

examination is helpful in detecting corneal abrasions, keratitis, and cataracts. Fluorescein dye may be used to improve visualization of eye disorders. Fluorescein dye coats the cornea and lines the border of a defect, such as an abrasion, or a foreign body lodged in the cornea, for example a piece of wood or metal. This dye fluoresces, or glows in the presence of a special light and highlights the defect or foreign body. Sometimes it allows the foreign body to be visualized without additional magnification. **Angiography** (AN-jee-**OG**-rah-fee; angio = vessel, graphy = procedure to record) is used by an ophthalmologist to discover vessel disease and problems with blood flow to the eye. Fluorescein dye is injected into a vein usually in the arm. After the dye fills the vessels of the eye, X-rays are made showing the vessels. Vascular disorders such as those caused by diabetic retinopathy can be visualized.

DIAGNOSTIC TESTS OF THE EAR

An **otoscope** (OH-toh-skope; oto = ear, scope = instrument to look) is the instrument used to examine the ear. During an otoscopy (oto = ear, scopy = procedure to look) or otoscopic examination (Figure 18–5), the external canal and tympanic membrane can be easily visualized. Otitis externa, otitis media, and a ruptured tympanic membrane can be diagnosed using the otoscope. Sometimes a small bulb can be attached to the otoscope that forces a puff of air into the auditory canal, allowing the examiner to evaluate movement of the tympanic membrane.

The basic test for hearing is called **audiometry** (AW-dee-**OM**-eh-tree; audio = sound, metry = measure). During the test, sound is delivered in varying levels or decibles through a headset. Each ear is tested separately. The greater the amount of sound needed for the individual to hear or recognize it, the greater the amount of deafness or hearing loss.

COMMON DISEASES OF THE EYE

The most common problem of the eyes is a decrease in visual acuity or the inability to see clearly. The most common cause of poor visual acuity is refractive error. Other

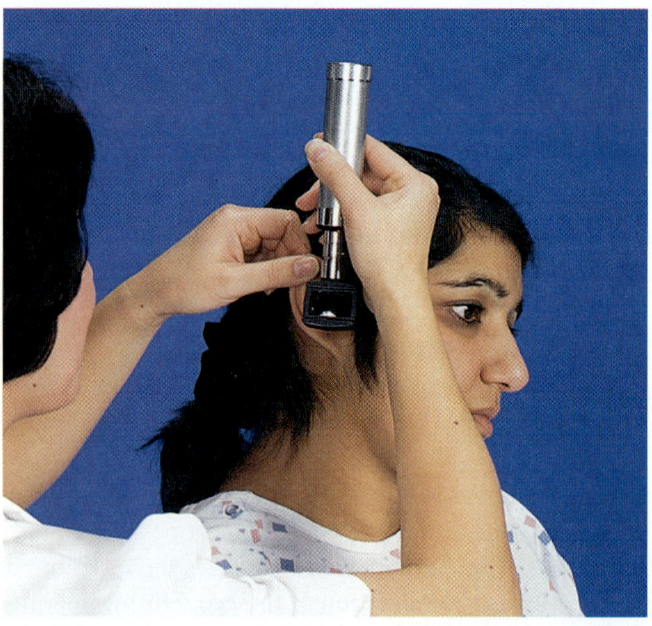

Figure 18–5 Otoscopy.

common problems include those related to inflammation or infection. Infection usually affects the outer eye because of its contact with the environment. Other eye disorders are clouding of the lens (cataract), increased inner eye pressure (glaucoma), and altered eye movement (nystagmus).

Refractive Errors

Refractive errors are those caused by the eye's inability to correctly focus images on the retina. Approximately one-third of the population is affected by refractive errors. The cause of refractive errors is unknown, although some run in families, suggesting an inheritance pattern. While these disorders affect individuals of all ages, incidence increases with age. There are four common types of refractive errors:

1. Myopia (my-OH-pee-ah) is commonly called nearsightedness or shortsightedness. Individuals with myopia can see objects that are near but have difficulty seeing distant objects (Figure 18–6B).
2. Hyperopia (HIGH-per-**OH**-pee-ah) is commonly called farsightedness. Individuals with hyperopia can see objects that are far but have difficulty seeing close objects (Figure 18–6C).
3. Presbyopia (PRES-bee-**OH**-pee-ah) is a type of hyperopia that is age (presby = old age) related. Presbyopia is not caused by the shape of the eyeball, but is related to the inability of the aging lens to properly focus light rays (Figure 18–6D). Presbyopia usually affects individuals aged forty or older. Presbyopia may be corrected by the use of reading glasses or bifocals.
4. Astigmatism (ah-STIG-mah-tizm) is an irregularity in the surface of the cornea causing light rays to spread over the retina rather than focusing properly on a part of the retina (Figure 18–6E). This refractive error may lead to blurred or fuzzy vision often described as seeing "halos" around objects.

Common symptoms of refractive errors include squinting, blurred vision, headaches, and rubbing of eyes. Tests for visual acuity include reading a Snellen chart and an ophthalmoscopic examination to look inside the eye. Refractive errors are commonly corrected by use of prescriptive eyeglasses or contact lenses.

Inflammation and Infection

Inflammation of the eye and related structures is commonly caused by infectious microorganisms. Internal infections, or infection affecting the inside of the eye, are

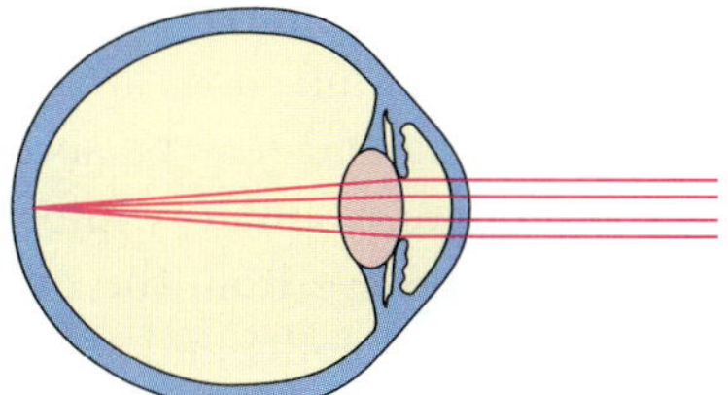

(A) Normal eye
Light rays focus on the retina

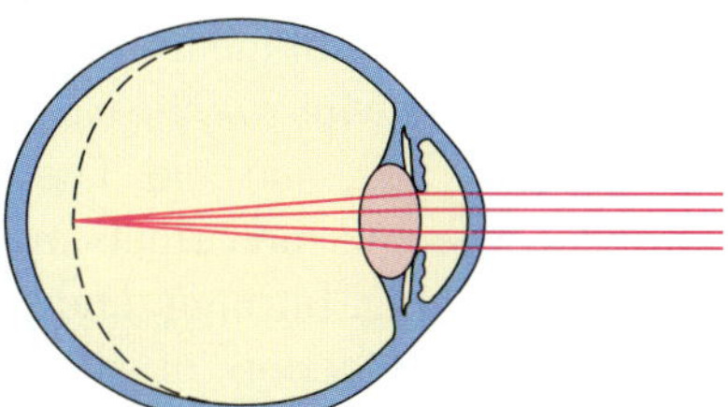

(B) Myopia (nearsightedness)
Light rays focus in front of the retina

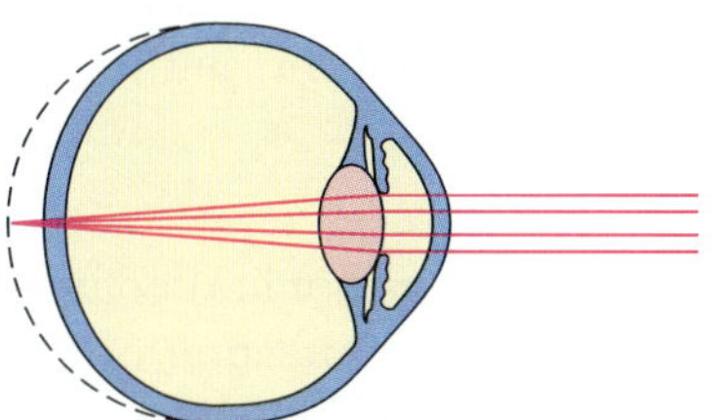

(C) Hyperopia (farsightedness)
Light rays focus beyond the retina

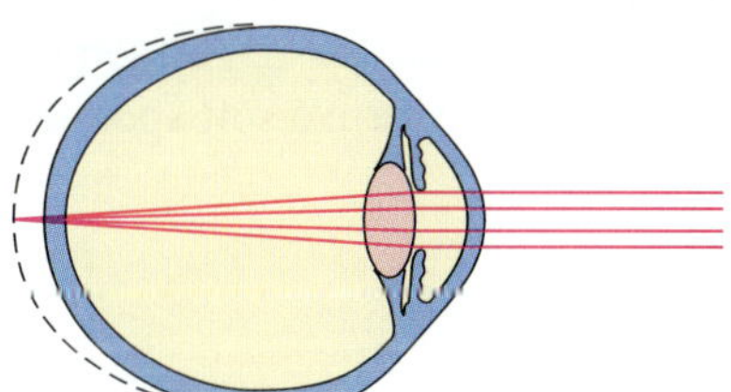

(D) Presbyopia
Light rays focus behind the retina

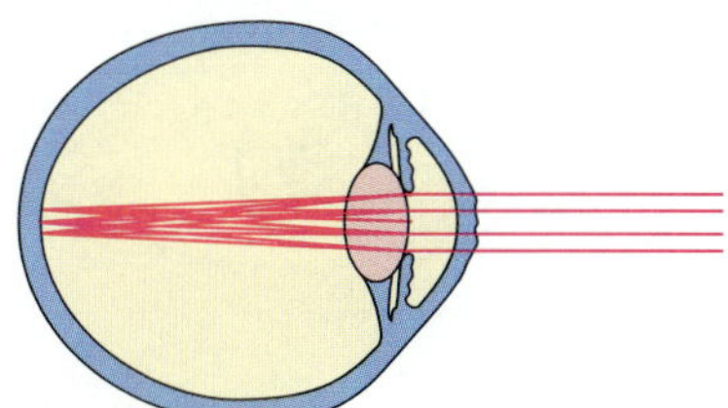

(E) Astigmatism
Light rays focus on multiple areas of the retina

Figure 18–6 A. Normal eye vision. B. Myopia. C. Hyperopia. D. Presbyopia. E. Astigmatism.

rare and are usually related to trauma. More common are inflammation or infections of the surface of the eye and its related structures. Eye infections are commonly caused by viruses and bacteria and may be secondary to allergies, trauma, and upper respiratory infections. Microorganisms may reach the eye from the individual's hands and contaminated washcloths and towels. Good hand washing and cleanliness are preventive measures.

Conjunctivitis. Conjunctivitis is an inflammation of the conjunctiva, the pink membrane lining the inner eyelids (Figure 18–7). Conjunctivitis may be caused by excessive exposure to wind, sun, heat, and cold. The eyelids become red and swollen. Affected individuals may complain of excessive tearing, itching, burning, and pain. An acute, contagious bacterial infection of the conjunctiva is called *pinkeye*. Pinkeye may become epidemic among school-aged children. Treatment includes warm compresses, anti-inflammatory medications, and analgesics to relieve pain. If infection occurs, cultures to identify the microorganisms followed by antibiotic ointment or drops may be needed.

Stye (Hordeolum). A stye or hordeolum (hor-DEE-oh-lum) is an inflammatory infection of a sebaceous (oil-secreting) gland of the eyelid (Figure 18–8). This gland is at the base of a hair follicle or eyelash. Styes resemble pimples, are commonly caused by staphylococcus bacteria, and are often seen in blepharitis. Warm compresses may relieve pain, help localize the infection, and promote drainage. Styes usually form a soft spot, open, and drain and heal without further treatment. In some cases, styes may need to be incised to promote drainage and healing. In chronic conditions, **topical** (placed on the skin) antibiotic or systemic (taken by mouth or injection) antibiotic may be needed.

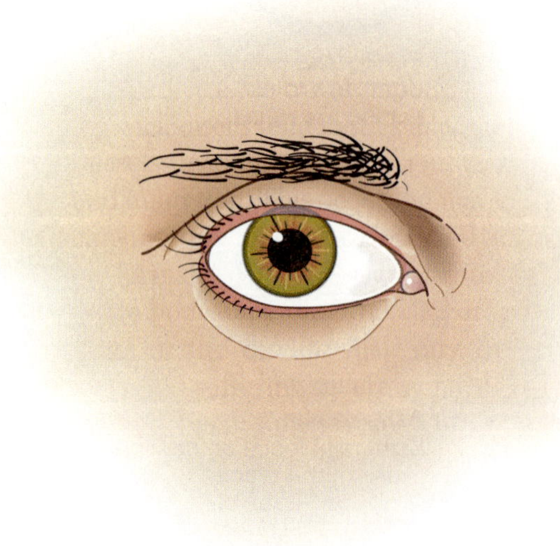

Figure 18–7 Conjunctivitis.

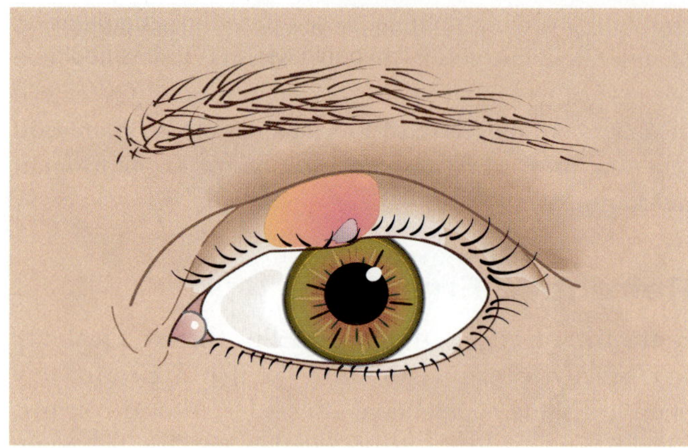

Figure 18–8 Stye (hordeolum).

Cataract

A cataract is a clouding of the lens of the eye (Figure 18–9). Cataracts develop from a change in metabolism and nutrition within the lens. The most common cause of cataract development is aging. Approximately sixty percent of all individuals seventy years of age or older will have clouding of a lens. Cataracts may also be caused by trauma, birth defects, and other diseases such as diabetes mellitus. Cataracts usually develop very slowly in one or both eyes. The main symptom is a decrease in visual acuity or a complaint about not being able to see clearly. Other symptoms include blurred vision, glare, and a decrease in color perception. In advanced cases, the

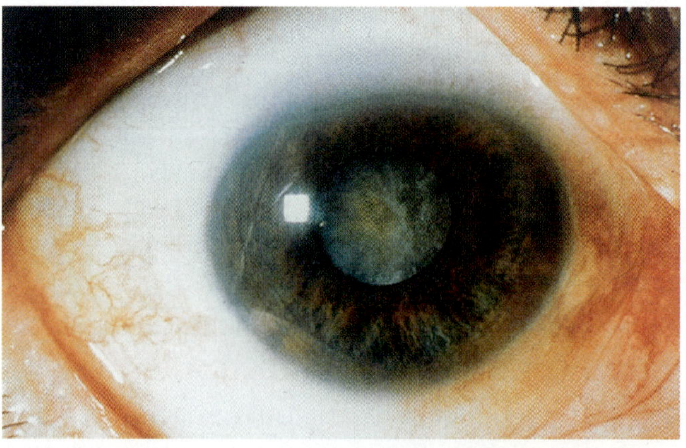

Figure 18–9 Cataract. (Courtesy of National Eye Institute.)

cataract can be seen through the pupil giving the pupil a white cloudy appearance. Diagnosis is confirmed by slit-lamp examination. Cataracts are commonly treated with surgery.

Glaucoma

Glaucoma is a common condition characterized by excessive pressure inside the eye. The fluid inside the front chamber of the eye, known as aqueous humor, is produced constantly by cells surrounding the lens. It circulates through the eye and is reabsorbed into the bloodstream. Excessive pressure inside the eye occurs if too much fluid is produced or does not drain properly. There are several forms of glaucoma. Generally speaking, glaucoma progresses slowly, may or may not be symptomatic, and rarely affects individuals under age forty. Increased pressure inside the eye for a continued period of time may lead to damage of the optic nerve and blindness. Permanent damage is often done before symptoms occur. For this reason, intraocular pressure should be checked on an annual basis.

Acute glaucoma, in contrast, develops rapidly, over a matter of hours to days. Patients who have a smaller angle between their cornea and iris (see Figure 18–1) are more likely to develop acute glaucoma. Signs and symptoms of acute glaucoma include corneal redness, a nonreactive or mildly reactive pupil, a significant elevation in intraocular pressure, haziness of the cornea, decreased visual activity, intense pain, and nausea. Treatment in the emergency department for acute glaucoma includes eye drops and systemic medications to quickly lower the pressure. Laser surgery to promote drainage and relieve the pressure may also be performed by an ophthalmologist on an emergent basis.

Diagnosis is made on the basis of an ophthalmic examination and tonometry revealing an increase in intraocular pressure. Early treatment is essential to prevent permanent blindness. Depending on the form of glaucoma, treatment may include use of eye drops or laser surgery. Both are directed toward either reducing the amount of aqueous humor produced or improving the drainage.

Nystagmus

Nystagmus (nis-TAG-mus) is a constant, involuntary movement of the eyes. Movement may be unnoticed by the affected individual. Movement may be vertical, horizontal, circular, or a combination of these. One or both eyes may be affected. Nystagmus may be the result of brain tumors, disease, alcohol abuse, and congenital defects. Diseases that cause nystagmus include Ménière's disease and multiple sclerosis. Treatment is directed toward correction of the underlying cause. Congenital nystagmus is often untreatable and permanent. Nystagmus may occur when the EMS provider's finger is held in the most lateral position while testing the extraocular muscles. Two or three beats is considered a normal finding; sustained beating may be pathologic and should be reported to the emergency department.

COMMON DISEASES OF THE EAR

The common diseases of the ear include infections and conditions of decreased hearing or total hearing loss. Gradual hearing loss may be caused by a primary ear disorder, such as an infection, or secondary to another disease or injury.

Infection

The ear and related bony structures are commonly subject to infection. The middle ear is connected to the nasopharynx by way of the eustachian tube making it easily accessible to bacteria that cause throat and respiratory infections. The external ear is open to the external environment, allowing infection from air and water. The bony mastoid process connects with the middle ear and is subject to infections affecting the middle ear. Ear infections are more common in infants and children.

Otitis Media. Otitis media is inflammation in the middle ear. It usually affects infants and young children and is commonly called middle ear infection, but it may not necessarily be an infection. The middle ear is normally air filled, but when this area fills with fluid inflammation occurs. For this reason, otitis media is classified by the type of fluid that fills the ear. Fluid types are:

1. Serous—may be caused by an eustachian tube obstruction, allergy, or change in middle ear pressure, as occurs with air flight, that allows clear serous fluid to accumulate in the middle ear. This fluid accumulation causes inflammation of the middle ear, but there is no infection. Symptoms are usually mild and include a feeling of fullness in the ear and conductive hearing loss.
2. Suppurative—an infection in the middle ear. The fluid is pus filled because of the presence of bacteria. The **suppurative** (SUP-you-**RAY**-tive; formation of pus) form of otitis media is often caused by bacteria entering the middle ear usually from the eustachian tube during an upper respiratory

infection. Blowing the nose forcefully often drives respiratory bacteria through the eustachian tube into the middle ear. Swimming in contaminated water may be another cause of suppurative infection. Symptoms include varying degrees of **otalgia** (oh-TAL-gee-ah; ot = ear, algia = pain), nausea, vomiting, fever, chills, **vertigo** (VER-tih-go; dizziness), and conductive hearing loss.

The structure and position of the eustachian tube is an important factor with either type of otitis media. If the eustachian tube is more narrow, shorter, and/or more horizontally placed than normal, the individual is more prone to otitis media. Infants and young children normally have more horizontally placed and narrow eustachian tubes, thus predisposing them to otitis media. As the child grows, the tube becomes more vertical explaining why children often "outgrow" ear infections.

Diagnosis is made on the basis of otoscopy revealing a bulging and nonmobile tympanic membrane (Figure 18–10). The normally pearly colored tympanic membrane is red and swollen. If the tympanic membrane is ruptured, a culture of the fluid may be performed, otherwise cultures are generally not obtained. An elevated WBC, white blood cell count, is also indicative of infection. Treatment for both types of otitis media includes analgesics for pain and decongestants to promote drainage. Suppurative otitis media will require antibiotic therapy.

Chronic otitis media, both forms, may need surgical removal of fluid by **myringotomy** (MIR-in-**GOT**-oh-me; myringo = eardrum, tomy = incision into) to prevent rupture of the tympanic membrane, permanent hearing loss, and possible mastoiditis. To prevent further accumulation of fluid and to relieve pressure, **tympanostomy** (TIM-pan-**OSS**-toh-me; tympano = eardrum, ostomy = new opening) tubes, commonly called PE tubes or pediatric ear tubes, may be placed through the tympanic membrane during a procedure called a **tympanoplasty** (TIM-pah-no-**PLASTY**; tympano = eardrum, plasty = surgical repair) (Figure 18–11). Tubes commonly fall out after several months, but may be removed after six to twelve months. Prognosis for both types of otitis media is good if given prompt treatment. Chronic untreated otitis media may lead to severe ear damage and permanent hearing loss. Prevention of complications is directed toward prevention and prompt treatment of upper respiratory infections and otitis media.

Otitis Externa. Otitis externa, also called swimmer's ear or external otitis, is an inflammation of the external ear canal. This disease commonly affects swimmers who spend many hours in the water. Other causes include trauma to the ear canal, as can occur when attempting to scratch or clean the ear canal and when swimming in contaminated water. The condition often is caused by bacterial or fungal infection. Symptoms of otitis externa include an inflamed ear canal with extreme pain, fever, **pruritis** (proo-RYE-tus; itching), and hearing loss. The ear may also drain clear or **purulent** (PYOU-roo-lent; containing pus) fluid. Diagnosis is made on the basis of an otologic examination. If an infection is suspected, a culture and sensitivity test may be needed. Treatment includes keeping the ear canal clean and dry, analgesics for pain, and antibiotics if an infection is detected. Prevention includes wearing earplugs while showering or swimming in order to keep the external canal clean and dry. Keeping foreign objects out of the ears may also be helpful. Otitis externa tends to be a recurring disease that may eventually become chronic and cause hearing loss.

Mastoiditis. Mastoiditis (MAS-toy-**DYE**-tis) is inflammation of the mastoid process, the part of the skull directly behind and slightly below the ear. This bone is porous or honeycombed in appearance and is located behind the ear. Acute mastoiditis is usually the result of

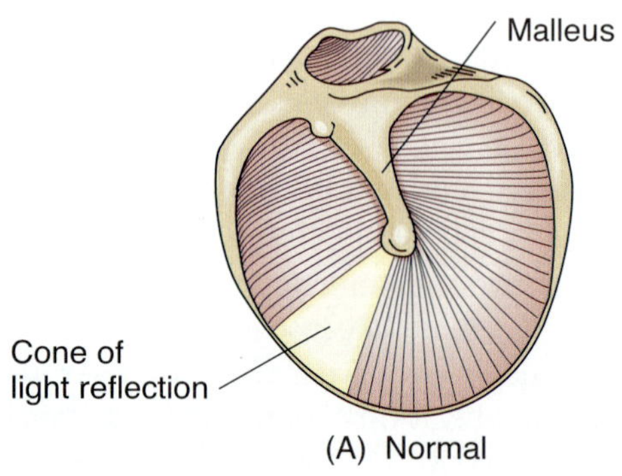

(A) Normal

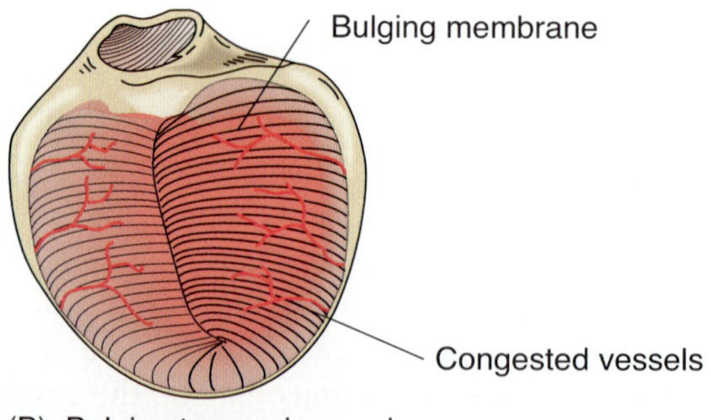

(B) Bulging tympanic membrane

Figure 18–10 Bulging tympanic membrane indicative of otitis media.

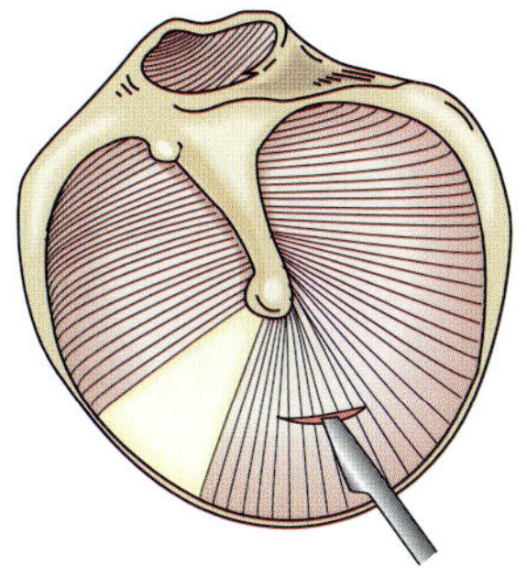

(A) Tympanic membrane incision

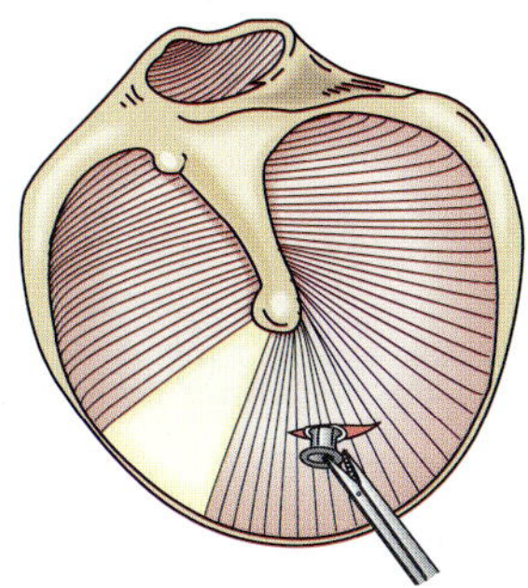

(B) Tube placement

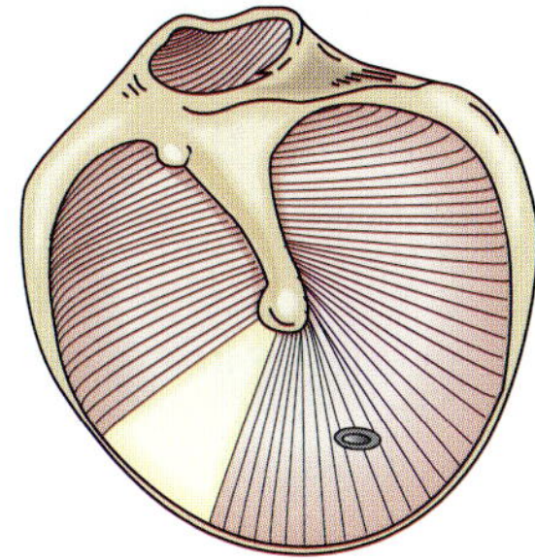

(C) Tympanoplasty completed

Figure 18–11 Tympanoplasty.

a middle ear infection. Infection in the mastoid bone is commonly caused by *Streptococcus*. Symptoms include **tinnitus** (tin-EYE-tus; ringing in the ears) and otalgia (oh-TAL-gee-ah; ot = ear, algia = pain). The mastoid may also become swollen and painful. Diagnosis is made on the basis of otoscopy (OH-**TOS**-koh-pee; oto = ear, scopy = procedure to look into), cultures, and X-ray of the mastoid bone. Mastoiditis generally responds to antibiotic therapy. Severe or chronic mastoiditis may need surgical treatment with a **mastoidectomy** (MAS-toy-**DECK**-toh-me; ectomy = removal or excision) to prevent complications and preserve hearing.

Ménière's Disease

Ménière's disease is a chronic disease of the inner ear characterized by tinnitis, vertigo, progressive hearing loss, and a feeling of fullness in the ear. Acute attacks may last from a few hours to several days, with symptoms of nausea, vomiting, diaphoresis, and vertigo. Ménière's usually affects individuals between the ages of forty and sixty. The cause is unknown, although predisposing factors appear to include middle ear infections and head trauma. Patients with Ménière's disease may lose their ability to maintain balance during their attacks, predisposing them to falls. Treatment for acute attacks includes medications to control nausea and vomiting. A low salt diet, diuretics, antihistamines, and cessation of smoking are usually effective for long-term treatment. Surgery may be performed if the disease does not respond to treatment, but a major complication of surgery is permanent deafness.

Labyrinthitis

Labyrinthitis is an inflammation of the apparatus on the semicircular canals of the inner ear that is responsible for maintaining balance and reporting head position and velocity to the brain. The inflammation results in a mismatch of information sent to the brain causing vertigo, nausea, and vomiting. These symptoms are not associated with hearing loss or change in hearing and labyrinthitis can occur in any age group. Patients will generally report an upper respiratory viral type illness within a week or two preceeding the onset of vertigo. Other findings upon assessment include an increase in vertigo with head movement and nystagmus.

This condition is rarely dangerous, but can induce dehydration from vomiting. In the acute stage, compazine and other antiemetics can be helpful in reducing nausea and meclizine can be used to decrease the vertigo sensation. Sometimes a scopolamine patch is used for vertigo. In general, this is a self-limiting condition that will resolve without deficits.

TRAUMA

Trauma to the eye and ear make up a small percentage of trauma treated in the pre-hospital setting. Trauma can be isolated, as in the case of a corneal abrasion or traumatic retinal detachment, but often occurs with other head and facial trauma. Eye trauma will generally not be life-threatening, but can result in tragic consequences for a patient who has lost his sight. Trauma to the ears can go along with serious brain injuries or skull fracture, with the signs surrounding the ears as the only clue to a more serious, underlying injury. This section covers the common injuries to the eye and ear that you will encounter as an EMS provider.

Corneal Abrasion

The cornea, the transparent outer layer of the eye, is subject to trauma because of its position. Corneal abrasions may be caused by:

- trapping a foreign object such as sand or sawdust between the eyelid and the cornea
- contact lenses that do not fit properly, are dirty or scratched, or are worn for too long a time period
- accidentally poking a finger in the eye
- extreme light, as with welding

Symptoms are often delayed, occurring twelve to eighteen hours after the trauma and include severe pain, tearing, and **photophobia** (photo = light, phobia = fear; an extreme sensitivity to light). Diagnosis is made on the basis of history and visual examination. Abrasions may be easily stained with fluorescein and viewed with a slit lamp. Treatment includes removal of the foreign body and antibiotic ointment or drops to prevent infection. Analgesic medications for pain may be prescribed. A pressure dressing may be applied to the eye to keep the eyelid from moving against the cornea and to reduce the pain of photophobia. Interestingly, the pain caused by corneal abrasion comes from the inside of the eyelid rubbing over the abrasion on the cornea. The cornea does not have sensory nerves. Abrasions can often be avoided by use of protective eyewear.

Conjunctival Hemorrhage

The conjunctiva is normally a clear membrane covering the eye (see Figure 18–1). The conjunctiva is filled with many microscopic blood vessels that can rupture or bleed from direct trauma to the eye, conjunctival irritation, or from a sudden increase in pressure within the vessels as can occur with sneezing, vigorous coughing, or a Valsalva maneuver. Generally, a small amount of blood is not a problem and will resolve on its own. However, a large amount of dense bleeding should be evaluated further at the emergency department as it may indicate a rupture of the globe.

Hyphema

A hyphema is a collection of blood that pools in the anterior chamber of the eye (see Figure 18–1). Hyphemas generally develop as a result of trauma to the eye but may develop spontaneously. There is danger that the iron in the red blood cells within the hyphema may stain the cornea and affect the patient's vision if the blood is left in contact with the cornea. The blood may also clog up the meshwork of the suspensory ligaments that support the lens. The patient should be transported with the head elevated to a 45 degree angle, unless contraindicated by other injuries, to minimize contact between the blood and the cornea. Patients with a history of sickle cell anemia are at an increased risk for complications.

Ruptured Globe

A ruptured globe is an actual full thickness tear or rupture of the eyeball. This is an emergent situation, as the function of the involved eye is in jeopardy. Signs and symptoms include a significant reduction in visual acuity, a change in shape from a round shape to a teardrop shape, leakage of eye contents, and a large hyphema or conjunctival hemorrhage. Movement of the globe should be avoided and the patient transported to a facility that has the ability for a rapid ophthalmologic consult.

Orbital Fracture

Orbital fractures generally involve the facial bones that form either the inferior wall of the orbit or the nasal wall of the orbit. Patients who have sustained an orbital fracture may or may not have a globe rupture or other eye trauma. Unless rupture of the globe is suspected, the fracture does not require emergent surgery. With an inferior wall fracture, the inferior rectus muscle may become entrapped, limiting the patient's ability to look upward with that eye. Fractures of the medial wall of the orbit may cause subcutaneous emphysema because the air-filled ethmoid sinus is located on the other side of the orbital wall.

Chemical Trauma

Chemical trauma to the eye may involve a splash injury of either an acidic or alkaline material. Immediate flushing with a copious amount of water or normal saline (at least one to two liters) is key to minimizing injury. The affected eye should continue to be flushed during transport and after arrival at the emergency department. The patient should be positioned in a lateral recumbent position on the side of the affected eye, and the eye should be flushed from the bridge of the nose outward. This is done to prevent flushing the irritant chemical into the unaffected eye. The EMS provider may need to carefully retract and hold the patient's eyelids open to allow adequate flushing. Use of a Morgan lens or oxygen tubing can be used to ensure the flush fluid is applied to the eye and not just the ambulance stretcher.

Retinal Detachment

Retinal detachment often occurs with trauma, diabetes, and other retinopathies that cause an opening or hole in the retinal layer. This opening allows fluid from the vitreous humor to leak between the retina and choroid layer. The fluid lifts or floats the retina away from the choroid (Figure 18–12). As this process occurs, the individual

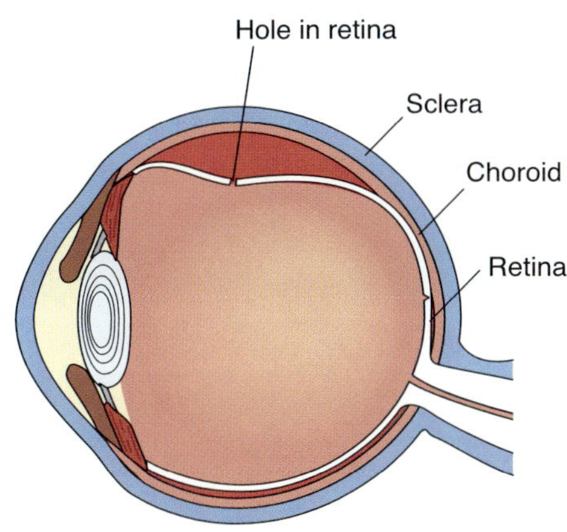

Figure 18–12 Retinal detachment.

experiences loss of vision in the detached area. Often symptoms of retinal detachment include blurred vision, flashes of light, and floating spots. Retinal detachment is painless, but needs immediate medical attention. Ophthalmoscopic examination will readily show the detachment. Surgery is the usual treatment to seal the opening and reattach the retina to the choroid layer. The retina usually regains function unless extreme detachment has occurred.

Ruptured Tympanic Membrane

The most common causes of a ruptured tympanic membrane are a severe middle ear infection or sticking a sharp object, such as a pencil, in the ear canal. The tympanic membrane can also rupture after an explosion or other blunt trauma to the outer ear. Symptoms include pain, partial loss of hearing, and usually bloody or purulent drainage. The main complication of a ruptured membrane is risk of infection. Diagnosis can be confirmed by otoscopy. Treatment may include antibiotics to prevent infection and surgical patching of the membrane with a tissue graft. Minimal hearing loss is associated with a ruptured tympanic membrane.

Basilar Skull Fracture

The base of the skull is the portion of the skull that the brain rests on. A portion of the skull base forms the superior wall of the middle ear and external ear canal. Fractures to the base of the skull, as can occur with a significant force applied to the head, may cause leakage of the cerebrospinal fluid and blood from the brain to leak into the middle ear or external ear canal. All head trauma patients should be assessed for blood or clear fluid flowing from the ears. If a basilar skull fracture is suspected, nasal airway adjuncts and nasal intubation should be avoided to prevent placement of the adjunct directly into the cranial cavity.

Separation of Ear Cartilage

The auricle of the ear is made up of cartilage, allowing it to retain shape but also flexible enough to allow some movement. Cartilage has a very poor blood supply, and is prone to poor healing. In the case of a partial separation, brush off any gross material with a sterile gauze, attempt to approximate the edges of the laceration and wrap the ear with a sterile dressing to control bleeding. If the auricle is completely separated, control bleeding and dress the wound, place the auricle in a plastic bag and place it on ice and transport the patient to the emergency department.

EFFECTS OF AGING ON THE SYSTEM

The effects of aging on the sensory organs are significant. Changes in vision begin in middle age and progress through the older adult years. The change is obvious in most people beginning with the inability to read small print or to see well in low light. These changes affect the older adult's ability to function well in society and often cause social isolation and dependence on others.

Vision changes begin around age forty and continue through the life span. Focusing on near objects, color perception, some sensitivity to light, and decreased visual acuity are all normal physiologic changes that occur during the aging process. Although the changes vary among individuals, most persons have about a 20/70 visual acuity by age sixty-five. Glaucoma and cataracts are common problems of the older adult, reducing the ability to see even further. In the diabetic older person, retinopathy is a very common problem that often eventually leads to blindness.

Hearing changes in the older adult affect the ability to perceive what is heard and may also affect behavior, personality, and attitudes. Many hearing problems can be corrected, but may not be because of financial constraints or social concerns. The inability to hear often affects the individual's ability to communicate and interferes with one's social life and independence. In some instances, speaking in a clear concise manner is more beneficial than raising one's voice.

As the individual ages, the tympanic membrane becomes thinner and less flexible, reducing the conduction of sound. This is a "conductive" hearing loss associated with aging. If there has been damage to the eighth cranial nerve, the individual has a sensorineural loss. If both types are present, it is called a "mixed" hearing loss.

The slow but gradual loss of hearing called presbycusis, affects more men than women. This type of hearing loss is caused by degenerative changes in neurons, the bones of the middle ear, and the cochlea. High-pitched sounds become the most difficult to hear at first, but gradual loss of low-pitched sounds also occurs eventually.

Other hearing conditions seen in the older adult include otosclerosis, tinnitus, and Ménière's disease. Although some of these may begin in younger life, they are most commonly detected in later years.

SUMMARY

The sensory organs of the body are often regarded as the most important to the individual to maintain a quality life. Visual and hearing impairments are often correctable, especially if diagnosed early in the degenerative period. Other system diseases, such as diabetes, often affect the sensory organs and can destroy their ability to function. Some of the most common disorders of the eyes include myopia, presbyopia, hyperopia, and glaucoma. The most common diseases of the ear include tinnitus, otitis media, conduction loss, otosclerosis, and Ménière's syndrome. In the older adult, sensory organ disorders are common. Some losses of vision and hearing occur naturally through the aging process while others are a result of other system diseases. Diagnosis and treatment of vision and hearing losses should be implemented early to prevent some of the complications of sensory dysfunction.

REVIEW QUESTIONS

Short Answer

1. What are some of the most common problems affecting the eyes?

2. What are some of the most common problems affecting the ears?

3. What diagnostic tests are used to diagnose or evaluate eye disorders?

4. What diagnostic tests are used to diagnose or evaluate ear disorders?

Fill in the Blanks

5. The lay term for ___________ is "pink eye."
6. Extreme sensitivity to light is called ___________.
7. Another term for nearsightedness is ___________.
8. Farsightedness is also called ___________.
9. A common eye disorder that occurs with aging is called ___________.
10. The main symptom of a cataract is the gradual ___________ of vision.
11. In ___________, aqueous humor is produced faster than it can be drained.
12. Sudden flashes or spots before the eyes may be a sign of ___________.

13. The cranial nerves that control the muscles of eye movement include ___________, ___________, and ___________.
14. Within the ear the organ of hearing is the ___________.
15. The major symptom of ear disorders is ___________.
16. Buzzing or ringing in the ear(s) is called ___________.
17. ___________ is also commonly called "swimmer's ear."
18. Vertigo is the common complaint of an individual with ___________.
19. Chronic otitis media may result in perforation of the ___________.
20. Blood that has pooled in the anterior chamber of the eye is known as a ___________.
21. You are presented with a patient who sustained trauma to his left eye. You note a significant reduction in visual acuity, a teardrop shaped eye ball, and a large hyphema. You should suspect a ___________ until proven otherwise.
22. Conjunctival hemorrhage may result from ___________.
23. Pain and extreme sensitivity to light is called ___________.
24. You are assessing an unconscious patient who sustained blunt trauma to his head. During your assessment, you note blood and clear fluid dripping from his right ear. You should immediately suspect ___________.
25. What treatment(s) are contraindicated for the patient in question 24? ___________

CASE STUDY

During your night shift, you respond to the scene of an altercation at the park. A police officer directs you to your patient, who is a 14-year-old male who has been struck in the face with a baseball bat. While assessing him, you note that he is conscious, his airway is patent, he has blood in the anterior chamber of his left eye, and his left eye appears sunken compared to the right. What is the blood in the anterior chamber called? What is the likely reason for the sunken left eye? How should you proceed with your assessment? What other injuries should you be concerned about?

BIBLIOGRAPHY

Bennett, D. (1997). Communication screening in older adults with vision loss. *Perceptual and Motor Skills, 84*(6 pt 1), 1097–1098.

Bentley, B. (2000). Ocular Emergencies. In D. M. Cline (Ed.), *Emergency medicine: A comprehensive study guide companion handbook* (5th Ed.). Dallas, Texas: American College of Emergency Physicians.

Berman, E. L. (1995). Clues in the eyes: Ocular signs of metabolic and nutritional disorders. *Geriatric, 50*(7), 34–36.

Blood, I. M. (1997). The hearing aid effect: Challenges for counseling. *Journal of Rehabilitation, 634*, 59–62.

Brody, J. E. (February 7, 1996). Using the mind's eye to combat eating disorders. *New York Times*, C9.

Brody, J. E. (January 20, 1998). For glaucoma risk group, ignorance is blindness. *New York Times*, F9.

Brody, J. E. (October 21, 1997). When eyes betray color vision. *New York Times*, F9.

Bron, A. J. (1997). Loss of vision in the ageing eye; research into ageing workshop. *Age and Ageing, 26*(3), 159–162.

Colorblindness, Lyme disease. (1997). *Flying, 124*(9), 85.

Dowler, D. L. (1996). Accommodating specific job functions for people with hearing impairments. *Journal of Rehabitation, 62*(3), 35–43.

Embil, J. M. (July 19, 1997). A blinding headache. *Lancet, 350*, 182.

Gentry, B. (1997). Failure rates of young patients with sickle cell disease on a hearing screening test. *Perceptual and Motor Skills, 84*(4), 434.

Gilbert, C. (July 5, 1997). Retinopathy of prematurity in middle-income countries. *Lancet, 350*, 12–14.

Hodson, S. (May 29, 1997). Cultivating a cure for blindness. *Nature, 387*, 449.

Morfid, L. (1997). REM sleep behavior disorder: A treatable cause of falls in elderly people. *Age and Ageing, 26*(1), 43–44.

Tesch-Romer, C. (1997). Psychological effects of hearing aid use in older adults. *Journals of Gerontology, Series B: Psychological Sciences and Social Sciences, 52B*(5), P127–P138.

White, R. (1997). "Hey Mr. White, that's the wrong color for that." *Smithsonian, 28*(10), 158.

Wright, K. J. (1997). Dietitians can and should communicate with older adults with hearing and vision impairments and communication disorders. *Journal of the American Dietetic Association, 97*(2), 174–176.

CHAPTER

19

Environmental Diseases and Disorders

CONTENT OUTLINE

- Heat Emergencies
  - Physiology of the Rhermoregulatory Mechanism
  - Fever
  - Heat Cramps
  - Heat Exhaustion
  - Heat Stroke
- Cold Emergencies
  - Hypothermia
  - Frostbite
- Water Emergencies
  - Near Drowning
  - Diving Emergencies
- Altitude Emergencies
  - Physiologic Response to Altitude
  - Acute Mountain Sickness
  - High Altitude Cerebral Edema
  - High Altitude Pulmonary Edema

KEY TERMS

Boyle's law
Conduction heat loss
Convection heat loss
Dalton's law
Dry drowning
Evaporation heat loss
Fever
Frostbite
Frostnip
Heat cramps
Heat exhaustion
Heat stroke
Henry's law
Hyperthermia
Hypothermia
Hypoxic ventilatory response (HVR)
Immersion foot
Piloerection
Pyrogeus
Radiation heat loss
Solubility
Thermogenesis
Thermolysis
Thermoreceptors
Trench foot
Wet drowning

LEARNING OBJECTIVES

Upon completion of this chapter, the student should be able to:

1. Describe the normal physiology of the thermoregulatory mechanism.
2. Describe the signs, symptoms, and pathophysiology for heat related conditions.
3. Describe the signs, symptoms, and pathophysiology for cold related conditions.
4. Describe the signs, symptoms, and pathophysiology for near drowning and diving emergencies.
5. Describe the normal physiologic changes that occur when an individual is exposed to high altitudes.
6. Describe the signs, symptoms, and pathophysiology for altitude related conditions.

OVERVIEW

Every year, millions of Americans head to the outdoors for recreation or employment. Even those who do not seek the outdoors are exposed to the environment and may succumb to changes in the environment. Risk factors for developing an environmental related condition include age (very young and very old populations are at increased risk), general health, fatigue, predisposing medical conditions, and certain medications. In this chapter, we will discuss the pathophysiolgy, signs and symptoms, and management of environmental emergencies.

HEAT EMERGENCIES

According to statistics, between 1979 and 1998 there were approximately 7,400 heat related deaths in the United States. Heat related conditions can easily present in any weather while individuals are engaged in activities where they are clothed in heavy personal protective equipment, for example, vehicle extrication, fire fighting, and hazardous materials operations. EMS providers who participate in these incidents should be aware of the signs of heat related emergencies, assess personnel involved in the incident regularly, and ensure adequate rehydration during and after the event.

Physiology of the Thermoregulatory Mechanism

The human body has an elegant and complex mechanism designed to maintain the core body temperature to within ±1° F (±0.6°C). This mechanism is centrally controlled and has both central and peripheral **thermoreceptors** that sense either heat or cold. Central thermoreceptors, located in the anterior portion of the hypothalamus in the brain, are more responsive to heat than cold, and work to prevent **hyperthermia**. Peripheral thermoreceptors are more responsive to cold than heat, and help to prevent **hypothermia**. Peripheral thermoreceptors are located in the skin and deep within the body surrounding the gut, great veins of the thorax and abdomen, and around the spinal cord. The signals from the central and peripheral thermoreceptors are received by the posterior hypothalamus in the brain, which controls the body's response to the outside environment (Figure 19–1).

The process of heat production is called **thermogenesis**. Thermogenesis occurs when the core body temperature falls below normal. Mechanisms used in thermogenesis include constriction of blood vessels in the skin, piloerection, and increased heat production. **Piloerection** is the elevation of the small body hairs to provide a layer of insulation between the environment and the skin. This mechanism of thermogensis is not as important in humans as it is in other animals. The body produces heat via three mechanisms, shivering, sympathetic stimulation, and thyroxine secretion. Shivering produces

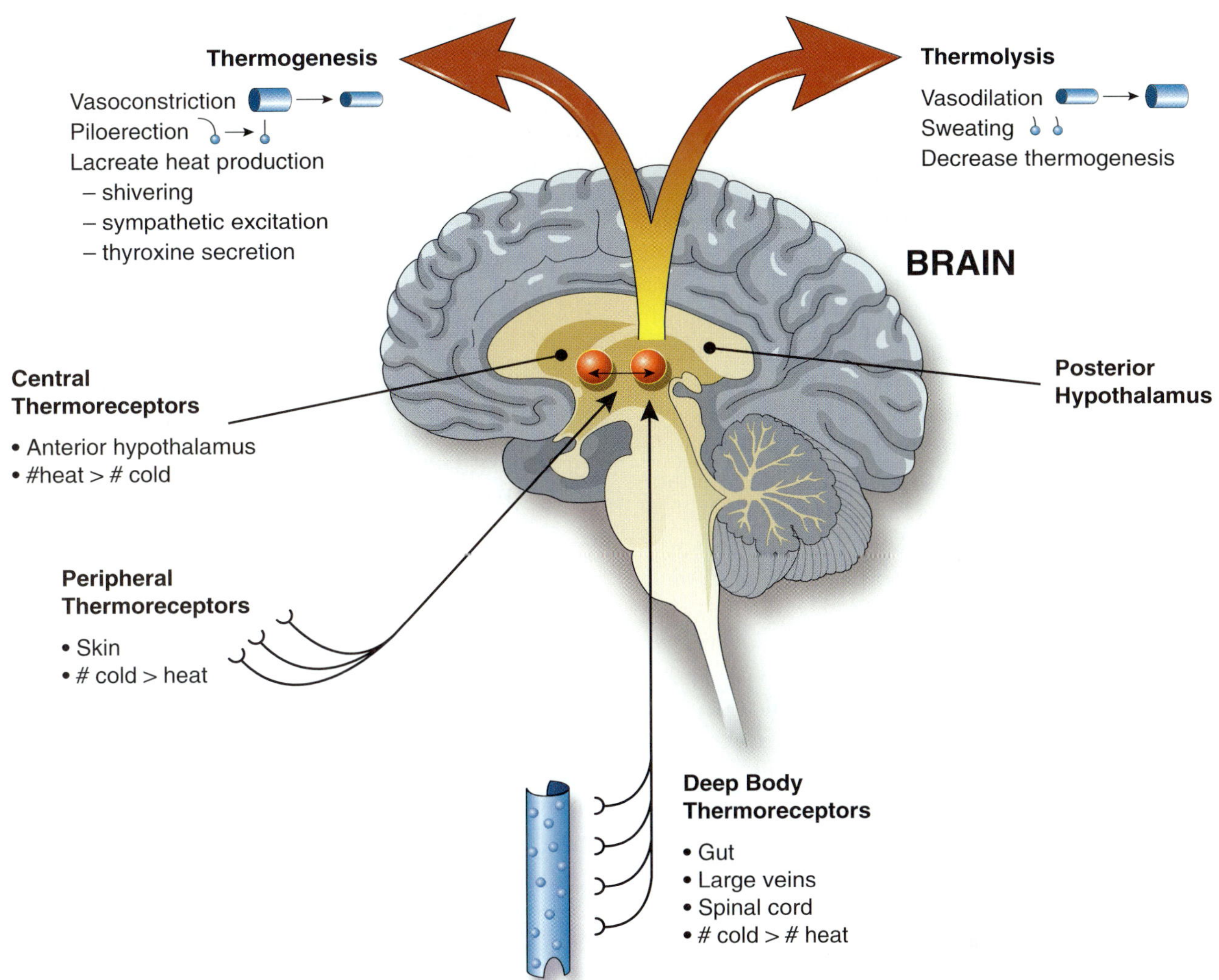

Figure 19–1 The thermal regulatory mechanism.

heat by increasing energy usage and movement in the muscles. Sympathetic stimulation produces peripheral vasoconstriction and helps release energy stores to allow increase of conversion of stored energy into heat. Increased production of thyroxine increases the body's metabolism and produces additional heat.

Thermolysis is the dissipation of heat from the body and occurs through three mechanisms. The first is peripheral vasodilation. Peripheral vasodilation allows more blood to reach the skin surface, thereby allowing more heat to be removed via convection. Production of fluid by the sweat glands allows heat to be removed from the body by evaporation. Dehydration can occur rapidly if the individual does not maintain adequate fluid intake. Finally, a feedback system exists where thermogenesis is decreased.

Fever

Fever is defined clinically as a body temperature greater than 100°F (37.8°C) and is a normal physiologic response to infection. In young and middle-aged adults without significant medical conditions, the fever response to infection is generally robust and can be used as an indicator for systemic infection as opposed to a localized infection. However, in the very young and the elderly, two age groups with a decreased physiologic reserve, a systemic infection can be present without a fever. In these age groups, systemic infections can be present and the patient presents with a decreased body temperature because the physiologic mechanisms have been overcome by the infection. Fever can occur for other reasons, for example, brain abnormalities that change the balance point in the thermoregulatory system, or when certain toxic substances are present.

A fever in the setting of infection is caused as a response to bacterial cell destruction by the body's immune system. Byproducts released by bacterial destruction and tissue damage, called **pyrogens**, cause an increase in the normal temperature set point in the posterior hypothalamus, similar to turning up the wall thermostat in a house. Rapid changes in the set point caused by pyrogens produce the chills and the flush described by patients during their infection. Chills are caused by a rapid increase in the temperature set point, tricking the body into thinking that thermogenesis is required. The patient reports feeling cold because body temperature is below the new set point on the thermostat in the hypothalamus. When the fever breaks, the set point is rapidly decreased, the body feels overly warm because the body temperature is now above the set point, and profuse sweating and vasodilation occur. This corresponds to the "flush" reported by patients as their fever breaks.

Definitive treatment of fever is identification and treatment of the source of infection. For symptomatic treatment, most patients respond to either acetaminophen or ibuprofen. Some patients may benefit from rehydration as many patients have poor fluid intake during an infection; however, intravenous replacement is preferred over oral fluid replacement only in the setting of a patient who is unable to drink liquids.

Heat Cramps

Heat cramps are caused by muscle spasm secondary to the loss of electrolytes. Heat cramps occur in individuals who are sweating profusely and who do not replenish electrolytes lost in the perspiration. These individuals may be replacing water lost, but not the electrolytes lost in the perspiration. The muscle spasm is caused by the loss of sodium, which works to allow muscles to relax after contraction, which is mediated by calcium. Heat cramps are generally not a life-threatening condition, and usually resolve with time; however, they can be very painful.

Treatment of heat cramps includes moving the patient to a cool environment and replacing fluids and electrolytes lost. Replacement can be oral, and many of the commercially available sports drinks contain a sufficient amount of electrolytes to replace what has been lost. Salt tablets should be avoided because they tend to irritate the stomach lining; however, they can be dissolved in water as directed by the packaging instructions. In very severe cases, rhabdomyolysis can occur from sustained muscle contraction.

Heat Exhaustion

Heat exhaustion is a condition where the body has lost a significant amount of fluid and electrolytes. The patient is symptomatic and can progress to heat stroke if not treated. Signs and symptoms of heat exhaustion include dizziness, weakness, vomiting, malaise, headache, and orthostatic hypotention. Patients are also often tachycardic, tachypnic, and can exhibit a body temperature of up to 104°F (40°C).

As with heat cramps, the EMS provider should remove the patient to a cool environment, assess the airway, breathing, and circulation, and begin rehydration. These patients are more likely to require intravenous fluid rehydration, but may be able to tolerate oral rehydration. If the patient presents in shock, rapid rehydration with two liters of normal saline is indicated.

Heat Stroke

Heat stroke is a life-threatening emergency. The patient's body temperature has increased to a dangerous level and the ability of the body to compensate has been exhausted. Heat stroke is defined as a body temperature of 104.9°F (40.5°C), signs of central nervous system dysfunction, and a lack of perspiration. The key differentiation between heat exhaustion and heat stroke is the presence of neurologic symptoms. Once the core body temperature rises above 105°F, the thermoregulatory ability of the hypothalamus is significantly altered, and the body totally loses its ability to compensate. CNS dysfunction can include altered mental status, posturing, seizures, or coma.

Treatment of a patient with suspected heatstroke is focused on reducing body temperature. The high mortality associated with heatstroke is believed to be associated with a delay in cooling. Once the airway, breathing, and circulation are secured, rapid infusion of normal saline should be initiated. Cooling can be accomplished by spraying the patient with water and fanning with a fan or towel, taking advantage of evaporative cooling. Another method of cooling involves placing ice packs in the groin and axillae, both highly vascular areas closer to central circulation. Cooling efforts should be stopped when the body temperature reaches 104°F (40°C) to avoid developing hypothermia.

COLD EMERGENCIES

Cold emergencies are commonly thought of as only occurring in northern climates and in the winter; however, they can occur in relatively warmer climates almost year round given the proper conditions. Nighttime temperatures in warmer climates can fall well below normal body temperature of 98.8°F (37.1°C). Sleeping outdoors on an uninsulated surface can provide a means for heat loss and development of a cold related condition.

Heat can be lost via several mechanisms (Figure 19–2). **Conduction heat loss** occurs from heat loss between objects that are in contact with each other. **Convection heat loss** occurs when air currents flow over a warmer object, transferring heat to the air and away from the object. **Radiation heat loss** occurs as heat waves are transmitted from an object into the air without air movement. **Evaporation heat loss** occurs when the energy from the warm object causes the liquid on the surface to evaporate.

Hypothermia

Hypothermia is defined as a decrease in core body temperature. This can occur as a result of inadequate thermogenesis, excessive cold stress, or from a combination of both factors. Both the pediatric and geriatric populations are predisposed to hypothermia because their natural thermoregulatory mechanism does not respond as well to temperature changes as the younger adult. Prior medical conditions such as hypothyroidism and hypoglycemia can also predispose an individual to hypothermia. Certain medications or substances, for example, alcohol, antihistamines, narcotics, NSAIDs, and antiseizure medications, can interfere with the thermoregulatory mechanism and predispose an individual to hypothermia. Other factors that can predispose an individual to hypothermia include fatigue, malnutrition, length of exposure and intensity of exposure.

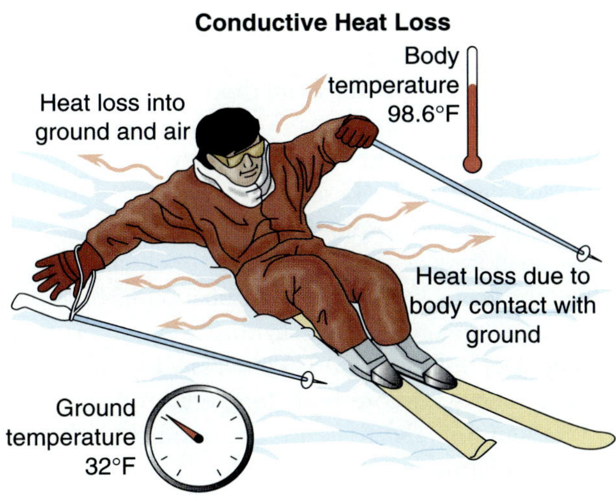

Figure 19–2 Methods of heat loss. (A) Conduction

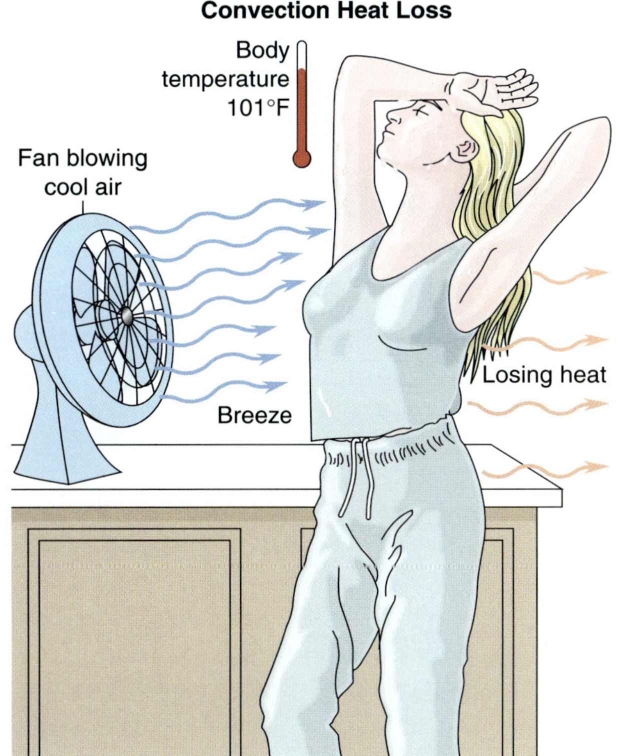

Figure 19–2 Methods of heat loss. (B) Convection

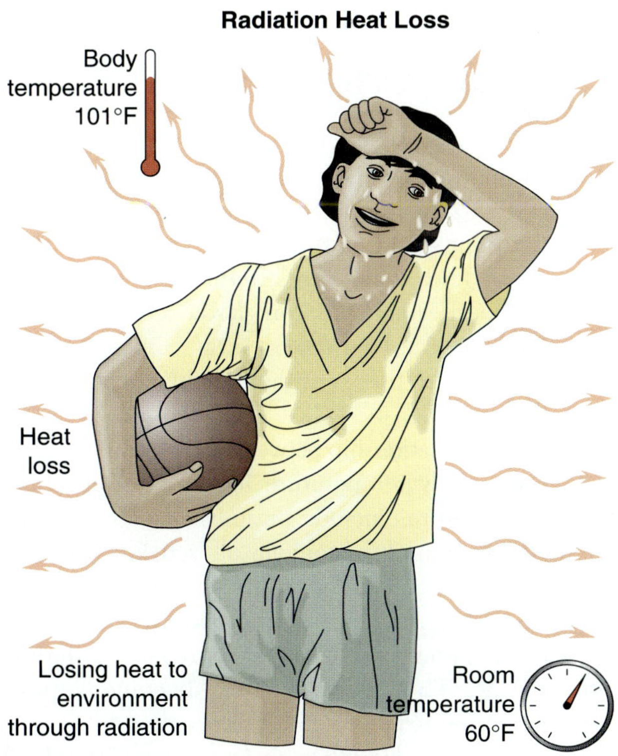

Figure 19–2 Methods of heat loss. (C) Radiation

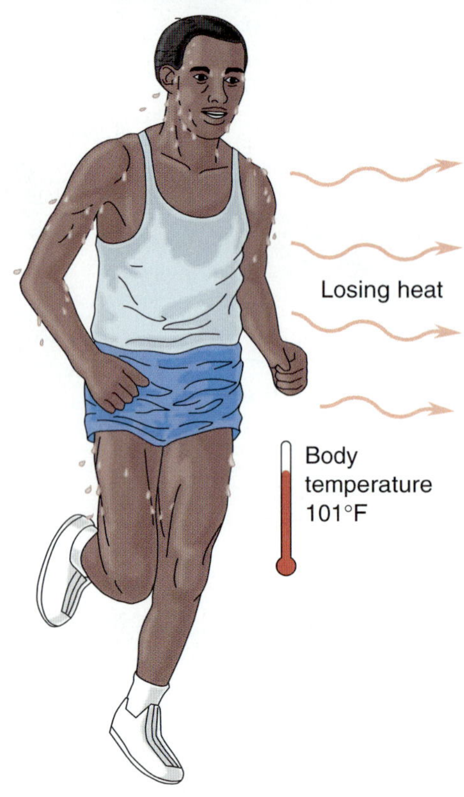

Figure 19–2 Methods of heat loss. (D) Evaporation

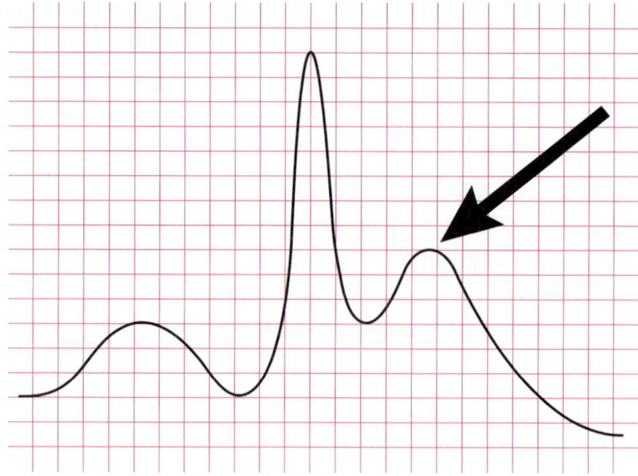

Figure 19–3 An Osborne or "J" wave associated with hypothermia.

Hypothermia can be broken down into three categories of severity: mild, severe, and compensated. Mild hypothermia is defined as the presence of signs and symptoms with a core body temperature greater than 90°F (32.2°C). Hypothermia is classified as severe when signs and symptoms are present with a core body temperature less than 90°F (32.2°C). Hypothermia is considered compensated if signs and symptoms are present with a normal core body temperature. In the situation of compensated hypothermia, the core body temperature is maintained by increased thermogenesis. Once glycogen stores are depleted, however, the individual's core body temperature will fall.

No reliable relationship between signs and symptoms and the core body temperature has been established. Signs and symptoms include diminished coordination, decreased psychomotor function, altered level of consciousness, shivering, and decreased core body temperature. An Osborne or J-wave may be present on the patient's ECG; however, this is not as reliable a finding (Figure 19–3). The myocardium can become irritable producing either atrial or ventricular ectopy.

Management of hypothermia involves stopping heat loss and rewarming the patient. If possible, the EMS provider should remove the patient from the cold environment, remove wet clothing, dry the patient, and then provide insulation in the form of blankets and a moisture barrier. The patient's head should be covered as a significant amount of heat is lost through the head. The patient should be handled gently to avoid producing ventricular fibrillation.

Rewarming can be accomplished in a passive or active manner. Passive rewarming includes insulation and moisture barrier. Active external rewarming utilizes a source of warmth, for example, heat packs or lights, to warm the patient. If heat packs are used, they should be insulated from direct skin contact to avoid burns and placed over areas of the body with high rates of heat transfer, namely, the base of the neck, the axilla, and the groin. Water immersion can be used; however, it can induce rewarming shock and may not be as applicable in the EMS environment. Active internal rewarming can be accomplished by providing warmed and humidified oxygen and warmed IV fluids. It is not clear how much heat transfer is accomplished by these methods.

Hypothermia presents some challenges to assessment and resuscitation. Additional time may be required to assess vital signs, up to 45 seconds for assessing for presence of a pulse and respirations. CPR may be required to assist an individual who is profoundly bradycardic caused by hypothermia. Endotracheal intubation has not been found to precipitate ventricular fibrillation if performed carefully. Defibrillation for VF/Pulseless VT should be limited to 3 shocks for core body temperature below 86°F (30°C). ACLS medications are also withheld if the core body temperature is below 86°F (30°C) because of concerns of buildup to toxic levels of medications. If medications are administered, they should be spaced at longer intervals than the 3–5 minutes for a normothermic arrest. Lidocaine and procainamide can paradoxically lower the fibrillation threshold, predisposing the patient to ventricular fibrillation. Bretylium and magnesium sulfate may be effective in hypothermia; however, bretylium was removed from the VF/Pulseless VT algorithm in the 2000 ECC changes and its use during hypothermic VF/Pulseless VT arrest was not addressed in the scientific consensus statement. Because of variance in local practice, the EMS provider should follow local protocol for rewarming, BCLS, and ACLS management of the hypothermic patient.

Frostbite

Frostbite is a condition in which there is local tissue damage caused by exposure to decreased temperatures. As the temperature of water decreases toward freezing, water expands. This expansion of intracellular fluid causes damage to the cells affected by frostbite. Frostbite can be classified as either superficial or deep. Trench foot is another condition related to localized exposure to cooler temperatures.

Superficial frostbite is commonly called **frostnip** and covers first and second degree frostbite (Figure 19–4). In first degree frostbite, the freezing is confined to the superficial epidermal tissues. The affected area initially appears red and swollen and there may be transient stinging, burning, or pain. Second degree frostbite involves freezing of the full thickness of the skin and involves redness, vesicles or blisters, numbness and throbbing.

Deep frostbite can be either third or fourth degree frostbite (Figure 19–5). Third degree frosbite involves full thickness and subcutaneous freezing and tissue damage. Purple colored blisters are often present along with a blue-gray discoloration of the skin. Sensation is often lost at this stage with shooting pains, throbbing, and aching as surrounding tissues are affected. Fourth degree frostbite involves the full thickness of the skin, subcutaneous tissue, muscle, and bone. There is often little edema and the skin has a mottled or cyanotic appearance. Eventually, the affected tissues take on a black or mummified appearance. Pain sensation is lost in the immediate area, but pain or aching can originate in the nearby tissues.

Trench foot, also called **immersion foot**, is very similar to frostnip and frostbite, but is related more to chronic exposure to a moist environment rather than to the cold. The name was derived from soldiers who slept with their combat boots on their feet instead of allowing them to air out. The signs and symptoms are similar to frostbite except that pain is usually present with this condition. Blisters may form during rewarming periods, burst and serve as a site of infection.

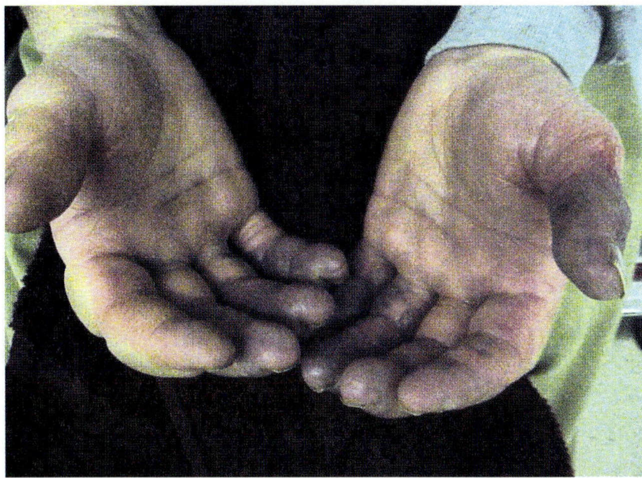

Figure 19–4 Superficial frostbite can be quite painful. (Courtesy of Kevin Reilly, M.D. Albany Medical Center, Albany, NY.)

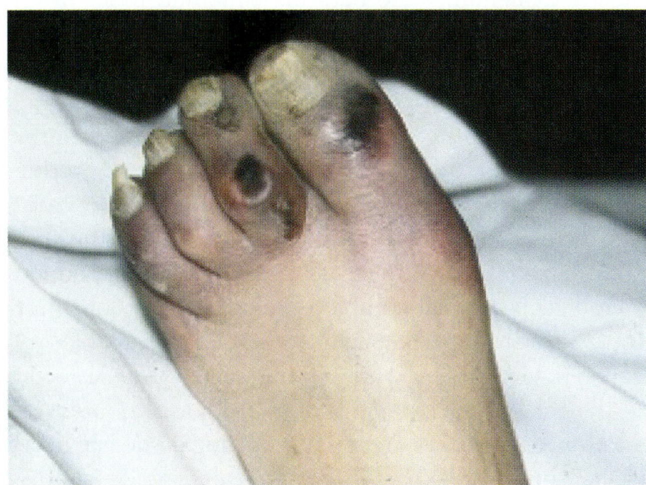

Figure 19–5 Deep frostbite results in permanent damage to tissue. (Courtesy of Deborah Funk, M.D., Albany Medical Center, Albany, NY.)

Management of frostnip and frostbite generally involve rewarming by immersion at the hospital. If transport is extended or delayed, and if there is not risk of refreezing, then rewarming in the field should be considered. Analgesics may be necessary for pain control. Trench foot can be treated by removing moist socks, allowing the affected foot to dry in warm air with aeration provided. Analgesics may also be required for pain control.

WATER EMERGENCIES

Each year, millions of Americans take to the water for recreation and several hundred thousand work on or under the water. The types of water emergencies the EMS provider may encounter include near drowning, and dive emergencies. EMS providers should remember that as water temperature is usually well below normal body temperature, hypothermia should also be considered when treating patients involved in water emergencies.

Near Drowning

According to the National Center for Health Statistics, in 1998, approximately 4,400 people died from drowning, with almost 25% of those being children under the age of 15 years old. Drowning is also the second leading cause of injury-related death for children aged 1 through 14. Alcohol use is also a major contributing factor in almost half of drownings of adolescent males. Most children drown in swimming pools, not in open bodies of water. Near drowning incidents can occur in any body of water, including the bathtub, sink, and toilet in the home, and at any time of the year.

There are two types of drowning, known as wet and dry drowning. As its name implies, a **wet drowning** involves filling the lungs completely with fluid, interrupting oxygen diffusion across the alveoli and producing a profound hypoxia. In contrast, in a **dry drowning** there is very little fluid in the airway. When the fluid comes in contact with the posterior pharynx, it produces a laryngospasm that completely closes off the lower airways. Severe hypoxia occurs after all the available oxygen in the lungs is used up. Aspiration of water may occur in the unconscious patient after the spasm relaxes. In addition to hypoxia, direct injury to lung tissue can occur after aspiration of bacteria, chemicals, vomit, or other organisms present in the aspirated water. There is no physiologic difference between fresh water and salt water drowning, as the cause of death is profound hypoxia and not electrolyte disturbances.

Treatment of the near drowning victim includes removal from the water using cervical spine precautions and assessing the airway, breathing, and circulation. Most long back boards will float, and can be placed under the drowning victim to assist both cervical spine stabilization and extrication from the water. A patent airway should be maintained, and positive pressure ventilation may assist in breaking the laryngospasm associated with drowning. CPR should be initiated and IV access obtained as needed. Even in warmer climates, the patient should be quickly moved to a warm, sheltered area, the wet clothing removed, and the patient covered with dry blankets to preserve heat. Resuscitative efforts should be continued until the victim is warmed, even in cases of prolonged submersion. All victims should receive supplemental oxygen and transport to the emergency department for evaluation, even if the incident was short and the patient is alert when EMS arrives. Aspiration pneumonia, non-cardiogenic pulmonary edema, and ARDS may develop in victims of near drowning.

Diving Emergencies

It is estimated that there are over four million recreational divers in the United States, in addition to the countless commercial or work related divers. In addition to dive physiology, there are four specific diving related emergencies that are discussed: decompression illness, pulmonary over-pressure accidents, arterial gas embolism, and nitrogen narcosis.

The Diver's Alert Network (DAN) is a non-profit organization formed in 1980 to assist with medical consultation and provide information about diving. DAN has an emergency hotline that can be accessed 24 hours a day for consultation on the treatment of dive related emergencies. The hotline in the United States is (919) 684-8111 for emergencies and (919) 684-2948 for nonemergency questions or information about the organization.

Dive Physiology. Both in dive and altitude physiology, air pressure is measured relative to the pressure at sea level. The pressure of the air acting on all objects at sea level is given a value of one atmosphere of pressure. As an individual is submerged in water, the weight of the water applies a certain amount of pressure on the individual. For each 33 feet of depth a person dives, the equivalent of one extra atmosphere of pressure is exerted on the diver. Thus, a diver at 66 feet has the equivalent of three atmospheres of pressure (1 at sea level plus 2 for depth of water). In contrast, the atmospheric pressure at the top of Mount Everest at over 25,000 feet in altitude is roughly one-third the pressure at sea level.

Dive physiology is based upon three laws that describe how gases interact with each other and the environment. **Boyle's law** states that the pressure of a gas multiplied by its volume is equal to a constant number. This means that if we take a gas and increase its pressure, we will decrease its volume, thus compressing the gas (Figure 19–6). If we take that same gas and place it in a larger volume, the pressure will decrease in proportion to the increase in volume. In terms of dive physiology, if a diver were to take a deep breath at depth and then surface while holding his breath, the air in the diver's lungs would expand and potentially rupture the lung

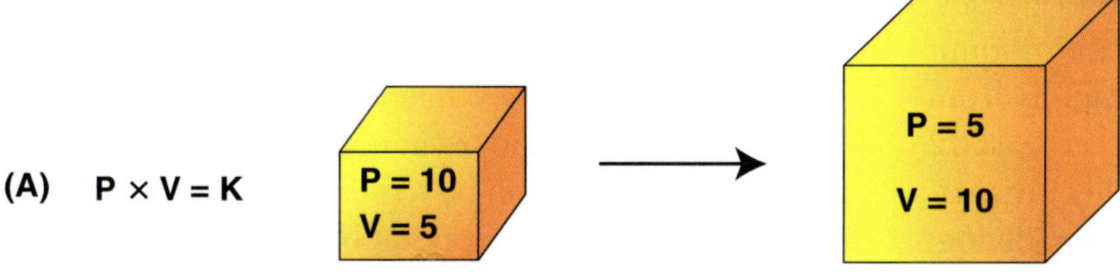

(B) $P_{mix} = P_{N^2} + P_{O^2}$ for same volume

V = 10 P = 30 P_{mix} = V = 10 P = 20 P_{N^2} + V = 10 P = 10 P_{O^2}

(C) Concentration = Pressure × Solubility

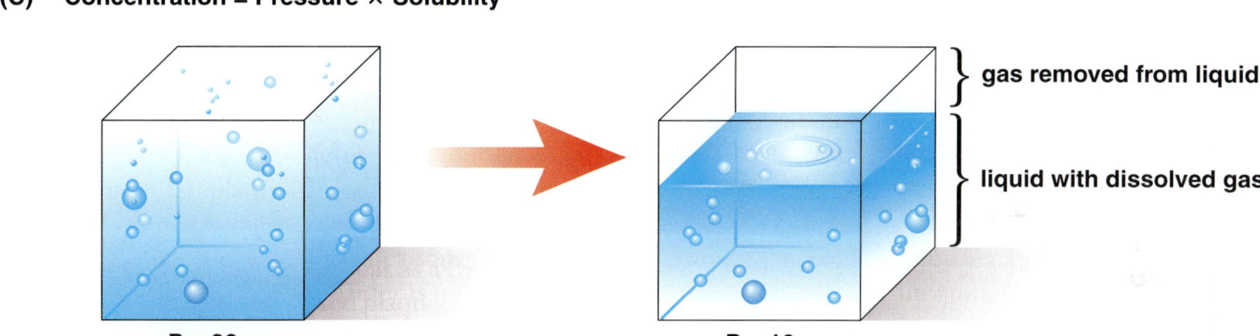

Figure 19–6 The three gas laws that define dive and altitude physiology. (A) Boyle's law (B) Dalton's law (C) Henry's law.

because of the decreased pressure relative to where the breath was taken.

Dalton's law states that the pressure of a gas made up of a mixture of several gasses is the same as the sum of the individual gas pressures if each gas occupies the same volume (Figure 19–6B). This means that the total gas pressure of a mixture is equal to the sum of the partial pressures of the individual gasses in that mixture. In terms of dive physiology, this means all gasses in the mixture are affected by the change in pressure associated with the dive.

Henry's law states that the amount of a gas that is dissolved in a liquid is proportional to the pressure of the gas (Figure 19–6C). Thus, if the pressure on a gas and liquid mixture increases, more gas will dissolve into the liquid, and if the pressure is decreased, more gas will come out of mixture with the liquid. Henry's law is dependant upon a constant called the **solubility**, which is different because of the chemical properties for each specific gas. Therefore, if a gas mixture that is dissolved in a liquid at a certain pressure is subjected to a change in pressure, the amount of gas that will come out of solution will differ based upon the solubility of the gas. Certain gasses will go into solution with increased pressure and come out of solution more readily than oxygen does. In terms of dive physiology, this means that gasses like nitrogen dissolved in the blood will come out of solution more readily than oxygen, potentially producing problems caused by the gas bubbles in the blood or other tissues. This is the reason divers should spend a specific amount of time out of the water and not ascend too rapidly from depth. Divers are also advised not to fly for at least 12 hours in commercial aircraft, which are usually pressurized to the equivalent of 8,000 feet, after diving. Patients with diving related illnesses should also not be flown for treatment unless the patient is flown in a low flying helicopter or an aircraft capable of pressurizing the cabin to a sea level pressure.

Decompression Illness. Decompression illness occurs when the gas nitrogen comes out of solution in the blood, synovial fluid in joints, cerebral spinal fluid in the spinal cord and brain, the skin, and the endolymph in the inner ear. The gas comes out of solution during a rapid ascent to the surface or if a diver flies or hikes to an altitude too soon after diving before the body can blow off the excess gas. The signs and symptoms of decompression illness can include joint pain, itching, subcutaneous emphysema, fatigue, paresthesias, and CNS disturbance. Relief of pain from inflating a blood pressure cuff around an affected joint virtually confirms a suspicion of decompression illness. There are two subclassifications of decompression illness. Type I refers to minor decompression illness composed of musculoskeletal, skin, and lymphatic manifestations, also referred to by divers as "the bends." Type II decompression illness includes neurologic disturbances and is the more severe form.

EMS treatment includes administering high flow oxygen, placing the patient in a supine position, and treating shock. The patient may need referral to a facility with a dive chamber for hyperbaric oxygen therapy. Hyperbaric oxygen therapy consists of placing the patient inside a chamber filled with 100% oxygen and increasing the pressure until symptoms are relieved. The pressure is then decreased to ambient pressure at a controlled rate to allow the body to eliminate any gas that comes out of solution.

Pulmonary Over-pressure Accidents. In a pulmonary over-pressure accident, air at depth is trapped in the lungs and, as described above under Boyle's law, expands as the individual returns to the surface. If the trapped air expands significantly, the lung can rupture producing a pneumothorax (Figure 19-7). Air can become trapped in the lung by holding one's breath too long, mucus plugging, or bronchospasm. The signs and symptoms of a pulmonary over-pressure accident include chest pain, dyspnea, and diminished breath sounds in addition to the other signs and symptoms of a pneumothorax. EMS treatment involves assessing the airway, breathing, and circulation, providing high flow oxygen, and treating a tension pneumothorax by needle decompression. In this condition, hyperbaric oxygen is usually not required, as the pneumothorax can be treated externally as in the case of a traumatic tension pneumothorax.

Arterial Gas Embolism. Arterial gas embolism (AGE) is the worst complication of diving and is feared by all divers. The gas embolism occurs when air trapped in the lungs passes through ruptured pulmonary veins, allowing a significant amount of air to pass from the smaller airways directly into the central circulation. These air bubbles can occlude the smaller arteries, and can produce cardiovascular collapse, pulmonary collapse, or cerebral collapse. The symptoms of an AGE most often are evident within two minutes of ascent; however, they can occur immediately or up to ten minutes after ascent. The most common presentation of AGE is similar to that of a cerebrovascular accident, including vertigo, confusion, ataxia, and visual disturbances. In severe cases, the patient may become unconscious or lapse into cardiac arrest. An AGE should be suspected in any patient who has a syncopal episode shortly after diving. Treatment includes securing the airway, breathing, and circulation, administering high concentration oxygen, and transport in a supine position. Hyperbaric oxygen therapy is the definitive treatment and the patient should be transferred to a facility with hyperbaric oxygen capability without subjecting the patient to high altitudes.

Nitrogen Narcosis. Nitrogen narcosis is caused by the anesthetic effect of nitrogen when the excess nitrogen is dissolved in the blood. The nitrogen is very lipid soluble and produces a state similar to alcohol intoxication in the diver. Nitrogen narcosis commonly occurs in dives from 70 to100 feet and unconsciousness can occur at depths below 300 feet. While not directly life-threatening, many accidents are the result of impaired judgment that occurs with nitrogen narcosis. This condition is generally resolved after returning to the surface.

ALTITUDE EMERGENCIES

When altitude related conditions are discussed, one generally thinks of the physiologic extremes encountered on Mount Everest, K2, Aconcagua, Mount McKinley or Denali. However, individuals can experience mild to severe symptoms at lower altitudes found in some of the popular ski resorts in Colorado and along the Western coast of the United States.

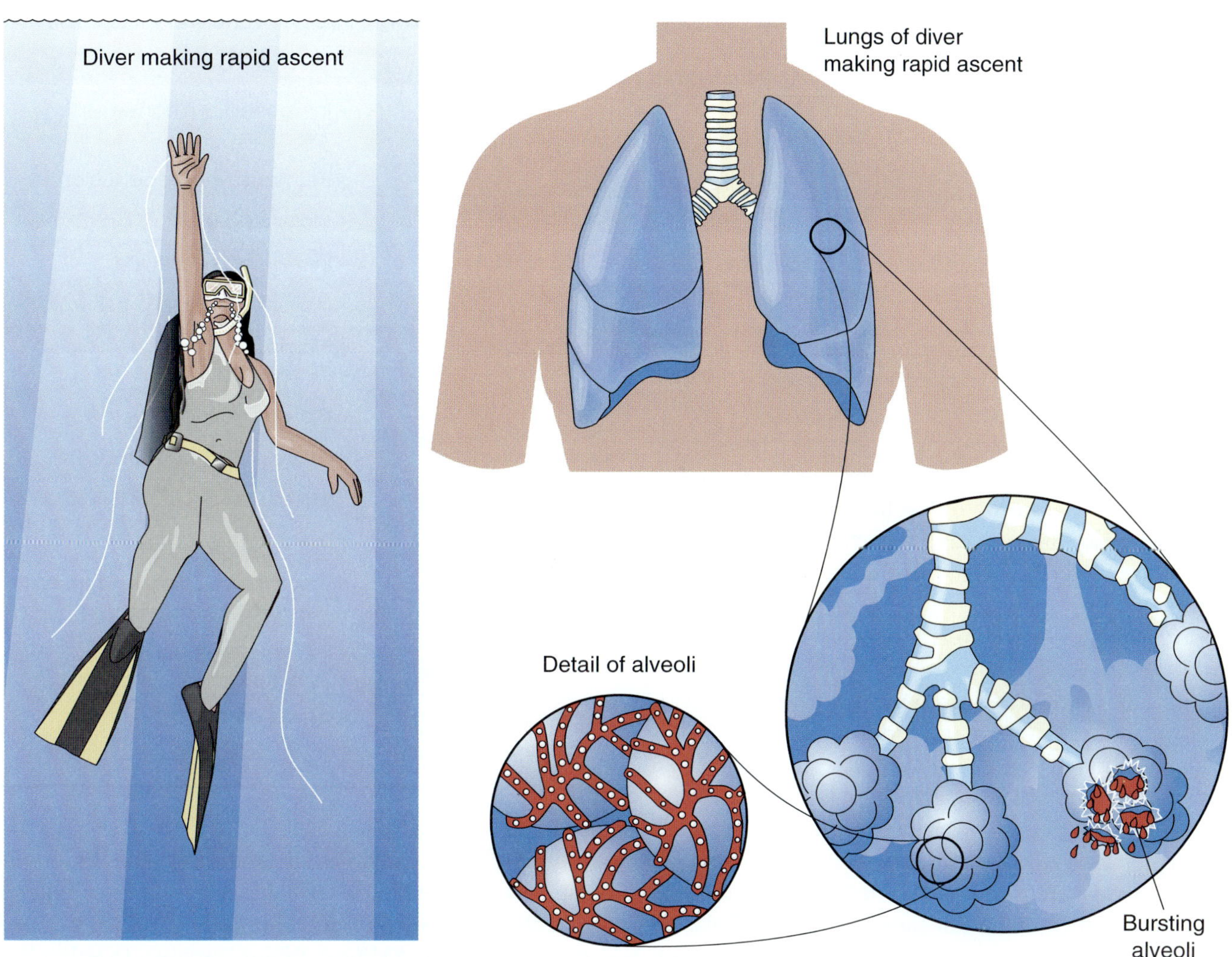

Figure 19–7 Expanding air can rupture a lung if not allowed to properly escape during ascent from a dive. Air can rupture into a pulmonary blood vessel during ascent from a dive.

Many activities include ascent to high altitude, including climbing, skiing, and backpacking. Most individuals can easily acclimate to an altitude up to 8,000 feet above sea level without symptoms. Between 8,000 and 12,000 feet altitude, some individuals will experience symptoms related to altitude. Above 12,000 feet is considered high altitude, and gradual ascent is essential for preventing altitude related conditions.

In this section we discuss the normal physiologic response to changes in altitude, acute mountain sickness, high altitude cerebral edema, and high altitude pulmonary edema.

Physiologic Response to Altitude

As with dive physiology, altitude physiology is governed by Boyle's, Dalton's and Henry's laws as described previously. As altitude increases from sea level, the atmosphere thins and fewer gas molecules are available. Even though the composition of the air maintains 21% oxygen, the partial pressure of oxygen, which is related to atmospheric pressure, is markedly decreased from sea level values. As hemoglobin saturation is decreased with a decrease in partial pressure of oxygen, individuals accustomed to living at higher altitudes can have lower blood oxygen saturation than an individual living at sea level. The **hypoxic ventilatory response** (HVR) is a normal physiologic response to hypoxia, and occurs in individuals who travel or live at high altitude. Table 19–1 compares the HVR among certain groups.

When an individual becomes hypoxic, the respiratory rate increases in an effort to provide sufficient oxygen to the body. This increase in ventilatory rate decreases the pCO_2, alkalinizing the blood. After a few days, the kidneys

TABLE 19-1 Comparison of the Hypoxic Ventilatory Response Among Different Groups

Increased in:	Decreased in:
Women	Men
Adults	Pediatrics Geriatrics
Non-natives	Natives

TABLE 19-2 The Hypoxic Ventilatory Response

System	Effect
Pulmonary	• Increased pulmonary artery pressure • Pulmonary hypoperfusion • Increased work of breathing
Circulatory	• Increased heart rate • Increased blood pressure
Hematopoietic	• Hematocrit and hemoglobin increase • Plasma volume decreases • Blood viscosity increases
CNS	• Increased cerebral blood flow • Vasoconstriction • Decreased vision, fine motor, memory
Endocrine	• Increased aldosterone, ADH (promotes fluid retention) • Anorexia • Weight loss

will respond by excreting more bicarbonate, compensating for the hypoxia induced respiratory alkalosis. This process causes changes in several body systems.

Changes in the respiratory system include an increase in pulmonary artery blood pressure and a decrease in the perfusion of the lung tissue. The work of breathing also increases as the partial pressure of oxygen, and indirectly the oxygen saturation, decreases. Circulatory system changes are secondary to an initial increase in epinephrine levels and include an increase in heart rate and blood pressure. After approximately 7 days the heart rate should return to normal for that individual and the blood pressure should drop slightly. A persistent elevation of the resting heart rate may indicate an early manifestation of high altitude pulmonary edema.

Hematopoietic system changes include an increase in hemoglobin production with extended exposure to high altitude. In the more immediate time period, there is an increase in the hematocrit caused by a loss of plasma volume secondary to increased urination. This increase in blood viscosity increases the amount of work the heart must perform and puts the individual at a slightly higher risk for pulmonary embolism or deep vein thrombosis.

The CNS changes occur fairly rapidly. There is an increase in cerebral blood flow caused by the initial increase in carbon dioxide. Then as the respiratory rate increases and the pCO_2 falls, the cerebral vessels vasoconstrict, decreasing the amount of oxygenated blood to the brain. This can affect vision, fine motor skills, and memory for up to a year after the climb.

Changes in the endocrine system include an increase in the hormones aldosterone and anti-diuretic hormone (ADH). Both of these hormones are involved in the regulation of body fluid. An increase in the levels of these hormones encourages fluid retention.

Table 19–2 summarizes the physiologic changes that occur in response to altitude.

Acute Mountain Sickness

Acute mountain sickness (AMS) is a disorder involving symptoms associated with an ascent to altitude that occurs too rapidly. Its incidence is related to the altitude and rate of ascent. AMS in its mild form is almost completely and rapidly relieved by descent to a lower altitude. Moderate and severe AMS can rapidly progress to either high altitude pulmonary edema or high altitude cerebral edema. AMS can be prevented by a gradual climb allowing the body to become accustomed to the change in altitude.

Symptoms of AMS may include headache, dizziness, fatigue, dry cough, loss of appetite, nausea, vomiting, malaise, and disturbed sleep. A decrease in urinary output instead of the increase in output that normally accompanies acclimatization to altitude is associated with the development of acute mountain sickness. If ataxia, or an unsteady gait, is present, this is an ominous sign that the patient may be progressing toward high altitude cerebral edema. Symptoms will normally present within twelve to twenty-four hours after the climb and should decrease gradually over the next several days. Children and the elderly are more prone to developing acute mountain sickness than younger and middle-aged adults.

Treatment of AMS includes descent to an altitude 2,000 to 3,000 feet below the altitude of onset and administration of supplemental oxygen, as little as 2 liters per minute oxygen for at least 15 minutes can have a beneficial effect. Encouraging the individual to breathe deeply for several minutes can also improve oxygenation sufficiently to lessen the effects of AMS. Pharmacologic agents that can be used for treatment or prevention of AMS include acetazolamide, aspirin, prochlorperazine, and dexamethasone. Acetazolamide, a carbonic anhydrase inhibitor that acts in the kidneys, can also be administered prophylactically to prevent or to reduce the severity of AMS. Aspirin can be used to treat the headache associated with AMS and prochlorperazine can be used to treat nausea. Dexamethasone can be used for severe AMS that develops rapidly or is refractory to treatment. Many other conditions can mimic AMS and descent to a lower altitude should facilitate evacuation if the signs and symptoms do not resolve at the lower altitude.

High Altitude Cerebral Edema

High altitude cerebral edema (HACE) is an altitude related condition that produces cerebral edema and an increase in intracranial pressure. This is a continuum related to worsening acute mountain sickness that occurs in a small percentage of individuals who ascend to an altitude greater than 12,000 feet. The actual pathophysiologic changes have not been clearly described; however, fluid retention is a feature of both HACE and AMS. In general, HACE can be reversed by descent and treatment, but on occasion may produce permanent brain injury or rapidly progress to a life-threatening increase in intracranial pressure and result in death.

Signs associated with HACE are similar to those of AMS with the hallmark signs of ataxia and a persistent headache. Additionally, the patient may experience confusion, poor judgment, and memory changes. In more severe cases, HACE can also produce sensory, motor, and reflex changes, hallucinations, psychotic episodes, or coma and death.

Treatment of HACE is similar to that of AMS. Mannitol and diuretics are not recommended, even after descent, as the edema may have resolved with descent and the additional diuresis can produce a decrease in blood flow to the brain, exacerbating any damage present.

High Altitude Pulmonary Edema

High altitude pulmonary edema (HAPE) is the most serious altitude related condition, but it also occurs infrequently in less than 0.2% of a general alpine mountaineering population and 0.1% of visitors to ski resorts in the Rocky Mountains of Colorado. HAPE is a noncardiogenic pulmonary edema caused by an increase in pulmonary artery pressure. Hypoxia (including sleep hypoxia), high altitude, and heavy exercise all increase the pressure in the pulmonary artery. Normally, when the pulmonary arterioles are presented with hypoxic blood, the arterioles will constrict and shunt the blood toward areas of the lung that are better oxygenated. This constriction helps maintain a lower pressure and less shear force on the walls of the blood vessels. In HAPE, these arterioles do not constrict and the increased pressure and shear forces promote fluid leakage across the capillary walls into the alveoli. As in cardiogenic pulmonary edema, this fluid in the alveoli impedes oxygen diffusion from the alveoli to the pulmonary capillary and worsens the patient's hypoxia. Severe HAPE can be complicated by the development of adult respiratory distress syndrome (ARDS), pulmonary embolism, pneumonia, or development of cardiogenic pulmonary edema.

Symptoms and signs of AMS generally precede signs and symptoms of HAPE. Dyspnea on exertion is often an early sign of HAPE, followed by a dry cough and reduced exercise performance. Orthopnea, dyspnea at rest, and a worsening of the cough indicate worsening HAPE. As in advanced cases of cardiogenic pulmonary edema, a patient with severe HAPE will produce pink, frothy sputum. HACE may also occur in conjunction with HAPE, and ataxia, decreased mental status or coma may also be present. It is important to assess patients who are unconscious for HAPE.

Primary treatment for HAPE includes immediate descent by 3,000 feet or administration of low flow supplemental oxygen. If neither is possible, nifedipine, a calcium channel blocker that decreases pulmonary artery pressure and pulmonary vascular resistance, can be administered every 6–8 hours. Nifedipine may also be used prophylactically by climbers with a prior history of HAPE. Morphine and furosemide may be used for severe HAPE to draw the fluid off the lungs and promote diuresis. Intubation and mechanical ventilation may be required if the patient tires and is unable to perform the work of breathing. In a remote rescue setting, it may be difficult to manage long-term ventilation required during a protracted evacuation. Failure of the patient to improve after initial descent is an ominous sign that suggests another pathologic process, for example, ARDS or pulmonary embolism, is present and the patient should be rapidly evacuated to an appropriate medical facility if possible.

SUMMARY

Environmental emergencies can occur during any time of the year and include a variety of illnesses. The body's temperature is tightly controlled by the posterior hypothalamus after receiving input from the central thermoreceptors and the peripheral thermoreceptors. The posterior hypothalamus then signals the mechanisms for thermogenesis if the body temperature is below the set point or thermolysis if the body temperature is above the set point. Fever and the symptoms associated with a fever are caused by a change in the set point produced by the release of pyrogens from bacterial and tissue destruction. Heat related emergencies include heat cramps, heat exhaustion, and heat stroke, with heat stroke being the most severe and potentially life-threatening. Cold emergencies include hypothermia and frostbite. Hypothermia alters cardiac arrest management by withholding medications until the core temperature is above 86°F (30°C) and continuing resuscitation until the patient is warmed sufficiently. Water emergencies include near drowning and diving emergencies. The three gas laws discussed in the text, Boyle's law, Dalton's law and Henry's law, affect both dive physiology and altitude physiology. Hyperbaric oxygen is the treatment of choice for decompression illness and arterial gas embolism while nitrogen narcosis is a self limited condition and pulmonary over-pressure accidents often require intervention for a tension pneumothorax. Adaptation to altitude involves very complex physiologic mechanisms that affect oxygen delivery to the tissues. Acute mountain sickness is a mild form of altitude illness that generally resolves without lasting deficiencies if the condition is identified early and the patient descends rapidly. HACE and HAPE are two more life-threatening forms of severe acute mountain sickness that often result in permanent disability or death.

REVIEW QUESTIONS

Multiple Choice

1. Central thermoreceptors are more responsive to heat and are located:
   a. around the large veins in the abdomen.
   b. along the spinal cord.
   c. in the anterior hypothalamus.
   d. on the surface of the skin.
2. The mechanisms involved in thermogenesis include:
   a. Piloerection.
   b. Vasoconstriction.
   c. Thyroxine secretion.
   d. All of the above.
3. Mechanisms of thermolysis include:
   a. Sympathetic nervous system stimulation.
   b. Shivering.
   c. Peripheral vasodilation.
   d. None of the above.
4. General treatment principles of heat related emergencies include:
   a. Moving the patient to a cool, dry environment.
   b. Oral rehydration with electrolyte containing fluids.
   c. Active cooling with ice packs if the patient is not perspiring.
   d. All of the above.
5. Heat loss caused by contact with the snow is considered:
   a. Convective heat loss.
   b. Evaporative heat loss.
   c. Conductive heat loss.
   d. Radiation heat loss.

6. Your patient was found after a prolonged exposure to the cold. What is a common substance that can predispose an individual to hypothermia?
   a. Alcohol
   b. Oral hyperglycemic medication
   c. Hyperthyroidism
   d. None of the above
7. ACLS medications should be withheld if the hypothermic patient has a core body temperature below:
   a. 95°F (35°C).
   b. 91.4°F (33°C).
   c. 86°F (30°C).
   d. 82.4°F (28°C).
8. Signs of third degree frostbite include:
   a. Red and swollen area without vesicles.
   b. Mottled or cyanotic skin appearance.
   c. Blue-gray skin discoloration.
   d. Red skin discoloration with blisters.
9. The physiologic mechanism that produces a "dry drowning" is:
   a. Aspiration of fluid into the lungs.
   b. Direct tissue injury from chemicals and bacteria in the water.
   c. Laryngospasm leading to suffocation.
   d. Profound electrolyte disturbance.
10. The law that states that the pressure of a gas multiplied by its volume is equal to a constant is:
    a. Dalton's law.
    b. Myers' law.
    c. Henry's law.
    d. Boyle's law.
11. The condition commonly referred to as "the bends" is:
    a. Nitrogen narcosis.
    b. Decompression illness Type I.
    c. Decompression illness Type II.
    d. Arterial gas embolism.
12. The definitive treatment for an arterial gas embolism is:
    a. High concentration oxygen.
    b. Arterial catheterization.
    c. Fibrinolytic therapy.
    d. Hyperbaric oxygen.
13. Changes that occur during the normal hypoxic ventilatory response include:
    a. Bradycardia.
    b. Respiratory acidosis.
    c. Increased hemoglobin production.
    d. Decrease in cerebral blood flow.
14. Which of the following may indicate an individual at risk for developing high altitude pulmonary edema?
    a. Persistant tachycardia.
    b. A decrease in blood pressure.
    c. Respiratory alkalosis.
    d. Increased respiratory rate.

15. The two signs that differentiate acute mountain sickness from high altitude cerebral edema are:
    a. Dizziness and poor judgment.
    b. Disturbed sleep and headache.
    c. Persistent headache and ataxia.
    d. Psychotic episodes and disturbed sleep.

CASE STUDY

You respond to the fishing docks for a reported syncope. Upon arrival, you find a male in his early thirties seated on the side of the pier complaining of severe chest pain and shortness of breath. He also complains of numbness in his right hand and cannot walk because "my balance is off." He was unconscious for about 2 minutes and this happened suddenly about five minutes after ascending from a dive to a wrecked fishing boat 30 feet below. What condition do you suspect? What would you do for treatment? How and where would you transport this patient?

BIBLIOGRAPHY

Anooshiravani, M., Dumont, L., Mardirosoff, C., Soto-Deberf, G., & Delavelle, J. (1999). Brain magnetic resonance imaging and neurological changes after a single high altitude climb. *Medicine & Science in Sports & Exercise, 31*(7), 969–972.

Bartsch P. (1999). High altitude pulmonary edema. *Medicine & Science in Sports & Exercise, 31*(1 Suppl.), S23–27.

Boussuges, A., Molenat, F., Burnet, H., (2000). Operation Everest III: Modifications of cardiac function secondary to altitude induced hypoxia. *American Journal of Respiratory Care Medicine, 161*, 264–270.

Centers for Disease Control. *Extreme heat. http://www.cdc.gov/nceh/hsb/extremeheat/*

Divers Alert Network website. *http://www.diversalertnetwork.org/*

Diving Medicine Online. *http://www.gulftel.com/~scubadoc/*

Dumont, L., Mardirosoff, C., & Tramer, M. R. (2000). Efficacy and harm of pharmacological prevention of acute mountain sickness: quantitative systematic review. *British Medical Journal, 321*, 267–72.

Guyton, A. C., & Hall, J. E. (1996). Body temperature, temperature regulation, and fever. In *Textbook of medical physiology* (9th ed.). (pp. 911–922). Philadelphia: Saunders.

Hall, K. N., & Syverud, S. A. (1990). Closed thoracic cavity lavage in the treatment of severe hypothermia in human beings. *Annals of Emergency Medicine, 19*, 204–206.

High Altitude Medicine Guide website. *http://www.high-altitude-medicine.com.*

International Consensus on Science. (2000). Guidelines 2000 for cardiopulmonary resuscitation and emergency cardiovascular care. *Circulation, 102*(8 Suppl.), I-229–I-232.

Litch, J. A. (1999) Endotracheal intubation and mechanical ventilation following respiratory arrest from high altitude pulmonary edema. *Western Journal of Medicine, 170*, 174–176.

National Center for Injury Prevention and Control. *Drowning prevention fact sheet. http://www.cdc.gov/ncipc/factsheets/drown.htm*

Wilkerson, J. A. (Ed.). (1992). *Medicine for mountaineering & other wilderness activities* (4th ed.). Seattle, WA: The Mountaineers.

CHAPTER

20

Behavioral Diseases and Disorders

CONTENT OUTLINE

- Common Signs and Symptoms
- Diagnostic Tests
- Common Mental Health Disorders
  - Developmental Mental Health Disorders
  - Substance Related Mental Disorders
  - Organic Mental Disorders
  - Psychosis
  - Mood or Affective Disorders
  - Dissociative Disorders
  - Anxiety Disorders
  - Somatoform Disorders
  - Personality Disorders
- Trauma
  - Grief
  - Suicide
- Mental Health Disorders in the Older Adult

KEY TERMS

Abuse
Addiction
Affect
Anorexia nervosa
Bulimia
Circadian rhythms
Compulsion
Delirium tremens
Dependency
Hallucination
Intoxicated
Mania
Mood
Obsession
Organic
Tolerance
Withdrawal

LEARNING OBJECTIVES

Upon completion of the chapter, the student should be able to:

1. Define the terminology common to mental health disorders.
2. Identify common mental health disorders.
3. Identify the important signs and symptoms associated with mental health disorders.
4. Describe the common diagnostic tests used to determine type and/or cause of mental health disorders.
5. Describe the typical course and management of the common mental health disorders.
6. State the mental health disorders found in the elderly population and the effects of these disorders.

OVERVIEW

Mental health disorders are some of the most difficult diseases to diagnose and understand. Symptoms may range from mild behavior changes to severe personality disturbances. Because of the variety of symptoms, the difficulty in diagnosing some disorders and the lack of understanding of the physiologic cause, many mental health disorders are misdiagnosed and can go untreated for years. Although some mental health problems are not yet well understood, many more are relatively easy to diagnose and treat. It is important to note that many people without mental illness will exhibit some of the characteristics described in this chapter. The key criteria in assessing a mental illness is the impairment of normal functioning, for example, getting in the way of personal relationships or employment.

COMMON SIGNS AND SYMPTOMS

For mental health disorders there are only a few common signs and symptoms. Typically, symptoms of mental health problems begin with behavioral changes.

These are often slow to develop and very subtle, so symptoms might not be noticed early in the development of a disorder. Many of the symptoms, such as forgetfulness, anxiety, or temper tantrums, are attributed to age, stress, or other illnesses. Typical symptoms of each mental health problem are discussed with the specific disorder.

DIAGNOSTIC TESTS

There are a variety of diagnostic tests used to determine the specific mental health problem. When symptoms first appear, several physiologic tests are typically performed, such as laboratory tests, brain scans, EEGs, and MRIs to determine if the cause is an organic or medical problem. Secondly, an individual may be referred to a psychiatrist for psychological testing to determine a diagnosis. These tests may include an aptitude test, personality test, and several others depending on the symptoms presented and the severity of the symptoms.

COMMON MENTAL HEALTH DISORDERS

A serious mental health disorder will affect approximately one in every four Americans during a lifetime without regard to boundaries of sex, income, and race. Phobias are the most common mental health disorders, affecting approximately six percent of the United States population. Depression is the second most common mental health disorder affecting one in four American females and one in ten American males. Eating disorders affect up to four to five out of one hundred adolescents. Suicide is the third leading cause of death for fifteen- to twenty-four-year-olds and the sixth leading cause of death for five- to fifteen-year-olds.

A few disorders have a genetic basis or relationship, others are caused by behavior choices, and some are of unknown cause. Early diagnosis and treatment are essential to assist the individual to either overcome the disorder or to improve the quality of life.

Developmental Mental Health Disorders

Developmental mental health disorders are those that are usually discovered during infancy, childhood, or adolescence. These disorders may diminish or worsen as the child matures. Developmental disorders that are carried into adulthood may be mild, allowing the involved individual to function in an adult role, or may be so severe that institutionalization may be needed.

Mental Retardation. Mental retardation is a condition of decreased intelligence leading to a decrease in the ability to learn, socialize, and mature. Mental retardation varies in degrees from mild, moderate, severe, and profound. In the past, these degrees were described as feebleminded, idiot, imbecile, and moron, but these terms are no longer used. Affected children may not show signs of mental retardation until entry into school. Difficulty learning and keeping up with other children of the same age may be indicative of mental retardation. Diagnosis is confirmed on the basis of observation and IQ testing. The cause of mental retardation is often unknown. Known causes of mental retardation fall into two categories: genetic and acquired (Table 20–1). Some types of mental retardation can be avoided by providing prenatal care. Treatment of mentally retarded individuals varies with the amount of retardation. Many mildly retarded individuals grow up and find employment in a suitable occupation and lead a fairly normal life. Others may need special dependent living facilities, but very few are retarded to the level of needing institutionalization.

TABLE 20–1 Genetic and Acquired Causes of Mental Retardation

Genetic	Acquired
Down Syndrome	Prenatal Maternal Rubella
PKU—phenylketonuria	Prenatal Maternal Syphilis
Hypothyroidism—Cretinism	Blood Type Incompatibility
	Prematurity
	Anoxia
	Birth Injury
	Poor Nutrition
	Head Trauma

Autism. Autism is a severe type of developmental disorder characterized by a preoccupation with inner thoughts, daydreams, fantasies, and **delusions** (a false belief that is firmly adhered to although it is not shared by others). Symptoms of autism are usually apparent in infancy when the infant exhibits an eye to eye gaze and blank facial expression. Affected children are so involved with self that they become inaccessible to others, including parents. These children may happily play alone for hours and become angry if interrupted. The cause of autism is unknown, although there may be a physical cause. Diagnosis is confirmed on the basis of observation of behavior. Behavioral therapy to teach the child how to adapt to situations is beneficial. Prognosis is still relatively poor and affected children may require life-long assistance.

Attention-deficit Hyperactivity Disorder. Attention-deficit hyperactivity disorder (ADHD) is a mental health disorder characterized by an inability to concentrate, hyperactivity, and impulsiveness. This behavior may be apparent at any age, but is usually observed before the age of seven, becoming more obvious in school situations. Examples of ADHD behavior include forgetfulness, not appearing to listen, difficulty in remaining seated or waiting one's turn, squirming, excessive running, climbing, and talking, inability to complete detailed work, messy work, and an inability to organize. These behaviors tend to become more exaggerated in a group situation. The cause of ADHD is unknown but there does appear to be a familial pattern. Diagnosis is made on the basis of observation of the age inappropriate behavior. Treatment of ADHD with amphetamines, such as Dexedrine and Ritalin, has shown varying degrees of effectiveness. Behavior modification by rewarding appropriate behavior has also been successful.

Eating Disorders. Eating disorders currently affect approximately one in one hundred females. It is thought that a factor in eating disorders centers around the great emphasis Americans place on the thin, perfect, female body. In order to obtain this ideal figure, many females go to dieting extremes. Two common eating disorders are **anorexia nervosa** and **bulimia**. (These are also discussed in Chapter 23 as disorders of adolescents.)

Anorexia (AN-oh-**RECK**-see-ah; an = without, orexia = appetite) nervosa is a disorder of self-imposed starvation resulting from a distorted body image. The term anorexia is a misnomer as the appetite is not diminished, but the affected individual simply refuses to eat in fear of becoming fat. The typical characteristics of an individual with anorexia nervosa include:

- Adolescent female
- Meticulous, high achiever
- Body image distortion (feels fat no matter how thin)
- Intense fear of becoming fat
- Performs excessive exercise

Treatment is often difficult and lengthy and involves restoring normal nutrition and resolving psychological problems. Death from starvation is often caused by compromised cardiac function.

Bulimia (byou-LIM-ee-ah) is an eating disorder characterized by episodes of binge eating followed by activities to negate the calorie intake or purging. Purging behaviors include self-induced vomiting or excessive laxative use. Excessive vomiting often leads to electrolyte imbalances and erosion of the teeth. Individuals affected with bulimia are usually older than anorexics, more obese, and experience a wide fluctuation in weight. Bulimic individuals tend to have perfectionist personalities and a dreaded fear of becoming fat, both similar to anorexics. Treatment of bulimia is similar to anorexia including the use of antidepressant drugs and group therapy.

Substance Related Mental Disorders

Substance related mental disorders cost the health care industry over $90 billion a year. Common terms used in substance related mental disorders include abuse, addiction, dependency, tolerance, and withdrawal. Abuse is the term used to describe using a substance in a way other than it was intended, for example, drinking alcohol to excess or sniffing model glue. **Addiction** means a physical and or psychological dependence on a substance. **Dependency** is a psychological craving for a substance that may or may not be accompanied by a physical need. **Tolerance** is the ability to endure a larger amount of a substance without an adverse effect or the need for a larger amount or dose of the drug to have the same effect. **Withdrawal** is the unpleasant physical and psychological effects resulting from stopping the use of the substance after an individual is addicted.

Alcoholism. Alcoholism is a physical and mental dependence on a regular intake of alcohol. It is a chronic, progressive, and often fatal disease. Onset of alcoholism is often insidious beginning in the teen years. Excessive use may be related to stress or depression or some other stressful life event. Alcoholism is a major drug problem adversely affecting the physical, mental, social, and spiritual health of the affected individual. Chronic alcoholism causes physical damage to nearly every organ system. Some of the common problems include heart disease, hypertension, cirrhosis, pancreatitis, anemia, peripheral neuropathy, and gastrointestinal problems (including an increased risk of stomach and esophageal cancer). Mental disorders include anxiety, depression, insomnia, impotence, and amnesia. These physical and mental problems, along with the associated accidents, injuries, and violence associated with alcoholism, can be psychologically, socially, and economically devastating to the affected individual and his family.

The cause of alcoholism is unknown. There is not a universally accepted explanation for alcoholism although recent research points toward a biologic explanation or at least a genetic predisposition. Other causal factors may include depression, poverty, peer pressure, and condoning of substance abuse by peers and family members. Individuals raised in homes where both parents are alcoholics are at very high risk for also becoming alcoholics.

Alcohol is absorbed in the mouth and small intestine and is broken down by the liver. A normal sized individual can metabolize or break down approximately ten milliliters of alcohol or one ounce of whiskey every ninety minutes. If taken in higher amounts or consumed more frequently, alcohol causes a sedative effect and may depress breathing and lead to death. An individual is legally **intoxicated** when the blood alcohol level reaches 0.10 percent or more (0.08 percent in some states). Four to six hours after intoxication occurs, the individual experiences a hangover with symptoms of nausea, vomiting, fatigue, sweating, and thirst. The primary cause of a hangover is the accumulation of alcohol in the blood, dehydration, and hypoglycemia. Alcoholics become physically dependent on alcohol and may experience symptoms of withdrawal if alcohol is withheld for twenty-four to forty-eight hours. Symptoms of withdrawal include **hallucinations** (a false sensation of sight, touch, sound, or feel), tremors of the hands, mild seizures, and **delirium tremens** (**DTs**). Symptoms of delirium tremens may include agitation, memory loss, anorexia, seizures, and hallucinations. DTs usually last one to five days and may be fatal if not properly treated. Treatment for withdrawal includes tranquilizers, anti-convulsive medication, adequate nutrition, and anti-emetic (anti = against, emetic = nausea or vomiting) medications.

Marijuana. Marijuana, also called pot, grass, maryjane, and weed, is a mixture of dried leaves and flowers of an Indian hemp plant (Cannabis sativa). This mixture is crushed and rolled into cigarettes called reefers or joints. *Hashish*, a resin from the flowering top of the hemp plant, is thought to be four to eight times stronger than marijuana. Both marijuana and hashish usually produce a euphoric effect or sense of well-being. This effect is immediate and lasts approximately two to three hours. True tolerance does not develop with marijuana use, but chronic use may lead to a psychological dependence. Marijuana use has not been proven to lead to the use of hard drugs, but users often experiment with other drugs. Beneficial uses of marijuana include a lowering of intraocular pressure in glaucoma patients and relief of nausea and vomiting in individuals on chemotherapy.

Cocaine. Cocaine is a powerful stimulant that accelerates the central nervous system and an anesthetic that numbs whatever it touches. Cocaine is obtained from the leaves of the coca plant found in South America or may be produced synthetically. Cocaine is a pure white powder and may be referred to as "coke." This form of cocaine is commonly snorted from a spoon or straw. It may also be mixed with water, heated to help with the dissolving process, and injected. Drug paraphernalia not only includes syringes, spoons, and straws, but also may include a razorblade and mirror or piece of glass used to carefully divide the powder dose. Powder cocaine is quite expensive at $100 per gram. Snorting produces a slower response than injecting, with effects lasting approximately twenty minutes. Complications of snorting cocaine include disintegration of the mucous membrane of the nose and ulceration through the nasal septum. Injecting cocaine and sharing needles increases the risk of HIV. The anesthetic properties of powdered cocaine make it an ideal legal medication for patients undergoing nasal surgery.

Another form of cocaine is called "crack" or "free base." Crack cocaine is currently made by heating a mixture of powder cocaine, water, and ammonia, or baking soda, causing the material to precipitate into a hardened form of small chips or chunks. Historically this process involved the use of ether and other flammable bases. Processing with the ether method is very dangerous because of the flammability of this product. Crack cocaine is four to five times stronger and much more addictive than powder cocaine. Crack is smoked rather than snorted or injected. Manufacturing and smoking crack cocaine is called "free basing." When smoked, crack reaches the brain within seconds giving an intense high or rush to the body. The high lasts approximately five minutes then fades into a restless desire for more of the drug. Crack is sold in small vials (approximately two doses)at a cost that is initially less expensive than powdered cocaine, but the intense addiction this drug causes leads to increased use and cost. Addiction often leads to theft, prostitution, and "dealing" in order to obtain the money needed to purchase more cocaine. Crack cocaine is usually smoked with marijuana, tobacco cigarettes, or in a glass pipe. Overdosing with crack is more common than with powder cocaine. It is estimated that one in two Americans between the ages of twenty-five to thirty-five have tried cocaine and 1.4 million Americans are regular cocaine users. Infants born to cocaine-using mothers are often addicted and exhibit low birth weight, hyperactivity, tremors, and frantic sucking activities.

Caffeine and Nicotine. Two of the most common addicting substances in our society are caffeine and nicotine. Caffeine is a stimulant found in coffee, chocolate, tea, cola drinks, and some over-the-counter medications. Caffeine causes vasoconstriction and over a long period of time may lead to circulatory problems. Individuals addicted to caffeine often experience severe withdrawal headaches, anxiety, drowsiness, fatigue, and nausea. Caffeine tends to cause breast tenderness in females and intensify the symptoms of premenstrual syndrome (PMS). Caffeine is the cheapest and most abused drug in the United States.

Tobacco use in this country is on the rise especially among the teen population despite widespread knowledge of the devastating effects of nicotine on the cardiovascular and respiratory system. Nicotine is a stimulant that narrows blood vessels, and raises heart rate and blood pressure. It has been theorized that nicotine is as addictive as cocaine. Symptoms of withdrawal include depression, irritability, anger, anxiety, and an increase in appetite and weight gain. Smoking during pregnancy can result in spontaneous abortion and premature birth. Nicotine patches that reduce nicotine intake gradually have been successful in helping millions of affected individuals to quit smoking.

Sedatives or Depressants. Drugs in this category are commonly anti-anxiety medications (Librium or Valium), barbiturates (Nembutal and Seconal), and hypnotics (Dalmane and Placidyl). Individuals addicted to these medications may use as much as 65 milligrams of Valium or 600 milligrams of Seconal a day.

The most severely abused group of sedatives or depressants are the barbiturates. Street names for these drugs include downers, barbs, or may be known by the color of the capsules (reds, yellow jackets, or rainbows). These medications are often prescribed to treat insomnia, hypertension, and seizure disorders. Barbiturates distort mood leading to euphoria, slow down reaction times causing an increase in automobile and home accidents, and in some cases cause hallucinations. Taking barbiturates with alcohol potentiates or enhances the effect of alcohol. Addiction and tolerance to barbiturates are developed quickly. Tolerance commonly leads to overdosing of barbiturates, causing a slowing of the heart and breathing often resulting in death. Barbiturate use is one of the main causes of accidental death and is the most common method of suicide. Sudden withdrawal from barbiturates may be life-threatening. It is recommended that withdrawal be under the guidance of a physician. Affected individuals are usually hospitalized and the drug is withdrawn slowly to prevent nausea, delirium, and seizures.

A non-barbiturate sedative, methaqualone (Quaalude), was introduced in the United States in the mid-1960s and was marketed as having no effect on sleep patterns and little potential for abuse. Since that time it has been discovered that Quaalude, commonly called "ludes," does interfere with rapid eye movement (REM) sleep and does cause psychological and physical dependence. Withdrawal symptoms may last two to three days and may include insomnia, anxiety, nausea, hallucinations, and nightmares.

Amphetamines. Amphetamines are stimulant drugs that cause a release of the body's natural epinephrine, leading to an increase in heart rate and other body systems. Commonly, amphetamines are called "speed," "uppers," "bennies," and "pep pills." These drugs are often used by obese individuals to lose weight, by truck drivers to stay awake, and by college students to stay alert for studying. Amphetamines are addictive and do lead to tolerance. Chronic use often leads to an opposite effect causing drowsiness. Depression and suicide may occur following sudden withdrawal.

Hallucinogens. Hallucinogens, also called psychedelic drugs, commonly produce hallucinations. These drugs cause a heightened and distorted response to visual, auditory, and tactile stimuli. This heightened response allows the affected individual to see flat objects take on shape, stationary objects move, and colors become more vivid. Hallucinogenic drugs include LSD (lysergic acid diethylamide), Mescaline, and PCP. LSD is a colorless, tasteless, and odorless synthetic substance that is primarily produced in illegal laboratories. It may be added to the food or drink of an unsuspecting victim or may be added to chewing gum, hard candy, postage stamps, or stickers. LSD is a very potent drug. An amount of drug visible to the eye is enough to cause an eight-hour "trip." LSD causes abnormal thought process and may cause temporary or permanent mental changes. Controversy exists over the fact that LSD may also cause chromosomal damage. Suprisingly, LSD is not addictive. It appears that this drug is abused to escape reality rather than make an effort to cope with reality. Abusers of LSD do have a high tendency to abuse marijuana, barbiturates, and amphetamines. The danger of this drug lies in the fact that the activities of an individual under the influence of LSD are totally unpredictable. There may be attempts to "fly" or episodes of violence and self-destruction. Flashbacks (recurrence of a trip) may occur months after the drug was taken, as this drug is stored in fat tissue and may be released at a later time.

Mescaline is similar to LSD but much weaker. Mescaline is an active chemical found in the Mexican peyote cactus that may also be produced synthetically. The American Indians have used this cactus as part of their traditional religious ceremonies.

PCP, also known as "angel dust," "peace pill," and "peace weed," is a depressant that was introduced in the 1950s as an animal tranquilizer. Its use has since been abandoned because of unpredictable side effects. PCP is easily produced in illegal laboratories and may be taken as pills, injections, by snorting, or by smoking. Danger lies in the poor and varied quality of the product sold on the street. PCP may cause memory lapses lasting for several days. Other symptoms are coma, convulsions, and respiratory arrest.

Narcotics. Narcotics are depressants that are primarily prescribed as analgesics. Demerol, methadone, morphine, heroin, and opium are classified as narcotics and are commonly abused. Narcotics slow nerve and muscle action, slow the rate of the heart, slow breathing, and lower blood pressure. Physical and psychological dependence and tolerance rapidly develop with the use of narcotics. Overdose symptoms include slurred speech, confusion, staggering, coma, and respiratory arrest.

Opium is an air-dried milky residue obtained from the unripe opium poppy. References to opium smoking are common in Oriental history, with some Asian countries still smoking opium. The western countries, including America, prefer opium derivatives such as morphine and heroine. Opium contains approximately ten percent morphine. Heroin is a derivative of morphine but is approximately eight times stronger. Heroin is very addictive and is commonly called "smack" and "horse." Heroin is the narcotic most widely used by narcotic addicts today. Heroin is a fine white powder that is usually mixed with water and injected intravenously, called "main-lining." It may also be snorted or smoked. Heroin use usually gives a "rush" or intense feeling of well being, followed by a sleepy, drowsy state. Withdrawal from heroin without medical treatment is called "going cold turkey." Withdrawal is often uncomfortable, but usually not life-threatening. Symptoms of withdrawal include sweating, shaking, diarrhea, vomiting, and sharp pain and cramps in the stomach and legs.

Inhalants. Inhalants include over 1,000 legal substances, including glue, spray paint, hair spray, nail polish, lighter fluid, and gasoline. These substances commonly contain harmful hydrocarbons and an oily base, that when inhaled, coats the inner lining of the lungs. Inhalant abuse refers to intentionally breathing the vapors of a substance in order to get high. This intentional breathing in is commonly called "huffing," "snuffing," or "bagging." Bagging is the most dangerous as it entails placing a plastic bag over the head in order to get a longer effect. Using inhalants over a period of time may result in permanent brain, heart, kidney, and liver damage. Some products such as paint and gasoline contain lead and may lead to death from lead poisoning. Inhalant abuse is the third most common substance abused by individuals age twelve to fourteen years, surpassed only by alcohol and tobacco. Symptoms of inhalant abuse include spots or sores around the mouth, a glassy eyed look, fumes on the breath or clothing, anxiety, and loss of appetite.

Organic Mental Disorders

Organic mental disorders are those associated with some type of known physical cause. These disorders affect the cognitive abilities or the abilities to think, remember, and make judgments of the affected individual. These disorders may be temporary or permanent.

Dementia. Dementia is a progressive deterioration of mental abilities caused by physical changes in the brain. The cognitive or mental abilities include severe memory loss, disorientation, impaired judgment, and the inability to learn new information. Dementia may or may not be reversible depending on cause. Symptoms of dementia are usually severe enough to interfere with the individual's ability to care for self. Dementia is not a part of the normal aging process although most individuals with dementia are older. Factors important in determining whether dementia will occur in an individual include nutritional status, family history, chronic diseases, and general state of health. Onset of dementia may be slow or sudden, depending on the cause. Causes of dementia are listed in Table 20–2.

Delirium. Delirium is an acute condition that develops suddenly, often as a result of medications, alcohol, fever, or physical illness. The affected individual is often frightened, disoriented to place and time, has illusions, hallucinations, and incoherent speech. Individuals with delirium expend great amounts of energy continually wandering and performing aimless activities. Causes of delirium are also listed in Table 20–2.

Alzheimer's. Alzheimer's disease is a progressive and irreversible form of dementia. Alzheimer's accounts for fifty percent of all dementias and commonly occurs after age

TABLE 20–2 Physical Causes of Dementia and Delirium

Drugs
Prescribed medications
Alcohol
Abused substances
Metabolic Disorders
Endocrine gland disorders
Nutritional Disease
Vitamin deficiencies
Malnutrition
Infection
Meningitis
Encephalitis
Brain abscess
AIDS
Trauma
Head injury
Vascular Disorders
Cerebrovascular accidents (CVA)
Arteriosclerosis
Neoplastic
Brain tumors
Neurologic
Epilepsy

sixty-five, but may occur as early as age forty. Symptoms begin with mild memory loss and progress to impaired mental function, personality changes, and speech and language problems. In the final stage the affected individual is often depressed and paranoid and may have hallucinations. At this stage, the individual with Alzheimer's is dependent on another individual for total care and may need institutionalization. Death usually occurs in ten to fifteen years from onset and is usually caused by complications of immobility. The cause of Alzheimer's is unknown, but some theories include an inherited chromosomal defect, viral infection, a deficiency in neurochemicals in the brain, and an immunologic defect. Interestingly, postmortem studies have revealed a high level of aluminum in the brain and a higher incidence of a serious head injury. Physical changes noted during autopsy include brain plaques and neuronal tangles. Treatment is aimed at relieving symptoms and managing behavior problems. (See Chapter 9 for more information.)

Psychosis

Psychosis is a term describing conditions characterized by a disintegration of one's personality and a loss of contact with reality. Psychotic individuals have impaired communication skills, an inability to deal with life's demands, delusions, and hallucinations. These mental disturbances may or may not have a physical or structural change in the brain. One of the most common psychotic disorders is schizophrenia.

Schizophrenia. Schizophrenia, meaning "split mind," is a serious type of psychosis. Contrary to popular belief, it is not a split personality disorder. This disorder often appears in individuals age sixteen to twenty-five and is more common in females than males. Patients with schizophrenia lose touch with reality and act on imagined or fantasized reality. Various theories exist as to the cause of schizophrenia, including genetics, brain biochemical disorders, and structural alterations. It is generally agreed that patients with schizophrenia have a genetic vulnerability, as an individual with a schizophrenic parent, sibling, or other close relative, has an increased possibility of developing schizophrenia. Another theory suggests that patients with schizophrenia were deprived of meaningful relationships with family members during childhood years.

Delusional Disorders. Delusional disorders are characterized by a firm belief of a delusion in an otherwise normally adjusted and balanced personality. The delusions often center on feelings of persecution and grandiosity. Areas of delusion often involve romance, religion, and politics. These delusions often develop slowly and involve a false interpretative feeling of an actual occurrence. Delusional individuals become firmly convinced that something is true no matter how convincing evidence is to the contrary. Types of delusional disorders affecting the thinking of affected individuals include:

- Grandiose—an inflated sense of self worth, power, and knowledge
- Jealous—belief that a sexual partner is unfaithful
- Erotomanic—belief that someone of higher status is in love with them
- Persecutory—suspicious actions and feelings that people are spying on them with harmful intentions
- Somatic—belief that they have a physical disease or disorder

Mood or Affective Disorders

Mood or affective disorders are those that involve the emotions (**mood**) and the outward expression of those emotions (**affect**). Mood ranges on a spectrum with extreme depression at one end and extreme elation or happiness at the other. Individuals normally experience times of sadness and moments of joy. When these emotions are not appropriate to the events of life, last for an inappropriate length of time, or are extreme in nature, then mood disorders may be suspected. Individuals with mood disorders may have extreme depression while some individuals will exhibit both extreme depression and extreme elation at alternating times (bipolar disorder).

Depression. Depression is a prolonged feeling of extreme sadness or unhappiness, despair, and discouragement. Depression is different from grief, which is a realistic sadness related to a personal loss. Prolonged grief may become depression as depression is often associated with loss of a loved one, possessions, self-esteem, or youth. A depressed individual often exhibits the following characteristics:

- Feels rejected, helpless, and worthless
- Is indecisive and disinterested in surroundings
- Does not enjoy pleasurable events
- Has a low energy level, always feels fatigued
- Is unable to sleep or sleeps excessively
- May cry easily and often
- May have thoughts of suicide

Depression more commonly occurs during critical periods along the life cycle including adolescence, menopause, and old age. Depression is often untreated with only one in every three affected individuals seeking assistance. Treatment of depression may include psychotherapy and antidepressant medications. The majority of individuals with serious depression will show improvement in only a few weeks with medication.

Seasonal Affective Disorder. Seasonal affective disorder (SAD), also called winter depression, is a depressive condition that occurs more commonly during the winter months. Onset of depression typically begins in the fall, becomes progressively worse through the winter months, and clears or improves in the spring. SAD tends to recur each year with the change of seasons. Symptoms include chronic fatigue, excessive sleep, and excessive eating with weight gain. SAD occurs more commonly in women and those living at higher latitudes with shorter daylight hours. The cause of SAD is thought to be related to an increase in the hormone melatonin. This hormone is released by the pineal gland during dark hours and suppressed by light. Increased amounts of melatonin cause drowsiness and fatigue. It is thought that individuals with SAD are affected by high levels of melatonin. Medications to reduce melatonin secretion have been of some benefit. Another theory suggests that SAD is caused by a delay in the individual's **circadian rhythm** (a normal twenty-four-hour cycle of biological rhythms including sleep, metabolism, and glandular secretions) causing a type of hibernation. This theory is supported by the fact that daily exposure to bright light during the winter months has improved depression in individuals affected by SAD (Figure 20–1).

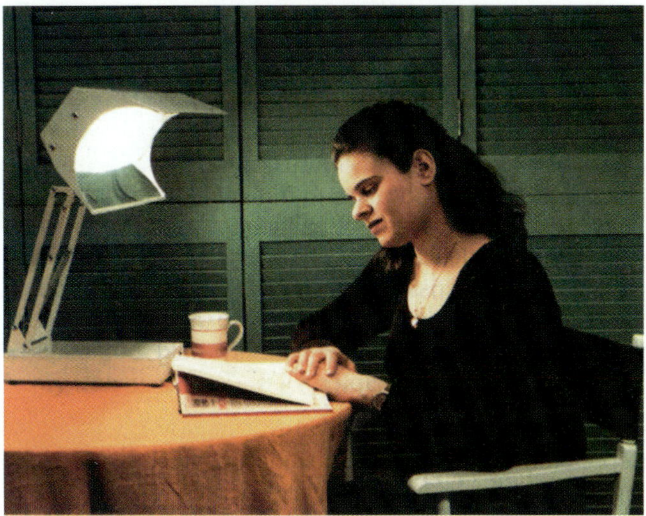

Figure 20–1 Seasonal affective disorder—many clients with seasonal affective disorder will find their spirits lifted when using light therapy. (Courtesy of Northern Light, Montreal, Canada.)

Bipolar Disorder. Bipolar disorder is a mood disorder in which extreme depression and **mania** (extreme elation or agitation) occur. The mania is not truly a state of happiness but rather a state of elated depression. Affected individuals have a normal state of depression but experience dramatic swings between this state and extreme depression and extreme mania. Symptoms of extreme depression have already been discussed. Symptoms of mania include:

- Feelings of euphoria
- Increased energy, activity, restlessness
- Rapid thoughts and racing speech
- Unrealistic beliefs in one's abilities
- Extreme irritability
- Unusual behavior and denial that anything is wrong

The cause of bipolar disorder is unknown. Current theories suggest genetics and a deficiency in certain biochemicals in the brain. Current treatment includes psychotherapy and lithium medication to control mood swings.

Dissociative Disorders

Dissociative disorders are characterized by changes in identity or consciousness. These disorders include psychogenic amnesia, psychogenic fugue, depersonalization disorder, and multiple personality.

- Psychogenic amnesia is characterized by a sudden loss of memory that is more than simple forgetfulness. This disorder tends to occur after a major stress and is considered to be a way of escape.
- Psychogenic fugue is characterized by suddenly leaving home, traveling some distance, forgeting one's identity and past, and often changing one's name. Fugue usually occurs after a major natural disaster such as an earthquake or during wartime. This disorder often lasts only a few days but may last for several months.
- Depersonalization disorders often occur following severe depression, stress, fatigue, or recovery from drug addiction. The affected individual feels disconnected from his mind and body, and may feel like he is viewing his life from a distance. Often the individual feels that he is losing his mind.

- Mutiple personality is a rare disorder characterized by an individual exhibiting two or more distinct personalities. The dominant personality determines the actions and activities of the affected individual. The dominant personality is usually not aware of the secondary personality(ies), but the secondary personality(ies) are aware of the dominant personality. Change from one personality to another usually occurs quite suddenly and usually follows a stressful event.

Anxiety Disorders

Normally, anxiety is a temporary response to stress, but for some individuals anxiety becomes a chronic problem. Affected individuals often experience anxiety that is exaggerated or of inappropriate proportion to the situation. Anxiety disorders represent the largest mental health disorder in the United States. The cause of anxiety disorders may be related to genetic factors, severe stress, biochemical alterations, and in some cases, physical causes such as hyperthyroidism. Treatment may include psychotherapy, hypnosis, stress reduction, relaxation therapy including biofeedback, and physical exercise. Types of anxiety disorders include generalized, panic, phobia, obsessive-compulsive, and post-traumatic stress disorder.

Generalized Anxiety Disorder. Generalized anxiety disorder, also called "excessive worry," is a continuous state of mild to intense anxiety. The anxiety is not related to a specific event and for this reason is often called "free-floating anxiety." This state of constant anxiety often leads to physical symptoms including dry mouth, nausea and vomiting, diarrhea, and muscle aches.

Panic Disorder. Panic disorder is a state of extreme uncontrollable fear. It is commonly called "panic attack." Onset of an attack is usually sudden and peaks in ten minutes or less and may include a feeling of impending doom and a need to escape. Other symptoms include diaphoresis, chest pain, increased pulse, nausea, and dissociation or the feeling that the incident is happening to someone else.

Phobia Disorder. Phobia disorder is the most common anxiety disorder. A phobia is an intense and irrational fear of an object, situation, or thing resulting in a strong desire to avoid the feared stimulus. The affected individual usually realizes that the phobia is irrational but is still unable to control the fear. There are over 700 known phobias. See Table 20–3 for a partial listing of phobias. Fear of spiders, snakes, and enclosed areas are some of the more common phobias.

TABLE 20-3 Phobias

Name of Phobia	Fear of
Acrophobia	high places
Algophobia	pain
Androphobia	men
Arachnophobia	spiders
Astrophobia	thunder, lightning, storms
Avioidphobia	flying
Claustrophobia	closed, tight, or narrow spaces
Hematophobia	blood
Hydrophobia	water
Iatrophobia	physicians
Kakorrhaphiophobia	failure
Lalophobia	public speaking
Monophobia	being alone
Ochlophobia	crowds
Olfactophobia	odor
Ophidophobia	snakes
Pathophobia	disease
Phasmophobia	ghosts
Phobophobia	fear
Ponophobia	work
Pyrophobia	fire
Sitophobia	food
Thanatophobia	death
Toxophobia	being poisoned
Traumaphobia	injury
Triskaidekaphobia	the number 13
Xenophobia	strangers
Zoophobia	animals

Obsessive-Compulsive Disorder. Obsessive-compulsive disorder (OCD), is an anxiety disorder with two distinct parts. **Obsession** is repetition of a thought or emotion. **Compulsion** is a repetitive act the affected individual is unable to resist performing. With OCD, the individual is unable to stop the thought or the action.

Behavior becomes ritualistic and thoughts or attempts to stop the thought or action bring about extreme anxiety. This behavior becomes very time consuming, usually taking more than an hour a day, and may become so disruptive that the individual is unable to perform daily activities or hold a job. Examples of compulsive activities include hand washing, cleaning objects, checking an object, and locking and unlocking locks.

Post-Traumatic Stress Disorder. Post-traumatic stress disorder (PTSD) develops as a response to a psychologically distressing event that could not be controlled and is outside the normal range of human experience. This disorder is a relatively new addition to anxiety disorders and is observed frequently in Vietnam veterans. In addition to war, individuals who are victims of rape, child incest or abuse, or survive natural disasters or acts of violence are often affected. Public safety workers are at great risk for PTSD. The feelings and fears associated with the trauma do not normally diminish with the passing of time. Affected individuals often experience a reliving of this trauma for weeks, months, or years in painful recollections or dreams. These individuals often go to extremes to avoid any reminder of the trauma, such as not sleeping or avoiding certain situations. Symptoms may occur immediately or may not arise for months after the trauma. Symptoms include:

- Flashbacks with the individual reliving the traumatic event
- Difficulty developing and maintaining relationships
- Irritability and agitation
- Depression
- Social withdrawal
- Drug dependency

Somatoform Disorders

Somatoform (somato = body) disorders are characterized by physical symptoms that lead one to believe in a physical disease, but no organic or physiologic cause can be found. Additionally, the physical symptoms appear to be associated with unconscious mental factors or conflicts. These symptoms are very real to the affected individual except in the case of factitious disorders (Munchausen and malingering). Individuals with somatoform disorders characteristically are described as frustrated, dependent, emotionally deprived, and resentful of family members and physicians.

Conversion. Conversion disorder, formerly known as hysterical neurosis, is a very striking disorder characterized by dramatic physical symptoms such as paralysis of an arm or leg, blindness, numbness, and deafness. The affected individual usually exhibits a calm, indifferent attitude about the situation. These physical symptoms enable the individual to avoid a stressful or unacceptable situation, and at the same time gain attention from others that may not usually give them attention. A diagnosis of conversion disorder should be a diagnosis of exclusion so as not to miss a non-psychiatric disorder such as a CVA or MI.

Hypochondriasis. Hypochondriasis is a condition characterized by an abnormal anxiety about one's body and health. These patients have an astounding knowledge of medical conditions and are constantly watchful of symptoms. Patients with hypochondriasis have an unrealistic fear that they are ill, despite medical assurance to the contrary. Affected individuals have difficulty establishing and maintaining relationships because so much of their energy and conversation revolve around their perceived illnesses.

Pain Disorder. Pain disorder may occur at any age, but commonly occurs in adolescent and young females. This pain causes interference with the individual's social, occupational, and basic activities of life. Long-standing pain may lead to depression and suicide. This disorder is characterized by pain that is sufficient to cause a clinical evaluation. Three subcategories exist, one where psychological factors are judged to have a major role in the pain, a second where both a psychological and medical component are present, and a third where a psychiatric role is not a major contributor to the pain. This pain is typically greater than that normally expected for the presenting physical findings on examination. Based upon the DSM-IV classification, acute pain is defined as pain present for less than six months and chronic pain is pain present for greater than six months.

Malingering. Malingering is the factitious display of symptoms in order to gain financial or personal reward. Symptoms are usually exaggerated and fraudulent. Diagnosis is often difficult as many of the symptoms are subjective and difficult to disprove.

Munchausen Syndrome and Munchausen by Proxy. Munchausen syndrome is a factitious disorder. The affected individuals simulate illness for no other apparent reason than to receive treatment. Often the individuals will go to extremes to present false tests, for example scratching or cutting themselves in order to add blood to urine specimens. An affected person may also self-inject a variety of substances into the blood or tissues in order to cause an illness. Generally, this individual has an extensive knowledge of diseases, medical treatments, terminology, and hospital routine. Affected individuals often present to emergency departments with reports of a variety of symptoms. Multiple tests and procedures are undergone willingly. When testing does not support the stated symptoms, the individual often reports different symptoms. There is usually a history of repeated hospitalizations with undetermined diagnosis. When the behavior is discovered, the confronted individual often becomes hostile and seeks attention at a different facility.

Munchausen by proxy is the same disorder except the patient projects the disorder to another person who is in their care, typically a child. The parent may inject the child or otherwise cause illness, then present the child for treatment. Illness tends to commonly be gastrointestinal or genitourinary in nature, and the parent denies any knowledge of the cause of the illness. Munchausen by proxy may be carried to the extreme and actually cause death of the child.

Personality Disorders

An individual's basic personality forms during the early years and depends in large part on how the individual learns to adapt to situations. This personality remains basically intact throughout life. A vast number of people have maladaptive patterns of seeing, relating to, and thinking about their environment. These individuals fit on a mental health spectrum at some point between mentally healthy and mentally ill. Most individuals with personality disorders have disturbances in emotional development and are maladjusted socially. Individuals with personality disorders often have incapacitating acute episodes of their mental disorder. Treatment of personality disorders includes psychotherapy and drug therapy. Hospitalization may be needed during acute episodes. Personality disorders include paranoid, schizoid, antisocial, narcissistic, and histrionic.

- Paranoid personalities are characterized by traits of jealousy, suspicion, envy, and hypersensitivity. These individuals exhibit extreme mistrust of others, and suspect the motives and intents as deliberately harmful to them. Paranoid individuals are often angry, hostile, cold, and unemotional.
- Schizoid personalities are loners. They lack warm or tender feelings for others and have few friends. The opinions of others have little effect on their feelings and they have difficulty expressing anger.
- Antisocial personalities usually are identified in the teen years by troublesome behavior including fighting, stealing, running away, and cruel behavior. The antisocial individual is selfish, irritable, aggressive, and impulsive. These individuals do not express feelings of guilt and do not learn from mistakes.
- Narcissistic personalities have an exaggerated sense of self-importance and self-love. They need constant attention and admiration. If criticized, they react with rage or humiliation and lack ability to express empathy.
- Histrionic personalities are overly dramatic with expressions of emotion. They exhibit theatrical mannerisms and overreact to events. This personality is vain and demanding and needs to be the center of attention while constantly seeking approval and reassurance.

TRAUMA

Grief

Almost every individual experiences grief and loss. The process of normal grieving is a healthy process that allows one to come to terms with the loss. However, some individuals have difficulty managing this process and may require assistance. As described earlier in this chapter, suicide is a significant problem as the third leading cause of death in the fifteen- to twenty-four-year-old age group and sixth leading cause of death in the five- to fifteen-year-old age group.

Grief is a natural process of coping with a loss. This may involve the loss of a family member, friend, or one's own impending death. The loss may be of lesser weight and include the loss of a body part or body function, a job, or a valued possession. No matter the cause, grief is real and is a natural part of life. Grieving is a healthy process. Those unable to grieve and complete the grieving process often have difficulty coping with life. People grieve differently in different cultures, and individuals in those cultures may also grieve differently. Some individuals are very emotional while others remain solemn. The normal grieving process passes through several stages. These stages were identified by Dr. Elisabeth Kubler-Ross in the 1970s and remain true today (Table 20–4). Not everyone is able to move through all the steps. Grieving individuals may stop

TABLE 20-4 Dr. Elisabeth Kubler-Ross' Five Stages of Grief/Death and Dying

Stage	Key ideas	Behavior
Denial	No not me	Refuses to believe, must be a mistake
Anger	Why me?	Envy those not dying or grieving, frustrated
Bargaining	If I could have one more chance	Becomes religious and good in an effort to bargain for time
Grief/Depression	Realizes bargaining is not working	Depressed, cries, gives up
Acceptance	OK, I give up but I may not like it	Expects death, may call family members near, completes unfinished business, prepares to die

in one stage and need assistance to move on or they may retreat back to a lower stage before moving forward again. The speed at which each individual moves through the grieving process is again very different. An important aspect of a funeral ceremony is to allow those who are grieving to say goodbye and to have closure in the situation. Individuals who were never allowed to say goodbye to a deceased or missing loved one, such as families of servicemen killed overseas or missing children or persons, may suffer with extreme depression. Inability to grieve and to complete the grieving process may lead to depression, poor coping skills, and the need for psychological counseling.

Suicide

Suicide is a common problem among those individuals with mental health disorders. Depression is a main cause of suicide. Suicidal individuals have feelings of depression, guilt, hopelessness, and helplessness. Changes in the life cycle, including aging, may lead to depression and suicide. It is estimated that over one third of people over age sixty-five try to commit suicide. Individuals diagnosed with a terminal illness often consider suicide as a means of living the remainder of life with dignity. Widowed, elderly white men, minority groups, and the unemployed are also at risk. It is important to ask *every* patient encountered for a mental health complaint about suicide in a professional and matter of fact manner. Asking patients if they are contemplating suicide will not encourage them to do so if they were not thinking about it in the first place. If the patient is considering suicide, the best indicator of intent is if the patient has a plan on how to carry out the suicide. If a person has a well-thought-out plan, he is at high risk for a suicide attempt. Again, asking a question about this plan will not encourage a patient to commit suicide. Other risk factors for suicide are listed in Table 20–5.

TABLE 20-5 Risk Factors for Suicide

- ✓ Recent depression
- ✓ Recent loss (e.g. death, financial, relationship)
- ✓ Thoughts of suicide
- ✓ Detailed plan
- ✓ Prior suicide attempts

MENTAL HEALTH DISORDERS IN THE OLDER ADULT

There are many mental health disorders that affect the older adult. Some of these may have begun early in life, while others occur very late in life. Some disorders of the neurologic system cause symptoms such as memory lapses, behavior changes, and confusion, that mimic symptoms of mental health problems but really are a physiologic or system specific disorder. Others, such as Alzheimer's disease, although a neurologic system problem, are also considered to be a mental health disorder. Many other disorders found in the older adult population are similar. Because of the changes that occur in the aging process, some symptoms seen in the elderly population may just be normal changes and not related to mental health disorders at all. Unfortunately, older adults are often labeled as having a mental health problem when they are merely dealing with the normal process of aging.

The most common mental health problems in the elderly population include depression, insomnia, isolation, stress, and disorders related to or caused by other system diseases. In addition, some individual medications or medication interactions may cause symptoms of mental health problems, such as confusion, forgetfulness, dizziness, and speech problems.

SUMMARY

Mental health disorders are some of the most misunderstood health problems. Although some are difficult to diagnose and treat, there are many more that can be either controlled or cured with proper diagnosis and intervention. Some of the symptoms of mental health problems are very slow to appear and are quite subtle, making it difficult to determine if a real problem exists. In the older adult, many neurologic disorders and the normal changes occurring in the aging process are often incorrectly attributed to a mental health disorder. Early diagnosis and treatment of any type of mental health disorder is important to assist the affected individual to live a quality life.

REVIEW QUESTIONS

Short Answer

1. What are some of the common signs and symptoms of mental health disorders?

2. What are some common tests used to diagnose mental health problems?

3. List some of the treatments used to control or cure mental health disorders.

Matching

4. Match the mental health disorder in the left column with the appropriate category in the right column. Items in the right column may be used more than once.

_____ Autism	a. developmental mental disorders
_____ Alcoholism	b. substance related mental disorders
_____ Depression	c. organic mental disorders
_____ Panic disorder	d. psychoses
_____ Dementia	e. mood disorders
_____ ADHD	f. anxiety disorders
_____ PTSD	g. somatoform disorders
_____ Obsessive-compulsive disorder	
_____ Drug abuse	
_____ Mental retardation	
_____ Munchausen	
_____ Schizophrenia	

CASE STUDY

You respond to a local supermarket where you find a young man in his early twenties pacing uncontrollably. He appears to be talking to himself, and knocks down food stacked in the aisles. His mother identifies herself to you and explains that her son's behavior has become more bizarre over the past week. She states that he seems suspect of everything she says or does and began acting this way after he thought she was going to harm him with some canned goods in the shopping cart. What do you suspect as a possible problem with this young man? What other causes (psychiatric and medical) should you also consider? How should you handle this situation?

BIBLIOGRAPHY

American Psychiatric Association (1994). *Quick reference to the diagnostic criteria from DSM-IV*.

Bower, B. (1997). Mysterious thoughts about phobias. *Science News, 152*, 315.

Bower, B. (1998). Genetic hint of psychosis. *Science News, 153*, 91.

Brems, S. (1997). Clinical implications of the co-occurrence of substance use and other psychiatric disorders. *Professional Psychology, Research and Practice, 28*(10), 437–447.

Brown, L. K. (November 1997). Adolescents with psychiatric disorders and the risk of HIV. *Journal of the American Academy of Child and Adolescent Psychiatry, 36*(11), 1609–1617.

Brown, R. A. (1996). Cigarette smoking , major depression, and other psychiatric disorders among adolescents. *Journal of the American Academy of Child and Adolescent Psychiatry, 35*(12), 1602–1610.

Cohn, C. K. (1997). Genetic risk for bipolar disorder. *The American Journal of Psychiatry, 154*(10), 1484.

DeMallie, D. A. (1997). Psychiatric disorders among the homeless: A comparison of older and younger groups. *The Gerontologist, 37*(2), 61–66.

Faraone, S. V. (1997). Attention-deficit disorder with bipolar disorder: A familial subtype? *Journal of the American Academy of Child and Adolescent Psychiatry, 36*(10), 1378–1387.

Kenny, J. T. (1997). Cognitive impairment in adolescents with schizophrenia. *The American Journal of Psychiatry, 154*(11), 1613–1615.

Kunzig, R. (1997). It kills horses doesn't it? *Discover, 18*(10), 96–105.

Markowitz, J. C. (1997). Dysthymic disorder in the context of other psychiatric disorders. *American Family Physician, 55(4)*, 1579–1580.

Marzuk, P. M. (June 18, 1997). Psychiatry. *Journal of the American Medical Association, 277*, 1892–1894.

Mental health informational statistics. http://www.mhsource.com/exclusive/mh.html.

Merkelbach, H. (1997). The etiology of childhood spider phobia. *Behaviour Research and Therapy*, 35(11), 1031–1034.

Subotnik, K. L. (1997). Depressive symptoms in the early course of schizophrenia: Relationship to familial psychiatric illness. *The American Journal of Psychiatry, 154*(11), 1551–1555.

Swartz, M. (1997). Family secret. *The New Yorker, 73*, 90–98.

Werner, A. (1997). Obsessive-compulsive symptoms in schizophrenia. *The American Journal of Psychiatry, 154*(11), 1635.

Zubenko, G. S. (1997). Mortality of elderly patients with psychiatric disorders. *The American Journal of Psychiatry, 154*(10), 1360–1368.

CHAPTER 21

Reproductive Diseases and Disorders

CONTENT OUTLINE

- Anatomy and Physiology
  - Female Anatomy and Physiology
  - Male Anatomy and Physiology
- Common Signs and Symptoms
- Diagnostic Tests
- Common Diseases of the Reproductive System
  - Female Reproductive System Diseases
  - Male Reproductive System Diseases
  - Sexually Transmitted Diseases (STD)
- Trauma
  - Rape
- Effects of Aging on the System

KEY TERMS

Bimanual examination
Cervicitis
Chancre
Cystoscopy
Digital rectal examination
Dysmenorrhea
Dyspareunia
Dysuria
Ectopic
Endometritis
Gumma
Laparoscopy
Leukorrhea
Menarche
Menopause
Oophoritis
Pyuria
RPR (Rapid Plasma Reagin)
Salpingitis
Septicemia
Sterility
VDRL (Venereal Disease Research Laboratory)

LEARNING OBJECTIVES

Upon completion of the chapter, the student should be able to:

1. Define the terminology common to the reproductive system and the disorders of the system.
2. Identify common disorders of the reproductive system.
3. Discuss the basic anatomy and physiology of the reproductive system.
4. Identify the important signs and symptoms associated with common reproductive system disorders.
5. Describe the common diagnostic tests used to determine type and/or cause of the reproductive system disorder.
6. Describe the typical course and management of the common reproductive system disorders.
7. Describe the effects of aging upon the reproductive system and the common disorders of the system.

OVERVIEW

The reproductive system is a complex system of structures with a variety of physiologic functions. Some parts of the reproductive system are endocrine glands (ovaries and testes) while other parts are strictly involved in procreation for a time during the individual's life span. Disorders of the system are common at all ages and may range from mild to severe, especially if not diagnosed early in the development of the disorder. Changes in the system during the aging process have both physiologic and psychosocial implications.

ANATOMY AND PHYSIOLOGY

The reproductive system is quite different between the male and female. Although the anatomy and physiologic features have a few commonalities, there are enough differences to discuss them separately.

Female Anatomy and Physiology

The female reproductive system consists of external structures—vulva, labia majora, labia minora, clitoris, vestibule, hymen, vaginal orifice, and vestibular glands, and internal structures—ovaries, fallopian tubes, uterus, cervix, and vagina (Figure 21–1). The ovaries secrete the female sex hormones estrogen and progesterone. The ovaries produce ova, the reproductive cells, within the graafian follicles (microscopic sacs). After a follicle releases an ovum, it develops into a corpus luteum. This structure is created by the leutinizing hormone from the

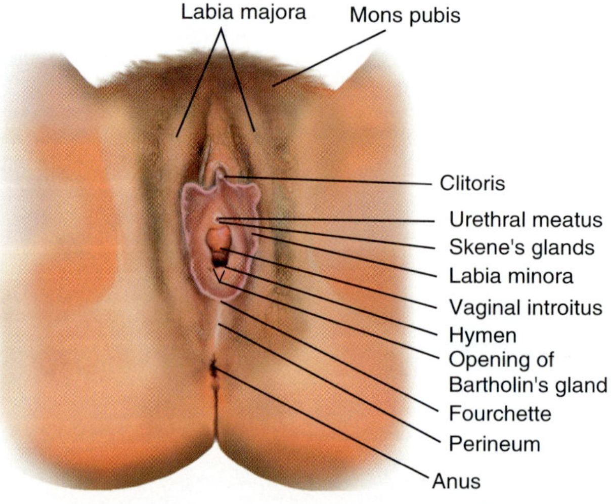

Figure 21–1 The female reproductive system.

pituitary gland. The corpus luteum secretes estrogen and progesterone. The fallopian tubes are ducts that carry the ova (eggs) from the ovaries to the uterus. The uterus is a pear-shaped muscular structure lying above the bladder in the pelvis. It is only about two inches by three inches in the non-pregnant state. The lower part of the uterus is called the cervix (neck). The inner layer of the uterus is the endometrium. During menstruation part of this layer is sloughed off and passed through the vagina and vaginal orifice. The vagina is the structure that receives the penis during intercourse and also becomes the birth canal during delivery of the fetus.

The hormones secreted by the ovaries are estrogens and progesterone. Secretion occurs in response to the effects of the follicle-stimulating hormone (FSH) and the luteinizing hormone (LH) produced by the anterior pituitary gland. Estrogens affect the development of secondary sex characteristics, characteristics occurring at puberty, changes in the endometrium, and growth of the uterus and vagina. Progesterone affects the development of the endometrium, assists the development of the placenta, causes enlargement of the breasts during pregnancy, prevents ova from being produced during pregnancy, and assists in the development of cells in the mammary glands.

The menstrual cycle is the process of secretion of hormones, the preparation of the endometrium for the implantation of the fertilized egg, and, if the egg is not implanted, the sloughing of the layer with bleeding from torn capillaries. The cycle runs for about twenty-eight days, but varies among individuals. The start of the menstrual flow is the first day of the cycle and usually lasts about four to five days. After that, estrogen is secreted until the graafian follicle matures and ruptures, about halfway through the cycle. Progesterone is then secreted by the corpus luteum. As the corpus luteum ages, progesterone levels go down causing menses and the beginning of the next cycle. Pregnancy will sustain progesterone levels maintaining the endometrium. **Menarche** is the first menstrual cycle that a young female experiences. The menstrual cycle may begin in females as young as ten years of age but typically begins at age eleven to twelve. The ceasing of the cycle is called **menopause**. This usually occurs between ages forty to fifty, but varies with the individual.

The female breasts are located between the second and seventh ribs over the pectoralis major muscle of the chest. Breasts are usually almost symmetrical and may be small or very large, depending on the individual's structure, body weight, and other factors. Endocrine secretions during menstruation and pregnancy affect the breast size and composition. The breasts show little sign of development until puberty. Over a two to three year period, the breasts change from the flattened preadolescent stage to the full breast maturity. As the female enters menopause, the breasts begin to atrophy and become more relaxed with a reduction in size.

The female breasts consist of three types of tissue: glandular, fibrous, and fat (adipose). The structure of the breast includes the nipple, areola, lactiferous ducts, lobules lined with milk-producing glands called acini, and fibrous dividers or septa. The breast also contains a network of lymph glands that drains the lymph and returns it to the circulatory system.

Male Anatomy and Physiology

The male reproductive system includes the external organs, scrotum and penis, and the internal organs, testes, epididymis, vas deferens, urethra, seminal vesicles, bulbourethral glands and the prostate (Figure 21–2). The penis houses the urethra, a tube that carries urine from the bladder and semen from the ejaculatory duct. At the tip of the penis is the prepuce or foreskin. The penis is composed of erectile tissue and arteries that dilate during sexual arousal. This causes the penis to become erect for the purpose of intercourse. The scrotum is a sac that hangs below the penis and holds the testes. The testes secrete testosterone, the male sex hormone, and produce sperm, the reproductive cells. Testosterone is responsible for changes occurring during puberty and secondary sex characteristics in the male.

The epididymis is the duct leading from each testis to the vas deferens, the excretory duct. The vas deferens from each testis extends up into the abdomen where it connects to create the ejaculatory duct that opens into the urethra. The seminal vesicles sit behind the bladder near the neck. They secrete fluid that is part of the thick white secretion called semen. The prostate gland and bulbourethral glands also secrete fluid that becomes part of the semen.

COMMON SIGNS AND SYMPTOMS

Common signs and symptoms of female reproductive system diseases and disorders include:

- Abdominal and pelvic pain
- Fever and malaise
- Abnormal vaginal drainage
- Burning and/or itching of the genitals

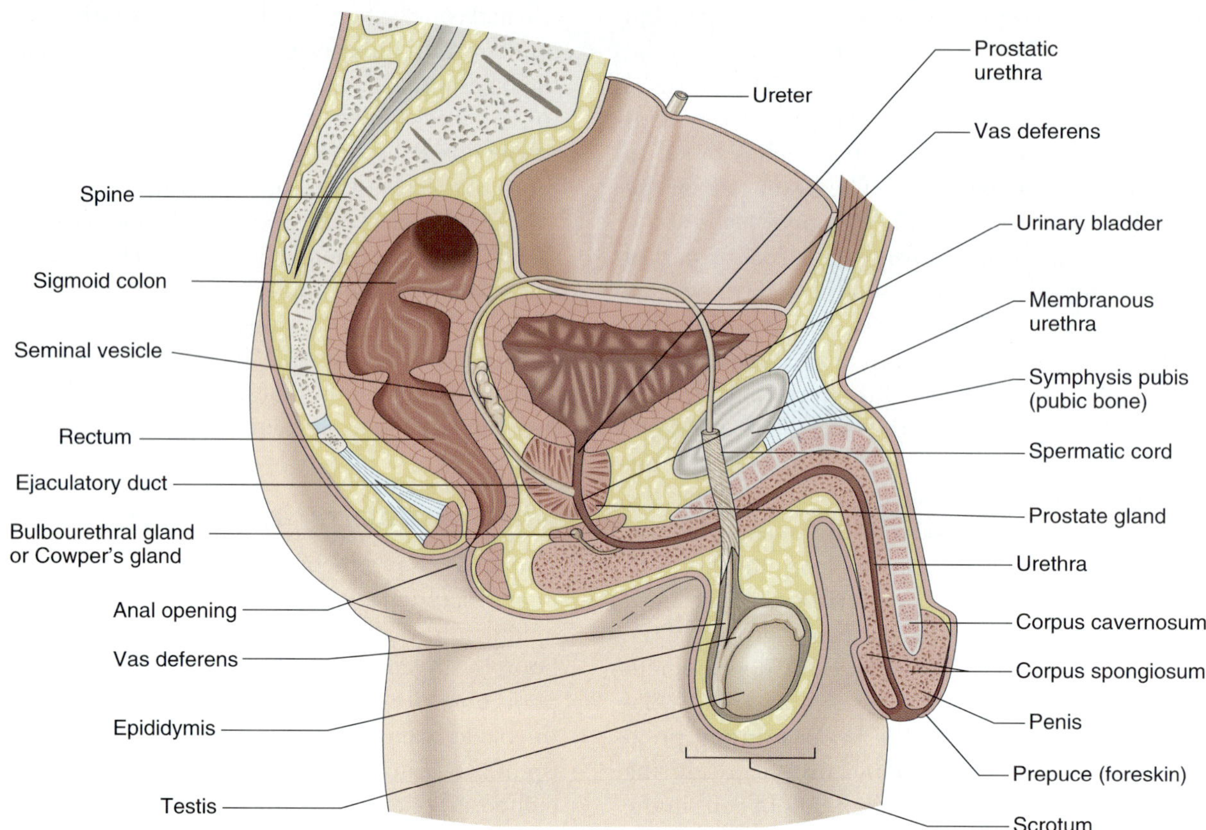

Figure 21–2 The male reproductive system.

- Pain during sexual intercourse
- Any change in breast tissue
- Abnormal discharge from the nipple

Common signs and symptoms of male reproductive system diseases and disorders include:

- Urinary disorders including frequency, dysuria, nocturia, and incontinence
- Pain in the pelvis, groin, or reproductive organs
- Lesions on the external genitalia
- Swelling or abnormal enlargement of the reproductive organs
- Abnormal penile drainage
- Burning and/or itching of the genitals

DIAGNOSTIC TESTS

Physical examination of the female reproductive system to aid in diagnosis of diseases begins with a pelvic examination. This exam includes inspection of the external genitalia, visual examination of the vagina and cervix through a speculum or instrument used to spread and hold the vaginal wall in an open position, and palpation of female internal organs by **bimanual examination**. A bimanual (two-handed) examination is so named because the physician places one hand on the abdomen and inserts fingers of the other hand into the vagina in order to feel the female organs between the two hands. A bimanual rectal examination allows palpation of the posterior aspect of the uterus and the rectum.

A **laparoscopy** (LAP-ah-**ROS**-ko-pee; laparo = abdomen, scopy = scope procedure), or looking inside the abdominal cavity with a lighted scope (Figure 21–3), is commonly used to view the female organs for abnormalities, to diagnose endometriosis, and perform a tubal ligation.

Laboratory tests to determine reproductive diseases include microscopic examination and culture and sensitivity of secretions or drainage from the vagina and genital lesions to determine the presence of infection. Blood tests to measure hormone levels including estrogen and progesterone levels are also common. Other blood testing includes **VDRL** (**Venereal Disease Research Laboratory**) and **RPR** (**Rapid Plasma Reagin**) test for syphilis.

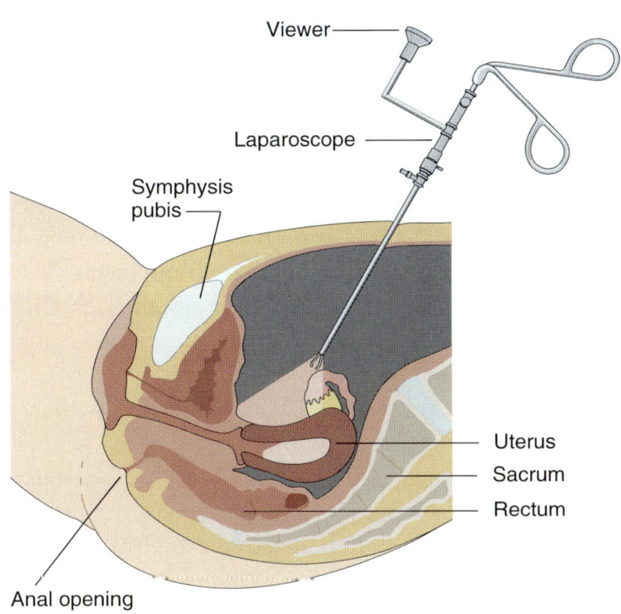

Figure 21–3 Laparoscopy.

Ultrasound may be performed on the pelvis to determine the presence of tumors and pregnancy and to visualize pelvic organ position and size. Benign breast cysts may be differentiated from solid tumors by ultrasonography.

Physical examination of the male reproductive system includes visual examination of the external genitalia for tumors, lesions, or penile drainage. The testes are palpated to determine presence of tumors. A **digital rectal examination** allows the physician to feel the prostate (Figure 21–4) for abnormal enlargement (hypertrophy or hyperplasia) and tumors. The rectal examination is also used in both males and females to detect bleeding from the gastrointestinal tract and during trauma or severe back pain to evaluate the nerves controlling the anal sphincter. If those nerves are compromised, the sphincter will relax.

Laboratory tests utilized in the determination of diseases of the male reproductive system include cultures and sensitivities of penile drainage, lesions, and urine to

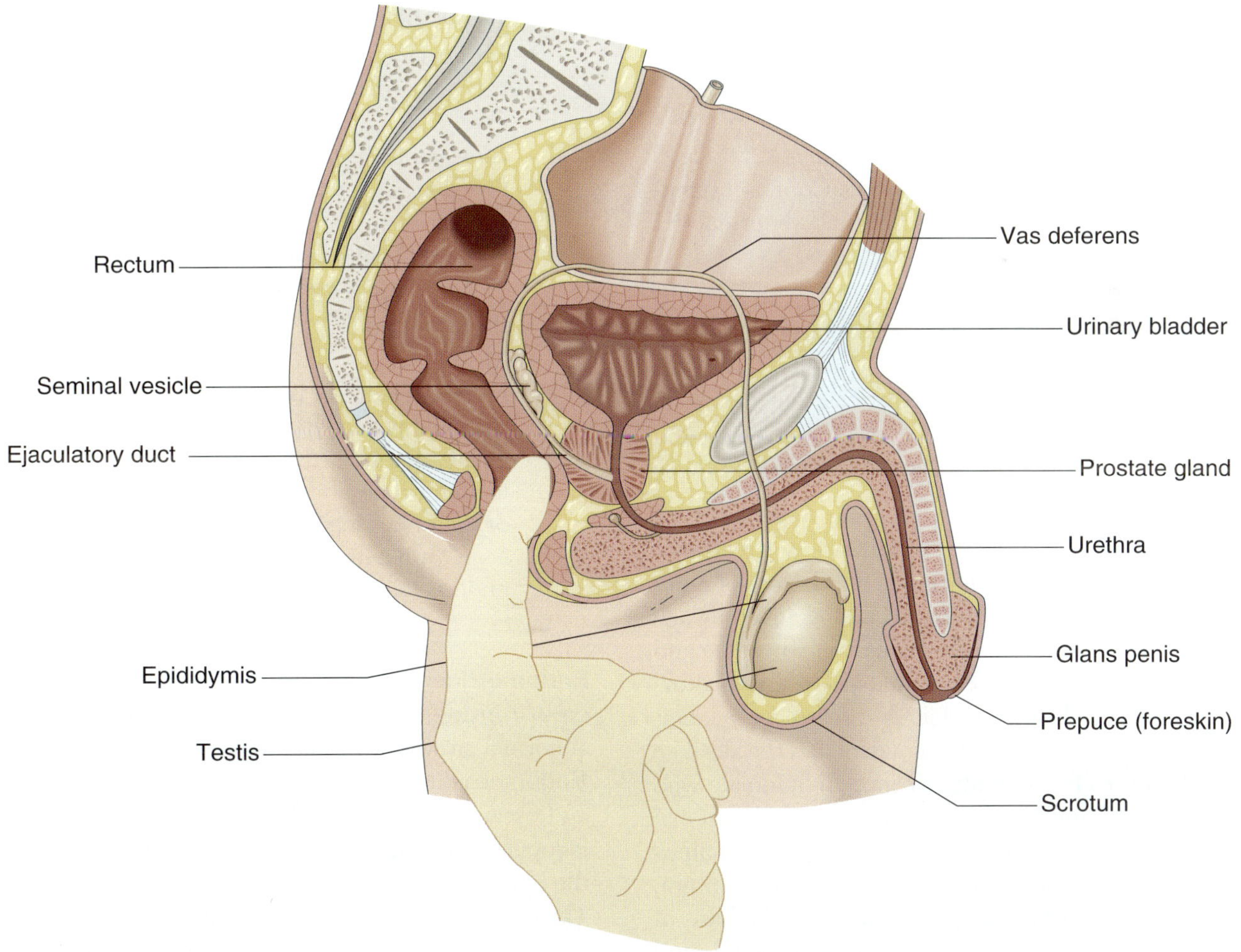

Figure 21–4 Digital rectal examination.

determine the presence of infection. A blood test called a prostate specific antigen (PSA) is helpful in the detection of prostate cancer. PSA levels also assist in determining effectiveness of prostate cancer treatment. Urine estrogen levels may assist in the diagnosis of testicular cancers.

Specific laboratory tests utilized for infertility testing include microscopic examination of semen to perform a sperm count, check sperm viability or ability to survive, and look for abnormally shaped sperm. Blood tests for the hormones testosterone and LH are also utilized.

COMMON DISEASES OF THE REPRODUCTIVE SYSTEM

Common diseases of the reproductive system involve those affecting both sexes. These diseases are divided into female reproductive system diseases, male reproductive system diseases, and sexually transmitted diseases.

Female Reproductive System Diseases

The female reproductive system is affected by numerous diseases and disorders caused by inflammation, infection, tumors, cysts, and hormonal imbalances. Diseases may range from mild to life-threatening. Common symptoms include abdominal or pelvic pain and abnormalities in the menstrual cycle.

Menstrual Abnormalities. Menstrual abnormalities are a common problem in the ovulating female. Causes of menstrual abnormalities vary as does treatment. Common abnormalities include amenorrhea, dysmenorrhea, menorrhagia, and metrorrhagia. A short description of these disorders follows.

- Amenorrhea (ah-MEN-oh-**REE**-ah; a = without, menorrhea = menstruation) is the absence of menstrual periods. If menses has not occurred by age 18, it is considered to be primary amenorrhea and may be caused by hormonal disorders, malformation or absence of female organs, pregnancy, or anorexia. Secondary amenorrhea is the absence of menses for 6 months or more in a female who has had regular cycles. Causes include hormonal imbalance, emotional upset, depression, malnutrition, excessive fitness training, ovarian tumor, and pregnancy. Diagnosis is made on the basis of a physical examination, hormonal blood and urine studies. Treatment depends on cause. If no abnormalities are present, hormone administration will usually begin the menstrual cycle in primary amenorrhea. Preventive measures include adequate nutrition, exercise, and stress reduction.
- Dysmenorrhea (DIS-men-oh-**REE**-ah; dys = difficult, menorrhea = menses) is painful or difficult menses and is one of the most common gynecologic disorders. Symptoms include dull to severe cramping pain in the pelvic area and low back pain. Pain may also radiate into the upper back, thighs, and genitalia. Causes of dysmenorrhea include pelvic infections, cervical stenosis, endometriosis, and unknown causes. Pain associated with cervical stenosis and endometriosis often occurs in females prior to childbearing and is often relieved after the birth of a child. Prognosis is good if the cause can be found and treated. Oral contraceptives may be effective in reducing dysmenorrhea as they regulate and decrease menstrual flow. Nonsteroidal anti-inflammatory medications are helpful in reducing inflammation and thus pain. Application of a heating pad to the pelvic area may also be helpful.
- Menorrhagia (MEN-oh-**RAY**-jee-ah; meno = menses, orrhagia = bursting forth, abnormal, excessive) is excessive or prolonged menstrual flow. Causes may be uterine tumors, pelvic inflammatory disease, and hormone imbalances. Treatment is related to cause and may include surgery to remove tumors, antibiotics to treat pelvic inflammatory disease and hormone therapy for hormone imbalances.
- Metrorrhagia (MET-roh-**RAY**-jee-ah; metro = uterus, orrhagia = bursting forth, abnormal, excessive) is abnormal bleeding between menstrual periods. Commonly, the cause is hormonal imbalance leading to an abnormal thickening and shedding of the endometrial tissue. Treatment may be a D & C (dilatation and curettage) returning the endometrium to normal and ending metrorrhagia.

Endometriosis. Endometriosis (EN-doh-ME-tree-**OH**-sis; endo = inside, metri = uterus, osis = condition of) is the abnormal growth of endometrial tissue outside the uterus. Endometrial tissue may flow retrograde during menses and escape into the abdominopelvic cavity through the fallopian tubes or, even worse, this tissue may escape into the blood supply and be carried to sites all over the body. The cause of retrograde flow is unknown, but use of tampons may be a causative factor. For this reason the use of tampons is discouraged. Common sites of endometrial implantation include the ovaries, fallopian tubes, abdominal wall, and intestine. Other sites of implantation include the urinary bladder, the diaphragm, nerves and ligaments of the back, and the vulva to name only a few (Figure 21–5). This endometrial tissue continues to act under the influence of hormones, thickening and bleeding with menstrual cycles. This action causes irritation and inflammation of normal tissue surrounding the implanted endometrial tissue thus causing the development of a special blood-filled cyst called "chocolate cyst," scar tissue, and adhesions. This bleeding of endometrial tissue in the abdominopelvic cavity and other **ectopic** (eck-TOP-ick, out of normal place) areas causes **dysmenorrhea** (DIS-men-oh-**REE**-ah; dys = painful, menorrhea = menses) beginning a few days before menses and extending several days into the menstrual cycle. There may be a constant cramping pain in the low back, pelvis, and vagina. Affected individuals, usually females of childbearing age, may also have heavy menses and **dyspareunia** (DIS-pah-**ROO**-knee-ah; painful sexual intercourse).

The primary complication of endometriosis is infertility. Other complications include ectopic pregnancy and spontaneous abortion. Diagnosis is made on the basis of history, pelvic examination, and laparoscopy, which will confirm the diagnosis and allow visualization of the extent of the condition. Treatment depends on affected individual's age and desire to have children.

Pelvic Inflammatory Disease (PID). Pelvic inflammatory disease is an inflammation of some or all of the pelvic reproductive organs. It may be mild to severe and may involve the cervix (**cervicitis**), the inner lining of the uterus (**endometritis**), fallopian tubes (**salpingitis**), and ovaries (**oophoritis**). This inflammation is commonly caused by infection by bacteria that ascend from the vagina and travel upward to the pelvic cavity. Bacteria can be introduced into the female reproductive system during childbirth, miscarriage, abortion, or other gynecologic procedures. The most common cause of PID is sexually transmitted disease, including gonorrhea and chlamydial infection. Young sexually active females and those who use IUDs are most at risk of developing PID. Symptoms are typical of an infection and include fever, chills, pain

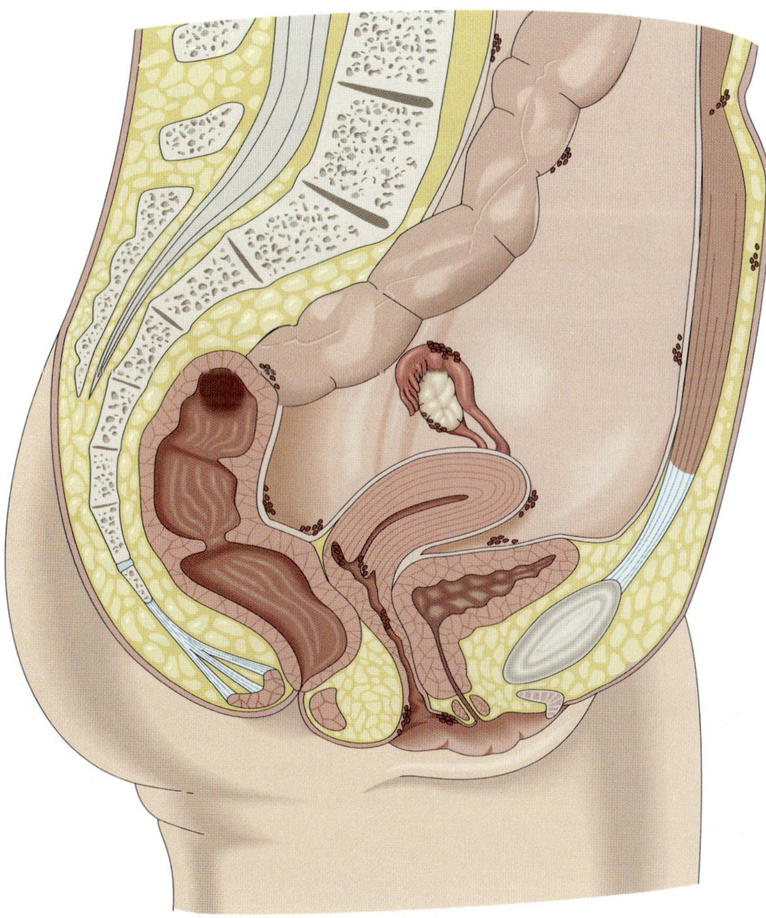

Figure 21–5 Endometriosis—common sites of endometrial implants.

in the pelvic area, and **leukorrhea** (LOO-koh-**REE**-ah; leuk = white, orrhea = flow or discharge), a white, usually foul-smelling vaginal discharge. Diagnosis is made on the basis of a pelvic examination including a positive culture or vaginal discharge. Treatment includes antibiotic therapy, analgesics, and bedrest. Without proper treatment an abscess may develop or the patient may develop **septicemia** (SEP-tih-**SEE**-me-ah; septic = dirty or contaminated, emia = blood), which may be life-threatening. Inflammation of the reproductive organs may lead to the development of scar tissue and adhesions. These adhesions may cause the complications of infertility and ectopic pregnancy.

Ovarian Cyst. Ovarian cysts are commonly benign fluid-filled sacs on or near the ovary (Figure 21–6). There are two types of cyst: physiologic, those caused by a normally functioning ovary, and neoplastic, an abnormal type not related to the function of the ovary. Physiologic cysts are the most common and may become very large, grapefruit size, before producing symptoms. Symptoms include low back pain, pelvic pain, and dyspareunia. Acute, extreme pain, nausea and vomiting may occur if the ovary becomes twisted because of the weight of the cyst. Diagnosis is made on the basis of history, pelvic examination, and ultrasound.

Treatment depends on the type and size of the cyst. Small physiologic cysts usually do not need treatment and often resolve spontaneously. Oral contraceptive medication may be given for several months to help resolve physiologic tumors of various sizes. Large cysts or those of questionable type are often viewed by laparoscopy. During laparoscopy the cyst may be removed or drained. Determination should be made as to the type of cyst as cancerous cysts need immediate treatment.

Fibroid Tumor. Leiomyomas, commonly called fibroid tumors, are benign tumors of the smooth muscle of the uterus (Figure 21–7). These tumors are the most common tumor of the female reproductive system, occurring in one out of five women over age thirty-five. The cause of fibroid tumors is unknown but it is known that these tumors are stimulated by estrogen, and thus tend to occur during reproductive years and regress or calcify after menopause. Fibroid tumors appear often in multiples and vary in size from small to quite large. Small fibroids are often asymptomatic. Symptoms include abnormal uterine bleeding, excessive menstrual bleeding, and pain. Diagnosis is made on the basis of pelvic examination and ultrasound. Treatment depends on the individual's age and desire for childbearing. Fibroids may be removed surgically, or in older individuals a hysterectomy is often the treatment of choice.

Toxic Shock Syndrome. Toxic shock syndrome (TSS) is a severe life-threatening illness characterized by sudden onset of high fever, vomiting, diarrhea, and a dropping blood pressure. TSS is found almost exclusively in menstruating females using tampons. It is thought to be caused by *Staphylococcus aureus*, a normal flora bacterium of the skin. This bacterium produces an increased amount of toxin when in contact with the synthetic fibers found in tampons. Diagnosis is made on the basis of history of tampon use and symptoms. Treatment includes intravenous fluids to counteract shock and antibiotics to treat the infection. Untreated or delayed treatment may be fatal. Prevention is good handwashing prior to tampon insertion to decrease the number of bacteria on the individual's hands. Tampons should be changed frequently to prevent infection.

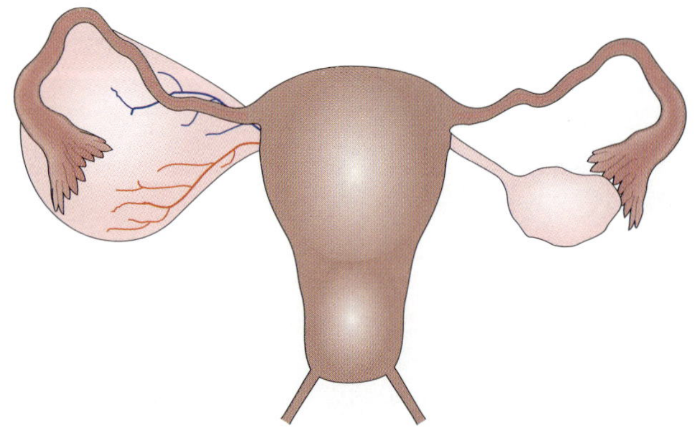

Figure 21–6 Ovarian cyst.

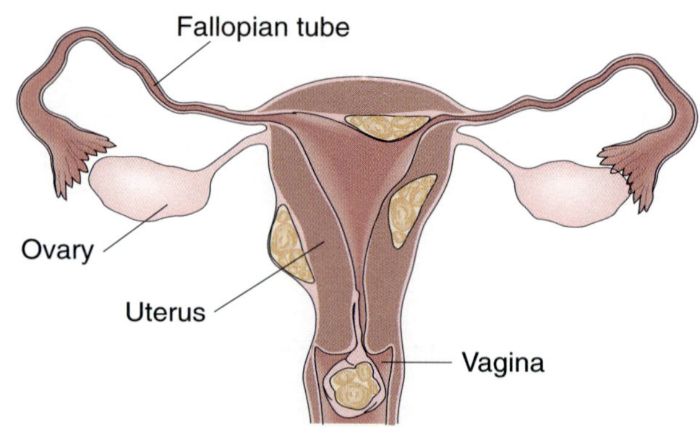

Figure 21–7 Fibroid tumors.

Male Reproductive System Diseases

The most common diseases affecting the male reproductive system include infection and diseases affecting the prostate. The positional relationship of the male urinary bladder and the prostate cause the male to experience urinary symptoms when the prostate is affected with disease.

Prostatitis. Prostatitis (PROS-tah-**TYE**-tis; prost = prostate, itis = inflammation) is inflammation of the prostate gland. This condition is more common in men over fifty years of age. Cause may be unknown or it may be the result of a urinary tract infection or infection by gonorrhea. Symptoms include **dysuria** (dis-YOU-ree-ah; dys-painful, uria – urination), **pyuria** (pye-YOU-ree-ah; py = pus, uria = urine), fever, and low back pain. Diagnosis is made on the basis of a urinalysis, urine culture, and digital rectal examination. Treatment is dependent on cause but often includes antibiotic therapy. Prognosis is good as prostatitis usually responds well to treatment.

Epididymitis. Epididymitis (EP-ih-did-ih-**MY**-tis; epididym = epididymis, itis = inflammation) is inflammation of the epididymis. Common causes include prostatitis, urinary tract infection, mumps, and sexually transmitted disease such as chlamydia, syphilis, and gonorrhea. Epididymitis is one of the most common diseases of the male reproductive tract and usually affects only one epididymis (unilateral). Symptoms include a swollen, hard, and painful epididymis often accompanied by severe scrotal pain and swelling. Scrotal discomfort makes walking difficult and the affected individual may walk straddle-legged in order to protect the scrotum.

Diagnosis is made on the basis of symptoms, urinalyis, and urine culture. Prompt, appropriate antibiotic therapy is usually very effective. A delay in treatment may lead to complications of scarring and **sterility** (inability to impregnate a female related to sperm quality or quantity). Other treatment includes bed rest, analgesics, use of a scrotal support, and avoidance of alcohol, spicy foods, and sexual stimulation. Prevention is aimed at cause and includes prompt treatment of causative infections, sexual abstinence, or use of condoms during sexual intercourse to decrease the risk of infection with sexually transmitted diseases.

Orchitis. Orchitis (or-KYE-tis, orch = testis, itis = inflammation) is inflammation of one or both testes usually caused by bacterial or viral infection or trauma. Viral mumps is the most common cause of orchitis in the adult male. Commonly orchitis occurs in conjunction with or as a complication of epididymitis. Symptoms include swelling, pain and tenderness of one or both testes, fever, and malaise. Diagnosis is made on the basis of symptoms, blood testing, and urinalysis. Treatment is dependent on cause.

Testicular Torsion. Testicular torsion involves the "spinning" of a testicle about the spermatic cord, causing blood flow to the involved testicle to be significantly reduced or completely disrupted. This can lead to an exquisitely painful testicle and permanent tissue damage within a few hours. The torsion occurs because there is a defect in the linings that surround the spermatic cord and testis that allows it the freedom to twist. Testicular torsions commonly occur around the time of puberty, although it can happen at any time during life. There is typically a history of some type of physical activity; however, torsions can occur while at rest. The pain is usually at the affected testicle, but it can radiate into the groin or abdomen. The affected testicle will be significantly elevated above the level of the unaffected testicle, lying in a transverse position; lifting the testicle up does not relieve the pain.

Definitive treatment will typically include surgery to reduce the torsion and repair the defect. The unaffected side may also be explored surgically because there is a high rate of bilateral defects. Occasionally, the torsion can be reduced in the emergency department by either the emergency physician or urologist. EMS treatment includes transporting in a position of comfort and an attempt to transport in a smooth fashion as the pain will increase with uneven roads. Pain medicine may be administered if allowed by local protocols or under medical control direction. The patient will typically not require any additional intervention; however, patient should be treated for other conditions as found during his history and physical exam.

Sexually Transmitted Diseases (STD)

Sexually transmitted diseases (STD) include a group of many diseases that are spread by intimate or sexual contact. The spread of STD is at an epidemic level in the United States. These infections are transmitted from one person to another by contact with infected skin, blood, semen, and vaginal secretions during vaginal, anal, and oral sex. Prevention is best achieved by avoiding intimate contact with infected individuals. Other precautions include use of a condom during sexual intercourse, avoiding multiple sex partners, avoiding sex with someone with an unknown sexual history, and avoiding the use of alcohol, which may impair judgment concerning a sexual encounter. Treatment of STDs commonly consist of identifying sex partners and treating the infected individuals concurrently to avoid reinfection or a "ping-pong" effect of passing the infection back and forth between involved individuals. Follow-up testing is needed after treatment to ensure the disease has been eradicated in all infected individuals.

Acquired Immunodeficiency Syndrome (AIDS). Acquired immunodeficiency syndrome (AIDS) is a blood-borne infection commonly transmitted sexually. Currently there is no cure for this immunodeficiency disease that predisposes the affected individual to a multitude of opportunistic diseases. Prevention is imperative and must include health and AIDS education. For more details about AIDS see Chapter 12.

Hepatitis. Hepatitis forms B and C may be spread by sexual intercourse and are thus considered STDs. For more information see Chapter 13.

Genital Herpes. Genital herpes is an extremely painful, recurring viral infection characterized by multiple blister-like lesions (Figure 21–8). The incidence of genital herpes in the United States is increasing at a frightening rate with one in every six individuals currently infected. Genital herpes is caused by herpes simplex virus (HSV) type II. This virus is closely related to herpes simplex virus type I, which commonly causes fever blisters or cold sores on the lips. Both herpes simplex viruses are highly contagious and are transmitted by intimate contact between two mucous membrane surfaces. HSV I may be spread by kissing an affected individual during the active phase of the disease. HSV II is commonly spread by sexual intercourse. HSV I may be spread to the genital area by oral-genital exposure and HSV II may be spread to the lips in the same manner. Self-infection with the hands is also possible. Touching an infected area followed by touching of the lips, genitals, or eyes may cause self-infection. Extreme care should be taken to avoid infection of the mucous membranes of the eyes.

Herpes disease cannot be cured. The virus remains dormant in the tissues until activated by stress or lowered immunity. Sunlight, fever, emotional stress, and menses are common activators of the herpes virus. Once activated the virus produces blisters that enlarge, rupture, and ulcerate. The lesions are extremely painful, especially during sexual intercourse. Severe itching and painful urination (dysuria) are common. Genital herpes infection in the male commonly produces blisters on the glans penis, the shaft of the penis, scrotum, and inner thighs. Lesions in the female commonly appear on the vulva, vagina, inner thighs, and rectal area. Childbirth in a female with active herpes infection is fatal to the infant fifty percent of the time. If the infant survives, major neurologic

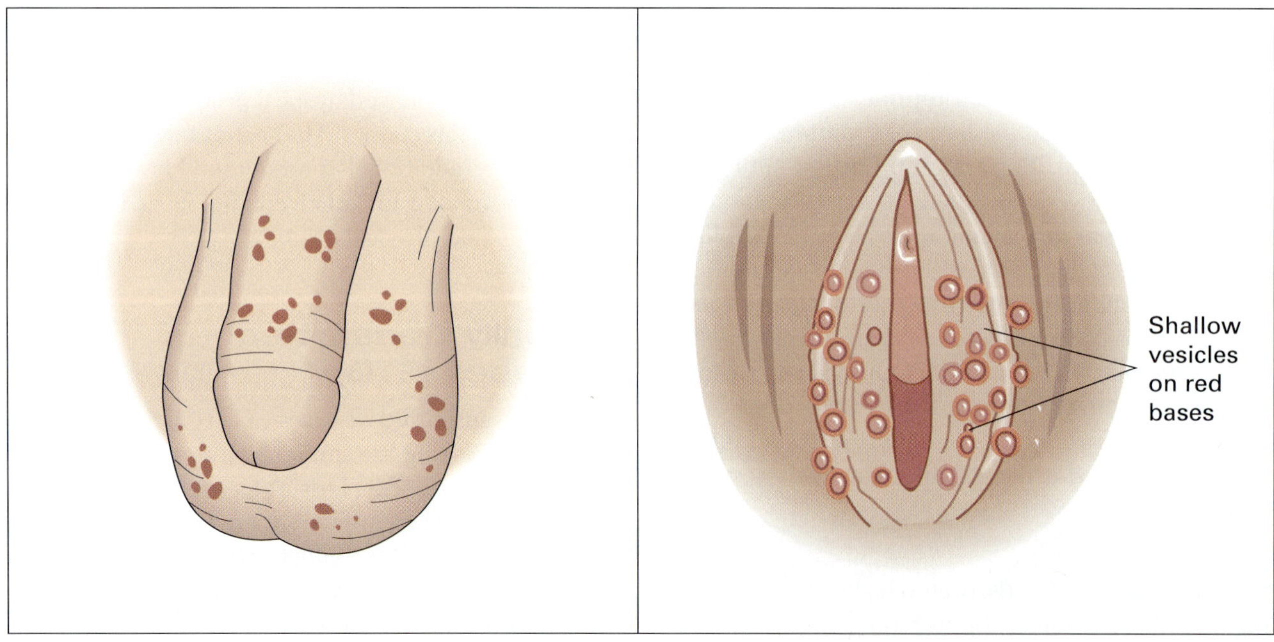

Figure 21–8 Genital herpes.

and ophthalmic complications usually occur. For this reason, delivery by cesarean section is performed in mothers with active genital herpes.

Herpes lesions generally last between one to three weeks but may re-occur weekly, monthly, or yearly. Diagnosis is made on the basis of presence of characteristic lesions and a positive viral culture of active lesions. Treatment is symptomatic and involves anti-viral medications to reduce symptoms.

Gonorrhea. Gonorrhea, also known as "clap," is a highly contagious sexually transmitted disease caused by the bacteria *Neisseria gonorrhoeae*. It is one of the most common STDs in the United States. This bacterial infection causes inflammation of mucous membranes of the genital and urinary systems in both males and females. Gonorrhea commonly causes urethritis in the male with symptoms of purulent discharge from the penis, dysuria, and urinary frequency. Females commonly show signs of cervicitis with purulent vaginal discharge, dysuria, urinary frequency, genital itching and a burning pain. The transmission of gonorrhea is often difficult to control as the infected individual, either male or female, may be asymptomatic. In this case the infected individual is a carrier of the infection and may unknowingly spread the infection. Infants born to mothers with gonorrhea run the risk of developing gonorrheal eye infection, which can lead to blindness. In order to prevent infant blindness, it is a common practice, and is state law in some instances, that all newborns' eyes are treated with prophylactic antibiotic at birth.

Diagnosis of gonorrhea is made on the basis of a culture of secretions. Treatment with antibiotics including penicillin, tetracycline, and ceftriaxone is usually effective. Untreated gonorrhea may lead to life-threatening systemic infections such as meningitis and endocarditis. Arthritis and sterility are also common in both the untreated male and female.

Syphilis. Syphilis is a serious sexually transmitted infection caused by *Treponema pallidum* bacteria. It is spread by sexual or intimate contact with contagious lesions. As soon as exposure occurs, bacteria rapidly penetrate the skin or mucous membrane and gain access to the vascular system, producing a systemic infection. Diagnosis is made on the basis of blood tests. Syphilis has a much lower incidence than gonorrhea and is more easily treated. Antibiotic treatment with penicillin or tetracycline is very effective. Untreated syphilis has a much worse outcome than gonorrhea, as it may become a chronic life-threatening disease. Untreated, syphilis progresses through three distinct stages with characteristic signs and symptoms. The stages are primary, secondary, and tertiary.

1. Primary—This stage is marked by the appearance of a painless, highly contagious lesion called a **chancre** (SHANG-ker) (Figure 21–9). This lesion occurs at the site of bacterial entry and usually appears several weeks after contact. It may vary in appearance from pimple-like to an ulcerated sore. In the male the chancre usually appears on the head of the penis. In the female the chancre commonly appears on the vulva, although it may occur inside the vaginal cavity and thus be hidden and go unnoticed. The chancre may appear at other sites in both sexes including the lips, fingers, anus, and tongue. Even without treatment the chancre commonly disappears in ten to thirty days, often leading to the false conclusion that the disease is cured. Lymphadenopathy, or sore swollen lymph nodes, is common. The disease is highly contagious during this stage but is easily cured with antibiotic therapy.
2. Secondary—After the chancre heals, a period of rest occurs that may last from six weeks to one year. During this time the bacteria rests then rapidly grows and multiplies causing the characteristic rash of secondary syphilis. This rash may appear in any area of the body: the palms, soles of the feet, mouth, or it may spread over the entire body. The rash does not itch and may be erroneously diagnosed as mumps, chickenpox, or ringworm. The individual is highly contagious during this stage. If mouth sores are present, kissing may spread the

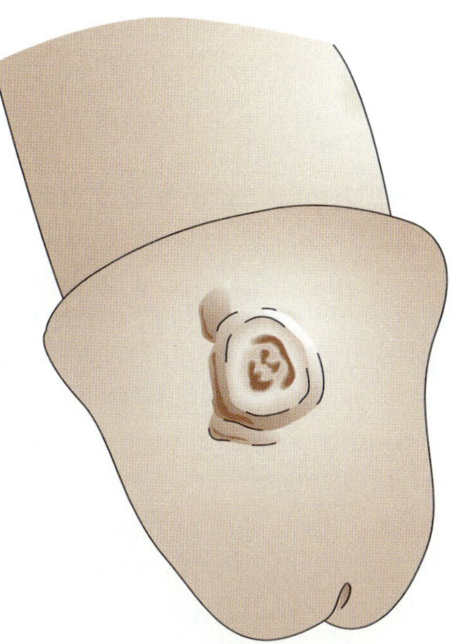

Figure 21–9 Syphilis chancre.

disease. Syphilis can be easily diagnosed, based on a blood test, during this stage and easily treated with antibiotics. The primary and secondary stages are often combined and called *early syphilis*.

3. Tertiary (Late or Latent)—If secondary syphilis is untreated, the bacterial organisms withdraw into single or multiple sites in the body and become dormant. The length of this dormant time ranges from one to twenty years. During this time the infected individual may be unaware of the infection. Blood testing may even show negative results. The disease at this time is less contagious to others, but is dangerous for the infected individual. Bacteria invade organs throughout the body producing a characteristic soft gummy lesion called **gumma** (GUM-mah). Symptoms vary depending on the organs attacked. Common problems include aortic aneurysm, heart failure, mental disorders, insanity, deafness, blindness, paralysis, and death. Tertiary syphilis can be cured with antibiotic treatment, but the effects of the lesions are irreversible.

Syphilis in pregnant females may cause spontaneous abortion or death of the infant. Infants that survive commonly have numerous defects including physical and mental deformities, blindness, and deafness. Pregnant females should be tested for syphilis early as syphilis can be cured with antibiotic treatment during the first five months of pregnancy thus preventing infection in the unborn child.

Chlamydial Infection. Chlamydial infection, caused by the bacteria *Chlamydia trachomatis*, is very common in the United States and is one of the most damaging of the STDs. Chlamydial infection is often called the "silent" STD as infected individuals may be asymptomatic until dangerous complications occur. Chlamydial infection is the leading cause of PID and thus a major cause of female infertility. Males with chlamydial infection are usually symptomatic with drainage from the penis, burning and itching with urination caused by urethritis, and epididymitis. Symptomatic females experience vaginal drainage with burning and itching of the genital area. Abdominal pain and dyspareunia may be indicative of PID. Diagnosis is made on the basis of cytologic examinations. Treatment with antibiotic therapy is effective. Prognosis is good if treatment occurs prior to the onset of complications. Untreated females may suffer with PID and infertility. Untreated males may suffer with severe epididymitis causing sterility.

Trichomoniasis. Trichomoniasis is an infection by a protozoan, *Trichomonas vaginalis*. Trichomoniasis is a fairly common STD, affecting approximately ten percent of all sexually active individuals. Most infected individuals are asymptomatic, resulting in extensive spread of the infection. If symptoms occur in the male they commonly include urethritis, epididymitis, and prostatitis. Infected females, when symptomatic, have itching and burning of the genital area with a green frothy vaginal drainage. Diagnosis is made on the basis of microscopic examination of vaginal or penile secretions revealing the presence of the causative organism. Treatment with an anti-parasitic medication is usually very effective.

Genital Warts. Genital warts are cause by a virus commonly spread during sexual contact (Figure 21–10). Warts may be asymptomatic or may cause tenderness in the affected area. The amount of discomfort is related to the size, location, and number of warts present. These viral lesions commonly appear one to six months after exposure to an infected individual. In the male, warts are usually located on the head of the penis, but may also be found along the penile shaft and around the anus. In the female, these lesions commonly appear around the vaginal opening and may spread to the perianal area. Size of genital warts may vary from very small to three or four inches in diameter. They may appear singly or in clusters. Pregnancy tends to cause the warts to grow more rapidly. Genital warts in a pregnant female may even reach a point of occluding the vaginal canal, thus making a cesarean delivery necessary. Cervical cancer is also

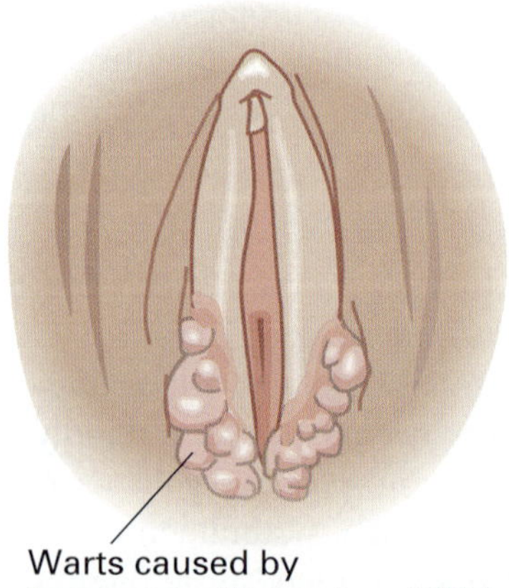

Figure 21–10 Genital warts.

more common in females with genital warts. Diagnosis is made on the basis of visualization of the warts and biopsy to rule out carcinoma. Treatment is commonly surgical or chemical removal of the infected tissue. Surgical removal does not mean cure, as recurrence of genital warts is common.

TRAUMA

Rape

Rape is sexual intercourse without consent or against the will of the involved individual. Victims of rape may be any age and of either sex, but it is primarily an act violating females. The crime of rape occurs at an alarming rate, but many cases are unreported as the victim often feels embarrassed, ashamed, and guilty. Rape is a crime of violence more than of sexual passion. An acquaintance, date, spouse, or an unknown individual may carry out rape. Recent publicity has been devoted to "date rape" drugs or medication that is placed in a drink and renders the individual unconscious to the point of becoming an easy victim. Signs and symptoms of rape may include, but are not limited to, torn clothing, disheveled appearance, bruises, and lacerations around the mouth, breasts, genitals, and rectum. Semen may be found on the inner thighs, in the vaginal cavity, and around the genital and rectal area if the victim has not bathed, showered, or douched after the act.

Diagnosis is made on the basis of history and physical examination. Special attention should be given to the emotional condition of the victim. Emergency guidelines are aimed at protecting the victim against disease and pregnancy and collecting legal evidence should the victim decide to allow legal action against the perpetrator. Gathering of criminal evidence is best if the individual has not bathed, showered, or douched, but often because the victim feels very "dirty and violated," these cleansing activities are performed immediately and prior to reporting of the crime. Sex crime evidence gathering may involve collecting samples of clothing, hair, scrapings from under fingernails, pubic hair, semen samples, and taking pictures of areas of trauma. EMS providers should assess and treat for life-threatening conditions. If possible, a female provider or officer should accompany the patient during the exam and transport. Allow the patient to direct the conversation and do not touch the patient without explaining what you are doing, even if it is something as common as checking a blood pressure. Visualize the genitalia only if you suspect a life-threatening injury. Any clothing worn by the patient during the attack should be placed in a paper bag and labeled with the patient's name, time, date, and the name of the person placing the items in the bag. Above all, EMS providers need to be professional and empathetic toward the victim. Recovery from rape is difficult. Crisis intervention counselors are needed and follow-up is very important. Individuals involved with the victim need to be nonjudgmental, confirm that the individual is a victim, and assure the individual that this act of violence was not deserved.

EFFECTS OF AGING ON THE SYSTEM

As the female ages, changes in the reproductive system may seem more distinct than in the male. The pubic hair becomes thin and gray, the external structures become less elastic and appear more wrinkled and sagging. The internal organs shrink in size, vaginal secretions diminish, and there is less elasticity of the vagina. Although sexual stimulation is still important, as in the male, it may take increased stimulation and the aid of a vaginal lubricant to enhance sexual intercourse. Some cancers of the female reproductive system, such as cancer of the uterus and ovaries, are more common in the older adult. Women over age sixty-five should be screened regularly for these disorders.

As the female enters menopause, the breasts also begin to atrophy and become more relaxed with a reduction in size.

As the male ages, there is a decrease in testosterone production and the formation of sperm. The size of the testes may also diminish, but the functional ability of the male for sexual intercourse and reproduction continues. There is some loss of elasticity of the penis and scrotum, causing them to appear more wrinkled and sagging. There is some thinning and graying of the pubic hair. Although the male is still able to have an erection, sometimes it takes greater stimulation to achieve this. The ejaculation amount may also be diminished. The prostate slowly enlarges in most men beginning around age fifty. This prostatic hypertrophy can cause problems with urination. The prostate is also a common site for cancer development in the older male. Routine rectal examination of the prostate and laboratory levels of PSA (prostate specific antigen) should be completed by all adult males over age fifty.

SUMMARY

The reproductive system is a highly complex multi-function system. It has important physiologic functions, but is also very important in social relationships between individuals. Both procreation and the relationship/intercourse aspect of the system can be altered when disorders develop in the system. Common disorders of the system in the female include infections, inflammation, STDs, and cancer. In the male, common disorders include infections, STDs, impotence, and cancer. Signs and symptoms of reproductive disorders in both sexes may include pain, discharge, lesions, and abnormal enlargement of tissue. Changes occurring in the system in the older adult often affect the individual's ability to perform sexual intercourse satisfactorily. Other changes include decrease in hormone secretion, loss of elasticity of tissues, diminished lubricating secretions, and increased risk for cancer development.

REVIEW QUESTIONS

Short Answer

1. What are some of the common reproductive system disorders:
   a. Female?

   b. Male?

2. What are the common signs and symptoms of reproductive system disorders:
   a. Female?

   b. Male?

True or False

3. T F Endometriosis is an ectopic occurrence of endometrial tissue.
4. T F Toxic shock syndrome is characterized by high fever.
5. T F Leiomyoma is a metastatic tumor of the uterus.
6. T F Epididymitis is usually caused by an infection from the bladder.
7. T F STDs are not common in the male reproductive system.
8. T F A testicular torsion typically requires surgical treatment to save the affected testis.
9. T F Pelvic inflammatory disease is a condition that involves inflammation without infection of one or more of the female reproductive organs.
10. T F Infection of the ovaries is called oophoritis.
11. T F Ovarian cysts are typically painless as they grow larger.
12. T F Gonorrhea is the most common STD in the United States.
13. T F A rape victim's torn clothing should be placed in a plastic bag and handed over to the authorities to look for evidence.

14. T F There is some loss of elasticity of the penis and scrotum during the aging process.
15. T F It may take increased stimulation and the aid of a vaginal lubricant to enhance sexual intercourse between the older adult male and female.

CASE STUDY

You are on standby at a local college football game when one of the players goes down after a minor exchange on the field clutching his groin. Upon your arrival you find a 19-year old male who is alert and oriented and complaining of pain in his groin. He denies any other injuries and gets up and hobbles over to the ambulance with your assistance. His pain worsened with movement, but now that he is on the ambulance stretcher, the pain is present, but still moderate. Upon assessment, you notice that his left testicle is markedly higher than his right testicle and he can localize his pain to the left testicle. What do you suspect? What is your plan? What can you tell your patient about the condition you are suspecting?

BIBLIOGRAPHY

Thomas, S. H. (2000). Male genital problems in *Emergency Medicine Companion Handbook* (5th ed.). (298–299) Dallas, TX: American College of Emergency Physicians.

CHAPTER 22

Disorders Related to Labor and Delivery

CONTENT OUTLINE

- Obstetric History
- Physiology of Normal Pregnancy
  - Reproductive System
  - Cardiovascular System
  - Respiratory System
  - Musculoskeletal System
  - Gastrointestinal System
  - Renal System
- Common Disorders of Pregnancy
  - Hyperemesis Gravidarum
  - Abortion
  - Ectopic Pregnancy
  - Placenta Previa
  - Abruptio Placenta
  - Disseminated Intravascular Coagulation
  - Pregnancy-induced Hypertension (PIH)
  - Chronic Medical Problems
  - Hemolytic Diseases
  - Multiple Pregnancy
  - Substance Abuse
  - Preterm Labor
- Physiology of Normal Childbirth
  - Onset of Labor
  - Maternal Systemic Responses to Labor
  - Variables Affecting Labor
  - Stages of Labor
- Complications of Childbirth
  - Preterm Labor and Birth
  - Premature Rupture of Membranes
  - Dystocia
  - Abnormal Duration of Labor
  - Prolapsed Cord
- Postpartum Care and Complications
  - Care of the Infant
  - Care of the Mother
  - Newborn Physiologic Changes
  - Maternal Physiologic Changes
  - Postpartum Complications
- Trauma in Pregnancy

KEY TERMS

Abortion
Abruptio placenta
Bloody show
Braxton Hicks contractions
Cephalopelvic disproportion (CPD)
Crowning
Dystocia
Eclampsia
Ectopic pregnancy
Effacement
Engagement
Estimated date of confinement (EDC)
Fetal attitude
Fetal lie
Fetal presentation
Fontanelle
Fundus
Gravida
HELLP syndrome
Hyperemesis gravidarum
Incompetent cervix
Involution
Kernicterus
Macrosomia
Mastitis
Mechanisms of labor
Metritis
Miscarriage
Nuchal cord
Oophoritis
Para
Placenta previa
Precipitate labor
Precipitate birth
Preeclampsia
Presenting part
Prolapsed cord
Puerperal infection
Salpingitis
Sutures
Thrombophlebitis

LEARNING OBJECTIVES

Upon completion of the chapter, the student should be able to:

1. Describe the physiologic changes that occur throughout pregnancy.
2. Describe the pathophysiology and management of the common complications of pregnancy.
3. Describe the four stages of labor.
4. List the common fetal presentations.
5. Describe the movements that occur during delivery.
6. Describe the common complications of delivery.
7. List the five areas and scoring system that comprise the APGAR score.
8. Describe the physiologic events that occur to the infant and mother in the postpartum period.
9. Describe the pathophysiology and management of the common postpartum complications.
10. Describe the complications of trauma in pregnancy.

OVERVIEW

The pregnant female goes through a significant number of physiologic changes from the moment of conception, through gestation, during labor and delivery, and in the postpartum time period. During the amazing process of pregnancy, labor, and delivery, and postpartum these physiologic changes affect every organ system in the female. It is important for the EMS provider to understand these changes, the common complications of pregnancy and delivery, common conditions that occur in the postpartum period, and the effects of trauma in order to confidently and properly manage pregnant patients.

OBSTETRIC HISTORY

A good obstetric history can help the EMS provider anticipate problems during contact with a pregnant or laboring patient. Questions to ask the pregnant patient include:

- **Estimated date of confinement** (EDC) or due date. The normal human gestation period is 40 weeks. The due date is determined by the last menstrual period and typically confirmed by ultrasound roughly halfway through the pregnancy. The EDC can be calculated using Naegele's rule by adding nine months and seven days to the date of the last menstrual period. For example, if a woman's last menstrual period were on January 13, her EDC would be calculated as October 20.
- **Gravida** or total number of times pregnant. A primagravida is a woman who is pregnant for the first time.
- **Para** or total number of deliveries. A nulliparous woman is a woman who has never delivered a baby.
- Complications with this pregnancy, for example diabetes or hypertension.
- Complications with past pregnancies.
- Complications with past deliveries as described later in this chapter.

- History of pre-term labor or "fast" labor.

The information in an obstetric history can help the EMS provider develop a specific plan for the patient and may affect transport and treatment decisions.

PHYSIOLOGY OF NORMAL PREGNANCY

The pregnant female goes through a significant number of physiological changes which have an effect on every organ system of the woman from the moment of conception and extending for months after delivery.

Reproductive System

The reproductive system goes through significant changes from the beginning of pregnancy. Once the body senses that an egg has implanted in the uterine wall, several hormones are made to halt menstruation and support the pregnancy. One hormone in particular, hCG, may be measured in the urine or blood soon after conception and is the basis for the pregnancy test. The uterus grows significantly in size to accommodate the growing fetus. Later in pregnancy, the breasts enlarge and become swollen as they get ready for the task of breast feeding after delivery.

Cardiovascular System

The volume of blood flowing through the uterus increases dramatically throughout pregnancy. As a result of the increased needs of the reproductive organs and the baby, the mother's cardiac output increases by 30% to 40% over the pre-pregnant cardiac output. The heart rate increases 10 to 20 beats per minute and most pregnant women have an audible murmur caused by the increased blood flow through the heart. The blood pressure can also decrease up to 15 mmHg during pregnancy.

The blood volume also increases by approximately 30%, providing the mother with an extra 1–2 liters of blood volume by term. This increased blood volume provides a safety factor for blood loss during the delivery. Along with the increased blood volume, the mother also increases production of blood components, especially red blood cells. It is therefore important for the mother to obtain the necessary iron and vitamins to support blood cell production. Even with an adequate amount of iron and vitamins, many women are slightly anemic during pregnancy.

Respiratory System

The mother's metabolic rate increases during pregnancy caused by both the addition of the developing fetus and the changes occurring in her own body. This results in an increased need for oxygen and an increased production of carbon dioxide. It is estimated that the minute ventilation (see Chapter 7) increases by almost 50% to support the increased metabolic demand. As the fetus gets larger and fills the abdomen, the mechanism of respiration is altered and the mother needs to breathe at a faster rate to maintain adequate respiration.

Musculoskeletal System

As the fetus grows, the pregnant woman carries additional weight in her abdomen in front of the center of gravity. To compensate for this shift in weight, the lumbar spine flattens out and the pelvis tips. These changes place an increased strain on the postural muscles, leading to low back discomfort during pregnancy.

Relaxin, a hormone secreted by the ovaries and placenta, allows the ligaments and the pubic symphysis to relax and stretch, providing additional room for the baby to maneuver during delivery.

Gastroenterologic (GI) System

As the developing fetus grows, the abdominal contents are displaced. This leads to gastric reflux, the need to take in smaller meals, decreased GI system motility, and constipation.

Renal System

The kidneys absorb additional water during pregnancy to help increase blood volume and aid in amniotic fluid production. The weight of the growing fetus tends to sit on the bladder and the ureters as the pregnancy continues. The pregnant female has to urinate more frequently with smaller amounts of urine as the pregnancy progresses. Also, the pressure on the ureters slows the flow of urine from the kidneys, producing a backup and setting up an environment for a urinary tract infection with a rapid progression to pyelonephritis. Pyelonephritis in a pregnant woman can produce preterm labor and potentially cause permanent damage to the kidneys.

COMMON DISORDERS OF PREGNANCY

It is truly impressive that most pregnancies have no complications. For those patients who do have complications, it can be a very frightening and guilt-ridden situation. Regular prenatal care is the best way to identify patients who have high-risk factors. These patients may then be assessed and monitored more closely, and signs and symptoms of complications detected as early as possible. Many of the causes of high-risk pregnancies are given in Table 22–1.

This section covers the common complications of pregnancy including etiology and EMS management.

Hyperemesis Gravidarum

Hyperemesis gravidarum is excessive vomiting during pregnancy. The cause is unknown but may be related to an increased estrogen level, gonadotropin production, or trophoblastic activity. Psychologic factors may also be involved. The vomiting progresses to the point that the woman vomits everything swallowed. It does not subside at about 12 weeks' gestation as does "morning sickness."

Dehydration leads to fluid and electrolyte imbalance and alkalosis from the loss of hydrochloric acid. As the situation becomes worse, the patient experiences tachycardia and may have hypovolemia, hypotension, an increase in hematocrit and blood urea nitrogen (BUN), and a decrease in urine output.

The starvation situation causes protein and vitamin deficiencies. Cardiac functioning may be disrupted by severe potassium loss. Untreated, the patient may experience metabolic changes or death. Embryonic or fetal death may occur.

The management goals are to control vomiting, correct dehydration, restore electrolyte balance, and maintain adequate nutrition.

After ensuring the ABCs are patent, the EMS provider should establish an IV and follow local protocol for shock if the patient is hypovolemic. Initial fluid resuscitation in the field is often with lactated ringers or normal saline and will likely be switched at the emergency department to another solution containing glucose and added electrolytes. An antiemetic, for example promethazine, may be administered intravenously if within protocols to control the nausea. The patient should be transported to a hospital with a labor and delivery area so the fetus may be checked and mother treated.

Abortion

Abortion is the spontaneous (natural) or induced (purposeful) termination of a pregnancy before viability of the fetus. A fetus is considered viable at 24 weeks' gestation. With medical intervention, a fetus between 20 and 24 weeks' gestation may survive. Some states have defined viability as 20 to 24 weeks' gestation and a weight of 500 g.

A spontaneous abortion is often called a **miscarriage**. Spontaneous abortions may be related to chromosomal abnormalities, faulty implantation, teratogenic substances, placental abnormalities, incompetent cervix, chronic maternal diseases, maternal infections, and endocrine imbalances. Clinically, spontaneous abortions are classified as:

- Threatened: Unexplained bleeding and cramping. The cervix is closed and membranes are intact (Figure 22–1A).
- Inevitable: Increased bleeding and cramping. The cervix begins to dilate and the membranes may rupture (Figure 22–1B).
- Incomplete: Some of the products of conception are expelled. Most often the placenta is not

TABLE 22-1 Causes of High-Risk Pregnancy

General	Obstetric	Medical	Other
Age (under 15 or over 35 years)	Previous problems	Chronic diseases	Smoking
Unmarried	Abortion	Diabetes	Drug abuse
Low socioeconomic group, little education	Excessive size of infant	Hypertension	Alcohol Abuse
Prenatal care begun 27 weeks or later	Cesarean birth	Sickly cell anemia	Nutritional deficit
	Postterm birth	Thyroid disease	
	Incompetent cervix	Sexually transmitted disease	
	Abnormal fetal presentation	Cervical neoplasia	
	Rh negative and sensitized	Urinary tract infection	
	Preeclampsia	Neurologic problem	
	Multiple pregnancy	Psychiatric problem	

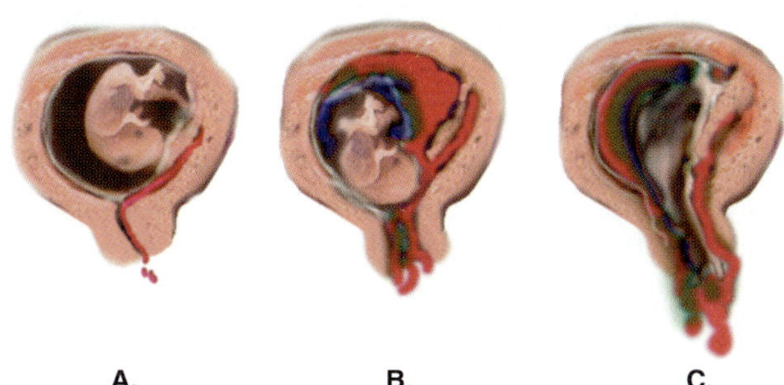

Figure 22–1 Types of spontaneous abortions: A. Threatened; B. Inevitable; C. Incomplete.

expelled. Bleeding is heavy and cramping severe (Figure 22–1C).

- Complete: All products of conception are expelled.
- Missed: Embryo or fetus dies but is retained. The cervix is closed. If the fetus is not expelled within 6 weeks, disseminated intravascular coagulation (DIC) may develop.
- Habitual: Any of the above occurring in 3 consecutive pregnancies. Most commonly, the cervix begins to dilate in the second trimester. This is called an incompetent cervix.

EMS management includes assessing the ABCs, assessing for and treating shock, and comforting the patient. Early in pregnancy, there is little that can be done to avoid the abortion, and the patient may require a surgical procedure to ensure all the products of conception have been passed.

Ectopic Pregnancy

An ectopic pregnancy occurs when a fertilized ovum implants outside the uterine cavity. The most common site is in the fallopian tube. This generally happens when the fertilized ovum is unable to move through the tube. Figure 22–2 illustrates other possible sites of implantation in an ectopic pregnancy.

More than 70,000 ectopic pregnancies occur annually in the United States. Risk factors include pelvic inflammatory disease, sexually transmitted diseases, pharmacologic treatment of infertility, and endometriosis.

The pregnancy appears normal at first with the usual signs and symptoms including the presence of hCG in the blood and urine. Symptoms of ectopic pregnancy begin gradually about 3 to 5 weeks after the first missed menstrual period. Pain is noted as the fallopian tube stretches with the growing embryo. The tube finally ruptures (a severe pain occurs) and bleeds into the peritoneal cavity. Some vaginal bleeding may be apparent. The patient may rapidly show signs of hypovolemic shock. The signs of shock are out of proportion to the apparent blood loss. Ectopic pregnancy is a significant cause of maternal morbidity and mortality, and is nearly always fatal to the embryo.

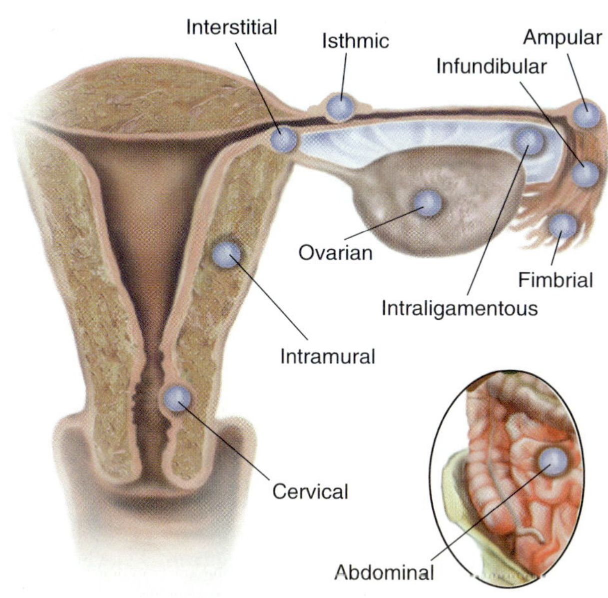

Figure 22–2 Possible sites of implantation in ectopic pregnancy.

EMS management of a suspected ectopic pregnancy includes assessing for a patent airway, adequate ventilations, and signs of shock. Treatment includes high flow oxygen and intravenous fluids for shock. Applying and inflating the MAST suit may help to tamponade the bleeding, although the use of the MAST suit in this particular situation has not been well studied. Definitive treatment generally involves a surgical procedure to remove the ectopic pregnancy. This may sometimes disrupt the ability for the affected fallopian tube to function properly after the surgery, affecting the woman's fertility. As the complications of a ruptured ectopic pregnancy may threaten the patient's life, the EMS provider should suspect an ectopic pregnancy for any woman of childbearing age that presents to EMS with abdominal pain.

Placenta Previa

Placenta previa occurs when implantation is in the lower uterine segment with the placenta lying over or very near the internal cervical os (Figure 22–3). The cause is unknown, but predisposing factors may be multiparity, uterine scarring from D & C or cesarean birth, or uterine infections.

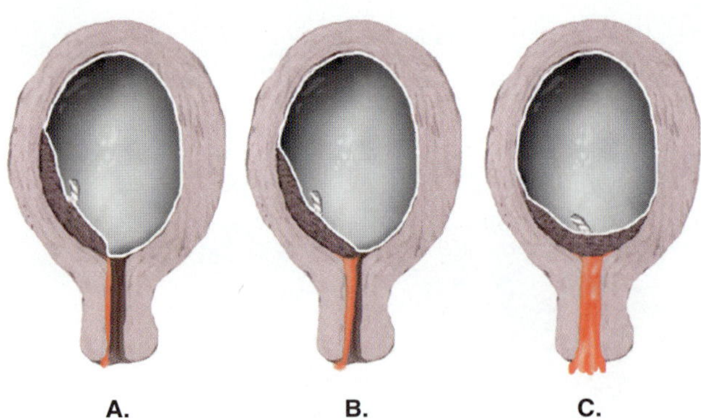

Figure 22–3 Placenta previa: A. Low implantation (marginal); B. Partial placenta previa; C. Total placenta previa.

The classic symptom is **painless bleeding** in the last half of pregnancy. There may be occasional bright red spotting or intermittent gushes of blood. Rarely is bleeding continuous. The uterus is relaxed and not tender. Bleeding is unrelated to maternal activity. Placenta previa is classified in three ways:

- Low-lying or marginal: Placenta is near the internal cervical os but does not cover any part of opening.
- Partial: Placenta covers part of internal cervical os opening.
- Complete or total: Placenta completely covers internal cervical os opening.

Toward the last part of pregnancy, the cervix effaces (thins). This movement of the cervix pulls away from the placenta, and the exposed placental sinuses begin to bleed. The earlier this happens the more serious the situation.

The gestational age of the fetus and the amount of bleeding determine the effects on the fetus/neonate. During profuse bleeding the fetus may suffer from hypoxia. After delivery, the neonate should be checked to see if the bleeding resulted in anemia.

Field management of a patient with a placenta previa is similar to that of a patient in normal labor, except vaginal birth is contraindicated because of the extreme blood loss and significant potential for maternal and fetal death. Women with a known previa are normally scheduled for a cesarean birth two to three weeks prior to the due date so as not to allow the patient to begin labor. If the woman does begin labor, she is instructed to meet her physician at the hospital so that either a cesarean delivery may be performed or the labor halted. Sometimes rehydrating the woman will stop labor that began because of slight dehydration. Most of the time, however, the patient will require a tocolytic (labor stopping) medication to cease labor. In the event a patient with a placenta previa is delivering in the field vaginally, one should be prepared for significant blood loss for both the mother and the baby and rapidly transport both patients to the closest facility.

Abruptio Placenta

The premature separation from the wall of the uterus of a normally implanted placenta is called **abruptio placenta**. It occurs spontaneously after the 20th week of gestation in one out of 75 to 90 pregnancies. The cause is unknown. Contributing factors may include: maternal hypertension, multiple pregnancy, smoking, use of alcohol, or use of cocaine. Generally, it occurs late in pregnancy or during labor. There are three types of abruptio placenta (Figure 22–4).

- Central: Center of the placenta separates with blood trapped between placenta and uterine wall; there is no apparent bleeding.
- Marginal: Edge of placenta separates and bright red bleeding is apparent vaginally.
- Complete: Entire placenta separates with profuse bleeding apparent vaginally.

A central abruption may progress to a complete abruption. In central and complete, blood invades the uterine muscle causing a rigid, painful abdomen. After delivery the uterus contracts poorly and the patient may require a hysterectomy to control the bleeding. The damage to the uterine muscle and the retroplacental clotting may cause a large release of clotting factors that can trig-

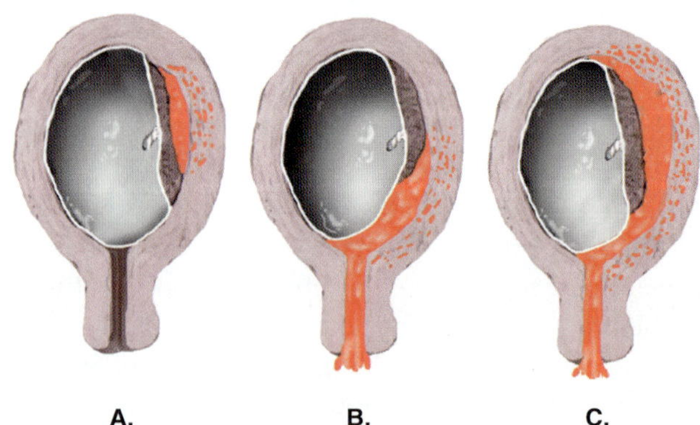

Figure 22–4 Abruptio placenta: A. Central abruption, concealed hemorrhage; B. Marginal abruption, external hemorrhage; C. Complete abruption, external hemorrhage (could also be concealed).

ger the development of disseminated intravascular coagulation (DIC). Maternal mortality is relatively low. Problems after the delivery depend on the severity of the bleeding. Table 22–2 compares placenta previa and the various types of abruptio placenta.

Perinatal mortality is about one-third of the cases of abruptio placenta. The outcome depends on fetal maturity and severity of the abruption. Preterm labor, hypoxia, and anemia are the most serious complications. Irreversible brain damage or fetal death may occur if hypoxia is not reversed quickly.

EMS management of a patient who is suspected to be abrupting includes maintaining the ABCs with high flow oxygen, airway management and ventilation as required, fluid replacement, and rapid transport to the closest facility. If the abruption is small and the patient is near term, the patient may be induced and normal labor and delivery accomplished. Most often, a cesarean delivery is required to save the baby and the mother.

Disseminated Intravascular Coagulation

Disseminated intravascular coagulation (DIC) is an overstimulation of the normal clotting process and occurs as a complication of a primary problem. Obstetrical problems that may precipitate DIC include: abruptio placenta, placenta previa, PIH, retained products of conception, amniotic fluid embolism, and infections. The primary problem may require immediate delivery of the fetus, even if preterm. The fetus may experience hypoxia to varying degrees. Fetal death can occur. The pathophysiology and management of DIC are discussed in Chapter 16.

Pregnancy-Induced Hypertension

Pregnancy-induced hypertension (PIH), the most common hypertensive disorder in pregnancy, appears after 20 weeks' gestation. The classic symptoms are hypertension, edema, and proteinuria. It is seen most often in primigravidas, especially those under 20 or over 35 years of age, who are in a lower socioeconomic group and have poor nutritional status. Diabetes, multiple pregnancy, or a family history of PIH also increase a patient's risk.

Peripheral arteriole vasoconstriction and vasospasm lead to increased blood pressure and decreased perfusion of the uterus and placenta. Renal blood flow is lowered, and protein spills into the urine. Cerebral edema causes headaches and visual disturbances. Deep tendon reflexes become hyperactive. The liver enlarges, putting pressure on the liver capsule which causes epigastric pain. The condition may progress to **eclampsia**, or convulsions.

Despite decades of research, the cause remains unknown. It was previously called *toxemia* because it was thought that a toxin was produced in a pregnant woman's body. This term is no longer used. The only cure is delivery of the baby. PIH is a progressive condition developing from mild to severe **preeclampsia** to eclampsia and HELLP syndrome.

Abruptio placenta and placental infarction may occur. Intrauterine growth retardation (IUGR) may occur as well as acute hypoxia and intrauterine death. A preterm infant may be born either because of spontaneous labor or obstetrical intervention.

Mild Preeclampsia. In mild preeclampsia the blood pressure increases 30 mmHg systolic *or* 15 mmHg diastolic over the patient's baseline blood pressure on two occasions at least 6 hours apart, or a BP of 140/90 is noted. For example, a patient with a baseline BP of 92/64 would be considered hypertensive at 122/80. Thus, it is very important to have a baseline BP early in pregnancy.

Edema may be noted in the face and hands. It is objectively defined as weight gain of more than 1 pound a week.

Urine may show 1+ or 2+ albumin on a dipstick or 300 mg/l in 24 hours. Proteinuria is usually the last of the three classic symptoms to appear.

TABLE 22-2 Comparison of Placenta Previa and Abruptio Placenta

Condition	Bleeding	Abdomen	Pain	BP
Placenta Previa	Bright red	No rigidity	None	Depends on amount of bleeding
Abruptio Placenta				
Central	None	Rigid	Acute	Decreased
Marginal	Dark red	No rigidity	Uterine tenderness	Decreased
Complete	Profuse	Acute	Rigid	Shock

Severe Preeclampsia. Blood pressure increases to 160/110 or higher on two occasions 6 hours apart in severe preeclampsia. Generalized edema is easily noted in the face, hands, sacral area, lower extremities, and abdomen. Weight gain may be 2 pounds in a few days to a week.

Urinary protein is high and urine output may drop. The patient may exhibit other symptoms such as: continuous headache, blurred vision, scotomata (spots before the eyes), nausea, vomiting, irritability, hyperreflexia, cerebral disturbances, pulmonary edema, dyspnea, cyanosis, and epigastric pain. Epigastric pain is often the last symptom identified before the patient moves into eclampsia.

Eclampsia. The grand mal seizure experienced by the patient has a tonic phase (pronounced muscular contractions) and a clonic phase (alternate contraction and relaxation of muscles). Then the patient slips into a coma lasting from minutes to hours. With no treatment, the seizure/coma sequence may be repeated one or more times and death may follow.

Seizure activity may trigger uterine contractions, but the patient in a coma is unaware of them and unable to let anyone know.

HELLP Syndrome. HELLP syndrome is PIH with liver damage. It is characterized by **h**emolysis, **e**levated **l**iver enzymes, and **l**ow **p**latelet count.

- Hemolysis is caused when intra-arterial lesions develop from vasospasm, causing platelets to congregate. The RBCs are forced through the smaller vessels and break apart.
- Elevated liver enzymes may be caused by microemboli in the vessels of the liver, resulting in ischemia.
- Low platelet count occurs when the platelets are entrapped at the intra-arterial lesions.

The result of this syndrome is ischemia and tissue damage. The patient may also show signs of hypoglycemia. A blood sugar of less than 40 mg/dl is often associated with maternal mortality.

The goals for treatment of PIH involve lowering the blood pressure and reducing patient stimulation. Once the ABCs are patent, and IV access is obtained, the patient may be quietly transported lying in a left lateral recumbant position to reduce stimulation and decrease the patient's blood pressure. Magnesium sulfate is commonly administered to patients with severe PIH to help prevent them from progressing to eclampsia. The side effects of magnesium administration include respiratory depression and a decrease in the patient's reflexes. Medical control may order an antihypertensive medication

Chronic Medical Problems

Conditions in this group include diabetes mellitus, chronic hypertension, and heart disease.

Diabetes Mellitus. Diabetic patients who wish to become pregnant should have their diabetes well under control before conception.

Gestational diabetes mellitus (GDM) is an abnormal glucose metabolism that appears only during pregnancy. Many women with GDM will have diabetes later in life. Whether the mother has chronic diabetes or GDM, the effects during pregnancy are the same.

Pregnancy and Carbohydrate Metabolism. Insulin production is increased in early pregnancy by the stimulation of the mother's pancreas by the increased levels of estrogen, progesterone, and other hormones. The tissue response to insulin is also increased along with increased storage of glycogen in the liver and muscles. An increased resistance to insulin develops in the last half of pregnancy caused by several factors. This effect of pregnancy occurs after about 20 weeks' gestation. Glucose from the mother provides the growing fetus with energy, thus putting stress on the balance of glucose production and utilization. Diabetes already present is more difficult to control. In a case where the pancreas has little insulin reserve, gestational diabetes occurs.

Effects of Pregnancy on Diabetes. The insulin requirements change throughout pregnancy. The need for insulin may decrease during the first trimester. The risk of hypoglycemia or hyperinsulinemia is increased if nausea and vomiting are present. Placental maturation and the increasing production of hPL cause the insulin requirements to rise during the second trimester, and they may be 4 times higher by the end of pregnancy. After the placenta is passed, removing the source of hPL, there is generally an immediate decrease in the amount of insulin required.

There is a physiological decrease in the renal threshold for glucose. The risk of ketoacidosis is greater during pregnancy, as is an acceleration of vascular disease.

Effects of Diabetes on Pregnancy. Pregnancy in a diabetic patient has a higher risk of complications than for a non-diabetic patient. If vascular changes already exist, the chance for PIH is greater.

Hydramnios, an excessive amount of amniotic fluid, may occur. This may lead to preterm labor or premature rupture of the membranes.

Hyperglycemia may result in ketoacidosis caused by increased fat metabolism. Often, ketoacidosis develops slowly, but may result in maternal and fetal death if untreated. Maternal complications are directly related to the degree of blood glucose control.

Effects on the Fetus/Neonate. **Macrosomia**, excessive fetal growth, results from maternal hyperglycemia. The hyperglycemia stimulates fetal insulin production to utilize the available glucose. After birth, there is no more maternal glucose, but the fetal pancreas continues to produce a high level of insulin. In 2 to 4 hours the neonate is hypoglycemic. Fetal insulin production gradually decreases to an appropriate level.

Intrauterine growth retardation (IUGR) may result when the mother has vascular changes. Vascular changes also occur in the placenta. This decreases perfusion of the placenta and the fetus does not receive adequate amounts of nutrients.

A high fetal insulin level inhibits the production of surfactant in the lungs, making the possibility of respiratory distress syndrome very high. The decreased ability of maternal glycosylated hemoglobin (hemoglobin with glucose attached) to release oxygen causes the fetus to have polycythemia (excessive number of red blood cells). The polycythemia is a direct cause of hyperbilirubinemia as the immature liver is unable to metabolize the increased amount of bilirubin.

Congenital anomalies are several times higher in diabetic pregnancies and may be caused by hyperglycemia in early pregnancy. Many anomalies involve the heart, central nervous system, and skeletal system.

Women with gestational diabetes may present to EMS for a variety of reasons, from DKA to labor. The EMS provider should treat the signs and symptoms similar to those signs and symptoms in a non-pregnant patient. If the patient is in labor, the EMS provider should understand that the baby will tend to be significantly larger and complications with delivery more frequent. Transportation to an appropriate facility before delivery will allow better management of delivery complications. Infants delivered from a mother with gestational diabetes will often become hypoglycemic during the first few hours of life and may appear to be listless or seizing. Management involves assessing blood glucose and administering the appropriate amount of glucose based upon the infant's weight. Unless transport times are significant, this problem typically does not present in the field.

Chronic Hypertension. A BP 140/90 or higher before pregnancy or before the 20th week of gestation that lasts longer than 6 weeks after delivery is termed chronic hypertension. A diastolic pressure of more than 80 mmHg in the second trimester may indicate chronic hypertension.

A patient with untreated or poorly controlled hypertension may show signs of hypertensive vascular disease such as arteriosclerosis and retinal hemorrhage. Renal disease may be present. The placenta may have infarcts, and placenta abruptio may occur. A placenta with infarcts has reduced perfusion. This may cause IUGR and fetal hypoxia.

Patients who have moderate to severe chronic hypertension are most at risk to develop PIH. In these women PIH develops rapidly and moves to a crisis state faster than in women without chronic hypertension. More stillbirths, abruptio placenta, and severe renal failure are found in patients with chronic hypertension. Any of the classic signs indicate PIH. These patients are often hospitalized.

As with diabetes, the pregnant woman with a history of chronic hypertension may present to EMS for a variety of reasons. The EMS provider should understand that PIH is more common in women who have chronic hypertension and that the progression from PIH to eclampsia may occur more rapidly than in patients who do not have chronic hypertension.

Heart Disease. The normal physiological increase in blood volume that peaks about 28 to 32 weeks' gestation, and the increased cardiac output and heart rate, may cause problems in the patient with heart disease. The heart compensates at first by tachycardia, and ventricular dilation and hypertrophy. When these mechanisms fail, the heart is no longer able to compensate and congestive heart failure occurs.

The results of having had rheumatic fever often restrict cardiac output and cause pulmonary congestion. The effects of congenital heart disease on pregnancy depend on the specific defect. Hypertension may cause cardiac insufficiency.

Hemolytic Diseases

There are two types of hemolytic diseases: Rh incompatibility and ABO incompatibility. Rh incompatibility may be very devastating to the fetus, but it may be prevented. ABO incompatibility is naturally occurring and much less severe, but cannot be prevented.

Rh Incompatibility. Rh incompatibility can happen only when the mother is Rh negative and the fetus is Rh positive. That is, the mother does not have the Rh factor and the fetus does have the Rh factor (see Chapter 16). In this case, the father must be Rh positive for the fetus to be Rh positive. If the father is Rh negative, there is no problem because the fetus will also be Rh negative.

The placenta keeps the mother's blood and the fetus's blood separated. In cases of ectopic pregnancy, abortion, infection of the placenta, abruptio placenta, birth, or at the time of placental separation, small tears may occur in the placenta and fetal blood may enter maternal circulation. The mother is then sensitized by the fetal Rh positive blood. She may also be sensitized by having a transfusion of Rh positive blood, even the smallest amount.

Fetal (Rh positive) blood in maternal (Rh negative) circulation stimulates maternal production of Rh antibodies. The Rh antibodies, like many other antibodies, pass through the placenta and destroy fetal red blood cells (Figure 22–5). Since this usually occurs at the time of birth, the first infant is usually not affected.

If a tear occurred and there was no treatment, the next Rh positive fetus will have red blood cells destroyed by the maternal Rh antibodies. This causes anemia which in turn causes fetal edema (hydrops fetalis). The next step is congestive heart failure and severe jaundice. Severe jaundice may cause neurologic damage called **kernicterus**.

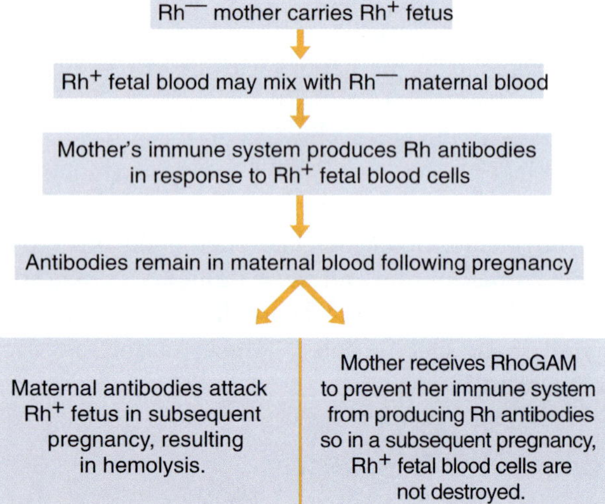

Figure 22–5 Rh sensitization and prevention.

This entire syndrome, the most severe of the two hemolytic diseases of the newborn, is called erythroblastosis fetalis.

At birth, the fetus' and mother's blood are tested and, if they have different Rh factors, the mother is given an intramuscular injection of RhoGAM, an immunoglobulin that binds to the antibodies created in the mother's blood against the fetus' red blood cells. This protects subsequent babies from the maternal antibodies. The mother must receive the RhoGAM with every pregnancy to prevent fetal complications.

ABO Incompatibility. In ABO incompatibility, the way in which a tear in the placenta may occur and fetal and maternal blood mix is the same as for Rh incompatibility. In this situation the problem occurs when maternal blood enters fetal circulation. Possible combinations for ABO incompatibility are given in Table 22–3. The most common type of ABO incompatibility occurs when the mother is type O and the fetus is either type A, B, or AB. The mother's plasma naturally contains anti-A and anti-B antibodies. These antibodies have a weaker hemolytic effect than Rh antibodies and only affect mature RBCs. The number of antibodies is limited to the amount of maternal blood that entered fetal circulation. There is not a continuous supply of antibodies. Since ABO incompatibility is naturally occurring, it may affect the fetus of the first pregnancy. The affected newborn will become jaundiced in the first 3 days of life.

Multiple Pregnancy

The first trimester proceeds much the same in a multiple pregnancy as with a single fetus except that maternal blood volume has a greater increase. Some women have more severe nausea and vomiting, as well as shortness of breath on exertion, dyspnea, and backache.

As the uterus grows, there is greater pressure on and displacement of the internal organs. Pressure on the ureters favors urinary infection. Digestive problems and constipation may be more disturbing, dependent edema

TABLE 22-3 Possible Combinations for ABO Incompatibility

Mother	Fetus
A	B
B	A
O	A, B, AB

more marked, and varicose veins more prominent. PIH is more frequent than with a single fetus.

Each fetus may have a decreased intrauterine growth rate (low birth weight). There is a greater risk of fetal anomalies, abnormal presentations, and preterm birth. Perinatal mortality is much greater for twins than for a single fetus.

Delivery in the woman who has a multiple pregnancy may be very complicated as at least one of the infants typically has a breech presentation (discussed later in this chapter). Labor often begins early, and there may be neonatal complications associated with premature births. If possible, the EMS provider should attempt to transport the patient to the nearest appropriate facility with enough resources to handle multiple pregnancy.

Substance Abuse

Drugs commonly abused include alcohol, cocaine, crack, marijuana, and heroin. The use of any of these substances is a threat to pregnancy. Substance abusers may not seek prenatal care, or seek prenatal care very late in pregnancy. Most substance abusers do not voluntarily admit their addiction. These mothers may have an increased rate of PIH, abruptio placenta, poor nutrition, and sexually transmitted diseases. They often use available money for the drug habit instead of food.

Alcohol may result in fetal alcohol syndrome, which manifests as both physical and mental abnormalities. Cocaine/crack increases the risk for IUGR, short body length, small head circumference, preterm birth, irritability, and low Apgar scores (an assessment of infant at 1 and 5 minutes after birth). Marijuana causes fine tremors and irritability. Heroin increases the risk for IUGR, hypoxia, preterm birth, irritability, and meconium aspiration.

Preterm Labor

Preterm labor is labor that begins after viability but before 38 weeks' gestation. The causes of preterm labor may be maternal, fetal, or placental. Maternal factors that may cause preterm labor include: PIH, diabetes, heart or renal disease, an incompetent cervix, premature rupture of membranes, and maternal infection. Fetal factors include: fetal infection, multiple pregnancy, and hydramnios. Placental factors are placenta previa and abruptio placenta.

Preterm labor may produce a neonate not able to cope well with extrauterine life.

The lungs are the last organ system to mature in the fetus, with most lungs maturing about 34 to 36 weeks' gestation. The maturity may be affected by a number of factors including IUGR and gestational diabetes. Premature infants may require aggressive airway management. Women who are in premature labor often receive a steroid to help the lungs mature.

PHYSIOLOGY OF NORMAL CHILDBIRTH

The process of labor and delivery has been occurring for thousands of years before the advent of monitors and prenatal care. Fortunately, in today's society, most of the time labor and delivery are uncomplicated events thanks to prenatal screening and care.

Onset of Labor

For 38 to 40 weeks the pregnancy has been advancing and the fetus developing. Now, as the fetus reaches maturity, the birth process begins. Researchers are still trying to determine exactly what causes the onset of labor. However, there are two theories relative to why labor begins.

The mechanical theory is based on the principle that as a hollow organ in the body becomes filled and distended, the organ tends to empty itself. Examples of this phenomenon are the bladder and sigmoid colon. This mechanism alone is not enough to fully explain the onset of labor since a woman can have a full-term 6½ lb baby with one pregnancy and full-term twins each weighing 5½ lb with the next pregnancy.

The hormonal theory of the onset of labor relates to the changes in maternal progesterone and estrogen levels, the maternal production of oxytocin and prostaglandin, and the increase in fetal production of cortisol. There seems to be a highly integrated relationship among these hormones.

As the pregnancy nears its end, the placental production of progesterone decreases, thus decreasing the relaxing effect of progesterone on the uterus. The estrogen level rises, causing an increased sensitivity of the myometrium to oxytocin. Oxytocin stimulates the uterus to contract. As the pregnancy nears 40 weeks of gestation, the uterus becomes more sensitive to oxytocin. Fetal cortisol production increases as the pregnancy nears term. It is believed to decrease the placental production of progesterone and stimulate the precursors of prostaglandin.

Signs of Impending Labor. There are several signs that indicate labor will soon begin. The signs are lightening, Braxton Hicks contractions, cervical softening, bloody show, rupture of membranes, and a sudden burst of energy.

Lightening is the descent of the fetus into the pelvis. This may occur as early as 2 weeks before labor begins in the primigravida patient but may not occur until a multigravida patient is already in labor. The downward movement of the fetus and thus the uterus makes the upper part of the abdomen flatter. This relieves pressure on the diaphragm, allowing the mother to breathe easier, but she may experience:

- Leg cramps from pressure now on pelvic nerves,
- Urinary frequency from pressure now on the bladder, and
- Increased venous stasis from pressure now on the veins, resulting in edema of the lower extremities.

Braxton Hicks contractions are irregular, intermittent contractions felt by the pregnant woman toward the end of pregnancy. The tightening sensation in the abdomen may become fairly regular and uncomfortable. The woman may go to the care provider's office or the hospital thinking she is in labor. If the cervix is not dilated and then the contractions stop, this is called false labor. Table 22–4 compares false labor and true labor.

At about 34 weeks of gestation, because of the changing ratio of estrogen to progesterone and the production of prostaglandin, the cervix begins to "mature" or "ripen." That is, the cervix becomes softer and more spongy. **Effacement**, thinning of the cervix, may begin, especially when the woman is a primigravida. These cervical changes increase during labor to allow delivery of the fetus.

Bloody show consists of cervical secretion, blood-tinged mucus, and the mucous plug that blocked the cervix during pregnancy. Labor often begins within 24 to 48 hours after the bloody show is noticed. However, a recent vaginal examination that includes cervical manipulation may result in a blood-tinged discharge. This may be confused with bloody show.

Rupture of membranes (ROM) usually occurs after labor has begun. However, in about 12% of women, the amniotic membranes rupture before the onset of labor. When this occurs, the pregnant woman should notify her physician and proceed to the birthing facility. If **engagement** (when the widest diameter of the fetal presenting part [head] enters the inlet to the true pelvis) has not yet occurred, there exists the danger that the umbilical cord will wash out with the amniotic fluid (prolapsed cord).

If labor does not begin spontaneously within 12 to 24 hours after the membranes rupture and the pregnancy is near term, labor is often induced to avoid infection.

It is sometimes difficult for the woman to determine whether the membranes have ruptured or whether urine has escaped from her bladder. A simple test may be performed in the physician's office or labor and delivery.

A few days before labor begins, some women will have a sudden burst of energy. The reason for this is unknown. The prospective mother should be careful not to tire herself. She will need the energy when labor begins.

Maternal Systemic Responses to Labor

Just as physiologic changes occur in the woman from the beginning of pregnancy, changes occur in response to labor.

TABLE 22-4 Comparison of False Labor and True Labor

False Labor	True Labor
Contractions often irregular but may be regular for a short time (1 to 2 hours).	Contractions occur at regular intervals.
Interval between contractions stays the same.	Interval between contractions gradually shortens.
Contraction intensity and duration remain the same.	Contractions increase in intensity and duration.
Contractions frequently stop when the client ambulates or changes position.	Contractions continue and often become stronger when the client ambulates.
Contractions eventually cease with controlled breathing or other relaxation techniques.	Contractions are usually not stopped with controlled breathing, other relaxation techniques, or sedation.
Cervix may soften but does not efface or dilate.	Cervix softens, effaces, and dilates.

Cardiovascular System. Cardiac output increases because 400 mL of blood is squeezed from the uterus into maternal circulation with each contraction. The patient's blood pressure increases during the first and second stages of labor because of the contractions. Blood pressure is highest during a contraction, so blood pressure should be taken *between* contractions. Anxiety and pain may also make the blood pressure increase. About 10% to 15% of women in labor will experience supine hypotensive syndrome, or decreased blood pressure when in a supine position.

Respiratory System. Oxygen consumption during labor is equal to that of moderate to strenuous exercise. As long as the respiratory center is not depressed by medication, the increased respiratory rate continues with oxygen consumption almost double the normal amount. If the mother develops hypoxia or acidosis, the fetus may be compromised. Hyperventilation may decrease the level of carbon dioxide in the mother's blood.

Renal System. When engagement occurs, the bladder, now an abdominal organ, is pushed forward and upward. A distended bladder may impede fetal descent. Pressure from the presenting part, especially during a contraction, may cause edema of the tissues because of impaired blood and lymph drainage. Urinary flow is decreased, especially when the woman is supine, because the uterus compresses the ureters. Often there is a lessened urge to void, so the patient must be encouraged to do so.

Gastrointestinal System. During labor, peristalsis and absorption decrease. Gastric emptying time is prolonged and gastric contents increase in acidity. The staff in many hospitals do not allow the patient in labor to eat solid food because there is always a possibility of an obstetrical emergency requiring surgery. Eating solid food would increase the risk of aspirating vomitus. The absorption of liquid is unchanged during labor. The lips and mouth become dry as a result of mouth breathing.

Fluid and Electrolyte Balance. Because of the muscular activity of labor, the mother's body temperature increases and she perspires profusely. The normal increase in respiratory rate and the tendency of women in labor to hyperventilate both cause an increase in fluid loss. The hyperventilation also affects electrolyte balance. To prevent dehydration, the staff in many hospitals routinely have intravenous fluids running on all patients in labor.

Immune System. The white blood count (WBC) increases, sometimes up to 25,000/mm3, during labor and stays elevated during the early postpartum period. The natural increase makes it difficult to identify any infectious process the woman may have.

Integumentary System. The vagina and perineum have a great ability to stretch. The degree of stretching varies with each patient. However, there may still be minute tears in the vagina and/or perineum after the birth of the baby.

Musculoskeletal System. The marked increase in muscle activity during labor is accompanied by increased body temperature, diaphoresis, and fatigue. The relaxation of pelvic joints, caused by the influence of relaxin, may result in backache. Leg cramps also may be experienced.

Neurological System. The patient may be euphoric at the beginning of labor. This often changes to seriousness and then to amnesia between contractions during the second stage of labor. Endogenous endorphins (a morphinelike chemical produced naturally by the body) increase the patient's pain threshold and have a sedative effect. Pressure on the perineum, by the fetus descending through the birth canal, causes physiologic anesthesia in the perineal tissues.

The discomfort and pain of labor and birth are individual, subjective, very personal, and have a wide range of expression. Visceral pain usually predominates the first stage of labor, with the stimuli originating in the uterus, cervix, adnexa, and pelvic ligaments. With fetal descent increasing during the late first stage and beginning second stage of labor, the traction and distention on the pelvic structures around the vagina are the primary stimuli for pain. The distention of the perineum is the stimulus for pain during the remainder of the second stage of labor and is transmitted primarily by the pudendal nerves. Figure 22–6 illustrates the intensity and distribution of discomfort during various stages of labor. Stages of labor are discussed later in this chapter.

The softness of pelvic tissues in parous women (women who have delivered at least one child) seems to cause less painful stimuli than in nulliparous women (women who have never delivered a child) during the first stage of labor. However, during the second stage of labor, parous women have increased painful stimuli because of the speed and intensity of fetal descent.

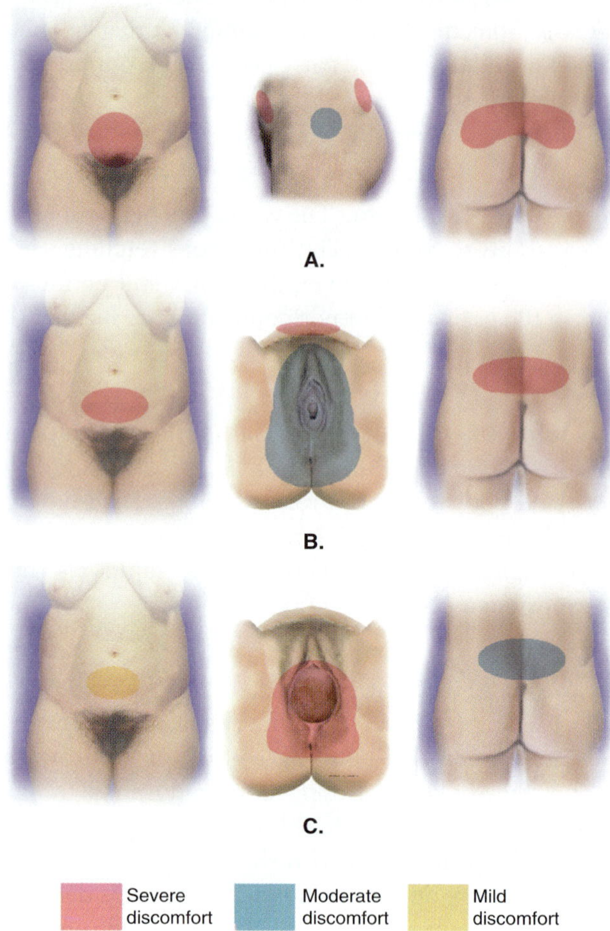

Figure 22–6 Intensity and distribution of discomfort during various stages of labor: A. First stage; B. Early second stage; C. Late second stage and birth.

Variables Affecting Labor

There are four major variables that affect labor: passage, passenger, powers, and psyche.

Passage. The passage consists of the bony pelvis, uterus, cervix, vagina, and perineum.

The size and shape of the true pelvis must be adequate for the fetal head to pass through for a vaginal birth.

The upper part of the uterus (fundus) becomes thicker with contractions and the lower section becomes thinner, forming a tube.

The uterine contractions put pressure on the fetus, which in turn puts pressure on the cervix, causing the cervix to efface and dilate.

The vagina sustains many changes throughout pregnancy. Various hormones cause an increase in vascularity, loosening of connective tissue, and hypertrophy of the smooth muscle cells. These changes allow the vagina to stretch enough for the fetus to pass through.

The pressure of the fetus on the perineum causes stretching and thinning of the perineum.

Passenger. The size of the fetus as well as the fetal attitude, fetal lie, fetal presentation, and fetal position affect how easily the fetus can advance through the passage.

The largest part of the fetal body is usually the head. Because the bones of the fetal skull are not fused, the bones can move and even overlap, as the fetus moves through the mother's bony pelvis. The shaping of the fetal head to adapt to the mother's pelvis during labor is called molding.

The major bones of the skull are two frontal bones, two temporal bones, two parietal bones, and the occiput. The bones are joined by thin, fibrous, membrane-covered spaces called **sutures**. Where the sutures meet, there are larger membranous areas called **fontanelles** (Figure 22–7). The largest is the diamond shaped anterior fontanelle. The posterior fontanelle is triangular and smaller. The two fontanelles and the suture connecting them can be palpated through the cervix to determine fetal position.

Fetal attitude is the relationship of fetal body parts to one another. The ideal attitude of the fetus at term is flexion, with the head flexed onto the chest, the arms flexed over the chest, and the hips and knees flexed on the abdomen. If any part of the fetus is extended, especially the head or the legs, labor is usually more difficult. The attitude is then called extension.

The relationship of the cephalocaudal (head to foot) axis of the fetus to the cephalocaudal axis of the mother is called the **fetal lie**. When the fetal cephalocaudal axis is parallel to the mother's, it is called a longitudinal lie. At term, the fetus has a longitudinal lie in 99% of pregnancies. When the fetal cephalocaudal axis is at a right angle to the mother's, it is called a transverse lie (Figure 22–8).

Fetal presentation is determined by the fetal lie and the part of the fetus that enters the pelvis first. The part of the fetus in contact with the cervix is called the **presenting part**. The most common type of presentation is cephalic (head), in 95% of deliveries, with breech (buttocks) being 4%, and shoulder 1% of deliveries (Figure 22–9).

Cephalic presentations may be further differentiated by the part of the head entering the pelvis first. They may be:

- Vertex—with the occiput as the presenting part,

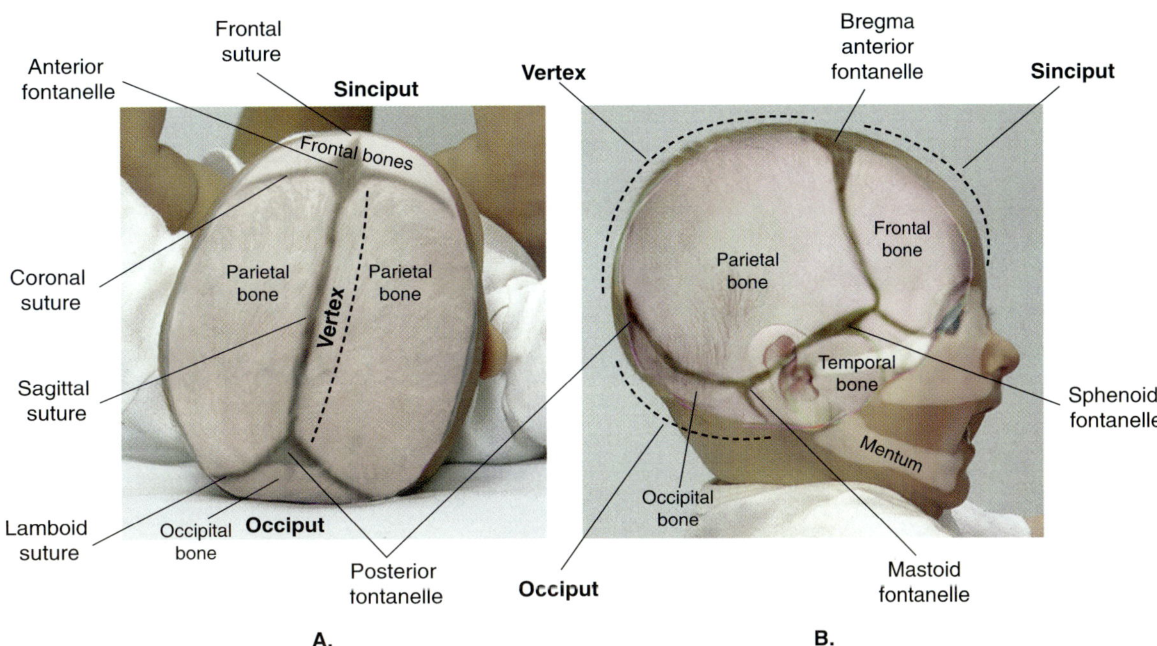

Figure 22-7 Fetal skull—sutures and fontanelles: A. top view; B. side view.

- Brow—with the sinciput as the presenting part, or
- Face—with the face as the presenting part.

Breech presentations are differentiated by the attitude of the fetus's legs. The various breech presentations are as follows:

- Complete breech: Hips and knees are flexed on the abdomen in an attitude of flexion, with the buttocks as the presenting part.
- Frank breech: The hips are flexed, but the knees are extended with the buttocks as the presenting part.
- Footling breech: The hips and knees are extended with the foot as the presenting part (may be single footling or double footling).

A shoulder presentation occurs in a transverse lie. The presenting part is usually the shoulder but may be the arm, back, abdomen, or side.

Fetal position refers to the relationship of the identified landmark on the presenting part to the four quadrants of the mother's pelvis (Figure 22–10). The identified landmarks on various presenting parts are shown in Table 22–5.

The brow presentation does not have an identified landmark. The brow usually changes either to a vertex or face presentation. Because the shoulder presentation cannot be delivered vaginally, a landmark to designate position is of no value.

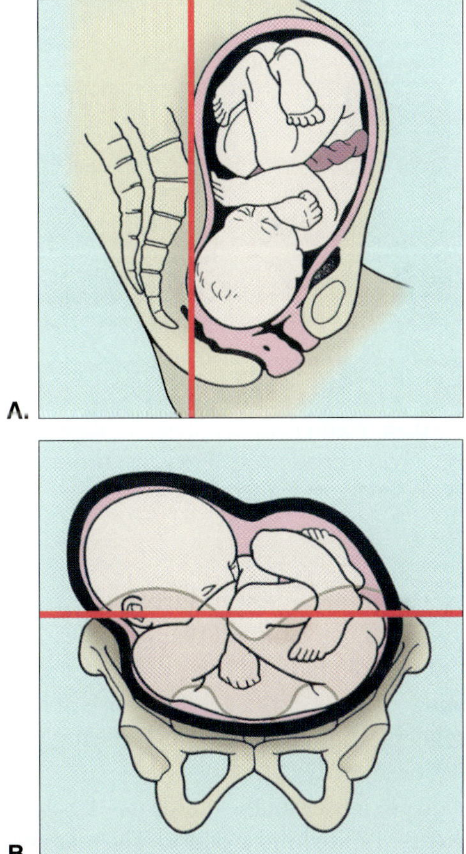

Figure 22-8 Fetal attitude and fetal lie: A. Fetal attitude flexion, fetal lie longitudinal; B. Fetal attitude flexion, fetal lie transverse.

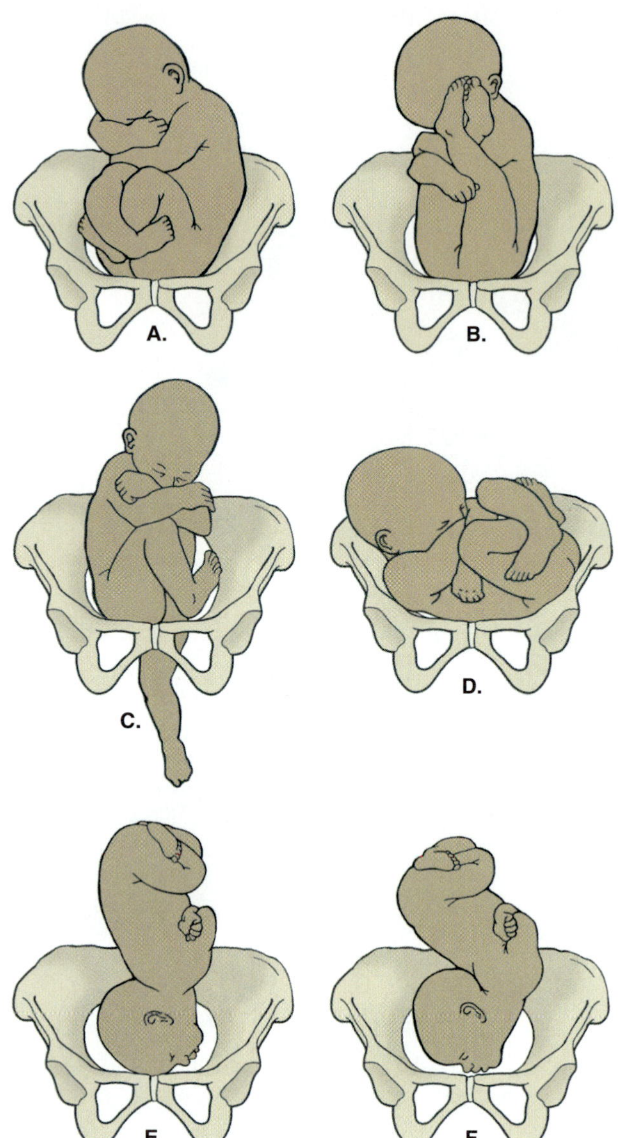

Figure 22–9 Fetal presentation: A. Complete breech; B. Frank breech; C. Footling breech; D. Shoulder; E. Brow; F. Face.

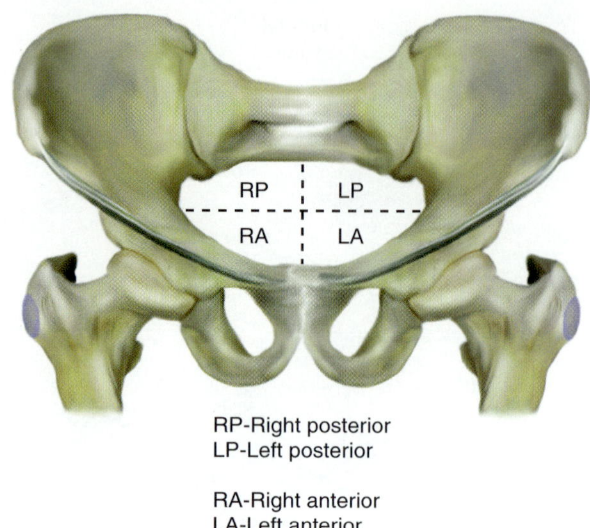

Figure 22–10 Pelvic quadrants.

TABLE 22-5 Identified Landmarks on Various Presenting Parts

Presenting Part	Identified Landmark
Vertex	Occiput (O)
Face	Mentum (M)
Breech (all)	Sacrum (S)

Powers. The primary power during labor is the involuntary contractions of the uterus, which cause cervical effacement and dilatation during the first stage of labor. The secondary power is the voluntary use of the abdominal muscles by the mother to push during the second stage of labor.

The smooth muscle of the uterus has the ability to contract and relax in a rhythmic manner. The relaxation period between contractions allows the muscles and the mother to rest. Uterine relaxation also restores uteroplacental circulation, which is important to fetal oxygenation and effective circulation in the uterus. Contractions begin in the **fundus**, top of the uterus, and spread over the uterus in about 15 seconds.

The muscle fibers of the uterus have the unique property of remaining permanently shortened to a small degree after each contraction. The shortening of the muscle fibers results in a gradual decrease in the uterine cavity size and a thickening of the muscle in the fundus. As the muscle fibers in the fundus retract, the lower uterine segment is pulled up. These two actions efface and dilate the cervix (Figure 22–11).

Each contraction has three phases:

1. Increment: increasing intensity of a contraction (the longest phase)
2. Acme: peak of a contraction
3. Decrement: decreasing intensity of a contraction

Contractions are described in terms of frequency, duration, and intensity. Frequency is the time from the beginning of one contraction to the beginning of the next contraction. It includes one contraction and one resting period between contractions (interval). Duration is the length of one contraction, from the beginning of the increment to the conclusion of the decrement. Intensity is the

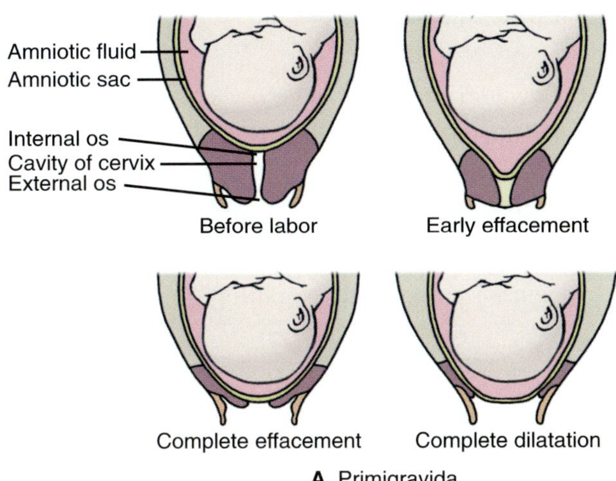

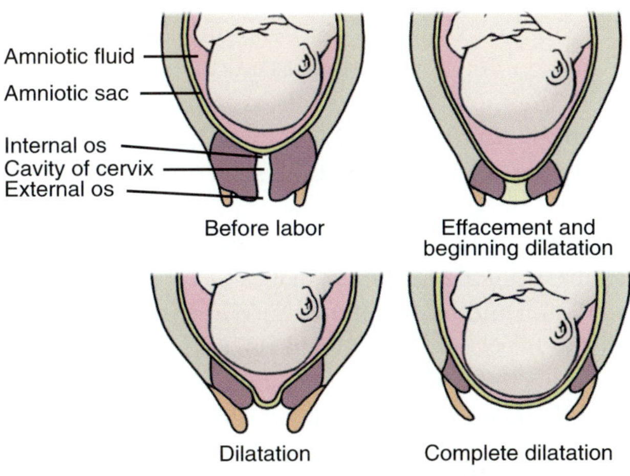

Figure 22–11 Effacement and dilatation: A. Primigravida; B. Multigravida.

strength of the contraction at the acme. Figure 22–12 illustrates these aspects of a contraction.

The duration of a contraction should not be longer than 90 seconds nor should the interval be less than 60 seconds. The uterus should completely relax between contractions. Contractions lasting longer than 90 seconds reduce uterine and placental circulation because of the prolonged compression of the blood vessels. This in turn compromises the fetus.

Contractions are affected by the mother's position. When the mother lies on her back the contractions are often more frequent but have less intensity. When she lies on her side, the contractions are usually less frequent but have greater intensity. Thus, a side-lying position improves progress in labor. Lying on the side also prevents supine hypotension syndrome in the mother and improves oxygenation of the uterus, placenta, and fetus because the heavy uterus is not compressing the inferior vena cava.

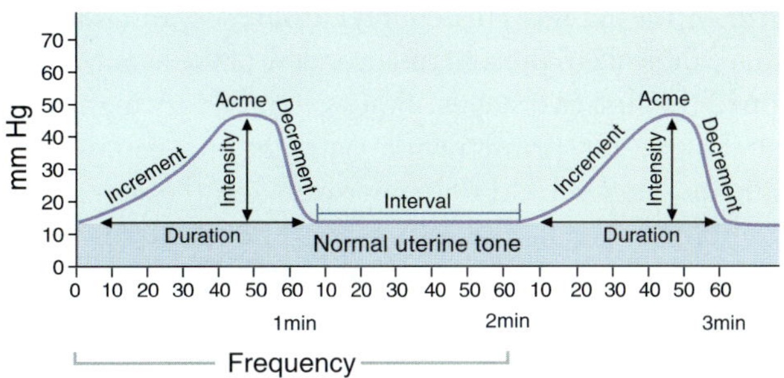

Figure 22–12 Aspects of a contraction (frequency 2 minutes, duration 60 seconds, intensity moderate)

Once the cervix has dilated completely, it is time for the fetus to navigate through the remaining mechanisms of labor. The accepted procedure has been for the mother to take a deep breath at the beginning of a contraction, hold her breath, and voluntarily push in a Valsalva-type bearing down throughout a contraction. This pushing technique is directed by the EMS provider.

The spontaneous onset of the urge to bear down is triggered when the presenting part reaches the pelvic floor where stretch receptors in the posterior vagina cause the release of oxytocin, which spontaneously increases the pushing sensation.

Psyche. Psyche refers to the mother's attitude toward labor and her preparation for labor. The mother's attitude toward labor is shaped by her experiences and expectations. Culture shapes values about and responses to childbirth. It provides the mother with ideas about how to behave during labor and how to interact with her baby.

Anxiety or fear causes the mother's body to secrete catecholamines, which can suppress uterine contractions and restrict placental blood flow. Relaxation increases the progress of labor. Childbirth preparation classes enhance the mother's ability to work with her body rather than working against it. When a woman has realistic expectations about childbirth, she is more likely to have a positive experience.

Stages of Labor

For many years, labor was divided into three stages. In each of these three stages, specific events can be identified. A fourth stage has been acknowledged as being critical to the birth process, the recovery period after the birth of the baby. This chapter discusses four stages of labor. Table 22–6 presents an overview of the average duration of the first two stages. Stages 1 and 2 vary in the average length for primigravida patients and multigravida patients. Stages 3 and 4 are approximately the same length for all patients and are not included in this table.

First Stage: Dilatation and Effacement. The first stage of labor begins with the onset of regular contractions and ends when cervical dilatation, the enlargement of the cervical opening (os), is complete (10 cm). This is usually the longest stage of labor and is divided into three phases: latent, active, and transition.

The latent phase of the first stage of labor ends when the cervix is dilated 4 cm. Contractions occur every 10 to 20 minutes at first and become more frequent, every 5 to 7 minutes. The duration of the contractions begin at 15 to 20 seconds and progress to 30 to 40 seconds. The contraction intensity begins as mild and gradually becomes moderate.

The active phase of the first stage of labor begins when the cervix is dilated 4 cm and ends when the cervix is dilated 8 cm. Contractions occur every 3 to 5 minutes with a duration of 40 to 60 seconds. They are of moderate intensity, progressing to strong. Patients perceive varying degrees of discomfort.

The transition phase of the first stage of labor begins when the cervix is dilated 8 cm and ends when the cervix is dilated 10 cm. Contractions occur every 2 to 3 minutes with a duration of 60 to 90 seconds. There is little rest for the patient between contractions. The intensity of the contractions is strong. The following are characteristics of the transition phase:

- Restlessness
- Hyperventilation
- Bewilderment and sometimes anger
- Difficulty following directions
- Focus on self
- Irritability
- Statements like "Don't touch me"
- Nausea, occasionally vomiting
- Very warm feeling
- Perspiration on upper lip
- Increasing rectal pressure

Second Stage: Birth of Baby. The second stage of labor begins when cervical dilatation is complete and ends with the birth of the baby. Contractions continue at a frequency of 2 to 3 minutes, duration of 60 to 90 seconds, and strong intensity. Now that the cervix is completely dilated, the mother can actively assist in the descent of the fetus by contracting the abdominal muscles and bearing down with each contraction.

As the fetal head descends, it puts pressure on the pelvic nerves and the mother has a greater desire to push. Pressure from the fetal head makes the perineum bulge, then flatten and move anteriorly. With each contraction the labia begin to separate and the baby's head is seen, but the head recedes between contractions. When the largest diameter of the fetal head is past the vulva (head can be seen between contractions), **crowning** has occurred and the birth is imminent (Figure 22–13). A few more contractions will push the head out, and a few more will deliver the body.

TABLE 22-6 Average Length of Labor Stages 1 and 2

	FIRST STAGE			
CHARACTERISTIC	Latent Phase	Active Phase	Transition Phase	SECOND STAGE
Primigravida	8 to 10 hours	6 hours	2 hours	1 hour
Multigravida	5 hours	4 hours	1 hour	15 minutes
Cervical dilatation	0 to 4 cm	4 to 8 cm	8 to 10 cm	
Contractions				
Frequency	10 to 20 progressing to 5 to 7 minutes	3 to 5 minutes	2 to 3 minutes	2 to 3 minutes
Duration	15 to 20 progressing to 30 to 40 seconds	40 to 60 seconds	60 to 90 seconds	60 to 90 seconds
Intensity	Mild progressing to moderate	Moderate progressing to strong	Strong	Strong

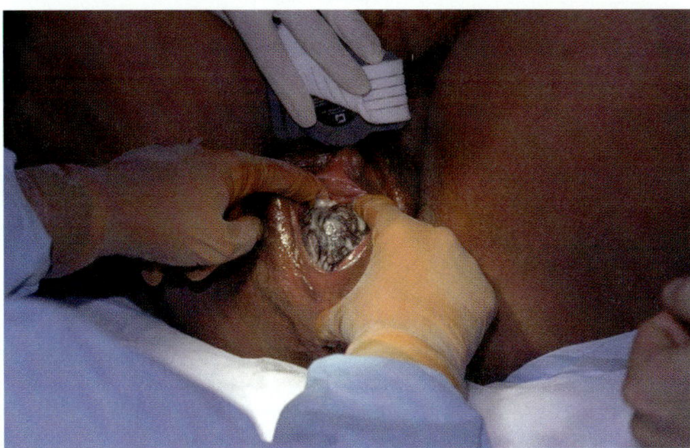

Figure 22–13 Crowning.

As the fetus moves through the pelvis and birth canal, several changes in position must occur. This series of movements is collectively called the **mechanisms of labor** or cardinal movements

The mechanisms of labor are engagement, descent, flexion, internal rotation, extension, external rotation, and expulsion (Figure 22–14). The first three generally occur during the first stage of labor.

As explained earlier, engagement occurs when the presenting part of the fetus (usually head) fully enters the true pelvis. It generally happens before labor begins in primigravidas and after labor begins in multigravidas.

Descent begins with engagement and continues with each contraction throughout the labor process.

The fetal head is bent forward as it meets resistance during descent, causing the chin to rest on the sternum. This allows the narrowest part of the head to enter the pelvic outlet.

Internal rotation takes place mainly during the second stage of labor. The head rotates so the occiput is next to the symphysis pubis.

As the fetal head continues to descend, the occiput pivots under the symphysis pubis and the fetal head becomes unflexed (extended) and pushes upward out of the vagina. The head is actually born at this time.

Once the head has emerged, it rotates back to be in normal alignment with the shoulders. Fetal position in the uterus may be identified by observing this turning of the head. The shoulders now rotate to be in an anteroposterior position under the symphysis pubis.

The EMS provider assisting with the birth applies gentle downward pressure on the baby's head to allow the anterior shoulder to emerge. Then the baby's head is gently raised so the posterior shoulder can be delivered. The rest of the baby's body then just slides out. This is called expulsion (Figure 22–15).

Third Stage: Delivery of Placenta. The third stage of labor begins with the birth of the baby and ends with the delivery of the placenta. This should occur in 30 minutes or less. After the baby is born, the uterus continues contracting, decreasing its capacity and thereby reducing the surface area of placental attachment. The reduced surface area causes the placenta to separate from the uterine wall. As it separates, bleeding occurs, causing the formation of a retroplacental (behind the placenta) hematoma. This hematoma facilitates the separation process. The membranes are peeled from the uterine wall as the placenta slides into the vagina.

Signs that the placenta has separated should be observed about 5 to 10 minutes after the birth of the baby. These signs are:

- Globular shape of the uterus,
- Gush of blood from the vagina, and
- More of the cord protrudes from the vagina (is visible).

When these signs of placental separation have appeared, the patient is asked to push one last time to deliver the placenta. The placenta is placed in a bag labeled with the patient's name so the obstetrician or pathologist can inspect the placenta to ensure the entire placenta was delivered. If the placenta does not deliver within twenty minutes, the EMS provider should package the patient and transport.

Fourth Stage: Recovery. The fourth stage of labor is the first 2 hours after the birth of the baby when the mother's body begins its physiological readjustments. Blood loss is usually between 250 ml and 500 ml. There is a moderate decrease in the systolic and diastolic blood pressure and an increase in pulse rate. The uterus should remain contracted to control bleeding and be positioned in the midline of the abdomen about midway between the symphysis and the umbilicus.

The new mother may be very hungry and thirsty. A shaking chill may be experienced in response to the ending of the physical work of labor. The patient may have urinary retention as the bladder sometimes loses its tone because of trauma during the second stage of labor.

COMPLICATIONS OF CHILDBIRTH

Most labors and births proceed as expected. However, there are complications that may be anticipated and some that happen unexpectedly. Young women under the age of 15 have a greater risk of preterm labor, prolonged labor,

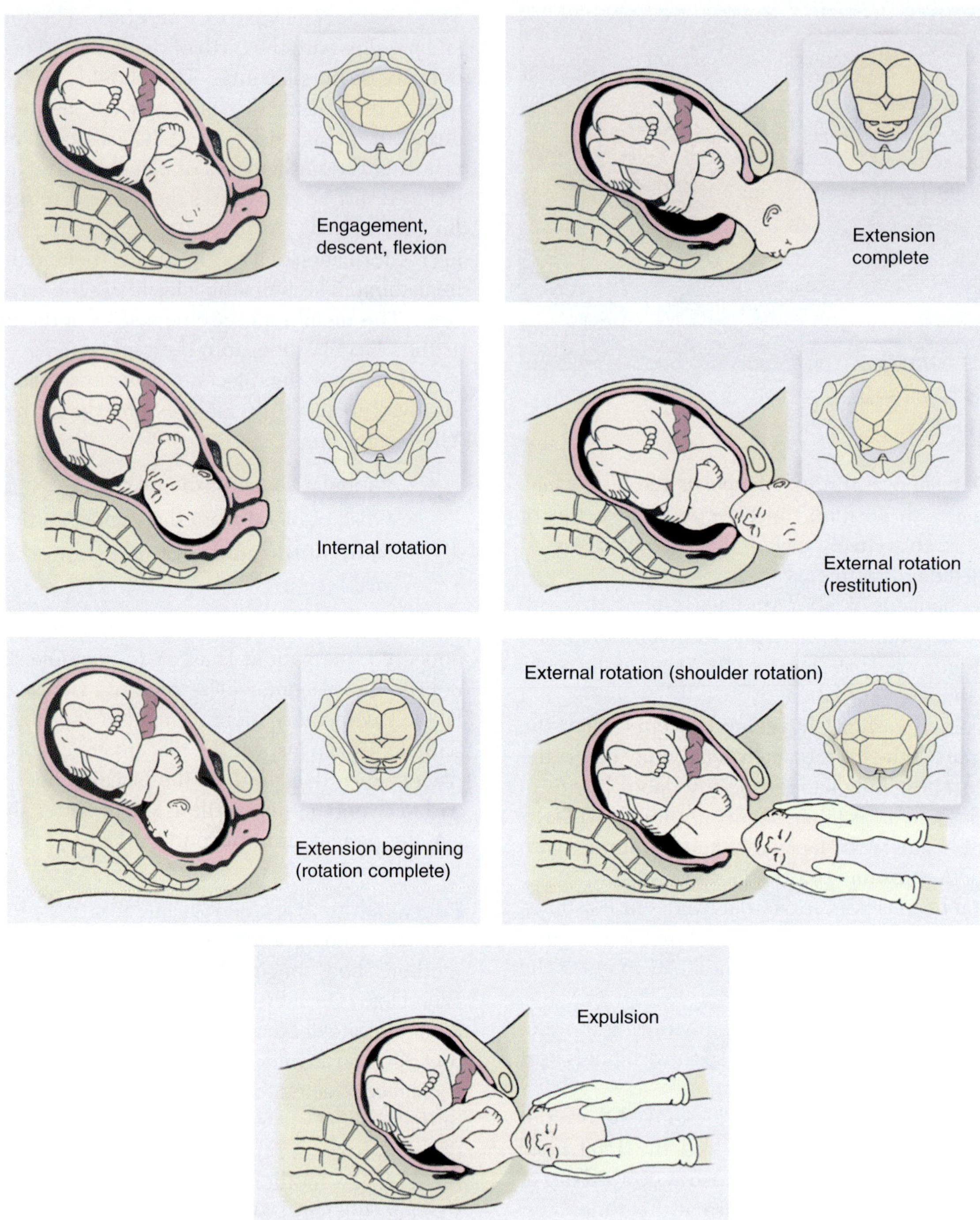

Figure 22-14 Mechanisms of labor.

and dystocia related to the small size of the pelvis because they have not yet reached skeletal maturity. Women over the age of 35 have a greater risk of preterm labor, longer labor, cesarean birth, and dystocia. The most common risks—preterm labor and birth, premature rupture of membranes, dystocia, abnormal duration of labor, and prolapsed cord—are discussed.

Preterm Labor and Birth

Preterm labor is the onset of regular contractions of the uterus that cause cervical changes between 20 and 37 weeks of gestation. Preterm birth is a birth that takes place before the end of the 37th week of gestation. Only about half of the time can a precipitating cause be identified. The single most important factor predisposing

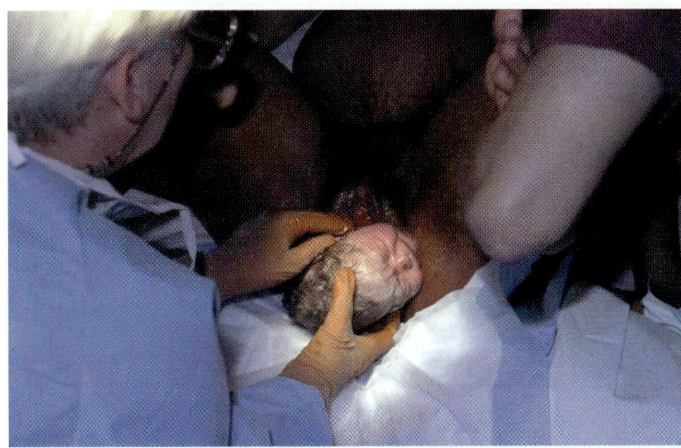

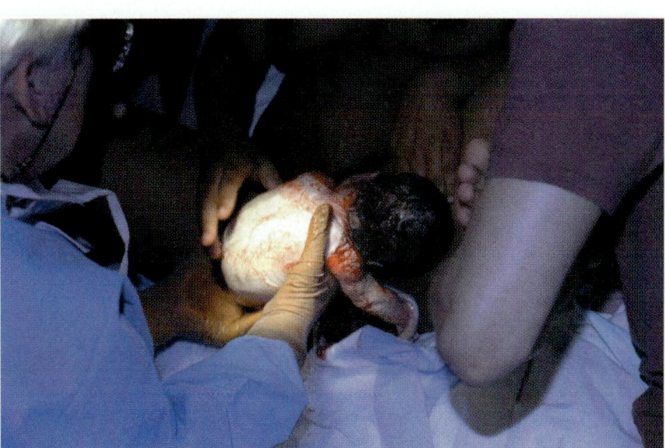

Figure 22-15 Birth of an infant.

to preterm labor and birth is having already had a preterm birth. Other factors often associated with preterm labor and birth include premature rupture of the membranes (PROM), multiple gestation, bacterial vaginosis, intra-amniotic infection, bleeding, and uterine/cervical abnormalities.

If contractions are continuing and cervical changes are occurring, tocolytic agents may be prescribed. Tocolytic agents are medications that inhibit contractions. The most commonly used in the hospital are ritodrine (Yutopar), terbutaline (Brethine), and magnesium sulfate. A corticosteroid may also be given to accelerate fetal lung maturation. There is greater fetal benefit if at least 24 hours elapse between the first dose and the birth.

If contractions subside and cervical dilatation and effacement remain the same, the patient may be discharged with instructions to limit activities and medication to prevent labor.

Premature Rupture of Membranes

When the membranes rupture before labor begins, it is called premature rupture of membranes (PROM). This is the most common cause of preterm labor and occurs in 2% to 18% of pregnancies. Contractions usually begin within 24 hours when the patient is at term. In pregnancies of 28 to 34 weeks' gestation, labor may not start for a week or more.

In most cases of PROM, the cause is unknown. Besides preterm labor and birth, PROM can result in prolapse of the cord and intrauterine infection. The patient may be hospitalized until after the birth of the infant, or if there are no signs of infections or fetal distress, she may be sent home.

Dystocia

Dystocia is a long, difficult, or abnormal labor caused by any of the four major variables that affect labor. The following may be causes:

- Dysfunctional labor: ineffective contractions or maternal pushing efforts (powers)
- Pelvic structure variations (passage)
- Fetal variations: anomalies, abnormal presentation or position, very large size, or number of fetuses (passenger)
- Mother's responses: related to preparation for childbirth, past experiences, culture, and support persons (psyche)

Dysfunctional labor is a labor with problems of the contractions or with maternal bearing-down efforts. The contractions may be hypertonic or hypotonic.

Hypertonic uterine contractions, usually occurring in the latent phase of labor, are very frequent and uncoordinated and have an increased resting tone. The mother has discomfort out of proportion to the intensity of the contractions, which do not dilate or efface the cervix. The excessive pain results from anoxia of the uterine muscle cells. A prolonged latent phase is generally the result.

Hypotonic uterine contractions usually occur in the active phase of labor. After normal progress through the latent phase of labor, the contractions become weak and inefficient in the active phase and may even cease. Common causes are cephalopelvic disproportion (CPD) (discussed later), malposition of the fetus, an overstretched uterus from multiple fetuses, a fetus of very large body size, hydramnios, or grandmultiparity (having delivered more than six infants).

The risks for the mother include intrauterine infection, especially if the membranes are ruptured and labor is prolonged; postpartum hemorrhage caused by inefficient uterine contractions after birth; exhaustion; and decreased coping ability. The fetus may experience distress because of the length of labor and sepsis from maternal pathogens ascending the birth canal.

A woman with a small or abnormally shaped pelvis may experience a long and difficult labor. Only about 50% of women have the pelvic shape most conducive to labor, fetal descent, and birth.

A distended bladder reduces the space available in the pelvis and is an obstruction to fetal descent. This greatly increases the patient's discomfort. Other, less common obstructions are uterine fibroids or pelvic cysts.

Variations of the fetus that may cause dystocia include the following:

- Anomalies
- Abnormal presentation or position
- Size
- Number of fetuses

Fetal anomalies such as hydrocephalus may prevent descent of the fetus. Anomalies are often discovered by an ultrasound during pregnancy. If a vaginal birth is not advisable or not possible, a cesarean birth is usually scheduled.

A cephalic presentation other than vertex makes a larger diameter of the fetal head move through the birth canal. Labor generally takes longer and is more difficult.

In a breech presentation, cervical effacement and dilatation are often slower because the buttocks are softer than the head and do not put firm pressure on the cervix to aid in dilatation. Following are risks to the fetus born in a breech presentation:

- Cord compression
- Aspiration of fluids in the vagina
- Head becoming stuck

It is not always possible to change the presentation of the fetus. Figure 22–16 illustrates the birth of a fetus in a complete breech presentation.

An infant weighing more than 4,000 g (8.8 lb) is said to be **macrosomic**—having a very large body size. This

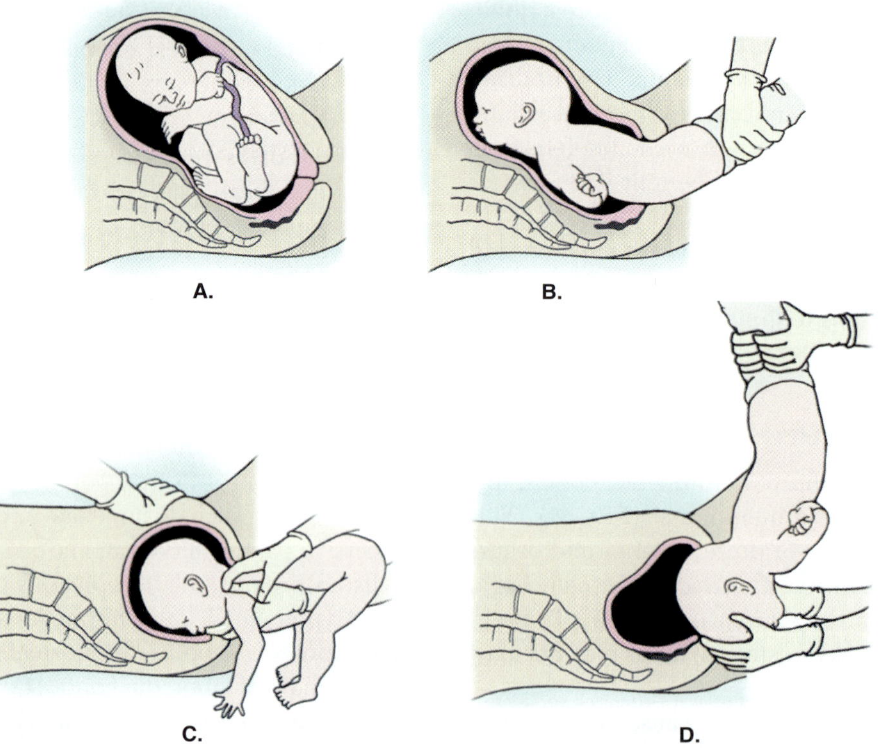

Figure 22–16 Birth of fetus in complete breech presentation: A. Descent and internal rotation; B. Extension of fetal back under symphysis (towel on legs used for traction); C. EMS provider maintains head flexion by putting pressure on lower face with fingers of left hand (suprapubic pressure is applied by assistant to keep fetal head flexed); D. Assistant holds fetal legs with towel while EMS provider assists the face and head over the perineum.

may cause problems for a vaginal birth. As long as the mother's pelvis is of a size and shape to accommodate an infant this size, there is no problem. When the fetal head will not fit through the mother's pelvis, it is called **cephalopelvic disproportion** (CPD). The cause may be either fetal or maternal. The fetal head may be abnormally large and the mother's pelvis of normal size and shape, or the fetal head may be of average size and the mother's pelvis small or abnormally shaped. Whatever the cause, a cesarean birth is required.

When more than one fetus is present, the uterus is overdistended. One or more of the fetuses may be in a presentation less desirable than vertex. Twins often have a cesarean birth, and when there are three or more fetuses, birth is almost always cesarean.

The mother's perception of labor is more important than her actual experience in labor. Tales from family and friends, a bad experience with a previous labor, and cultural expectations may add to the stress of labor. Excessive or prolonged stress experienced by the woman in labor may interfere with the progress of labor.

Abnormal Duration of Labor

Labor may be prolonged or abnormally short (precipitate).

Many of the conditions previously discussed, such as hypotonic uterine contractions, CPD, or abnormal fetal presentations or positions may cause prolonged labor. Labor progress in either the first or second stage may be prolonged or arrested (stopped).

When the active phase of the first stage of labor lasts more than 15 hours, the risk of fetal death increases sharply. With prolonged labor, maternal morbidity and mortality may result from infection, uterine rupture, serious dehydration, and postpartum hemorrhage.

A labor lasting less than 3 hours from the onset of contractions to the birth of the infant is considered a **precipitate labor**. Although a precipitate labor may end with a precipitate birth, they are not the same. Possible maternal complications during a precipitate labor include an increased risk of uterine rupture; lacerations of the cervix, vagina, and perineum; and postpartum hemorrhage. Possible fetal complications include hypoxia, distress, and cerebral trauma.

A **precipitate birth** is a birth occurring suddenly and unexpectedly. When a patient says "the baby's coming" or words to that effect, the EMS provider should always look to see whether she is correct. Most of the time a large part of the fetal head is visible, if not already crowning. In this situation the EMS provider should do the following:

- Stay on scene.
- Remain calm and reassure mother.
- Open emergency birth pack.
- If time permits, scrub hands, put on sterile gloves, and place a drape under mother's buttocks.
- As the head crowns, instruct mother to pant.
- If membranes are still intact, tear the sac, allowing amniotic fluid to flow out.
- Apply gentle pressure to the fetal head with one hand to prevent it from popping out. *Do not hold the head back with force enough to prevent it from being born.*
- With the mother still panting, check at the back of the fetal head for the umbilical cord. If there is a **nuchal cord** (umbilical cord around the neck) and it is loose enough, slip the cord over the baby's head. If it is too tight, place two clamps on the cord, cut the cord between the clamps, and unwind the cord from the neck.
- Suction the baby's mouth, then nose.
- With one hand on each side of the head, push gently downward until the anterior shoulder comes under the symphysis. Then gently raise the baby's head so the posterior shoulder is born.
- Ask the mother to push gently to assist in the birth of the rest of the infant's body.
- Hold the infant at the level of the uterus, being careful not to drop the slippery infant.
- Again, suction the mouth, throat, and nose of the infant.
- Dry the infant to prevent heat loss and place the infant on the mother's abdomen. Cover with a dry blanket.
- Document nuchal cord, time of birth, Apgar scores (addressed later in this chapter) at 1 and 5 minutes after birth, gender, time and method of placental expulsion, and mother's condition.

Prolapsed Cord

When the umbilical cord lies below the presenting part of the fetus, it is termed a **prolapsed cord**. Prolapse of the cord may occur anytime and may be hidden (occult, not visible) or visible (Figure 22–17). It most commonly occurs with ROM as the cord washes down with the amniotic fluid. This happens in 1 out of 400 births.

A cord below the presenting part is compressed between the fetus and the mother's pelvis, resulting in decreased blood flow to the fetus. Contributing factors

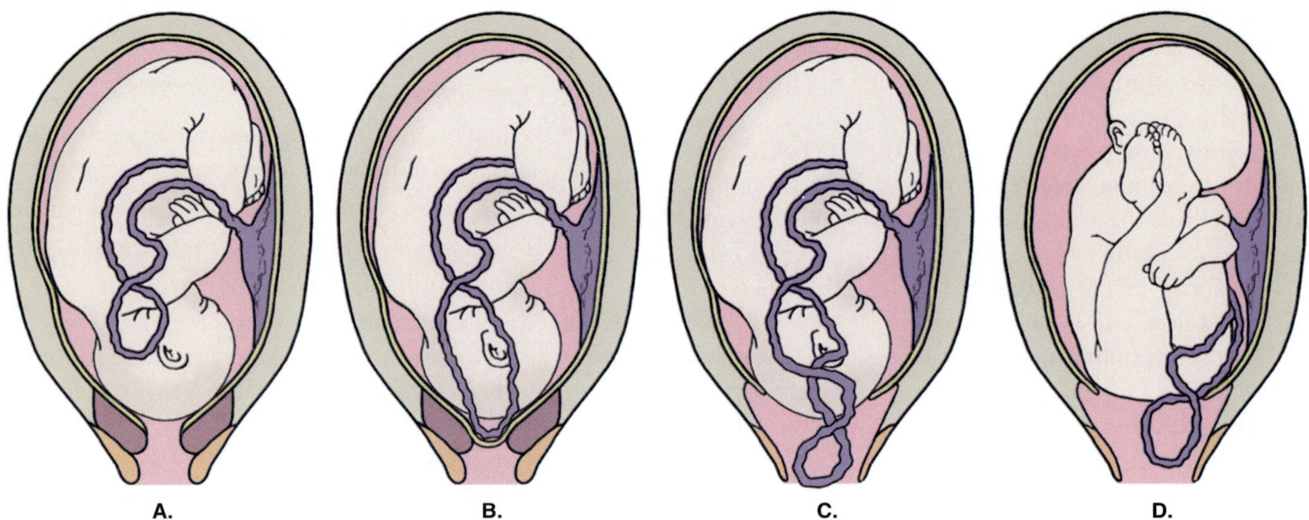

Figure 22–17 Prolapsed cord: A. Hidden (occult, not visible); B. Prolapse with membranes still intact; C. Cord may be seen in vagina; D. Breech with prolapsed cord.

include a long cord (greater than 100 cm or 40 in.), unengaged presenting part, breech presentation, or transverse lie.

When a prolapsed cord is identified, pressure on the cord must be relieved immediately. The EMS provider must don a sterile glove, insert 2 fingers into the vagina, and put pressure on the presenting part to relieve the compression of the cord. The patient can then be assisted into a modified Sims' position with her hips up on pillows, the knee-chest position, or the cot placed in Trendelenburg position. In these positions, gravity keeps the pressure of the presenting part off the cord (Figure 22–18). Generally a cesarean birth is required. The EMS provider must maintain pressure on the presenting part until the patient is in the delivery room or OR.

POSTPARTUM CARE AND COMPLICATIONS

During the first 20 to 30 minutes after the infant's birth, specific care is given to the infant and the mother.

Care of the Infant

Following are the immediate needs of the newborn infant:

- A—airway
- B—breathing
- C—circulation
- W—warmth

Airway. The EMS provider suctions secretions from the mouth then the nose of the infant at the time of birth. Shortly thereafter, the infant takes the first breath and may begin to cry. The mouth and nose of the infant are suctioned as needed to maintain an open airway. The bulb syringe must be compressed before inserting into mouth or nose of infant.

Breathing/Circulation. The infant's cardiopulmonary adaptation to extrauterine life is assessed by using the Apgar score (Table 22–7).

Each of the five items are assessed at 1 and 5 minutes after birth, providing a quick evaluation of how the heart and lungs are adapting. The five items to be assessed are arranged in priority from most important (heart rate) to least important (color). The infant is given a score, from 0 to 2, for each item. The five scores are then totaled.

When the Apgar score is 8 or higher, no special interventions are required. When the Apgar score is between 4 and 8, gentle rubbing of the infant's back for stimulation and administration of oxygen will usually result in an increase in the Apgar score at 5 minutes.

When the Apgar score is between 0 and 4, the infant requires resuscitation. Please refer to your PALS or NALS text for specific resuscitation steps.

Warmth. The infant must be dried to prevent heat loss by evaporation. It is extremely important to keep the infant warm, as the primary reason for decreased heart

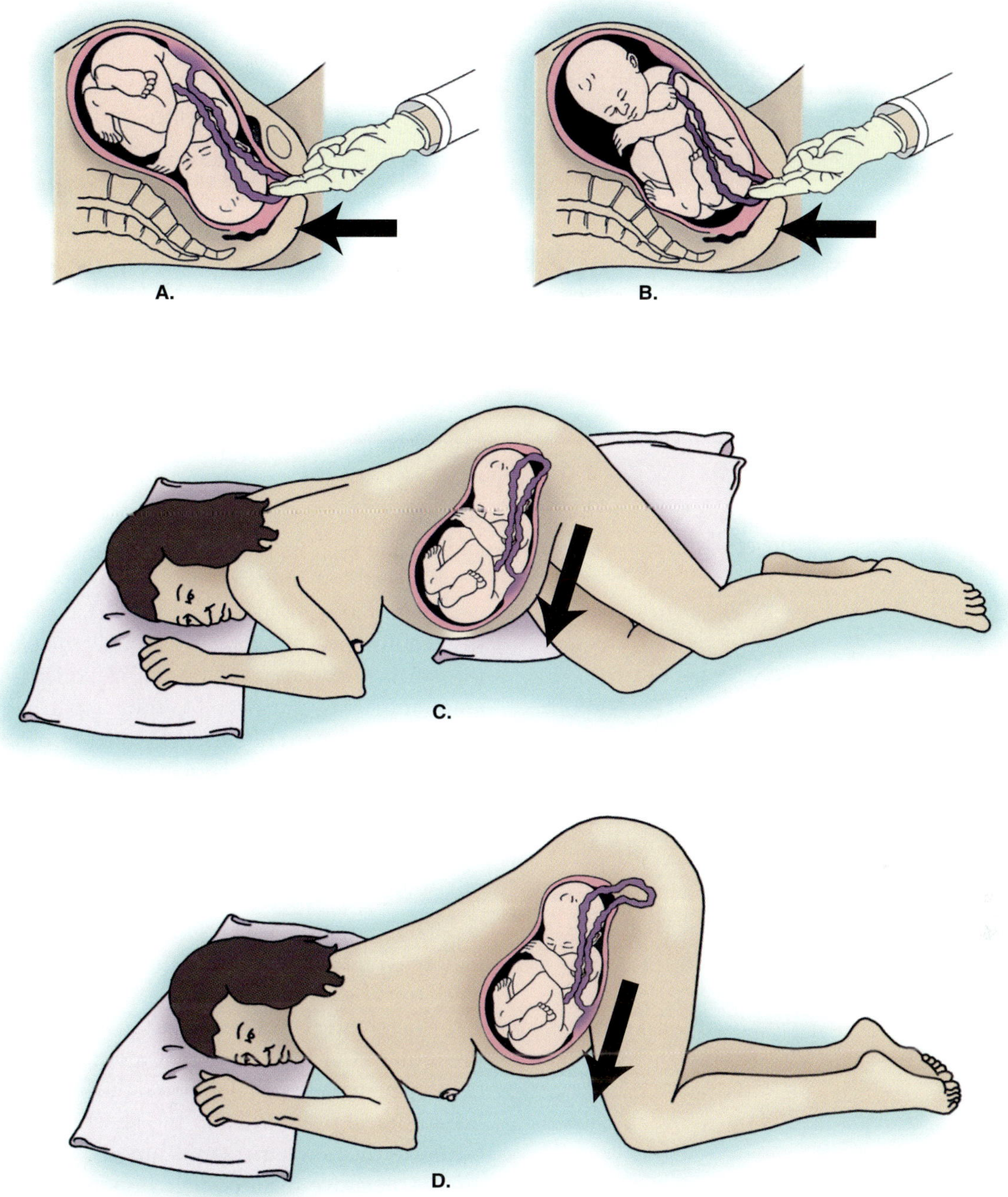

Figure 22–18 Examiner's fingers relieve pressure on prolapsed cord in (A) vertex presentation and (B) breech presentation; Gravity relieves pressure on prolapsed cord with mother in (C) modified Sims' position and (D) knee-chest position.

rate and respirations is a cold baby. Wrapping the infant in warm towels or blankets and placing the infant up against the mother will help keep the infant warm. Skin-to-skin contact with a parent may also be used to provide warmth. A stockinette cap on the infant's *dry head* also helps prevent heat loss.

Care of the Mother

The fundus of the uterus is palpated for firmness. It should be firm, about the size of a grapefruit, in the midline, below the umbilicus. The proper method of palpating the uterus is illustrated in Figure 22–19. Once the placenta is delivered, the mother's uterus can be

TABLE 22-7 Apgar Score

Item Assessed	Score 0	Score 1	Score 2
Heart rate	Absent	Slow (< 100)	Over 100
Respiratory rate	Absent	Slow, weak cry	Good cry
Muscle tone	Flaccid	Some flexion of extremities	Well flexed
Reflex irritability	No response	Grimace	Cry
Color	Blue, pale	Body pink, extremities blue	Completely pink (light skinned); absence of cyanosis (dark skinned)

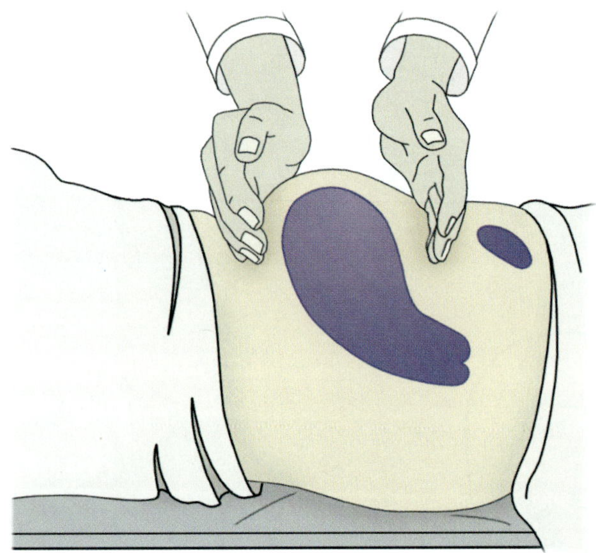

Figure 22-19 Palpation of uterus after delivery of placenta.

gently massaged to facilitate the postpartum contractions that stop bleeding.

Newborn Physiological Changes

Several changes occur in the newborn during delivery and in the first couple of days after delivery that allow the infant to adapt to its new environment. These changes transition the infant from obtaining all its oxygen, nutrients, and waste product removal from the mother via the umbilical cord to a self-sufficient organism. These transitions occur in both the respiratory system and cardiovascular system.

Respiratory. In utero, the fetus relied on the placenta and the mother's respirations for gas exchange. However, fetal breathing movements, from approximately 11 weeks' gestation, help develop the chest wall muscles and the diaphragm. By approximately 35 weeks' gestation, the surfactant produced by the alveoli is in sufficient amount to allow the alveoli to remain partially expanded when the newborn begins to breathe at birth.

For the lungs to function, two changes must happen:

- Pulmonary ventilation must be established with lung expansion at the first breath.
- Pulmonary circulation must greatly increase.

The initiation of breathing is influenced by four factors—physical, chemical, thermal, and sensory—that work together.

The physical or mechanical factors include the compression of the fetal chest as it moves through the birth canal, which squeezes fluid from the lungs and increases intrathoracic pressure; and the chest wall recoil, which occurs as the newborn's trunk emerges. The chest recoil creates negative intrathoracic pressure, which causes a small amount of air to replace the fluid that was squeezed out of the lungs and some of the lung fluid to move across the alveolar membranes into the interstitial tissue of the lungs. Because the protein concentration is higher in the capillaries, the interstitial fluid is drawn into them. All the alveolar fluid is absorbed within the first day after birth.

When the cord id clamped, placental gas exchange ceases, causing an increase in $PaCO_2$ and a decrease in PaO_2 and pH (a transitory asphyxia). These changes stimulate the carotid and aortic chemoreceptors, which send impulses to the respiratory center in the brainstem, which in turn stimulates respirations. A brief period of asphyxia stimulates respirations whereas prolonged asphyxia is a central nervous system (CNS) respiratory depressant.

The change in temperature from the intrauterine environment to the extrauterine environment, a decrease of more than 20°F, is also a stimulus to breathing. The colder temperature stimulates the skin nerve endings and the newborn breathes as a response. Cold stress and respiratory depression result from excessive cooling of the newborn.

The comfortable, relatively quiet uterine environment is left behind for an environment full of sensory stimuli. The auditory and visual stimuli associated with birth, along with the tactile stimulation of being handled, assist in the initiation of respirations.

Cardiovascular. Several circulatory changes are necessary for the successful change from fetal circulation to neonatal circulation. These changes involve the pulmonary blood vessels, ductus arteriosus, foramen ovale, and ductus venosus.

The dilation of these blood vessels begins with the first breath taken by the newborn. This results in lower pulmonary resistance, which allows the blood to freely circulate through the lungs to be oxygenated.

Within minutes after birth, the ductus arteriosis has a reversal of blood flow caused by the increased pressure in the aorta and the increase of oxygen in the blood. This results in more blood flowing through the pulmonary arteries for oxygenation. Closure of the ductus arteriosis is complete within 24 hours and is permanent in 3 to 4 weeks.

The foramen ovale also closes within minutes after birth because of the higher pressure in the left atrium than in the right atrium. The increased blood flow in the lungs decreases pressure in the right atrium and the return of blood from the lungs increases the pressure in the left atrium. Closure of the foramen ovale is permanent in approximately 3 months.

When the cord is clamped, the blood ceases flowing through the umbilical vein to the ductus venosus and into the inferior vena cava. Blood now flows through the liver and is filtered as in adult circulation.

Maternal Physiologic Changes

Many of the physiologic changes postpartum (following birth) are a reversal of the changes in the various body systems that occurred during pregnancy. The initiation of lactation and reestablishment of normal menstrual cycles also occur.

Reproductive System. Changes occur in the uterus, cervix, vagina, and perineum.

Uterus. **Involution** is the return of the reproductive organs, especially the uterus, to their pre-pregnancy size and condition. There are three processes involved in involution:

- Muscle fiber contraction: With the uterus now empty, the uterus firmly contracts to control bleeding from the area of placental attachment; the muscle fibers gradually regain their former size and shape.
- Catabolism: The enlarged muscle cells of the uterus experience catabolic changes in protein cytoplasm that reduce the size of each cell. Catabolic products are excreted as nitrogenous wastes in the urine.
- Regeneration: The endometrium is regenerated within 2 to 3 weeks, except for the placental site, which is healed and regenerated by approximately 6 weeks.

Following the birth, the uterus is about the size of a grapefruit with the fundus about halfway between the umbilicus and symphysis pubis. The fundus rises to the umbilicus in a few hours and stays there about 24 hours. Then the fundus descends about 1 cm, 1 finger breadth, each day for about 10 days when it is once again in the pelvis and unable to be palpated abdominally. A full bladder will push the uterus upward.

The contracting uterus may be a source of discomfort for some women after the infant's birth, especially for multiparas and those who are breastfeeding. Breastfeeding stimulates the release of oxytocin from the posterior pituitary, which stimulates strong uterine contractions as well as the "let down" reflex. These contractions are known as afterpains.

Lochia is the uterine/vaginal discharge after childbirth. It is initially bright red, then changes to a pink or pinkish brown, and then to a yellowish white. The odor of lochia is like a normal menstrual flow. A foul odor is indicative of infection.

Cervix. Within 18 hours after birth, the cervix has become firm, has shortened, and has regained its shape. By the end of 2 weeks the cervical os is closed, but after delivery the opening is more like a slit than a circle.

Vagina and Perineum. The vagina was greatly stretched during labor. It takes 6 weeks for the vagina to complete involution and regain the contour it had prior to pregnancy. It never does regain the size it had prior to pregnancy.

The stretching and thinning of the perineum during labor may cause edema and bruising of the perineum after the birth. Many women have an episiotomy (surgical incision of the perineum) before the infant's birth. Lacerations of the perineum also may occur. Even when the episiotomy or laceration is small, it can cause a great deal of discomfort because the muscles of the perineum are used when sitting, stooping, bending, squatting, walking, and defecating.

Endocrine System. After the expulsion of the placenta, the levels of the placental hormones estrogen, progesterone, human placental lactogen (hPL), human chorionic gonadotropin (hCG), and relaxin rapidly decline. The decrease in hPL, estrogen, and cortisol causes a reversal of the diabetogenic effect of pregnancy.

Lactation. The rapid decline of the estrogen and progesterone levels allows the prolactin to initiate milk production within 2 to 3 days after the infant's birth. Oxytocin causes the milk to be expressed into the lactiferous ducts. This is called "let down." The let-down reflex is a neurohormonal reflex; that is, either neuro (the mind) or the hormone (oxytocin) may initiate "let down." A breastfeeding mother hearing a baby cry or thinking about feeding her infant often stimulates the let-down reflex and milk will drip from the nipples (neuro). The release of oxytocin in response to the infant's sucking also stimulates the let-down reflex (hormonal).

Menstrual Cycle. There is a great difference when ovulation and menstruation are re-established based on whether the mother is breastfeeding or not breastfeeding. Ovulation in nonbreastfeeding mothers takes place as early as 27 days after the birth and usually has resumed by 2 months. Most nonbreastfeeding mothers resume menstruating within 3 months after the birth. The average time for ovulation to take place in breastfeeding mothers is approximately 190 days.

Gastroenterologic System. Most new mothers are hungry and thirsty after giving birth because of the energy expended during labor.

Mothers may encounter difficulty in having a bowel movement after giving birth. There are several reasons, including:

- Peristalsis has been decreased because of the effects of the increased progesterone level during pregnancy; this may take several days to become normal again,
- Prelabor diarrhea,
- Lack of food during labor,
- Dehydration,
- Perineal trauma, episiotomy repair, or hemorrhoids, and
- Mother's anticipation of discomfort.

Cardiovascular System. The increase in blood volume during pregnancy allows a significant loss of blood without any ill effects to the mother. In a vaginal birth, blood loss averages 500 ml, while a cesarean birth averages a 1,000 ml blood loss.

Vital Signs. The pulse, which increased during pregnancy, remains elevated or may even rise for up to 24 to 48 hours, but should not exceed 100 beats per minute. Periods of bradycardia may also be experienced. The pulse returns to the pre-pregnant rate in approximately 8 weeks.

The diaphragm descends when the uterus is emptied, making respirations much easier. In 6 to 8 weeks respiratory function will return to the pre-pregnant rate. The blood pressure may have a small increase in both the systolic and diastolic aspects that lasts about 4 days. The rapid decrease in intra-abdominal pressure after birth results in visceral blood vessel dilation, which may cause orthostatic hypotension.

Cardiac Output. Cardiac output, which increased during pregnancy, may increase even higher for up to 60 minutes following delivery. Cardiac output remains elevated for at least 48 hours, and then rapidly decreases in the first 2 weeks postpartum. The return of cardiac output to the prepregnancy level takes about 24 weeks.

Blood Volume. The changes in blood volume are rapid and dramatic. There are three physiologic changes that protect from excessive blood loss:

- Loss of the uteroplacental circulation (when the placenta is expelled) reduces the maternal vascular bed by 10% to 15%.
- Stimulus for vasodilation is removed with the loss of placental endocrine function.

- Movement of extravascular water, stored during pregnancy, into the blood vessels increases blood volume.

Blood Values. The white blood cell count, which increased slightly during pregnancy (to 12,000/mm^3), now increases to 20,000 or even 30,000/mm^3 during the first 10 to 12 days after the infant's birth. The neutrophil level increases the most for protection against invading organisms.

The large loss of plasma volume during the first 3 days after the birth results in a rise in both the hemoglobin and hematocrit levels by the seventh day, unless excessive blood loss has occurred.

Coagulation. The increased levels of clotting factors and fibrinogen during pregnancy remain elevated for a few days as protection against postpartum hemorrhage. Thus, there is an increased risk for thrombus (clot) formation. Mothers having varicose veins, a cesarean birth, or a history of thrombophlebitis are at greater risk for thrombus formation.

Urinary System. The hypotonia of the bladder and dilation of the ureters during pregnancy take approximately 2 to 8 weeks to return to the pre-pregnant state. Also, the bladder, urethra, and tissue around the urinary meatus may have been traumatized and become edematous during labor and birth, which may result in difficulty in urination.

The mother may have a problem with overdistention and incomplete emptying of the bladder and residual retention of urine because the diuresis causes the bladder to fill quickly. Those mothers who received a regional anesthesia are especially at risk for bladder distention and difficulty voiding until the anesthesia wears off.

Postpartum hemorrhage and urinary tract infection are two complications related to urinary retention and bladder overdistention. Urinary stasis provides the bacteria with enough time to multiply and cause an infection. A full bladder displaces the uterus up and to the side, resulting in uterine atony (inability of the uterus to contract). This is the primary cause of excessive bleeding.

Musculoskeletal System. The musculoskeletal changes that occur during pregnancy are reversed during the postpartum period.

Joints, Ligaments, and Cartilage. As the level of the hormone relaxin decreases, the ligaments and cartilage, especially of the pelvis, begin to revert to their pre-pregnant positions. Hip or joint pain may be noticed as these changes take place. Joints, cartilage, and ligaments are stabilized by 6 to 8 weeks after the birth.

All joints return to their normal pre-pregnant state except those in the feet. The new mother may discover a permanent increase in her shoe size.

Abdominal Muscles. It usually takes 6 weeks for the abdominal muscles to return almost to their pre-pregnant state.

Neurologic System. Any pregnancy-induced neurologic discomforts usually lessen after birth. However, fatigue, afterpains, muscle aches, episiotomy or abdominal incision pain, and breast engorgement all may give rise to maternal discomfort.

The mother who has a headache must be carefully assessed. If the mother had a regional anesthesia (epidural or spinal), the headache may be caused by a leakage of cerebrospinal fluid into the extradural space during needle placement; this is known as a spinal headache. This headache is generally more severe when the mother sits or stands and is relieved when she lies down. If the mother has blurred vision, photophobia, and abdominal pain with a headache, it may indicate that she is developing pregnancy-induced hypertension (PIH), or if she had PIH during pregnancy, that it is getting worse.

Postpartum Complications

The most common complications of childbirth are postpartum hemorrhage, infection, thromboembolic conditions, and disseminated intravascular coagulation.

Postpartum Hemorrhage. Postpartum hemorrhage is defined as a blood loss of more than 500 ml after the third stage of labor or 1,000 ml after a cesarean birth. The hemorrhage is identified as either early, within the first 24 hours, or late, generally occurring 1 to 2 weeks after the birth, but may occur up to 6 weeks after the birth.

Early Postpartum Hemorrhage. Early postpartum hemorrhage has several possible causes: uterine atony, retained placental fragments, lacerations of the birth canal, and hematomas. Predisposing factors for postpartum hemorrhage include the following:

- Overdistention of the uterus (large infant, multiple gestation, or hydramnios)
- Grandmultiparity (more than 5)
- Precipitate labor or birth
- Prolonged labor
- Use of forceps or vacuum extractor
- Use of tocolytic drugs
- Use of oxytocin to augment or induce labor,
- Cesarean birth
- Manual removal of the placenta
- Clotting disorders

Uterine atony is a lack of muscle tone in the uterus. The uterus feels soft and boggy. Hemorrhage from uterine atony is usually a steady flow.

Occasionally, small pieces of the placenta may not be expelled. These pieces prevent the uterus from contracting effectively, and bleeding continues.

Factors predisposing a woman to lacerations of the birth canal include the following:

- Nulliparity
- Forceps-assisted or vacuum cup-assisted birth
- Precipitous birth
- Macrosomia
- Epidural anesthesia

Lacerations may occur in the perineum, vagina, cervix, or around the urethral meatus. Most lacerations are identified and repaired immediately following the birth. Occasionally, a laceration is overlooked and bright red bleeding persists when the uterus is firmly contracted.

A hematoma forms when there is bleeding into the tissues; there is no external laceration. Spontaneous or forceps-assisted births may result in hematoma formation. The most common sites are the vulva, vagina, and retroperitoneal area. A hematoma is a bluish-purple mass that produces deep, severe, unrelenting pain and a feeling of great pressure. When the uterus is firmly contracted, the amount of lochia is within normal limits, and the mother has a falling blood pressure or tachycardia and persistently describes severe pain, a hematoma should be suspected.

Late Postpartum Hemorrhage. A late postpartum hemorrhage usually occurs 1 to 2 weeks after the birth because of subinvolution (incomplete return of the uterus to its prepregnant size and consistency) or retained placental fragments. Clots may form around the retained placental fragments immediately postpartum, thus keeping lochia within normal limits. Several days later, when the clots slough, excessive bleeding occurs. There is usually no warning of a late postpartum hemorrhage.

Infections. **Puerperal (postpartum) infection** is an infection following childbirth occurring between the birth and 6 weeks postpartum. It is defined as a temperature of 38°C (100.4°F) or more on 2 consecutive days during the first 10 days after the birth, not counting the first 24 hours.

Because all parts of the reproductive tract are connected to each other, it is easy for organisms to move from the vagina through the cervix, to the uterus, through the fallopian tubes, and out to the ovaries and peritoneal cavity. The increased blood supply to the reproductive tract during pregnancy provides more avenues for invading bacteria to be spread throughout the body with the possibility of causing a life-threatening septicemia.

Amniotic fluid and lochia are alkaline, so during labor and in the postpartum period the normal acidity of the vagina is reduced, which encourages bacterial growth.

Common postpartum infections are wound infection, metritis, mastitis, and urinary tract infection. Predisposing factors for puerperal infection are listed in Table 22–8.

The break in the skin from lacerations, episiotomies, and surgical incisions from cesarean birth provides an easy portal of entry for bacteria. Localized signs of infection (redness, warmth, edema, and tenderness) are assessed at the skin break, which, if untreated, will develop into generalized signs of infection, including an elevated temperature and malaise. Wound edges may separate and drainage may be evident.

Metritis, inflammation of the uterus, includes both endometritis (inflammation of the inside of the uterus, or endometrium) and parametritis (inflammation of the outside of the uterus, or parametrium, including the connective tissue of the broad ligaments). The usual causes are the organisms that normally inhabit the vagina and cervix. This infection easily spreads through the fallopian tubes (**salpingitis**) to the ovaries (**oophoritis**).

Mastitis is inflammation of the breast, generally during breastfeeding. The usual cause is *Staphylococcus aureus* but may also be *Candida albicans*. Symptoms appear between 2 and 4 weeks after birth. There is usually a crack or fissure in the nipple for the portal of entry. Nipple soreness may result in shorter breastfeeding times, allowing milk stasis, which is a good medium for bacterial growth.

Approximately 2% to 4% of new mothers will have a urinary tract infection (UTI). Trauma to the bladder

TABLE 22-8 Predisposing Factors for Postpartum Infection

Predisposing Factors	Description/Explanation
Antepartum	
Medical conditions	Ability to defend against any infection is decreased
• Diabetes	
• Alcoholism	
• Drug abuse	
• Anemia	
• Poor nutrition/malnutrition	
• Immunosuppression	
History of previous infections	Possibly more vulnerable to infections
Intrapartum	
Prolonged rupture of membranes	Provides direct access to interior of uterus
Chorioamnionitis	Organisms already in uterus
Prolonged labor	More time for bacteria to multiply
Excessive number of vaginal examinations	Increases opportunity for organisms from outside source or vagina to be introduced into the uterus
Internal fetal monitoring	Provides opportunity for introduction of organisms
Bladder catheterization	Possible introduction of organisms into bladder
Episiotomy, lacerations, and cesarean birth	Provide portals of entry for organisms
Postpartum	
Retained placental fragments	Good medium for bacterial growth
Hematoma	Makes tissues more susceptible
Hemorrhage	Infection-fighting components of blood are lost

and urethra during labor and birth, urinary stasis after the birth, and catheterization all contribute to the development of a UTI.

Thromboembolic Conditions. **Thrombophlebitis** refers to the formation of a clot in an inflamed vein. Superficial thrombophlebitis is more common when the mother had preexisting varicose veins. Deep vein thrombosis (DVT) may or may not be related to vein inflammation and is seen more in women with a history of thromboses. Pulmonary embolism may be a complication of DVT. Septic pelvic thrombophlebitis is more commonly found in a mother with metritis as the inflammation spreads to the pelvic veins.

The incidence of thromboembolic conditions has decreased over the past 20 years since early ambulation has become a standard practice after childbirth (Lowdermilk et al., 1999). Venous stasis and hypercoagulation, which are present during pregnancy, are the major causes. Other risk factors include maternal age over 35, cesarean birth, prolonged time in stirrups during second stage of labor, obesity, smoking, and a history of varicosities or venous thromboses.

Disseminated Intravascular Coagulation. Disseminated intravascular coagulation (DIC) is an abnormal stimulation of the clotting mechanism, which consumes clotting factors, causing small clots throughout the vascular system and widespread bleeding internally, externally, or both. This results in platelet and clotting factor depletion. DIC may result from a missed abortion, abruptio placenta, amniotic fluid embolism, severe preeclampsia, hemorrhage, and a dead fetus. It is a complication of a preexisting problem. See Chapter 16 for information on DIC.

TRAUMA IN PREGNANCY

Traumatic injury in pregnancy can be a devastating experience, not only for the patient and her family but also for the EMS, emergency department, and labor and delivery providers who care for the patient. Traumatic injury is the leading cause of non-obstetric death in pregnant women. It is important for the EMS provider to remember that when treating a pregnant patient, the EMS provider is in fact treating two patients, the mother and the baby. The survival of the fetus depends upon keeping the mother oxygenated and maintaining an adequate blood pressure.

As discussed in Chapter 6, during shock, the body diverts blood from low need areas, for example the skin and GI system, to high need areas, for example the heart and brain, in order to maintain life. Unfortunately, blood is shunted from the fetus and mother's reproductive system early on in shock, compromising the fetus. Maintaining an adequate blood pressure can help continue to perfuse the placenta and maintain the fetus.

The physiological changes that occur during pregnancy may make it difficult to assess for shock in the pregnant patient. With the increase in heart rate, it may be difficult to determine if the patient's tachycardia is normal for the pregnancy or in response to blood loss. The drop in blood pressure associated with pregnancy may also confuse the EMS provider. The increased blood volume by the third trimester can mask the effects of blood loss until a significant percentage of blood has been lost. Other complications of trauma in the pregnant female are preterm labor, spontaneous abortion early in gestation, or even placental abruption later in gestation.

Management of the pregnant patient in trauma can be challenging. Later in pregnancy, it may be impossible to immobilize the patient supine on a long spine board because of the supine hypotension that occurs when the weight of the uterus and fetus compresses the vena cava and drops blood return to the heart to almost zero. Immobilization may require creativity in order to meet the goal of minimizing spinal movement. One should aggressively treat the ABCs, as the viability of the fetus depends upon the mother. All pregnant patients should be encouraged to seek medical attention as some complications, for example placental abruption, may not show up for hours or days after the accident. Even if the woman refuses transport, advise her to call her obstetrician that same day for follow-up. Also advise her to seek emergency medical attention if any vaginal bleeding or contractions develop.

SUMMARY

The female body goes through a significant number of physiologic changes during pregnancy, through labor and delivery, and in the postpartum period. Most pregnancies and deliveries are uncomplicated and joyous occasions. Complications do occur and it is important for the EMS provider to understand the changes that occur and the pathophysiology of complications to effectively manage the pregnant patient in the field. Trauma is the leading cause of non-obstetric death in the pregnant population. The EMS provider should understand with any emergency, medical or traumatic, that there are two patients requiring treatment, and that the survival of the baby depends upon the survival of the mother.

REVIEW QUESTIONS

Multiple Choice

1. The term gravida in the obstetric history refers to:
   a. The number of times the patient had an abortion.
   b. The number of live children the patient has.
   c. The number of babies the patient has delivered.
   d. The number of times the patient has been pregnant.

2. The term para in the obstetric history refers to:
   a. The number of times the patient had an abortion.
   b. The number of live children the patient has.
   c. The number of babies the patient has delivered.
   d. The number of times the patient has been pregnant.
3. The average maternal cardiac output increases by ___ over the prepregnant cardiac output.
   a. 10%
   b. 20%
   c. 30%
   d. 40%
4. Maternal blood volume increases by ___ during pregnancy.
   a. 10%
   b. 20%
   c. 30%
   d. 40%
5. Judy is a 16-year-old primigravida who calls EMS because her membranes ruptured. She states that she is at 38 weeks, that she first saw a physician two weeks ago, and that she did not receive any prenatal care prior to that visit. She is contracting 8–12 minutes apart. Which of the following would be indicative of a high risk pregnancy?
   a. Lack of prenatal care.
   b. She is not considered high risk.
   c. The membranes rupturing spontaneously.
   d. The contractions at 8–12 minutes apart.
6. You are transporting a pregnant patient to a tertiary care center for preeclampsia. She is on a magnesium sulfate drip. During a reassessment, you find her respirations at 8 per minute and her reflexes are decreased. You should:
   a. Consider them to be the desired result.
   b. Record and monitor the vital signs to see if it continues.
   c. Stop the magnesium drip and contact medical control.
   d. Increase the drip rate as she is not receiving an adequate dose to treat her preeclampsia.
7. Fetal lie is:
   a. How deep the fetus' head has dropped into the pelvis.
   b. How long it takes for the fetus to move down the birth canal.
   c. The fetus' head being on the right or left side of the mother.
   d. The relation of the long axis of the fetus to that of the mother.
8. The patient in labor is encouraged to position herself on her side or with the head of the bed elevated to:
   a. Prevent maternal hypotension
   b. Prevent maternal hypertension
   c. Reduce the chance of nausea and backache
   d. Reduce the discomfort of contractions
9. In the first 24–48 hours after delivery, the woman's cardiac output will:
   a. decrease significantly.
   b. increase.
   c. stay the same.
   d. decrease then increase after 48 hours.

10. Disseminated intravascular coagulation in a pregnant or postpartum woman may be caused by:
    a. missed abortion.
    b. severe preeclampsia.
    c. dead fetus.
    d. all of the above.

CASE STUDY

You arrive at the scene of a two-car, five-patient motor vehicle collision and are assigned to a P2 34-year-old female patient who was a restrained back seat passenger. She states that she is having abdominal pain and cramping. From the bruises on her abdomen, it appears that she was not wearing her seat belt low and across her hips. She states she just had a prenatal visit and is at 33 weeks' gestation. What do you think is going on? To what kind of facility should you transport her? What principle about trauma in pregnancy should be in your mind as you treat this patient?

BIBLIOGRAPHY

Blackburn, S., & Loper, D. (1992). *Maternal, fetal, and neonatal physiology*. Philadelphia: W. B. Saunders.

Bougere, M. (1998). Action stat: Abruptio placenta. *Nursing 98*, 28(2), 47.

Bowes, W. (1996). Postpartum care. In S. Gabber, J. Niebyl, & J. Simpson (Eds.), *Obstetrics: Normal and problem pregnancies* (3rd ed.). New York: Churchill Livingstone.

Burroughs, A. (1997). *Maternity nursing* (7th ed.). Philadelphia: W. B. Saunders.

Cosner, K., & deJong, E. (1993). Physiologic second stage labor. *The American Journal of Maternal/Child Nursing, 18*(1), 38–43.

Cunningham, F. G., MacDonald, P. C., Grant, N. F., Leveno, K. J., Gilstrap, L. C., & Hankins, G. D. V. (1997). *William's obstetrics* (20th ed.). Norwalk, CT: Appelton & Lang.

Dickason, E., Silverman, B., & Schult, M. (1994). *Maternal-infant nursing care* (3rd ed.). St. Louis, MO: Mosby-Year Book.

Gorrie, T., McKinney, E., & Murray S. (1998). *Foundations of maternal-newborn nursing* (2nd ed.). Philadelphia: W. B. Saunders.

Guyton, A. C., & Hall, J. E. (1996). *Textbook of medical physiology* (9th ed.) (pp. 1039–41). Philadelphia: W. B. Saunders.

Hamadeh, G., Dedmon, C., & Mozley, P. (1995). Postpartum fever. *American Family Physician, 52*(2), 531.

Ladewig, P., London, M., Olds, S. (1998). *Maternal-newborn nursing* (4th ed.). Menlo Park, CA: Addison-Wesley Longman, Inc.

Lowdermilk, D., Perry, S., & Bobak, I. (1999). *Maternity nursing* (5th ed.). St. Louis, MO: Mosby-Year Book.

Lowe, N. (1996). The pain and discomfort of labor and birth. *Journal of Obstetric, Gynecologic, and Neonatal Nursing, 25*(1), 82–92.

Mechem, C. C. (2000). Trauma in pregnancy. In D. M. Cline (Ed.), *Emergency Medicine Companion Handbook*. (5th ed.). (pp. 821–824). Dallas, TX: American College of Emergency Physicians.

Minnick-Smith, K., & Cook, F. (1997). Current treatment options for ectopic pregnancy. *American Journal of Maternal Child Nursing, 22*(1), 21–25.

Simpson, K. (1997). Preterm birth in the United States: Current issues and future prospectives. *Journal of Perinatal Neonatal Nursing, 10*(4), 11.

Simpson, K., & Creehan, P. (1996). *AWHONN's Perinatal Nursing*. Philadelphia: Lippincott.

Varney, H. (1997). *Varney's midwifery* (3rd ed.). Sudbury, MA: Jones & Bartlett.

CHAPTER

23

Childhood Diseases and Disorders

CONTENT OUTLINE

- Infectious Diseases
  - Viral Diseases
  - Fungal Diseases
  - Bacterial Diseases
  - Parasitic Diseases
- Respiratory Diseases
  - Sudden Infant Death Syndrome (SIDS)
  - Croup
  - Asthma
  - Pneumonia
  - Respiratory Failure
- Digestive Diseases
  - Fluid Imbalances
- Cardiovascular Diseases
- Musculoskeletal Diseases
- Hematologic Diseases
  - Leukemia
- Neurologic Diseases
  - Reye's Syndrome
- Eye and Ear Diseases
- Trauma
  - Child Abuse
  - Suicide
  - Poisoning

KEY TERMS

Catarrhal
Dormant
Encephalopathy
Exudate
Incubation period
Inspiratory stridor
Koplik's spots
Malaise
Nits
Orchitis
Parotid glands
Paroxysmal
Patent
Prone
Pyoderma
Rhinitis
Supine
Vesicles

LEARNING OBJECTIVES

Upon completion of the chapter, the student should be able to:

1. Define the terminology common to childhood diseases.
2. Identify the important signs and symptoms associated with childhood diseases.
3. Describe the common diagnostic tests used to determine type and/or cause of the childhood disease.
4. Describe the typical course and management of the common childhood diseases.
5. State the common drugs abused by children, the effects of the drugs, and the potential health hazards of drug use.
6. List the immunizations available to prevent childhood diseases.
7. Identify the safety precautions for preventing poisonings in children.

OVERVIEW

Childhood diseases range from common infections such as tonsillitis and colds to more chronic and debilitating diseases such as Ewing's sarcoma and leukemia. In addition, traumatic events such as abuse and poisonings are very common in the young population. Childhood diseases can affect any body system. Even though immunizations against many of the common childhood diseases are available, thousands of children in this country have not been immunized at all or do not have adequate immunizations. This increases their likelihood of developing an acute infectious childhood disease.

INFECTIOUS DISEASES

More children are seen yearly by physicians for infectious disease diagnosis and treatment than any other problem. Infectious diseases of childhood fall into four categories: viral, bacterial, fungal, and parasitic diseases. Disorders in these categories include some of the most familiar diseases, such as colds, influenza, measles, pertussis, and tonsillitis. Several of the infectious diseases may be prevented by maintenance of a regular immunization schedule. Many of these diseases have an **incubation period**, the time between exposure to the disease and the presence of symptoms, which lasts several days. Signs and symptoms, in general, for the common infectious diseases include fever, **malaise** (a feeling of general discomfort), coughing, anorexia, nausea/vomiting, and/or rashes. Treatment varies with the specific disease. In many cases, treatment consists of symptom relief, good nutrition, and rest. Non-aspirin antipyretics are given to children with fever since aspirin has been linked with Reye's syndrome. Good hand washing is the primary means of preventing the spread of infectious diseases.

Viral Diseases

Viral diseases in children are usually treated symptomatically. Most children have mild cases of the disease and recuperate quickly. However, for some children, especially those who have other medical disorders, even a mild viral infection can become a critical health problem. Some viruses invade the host and remain dormant for long periods of time. The viruses activate when "triggered" by something. Although this concept is not well understood, it is known that stress is a common trigger for initiating the replication of a dormant virus.

Measles. Measles, also known as rubeola, is an acute viral disease. It is marked by fever, inflammation of the respiratory mucous membranes, runny nose, and a generalized dusky red maculopapular rash over the body trunk and extremities (Figure 23–1). Spots, called **Koplik's spots**, can be seen in the mouth early in the disease. These spots are rather unique to measles and are often the definitive symptom that confirms the diagnosis (Figure 23–2). Measles is transmitted by contaminated airborne particles. The incubation period is from seven to fourteen days. Treatment is usually directed at relief of symptoms and prevention of such complications as dehydration, pneumonia, or high fever. Having one episode of the disease should provide lifetime immunity, but all children should be immunized to prevent measles.

Rubella. Rubella is a type of measles also known as German measles or three-day measles. It is characterized by a rash similar to measles but lighter in color (Figure 23–3). Rubella is usually a very mild disease in children but can be quite serious in pregnant women. If it occurs during the first three months of pregnancy, there is an increased risk of fetal problems or congenital anomalies occurring. The incubation period is fourteen to twenty-one days. Rubella, like measles, is spread by contaminated airborne droplets. Symptoms include lymph node enlargement, rash, nasal discharge, joint pain, chills, and fever. Treatment is usually symptomatic with rest, good nutrition, and prevention of spread of the infection. All children should be immunized to prevent rubella.

Mumps. Mumps is an infectious disease characterized by inflammation of the **parotid glands** (the salivary glands located just in front of the ears). The incubation period is usually sixteen to eighteen days, but may be as long as twenty-five days. Symptoms include chills, fever,

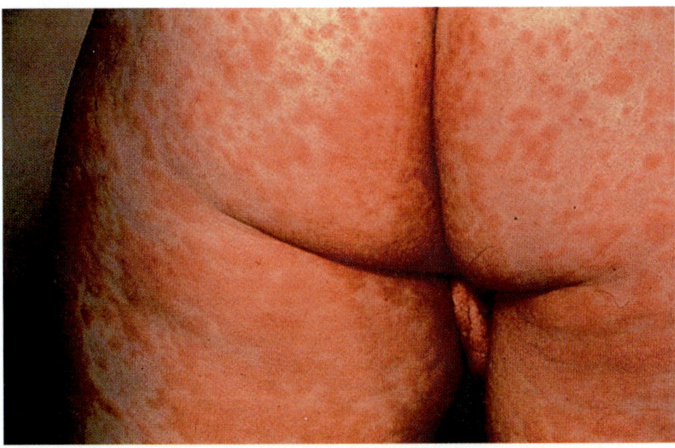

Figure 23–1 Maculopapular rash in rubeola. (Courtesy of the Centers for Disease Control and Prevention [CDC].)

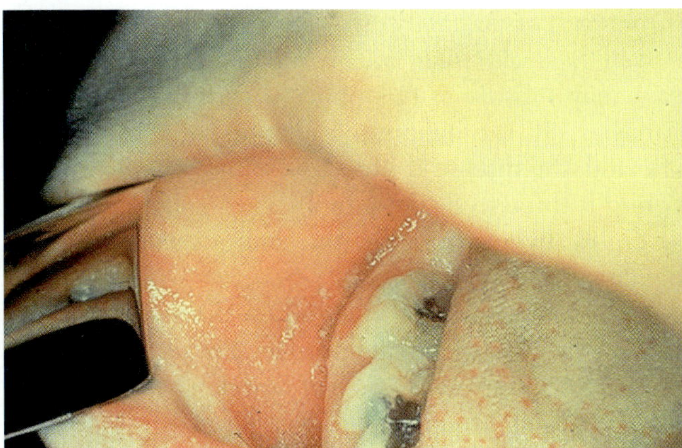

Figure 23–2 Koplik's spots in rubeola. (Courtesy of the Centers for Disease Control and Prevention [CDC].)

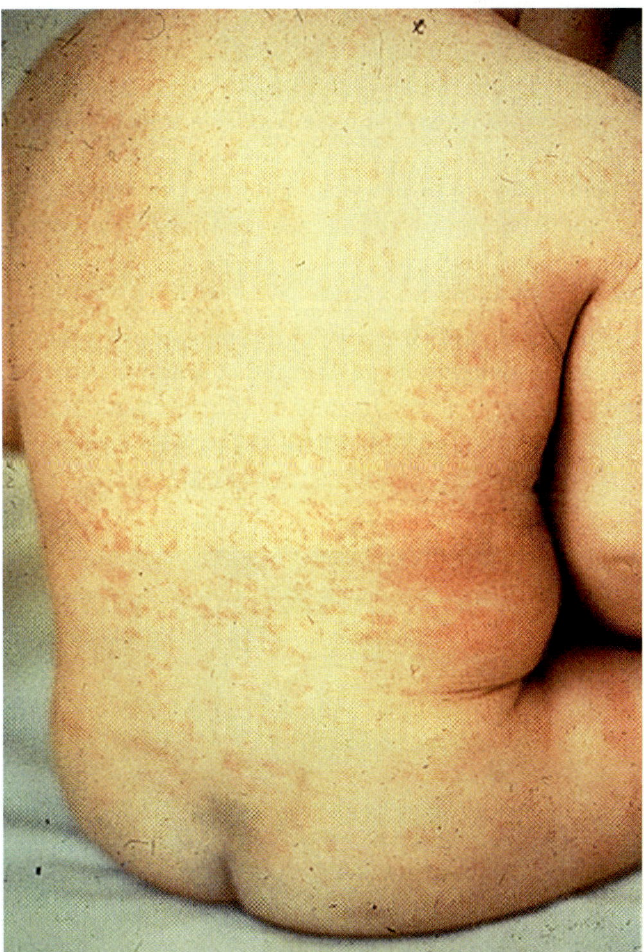

Figure 23–3 Rubella rash. (Courtesy of the Centers for Disease Control and Prevention [CDC].)

ear pain, and swelling of the parotid glands (one or both) (Figure 23–4). It is transmitted by airborne droplets and secretions of saliva. Treatment varies with the severity of the symptoms but is usually palliative (soothing or relieving symptoms). Complications of mumps includes **orchitis** (or-KYE-tis; inflammation of a testis) in males, and nerve conduction deafness. Although neither is common, they are a concern when mumps is diagnosed. Orchitis could result in sterility. All children should be immunized to prevent mumps.

Varicella. Varicella, more commonly known as chickenpox, is the result of infection with the varicella-zoster virus. This virus has an incubation period of ten to twenty-one days. Varicella can be transmitted by airborne particles or direct contact. It is one of the most common childhood infectious diseases. Symptoms of varicella include a macular rash over the face, trunk, and extremities (Figure 23–5). The rash may be quite limited or very widespread. The rash spots develop into **vesicles** (VES-ih-kuls; blister-like eruptions on the skin) in a few days causing intense itching. The vesicles break, dry, and become crusty. Treatment is usually symptomatic with care taken to prevent a secondary skin infection at the sites of the lesions. A vaccine has been available in the United States for several years and some pediatricians are recommending varicella vaccination to their patients.

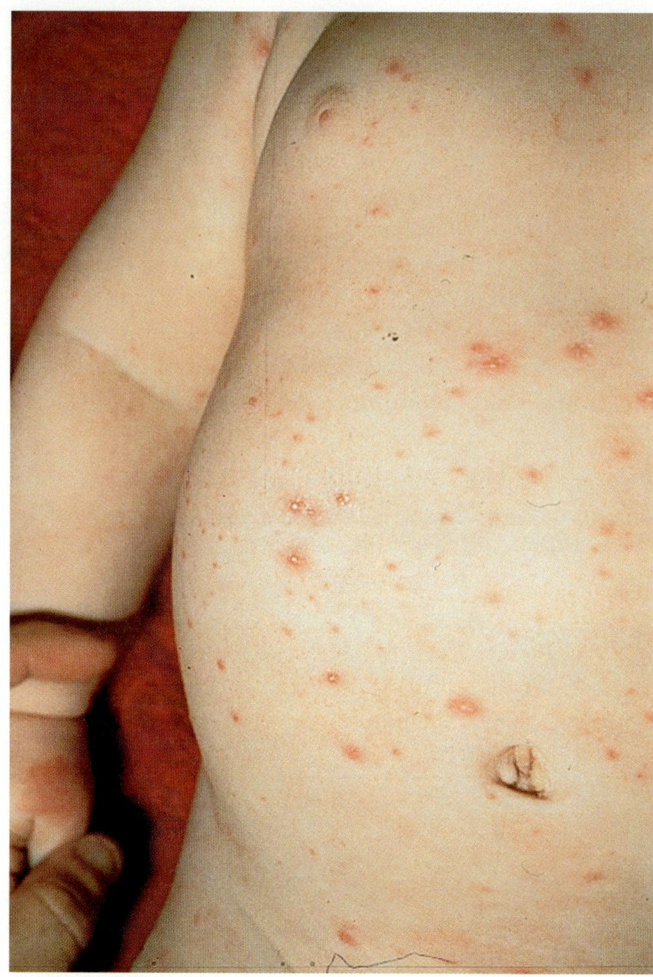

Figure 23–5 Macular rash in varicella. (Courtesy of Robert A. Silverman, MD, Clinical Associate Professor, Department of Pediatrics, Georgetown University.)

Poliomyelitis. Poliomyelitis, also called polio, is caused by the polio virus. It is spread through an oral route or fecal-oral route from an infected individual. Abortive poliomyelitis is a mild form of the disease that does not affect the central nervous system. In the more severe form of polio, early symptoms include fever, headache, sore throat, and abdominal pain. This may progress to stiffness of the neck, trunk, and extremities. Although the disease may subside at this point, it can also progress to paralysis. If the respiratory center of the brain is affected, the disease is life-threatening. The incubation period is three to six days for abortive poliomyelitis and seven to twenty-one for the more severe form of poliomyelitis.

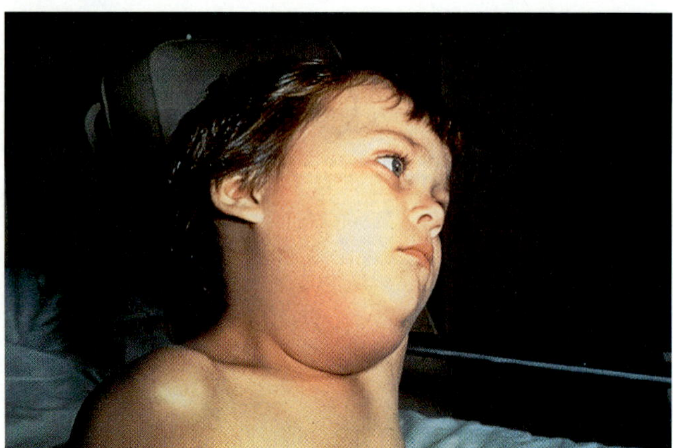

Figure 23–4 Mumps (parotitis). (Courtesy of the Centers for Disease Control and Prevention [CDC].)

Treatment of polio is based on the symptoms and severity but is usually supportive. Physical therapy is important to prevent wasting of muscles. Ventilator support is needed if the respiratory center is affected. Forty years of an aggressive immunization program in the United States has significantly reduced the threat of polio. However, it could still recur as a major health problem, so all children should be vaccinated against polio.

Influenza. Influenza, or the "flu," is an acute infectious respiratory disease. It is caused by viruses in the orthomyxovirus family. Influenza is characterized by chills, fever, headache, joint or muscle aches, runny nose, and a dry cough. It often develops very quickly, and in epidemic proportions in some communities. Very young children or children with other debilitating illnesses are at risk for severe illness. Generally, treatment in children is symptomatic with rest, hydration, and antipyretics if needed. Antiviral drugs may be given for some types of influenza. The American Association of Pediatrics recommends influenza vaccination for children aged 6 months to 16 years who either have chronic health conditions or are at risk for influenza infection. A new nasal spray vaccine is expected to be available in the near future, reducing the number of shots children at risk will receive for vaccination.

Common Cold. The common cold is one of the most frequently occurring diseases. There are numerous strains of viruses that can cause the common cold but the rhinoviruses are usually the causative agent. It is transmitted by direct contact and droplet contact. Good hand washing is the best preventive strategy for transmission of the cold virus. Symptoms of the common cold include **rhinitis** (RYE-**NIGH**-tis; inflammation of the nasal mucous membrane), nasal discharge, coughing, sneezing, fever, and watery eyes. Treatment is directed at symptom relief, getting adequate rest, hydration, and good nutrition.

Mononucleosis. Infectious mononucleosis is a condition where there are abnormally large numbers of mononuclear leukocytes in the circulating blood. Most cases of mononucleosis are caused by the Epstein-Barr virus but it can be caused by other viruses. The incubation period may be as long as four to seven weeks. Symptoms include sore throat, fever, malaise, fatigue, and enlarged lymph nodes. Treatment is directed at relief of symptoms. Rest and hydration are important.

Acquired Immunodeficiency Syndrome. Acquired immunodeficiency disease, commonly known as AIDS, has now affected thousands of children in the United States. It is caused by the human immunodeficiency virus (HIV). Early cases of pediatric AIDS involved children who received the HIV virus by blood transfusion. Many of these children had hemophilia and received transfusions or other blood products. Today, there are many more children diagnosed with an HIV infection or AIDS who were born with the infection as a result of maternal-fetal transfer through the blood. In addition, there are some cases in which HIV or AIDS was transmitted to them through sexual abuse. There are also increasing numbers of sexually active teens being diagnosed with HIV/AIDS.

The period of time between the HIV infection and development of AIDS is much shorter in infants and toddlers than in infected older children or adults. Many children do not experience symptoms of the disease and live a normal life for years. However, in those with severely compromised immune systems, opportunistic infections can be overwhelming, necessitating repeated hospitalizations to sustain life. Treatment of pediatric HIV infection and AIDS varies with the child and the severity of the symptoms. Therapy focuses on prevention and treatment of opportunistic diseases, good nutrition, antiviral drugs, and other support therapies as needed.

Bacterial Diseases

Bacterial diseases of childhood are caused by pathogens. There are millions of bacteria in the world, but not all bacteria are pathogenic (see Chapter 4 for more information). Some of the common infection-causing bacteria include *Staphylococcus, Clostridium, Haemophilus, E. coli*, and *Streptococcus*. Symptoms of bacterial infections may include coughing, fever, headache, difficulty breathing, and sore throat. Treatment is based on the causative agent, along with relief of symptoms. Some bacterial diseases can be prevented by immunizations.

Pertussis. Pertussis, also known as whooping cough, is an acute respiratory infection caused by *Bordetella pertussis*. It is characterized by (1) a **catarrhal** (inflammation of mucous membranes of head and mouth with increased mucous flow) stage, including cough, runny nose, and low-grade fever, (2) a **paroxysmal** (PAR-ock-**SIZ**-mal; spasm or convulsion) stage, including violent "whooping" coughing, cyanosis, distended neck veins, and some vomiting, and (3) a convalescent stage, including some periods of the "whooping" coughing but with gradually less frequent episodes. The incubation period is six to ten days but may be as long as twenty-one days.

Pertussis is transmitted by direct contact with respiratory droplets. It is treated with antibiotics and supportive therapy. Pneumonia is the most common complication of pertussis and can be life-threatening. All children should be immunized to prevent pertussis. Infants, prior to receiving vaccinations, are not immune to pertussis so it is a serious threat in this population.

Diphtheria. Diphtheria is an infectious disease caused by *Corynebacterium diphtheriae* and characterized by severe inflammation of the respiratory system. It produces a membranous coating of the pharynx, nose, and sometimes the tracheobronchial tree. This membrane becomes a thick fibrinous **exudate** (ECKS-you-dayt; fluid composed of protein and white blood cells that seeps from tissue) causing extreme difficulty breathing. The toxin can also produce degeneration in peripheral nerves, heart muscle, and other tissues. It is transmitted by direct contact with droplets from an infected person. The incubation period is two to five days. Treatment includes antibiotic therapy and diphtheria antitoxin. At one time, diphtheria had a high fatality rate, especially in children, but that is rare now. All children should be immunized to prevent diphtheria.

Tuberculosis. Tuberculosis (TB) is an infectious disease caused by the tubercle bacillus, *Mycobacterium tuberculosis*. For many years, the incidence of tuberculosis was decreasing, but in just the last few years it has been on the rise. Although the disease typically affects the respiratory system, it can also be found in the gastrointestinal system, the bones, brain, and lymph nodes. Tuberculosis is transmitted by contaminated droplets. Once the child is infected with the tubercle bacillus and the incubation period of four to twelve weeks is past, the skin test will be positive. Diagnosis is made by a positive skin test, positive sputum culture, clinical manifestations, and a chest X-ray. Signs and symptoms of TB include a persistent cough, bloody sputum, lymph node enlargement, fever, and malaise. (See Chapter 7 for more information about tuberculosis.)

Most children infected by the bacillus will not develop the symptomatic disease. The greatest percentage of cases of TB infection in children stay **dormant** (state of being inactive) and do not develop into the clinical disease. For those children who develop active tuberculosis, treatment consists of drug therapy, rest, good nutrition, and prevention of spread of the disease to other family members. Children at higher risk for developing TB are those who have other chronic diseases, are HIV positive or have AIDS, are malnourished, living in poor hygienic conditions, living with adults with TB, and/or are immunosuppressed.

Impetigo. Impetigo is a contagious superficial **pyoderma** (PYE-oh-**DER**-mah; inflammatory, purulent dermatitis), caused by *Staphylococcus aureus* or Group A streptococci. It is commonly found on the face in children (Figure 23–6). It is transmitted by direct contact between contaminated hands and the face. Good handwashing is the best preventive strategy, as impetigo is extremely contagious. Antibiotics are effective against impetigo (see Chapter 17 for additional information).

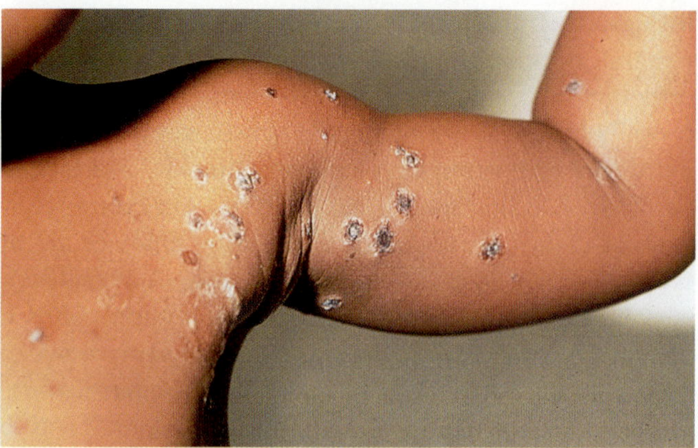

Figure 23–6 Impetigo. (Courtesy of Robert A. Silverman, MD, Clinical Associate Professor, Department of Pediatrics, Georgetown University.)

Otitis Media. Otitis media is an infection of the middle ear and is one of the most common diseases in children under the age of six years. It is believed that most of the cases of otitis media are caused by a virus or allergy and only a small percentage are caused by bacteria. If a bacterial otitis media is left untreated, a chronic infection or damage to the middle ear may result. It is most often diagnosed in very young children, ages six months to three years. Signs and symptoms include pain (in the infant this symptom may be indicated by the child pulling on the ear), fever, drainage, and upon otoscopic examination, a bulging reddish tympanic membrane. Treatment for bacterial otitis includes antibiotic therapy and acetaminophen or ibuprofen for fever and pain. If the condition persists, a myringotomy with tympanoplasty tubes may be the treatment of choice. (See Chapter 18 for more information.)

Fungal Diseases

Fungal diseases are usually seen on the skin or mucous membranes in children. These diseases may be seen in any age, but some, such as candidiasis, are more common in infants than in older children. Most fungal infections are not severe but can be very irritating to the child and need medical intervention to halt the spread of the infection.

Candidiasis. Candidiasis, or thrush, is an oral fungal infection common in infants. It is caused by an excessive growth of *Candida albicans* on the mucous membranes in the mouth. The organism can also cause a diaper rash if it passes through the intestine, since the continually wet diaper area is a good medium for growth of *Candida*. The infant may acquire the infection during delivery, or it may develop later from antibiotic therapy or from the use of unclean nipples on bottles. Diagnosis is made by visual exam of the mouth. White plaques are present on the mucous membranes and the tongue. The treatment of choice is usually swabbing the mouth with oral nystatin suspension.

Tinea. Tinea infections encompass a group of diseases commonly known as ringworm. Tinea capitis (scalp), tinea corporis (face, trunk, and extremities), tinea cruris (groin, buttocks, scrotum, also known as jock itch), and tinea pedis (feet, also known as athlete's foot) are caused by a group of fungi called dermatophytes. These are all common in children, especially tinea capitis. They are transmitted by direct contact, contact with infected articles (such as combs), or contact with infected animals. Tinea infections are usually diagnosed by visual examination. Treatment is usually the application of a topical antifungal agent. (See Chapter 17 for more information.)

Parasitic Diseases

Parasitic diseases include all disorders that are caused by an organism that feeds upon another organism, such as a worm that lives in the intestine of an individual. Parasites are common in areas where poor nutrition, contaminated water, and low socioeconomic conditions are widespread. The parasitic diseases common to children in the United States include giardiasis, pediculosis, and some helminth (worm) infestations.

Pediculosis. Pediculosis is the condition of being infested with lice. Lice are tiny wingless, blood-sucking parasites that are transmitted from human to human by direct contact. The type of lice that lives on human hair and feeds on the scalp is *Pediculosis humanus capitis*. Lice infestations reach epidemic levels in many school systems throughout the United States. Millions of dollars are spent on lice remedies each year. Lice infestations occur in all socioeconomic populations, and are more commonly found in females because they usually have more hair. An adult parasite produces about six eggs every twenty-four hours.

The diagnosis is by visual examination of the scalp and hair. The lice eggs (**nits**) can be seen on the hair shafts (Figure 23–7). Treatment typically involves a shampoo or solution designed to kill and a delousing comb to remove the parasite. Clothes and bedding should be laundered using very hot water and detergent.

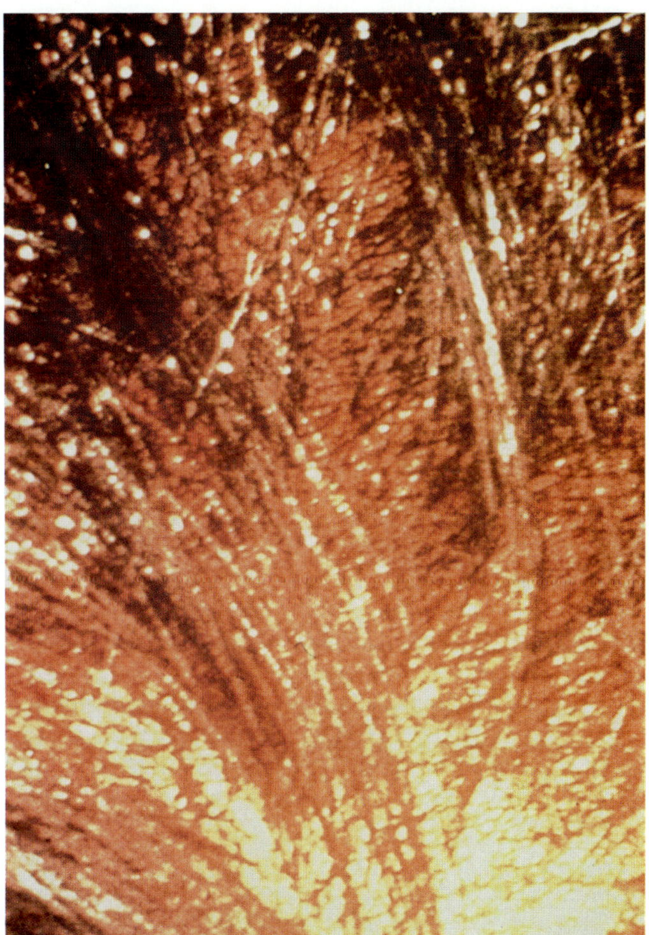

Figure 23–7 Head lice. (Courtesy of Reed and Carnrick Pharmaceuticals.)

RESPIRATORY DISEASES

Respiratory illnesses are the most common childhood diseases seen by physicians. Infants are extremely susceptible to upper respiratory problems since their immune systems are not fully developed. Infants also have very small air passages so even a minor amount of mucus can obstruct a passage and cause respiratory distress. Preschool and school-aged children are very vulnerable to the contagious respiratory diseases since they have a great deal of person-to-person and hand-to-mouth contacts. Several of the viral and bacterial respiratory diseases were covered earlier in this chapter.

Sudden Infant Death Syndrome

Sudden infant death syndrome, or SIDS, is the abrupt unexplained death of an infant under age one. It is also know as crib death since the infant is found dead after being put in bed to sleep. There are several theories about the cause of SIDS but none has been proven at this time.

It is now recommended that infants be placed in bed in the **supine** (SUE-pine; on the back) position rather than **prone** (on the stomach side) since more cases of SIDS have occurred in children lying in the prone position. Children at higher risk for SIDS include those with sleep apnea, siblings of SIDS infants, premature infants, and infants with respiratory problems. Diagnosis may be suspected when the child is brought to the emergency department, but SIDS can only be confirmed by autopsy and investigation. A diagnosis of SIDS is very traumatic to parents and families who experience not only loss and grief but also guilt. Counseling, along with further education, should be available for these families so SIDS might be prevented in future children.

Croup

Croup, also known as laryngotracheobronchitis, is caused by parainfluenza viruses 1 and 2. It is an upper respiratory infection characterized by a harsh barking cough, fever, **inspiratory stridor** (STRYE-dor; high-pitched sound during inspiration caused by blocked airways), laryngeal spasms, and increased difficulty breathing at night. It affects children from three months to three years. Diagnosis is made by physical examination. Complications may be serious if a **patent** (open) airway is not maintained. Emergency treatment for croup includes placing the child in a comfortable position (typically seated), administering blow-by humidified oxygen in small children or by mask in older children, an intramuscular or oral steroid to treat the inflammation, and nebulized racemic epinephrine if the child is not responsive or worsens.

Asthma

Asthma is a serious chronic respiratory system disease of unknown cause. It is characterized by acute episodes of coughing, wheezing, and shortness of breath. It is one of the leading causes of school absence for illness in children today. Approximately sixty-nine of every 1,000 children are affected by asthma and over 4.8 million children under the age of eighteen have been diagnosed with asthma. There are various stimuli (called triggers) of an asthmatic episode. Triggers may include cigarette smoke, dust mites, chemicals, pollen, animal hair and feathers, molds, cold air, and excessive exercise. In spite of the trigger, airway swelling and blockage result, causing the symptoms of respiratory distress.

Diagnosis is made by physical examination, chest X-rays, (although they usually show normal results except in severe cases), pulmonary function studies, and allergy tests. Treatment of asthma in the child includes avoidance of the triggers, medications such as bronchodilators and anti-inflammatory agents, and careful monitoring of the disease. Emergency treatment for a child experiencing an asthma attack is similar to emergency treatment in an adult (see Chapter 7). A peak flowmeter is used to monitor the breathing capacity of the child. This device measures the flow of air in a forced exhalation and reports it in liters per minute. The value of peak expiratory flow indicates the degree of airway obstruction. The data obtained from the peak flowmeter can help identify the onset of an asthmatic episode. The physician may use the information from the chart of measurements kept by the child to prescribe the appropriate medication regimen.

Education of the child and family is very important in effective asthma management programs. Effective management may allow the child to live a normal life with appropriate activity levels, may prevent acute asthmatic attacks, and may help the child avoid hospitalization for severe episodes. (See Chapter 7 for more information on asthma.)

Pneumonia

Pneumonia is an inflammation of the lung parenchyma. It may be of viral or bacterial origin. Pneumonia is characterized by the alveolar air spaces in the lungs being filled with exudate, inflammatory cells, and fibrin. The symptoms include cough, fever, wheezing, and malaise. Diagnosis is made by chest X-ray and auscultation of the chest. Field emergency treatment for a child with suspected pneumonia involves maintaining the airway and ventilation. Treatment is supportive in viral pneumonia but antibiotics may be used in bacterial pneumonia. Viral pneumonia usually runs its course in children in about five to seven days, but bacterial pneumonia may be more severe. (See Chapter 7 for more information.)

Respiratory Failure

Cardiovascular collapse in children under the age of eight is primarily caused by respiratory compromise. This age group is reasonably healthy and does not have the associated cardiovascular disease present in adults, where cardiovascular collapse and arrest is primarily caused by heart disease. Early recognition of respiratory distress allows the EMS provider to intervene earlier and prevent cardiovascular collapse in the majority of pediatric patients. Respiratory distress in children manifests differently from adults. In adults, the patient can usually tell you or a bystander that she is having difficulty breathing. Children, on the other hand, are not able to clearly express that they are having trouble breathing, if at all. The EMS provider must be aware of the signs of respiratory distress and failure, and quickly and accurately assess them in all infants.

The first impression is important in assessing a child. A young child who is sick will not make eye contact with the EMS provider when he or she enters the room. Children are curious about their surroundings and strangers and should at least briefly look at the EMS provider. A young child who is sick will also look sick, will not cry, and will not be active. An infant or young child who is crying and is active is usually doing well enough for the EMS provider to fully assess the situation.

The EMS provider should assess four key areas in determining the respiratory status of a child. These include respiratory rate, respiratory mechanics, air entry, and skin color and temperature. These four areas indicate to the EMS provider how well the child is getting oxygen into the blood. Tachypnea is generally a compensatory mechanism to allow the child to maintain an adequate minute-volume (see Chapter 7 for an explanation of respiratory values) or to compensate for an acid base alteration (Chapter 5). Tachypnea for no apparent reason should be a red flag and the child should be evaluated at the emergency department. A slow or irregular rate is generally a sign of impending respiratory arrest as the child does not have the energy available to breathe. Respiratory mechanics are another indication of the child's level of distress. Normally, the child should be able to breathe comfortably without using his or her accessory muscles. Accessory muscles of respiration include some of the muscles in the neck, abdomen, and between the ribs. These muscles are recruited during distress in an attempt to increase the amount of vacuum in the chest, allowing additional air to flow into the lungs. In severe distress, the child may exhibit intercostal retractions, where the muscles and tissue in between the ribs are drawn in with each breath, or sternal retractions, where the sternum is drawn in with each breath. This is a sign of impending arrest as the child cannot maintain accessory muscle use for an extended period of time before tiring. Air entry is assessed by evaluating the chest expansion and sounds associated with breathing. Breath sounds in children are transmitted easily throughout the chest so it may be difficult to determine if the sounds are decreased or absent over a particular portion of the chest. Stridor indicates a partial obstruction of the upper airway. The skin color and temperature not only indicate how well the child is getting oxygen into the blood but also indicate how well the cardiovascular system is performing to circulate the blood. In addition to the visible areas of skin, the EMS provider should also assess the mucous membranes in the mouth and the skin on the palms of the hand and soles of the feet. A very warm child may be feverish and an infection may be suspected as the cause of distress. A cold child should be warmed and then assessed for skin color.

Management of respiratory failure in children should be aggressive to prevent cardiovascular collapse. The Pediatric Advanced Life Support guidelines published by the American Heart Association outline initial care for the child in distress. Utilize the parents or caregiver by having them hold an oxygen mask near the infant's face to provide blow-by oxygen. Warm the child if he or she is cold and maintain warmth in children who have a normal body temperature. Be careful not to overheat a child that is feverish. Assist ventilations as needed with an appropriately sized bag valve mask with supplemental oxygen. A study published in 2000 in the *Journal of the American Medical Association* suggests that endotracheal intubation of children in the pre-hospital setting does not improve neurological outcome and implies that bag valve mask ventilation with a basic airway adjunct is sufficient for providing assistance to children. You should follow your local protocol and advice of on-line medical control for specific situations in your region.

DIGESTIVE DISEASES

Ingestion, digestion, absorption, and elimination are essential body functions. Children with digestive diseases may experience serious growth and development problems caused by lack of appropriate ingestion, digestion, absorption, or elimination. Fluid and electrolyte imbalances are frequently more severe in children, especially infants, than in adults. The imbalances may be caused by vomiting or diarrhea, or other digestive diseases that inhibit the child's ability to ingest or digest and absorb food and fluids. Other gastrointestinal conditions that are developmental in nature have been covered in Chapter 13.

Fluid Imbalances

Children have a higher metabolic rate than adults and thus have a higher exchange of fluids. This fact puts them at risk for serious complications if they experience bouts of vomiting or diarrhea. They can become dehydrated and be in severe electrolyte imbalance in a very short period of time. Dehydration is life-threatening in very young children and infants. Diagnosis is made by reported history of continued vomiting and/or diarrhea, physical examination, and laboratory data. Treatment focuses on replacement of the fluids and electrolytes. If the child cannot retain fluids because of vomiting, intravenous therapy is necessary. If fluids continue to be lost because of diarrhea, treatment focuses on correcting the cause of the diarrhea, administering medications to prevent the hyperactive bowel problems, and giving replacement fluids and electrolytes either orally or intravenously. Emergency treatment of a dehydrated child includes intravenous administration of a normal saline fluid bolus of 20cc/kg. Non-prescription oral electrolyte solutions are available for infants and young children (Pedialyte, Infanlyte) and for older children (Gatorade). Children who are active in sports in very warm weather should drink electrolyte replacement fluids frequently to prevent dehydration.

CARDIOVASCULAR DISEASES

Most cardiovascular diseases in children are related to genetic or developmental disorders. These are discussed in Chapter 8.

MUSCULOSKELETAL DISEASES

Musculoskeletal disorders in children are common because of their high activity levels and rapid growth patterns. Musculoskeletal problems range from soft tissue injuries and fractures to joint and bone deformities and degenerative muscle disorders. Musculoskeletal developmental disorders are discussed in Chapter 10.

HEMATOLOGIC DISEASES

One of the most common hematologic system disorders in children is leukemia, a type of cancer. Many of the other disorders diagnosed in children are chronic diseases, such as hemophilia and sickle cell disease. These, as well as acute disorders of the blood such as iron deficiency anemia, and some cancers, are discussed in Chapter 16.

Leukemia

Leukemia (leuk = white, emia = blood) is a malignancy of the blood-forming cells located in the bone marrow. It is the most common form of cancer in children. There are approximately 2,500 children diagnosed each year with leukemia (Childhood Leukemia Center, 1998). Leukemia is diagnosed more frequently in boys than in girls. The cause of the disease is unknown but factors that increase the risk for developing leukemia include exposure to radiation and the presence of genetic or immunologic disorders.

The most common type of leukemia in children is acute lymphoblastic leukemia (ALL). It is characterized by a proliferation of white blood cells that are still immature. As the marrow becomes filled with the diseased white cells, platelets, red cells, and healthy white cell production decrease causing symptoms to appear. Symptoms include pallor (pale skin); easy bleeding or bruising; fatigue; joint, bone, or abdominal pain; and fever. Leukemia is diagnosed by medical history, complete blood count, and bone marrow biopsy.

Childhood leukemias are now among the most curable diseases of all types of childhood cancers. Treatment for ALL in children is directed at killing all cancer cells. Chemotherapy is the treatment of choice. Radiation may also be used in some cases. Three or four chemotherapeutic agents are used in the first phase of treatment. Then, other combinations of the chemotherapeutic agents are given to prevent reappearance of the cancer cells. After this initial therapy, the child is placed on a maintenance schedule consisting of daily low-dose chemotherapy medications for two to three years. One of the complications of the therapy is the reduced ability to fight off infections. Children must be carefully monitored and protected during the initial treatment phase.

NEUROLOGIC DISEASES

There are many neurologic disorders in children. Some of them, such as meningitis and encephalitis, are covered in Chapter 9.

Reye's Syndrome

Reye's syndrome is an acute **encephalopathy** (en-SEF-ah-**LOP**-ah-thee; encephalo = brain, opathy = disease; disorder of the brain) seen in children under age fifteen who have had a viral infection. It is characterized by nausea, vomiting, liver enlargement, lethargy, seizures, coma, and in many cases, death. The cause is unknown, but a relationship has been found between the disease and the use of aspirin for febrile illnesses in children. Thus, it is recommended that aspirin not be given to children, but acetaminophen be used instead. Treatment is supportive.

EYE AND EAR DISEASES

Children are curious and use their senses even more than adults during the learning and growing process. Problems with the eyes and ears can have profound effects on the child's ability to learn and develop. Some of the common eye and ear problems are covered in earlier chapters, and in other sections of this chapter.

TRAUMA

Trauma in children is a major cause of disability and death. Child abuse is found at all ages but some types of trauma, such as drug abuse and suicide, are much more common in adolescents. Poisonings are at peak levels in toddlers.

Child Abuse

Child abuse is a serious problem in the United States. It is more common than most other pediatric illnesses and is frequently fatal. It has been difficult to define because "limits" of punishment, such as spanking, are hard to set. However, it is generally defined as purposeful (not accidental), significant, or demonstrable harm to a child. This may be in the form of physical, sexual, or emotional harm. It may also be in the form of neglect, which accounts for a major portion of the child abuse diagnosed. Neglect is defined as failing to provide basic needs, such as food, clothes, and schooling, for the child.

Physical child abuse, and sometimes neglect, is usually diagnosed by physical examination, review of verbal explanations from the child and parents, and investigation by authorities. It may be difficult to diagnose or prove at times because of conflicting stories reported by those involved. Many children try to cover up the abuse because of fear of retaliation by the abuser or because of shame. The most frequent instrument to inflict physical abuse is the hand. Belts, clubs, and other items are also used. Burns by cigarettes are also common, especially in very young children. Fractures in children under age three are suggestive of physical abuse. One of the most common injuries in infants is the shaken baby syndrome. This is a serious injury to the brain caused by vigorous shaking of the child. It may result in death.

Sexual abuse has become an epidemic problem. It is defined by specific acts, and may or may not include intercourse. Unfortunately, sexual abuse of children frequently occurs for years before being reported. The emotional effects are often more serious than the physical effects. The easiest way to identify sexual abuse is to listen to the child, ask open-ended questions, and report suspected abuse to appropriate persons.

Emotional abuse is the most difficult form of child abuse to recognize and diagnose. Constant stigmatizing, berating, or ignoring a child is considered emotional abuse. The effects of this abuse are manifested in symptoms such as failure to thrive, learning disabilities, eating disorders, social isolation, acting out behaviors, depression, and other behavior and personality disorders.

Recognizing child abuse early may save the life of the child. Licensed health care workers, such as physicians and nurses, are considered mandated reporters by most states where statutes exist that require these individuals to report suspected cases of child abuse to a state supported hotline and protect the reporter from any litigation from the report. The state is responsible for investigating the report, not the health care worker. Some states extend the mandated reporter status to EMS providers. Check with your local or state EMS authority to determine if you are a mandated reporter. When treating a child you suspect has been abused, do not confront the parents with your suspicions. Collect as much information as possible and report your findings to the emergency department staff. Confronting the parents about possible abuse may actually put the child's life in increased danger. You should discreetly alert the emergency department staff to your suspicion of abuse and call your state's abuse hotline to report the incident.

Suicide

Suicide was sixth in the ranking of cause of death for five- to fourteen-year-olds and third in the ranking of cause of death for fifteen- to twenty-four-year-olds in 1997. There were 233 suicides per 100,000 males aged five to fourteen and 3,559 per 100,000 males aged fifteen to twenty-four in 1997 (National Center for Health Statistics, 2001). The incidence is much lower for females of the same ages but is still significant. The suicide rate for males has increased significantly in the last two decades. It is thought that most teens who commit suicide do so during or immediately after a period of depression. The depression may be caused by a variety of factors, such as low self-esteem, chemical abuse, sociological make-up, family problems, and/or abuse. Alcohol abuse has also been found to be a contributing factor, as are other risky behaviors such as drug abuse and gang membership. Suicide attempts are highest in incarcerated youths. Females have a higher rate of suicide ideation and attempts than males, but a much lower incidence of death. Sexual abuse also contributes to suicide ideation and suicide attempts. Some children have been involved in suicide "pacts" with others but this is not common. Gay and bisexual youths have a higher suicide rate than heterosexual youths of the same age.

Early intervention is the key to preventing suicides in children. Recognition of problems in adolescents and involvement in treatment programs is imperative. Even casual statements about death or killing oneself need to be taken seriously by parents, counselors, teachers, and friends. These youths need to be referred to special counseling programs as soon as possible. In addition, early intervention in dysfunctional families, and prevention of sexual abuse, alcohol and drug abuse is extremely important.

Poisoning

Accidental poisoning can occur when a child ingests medications, cleaning products, alcohol, cosmetics, or other toxins. Parents and other adults frequently fail to recognize how toxic certain substances can be or do not even think about the consequences of leaving them in places accessible to children. Accidental poisoning is among the top five causes of death in children under ten years of age. About three-fourths of all poisonings occur in children under six years of age. Children are inquisitive and tend to put things in their mouths, a devastating consequence when the substance is toxic. Most poisonings are caused by common substances found in the home, such as cleaning products, medicines, and plants. Generally, the poisoning is an acute event and treatment is provided at a physician's office or emergency room. Symptoms and treatment depend on the substance ingested. With other substances, for example lead, toxicity builds up over a period of time because of chronic exposure. Lead poisoning in children may cause neurologic symptoms, chronic anemia, or difficulty with coordination. The diagnosis is made by checking the blood for lead levels. Chelation therapy treatment is instituted to remove the lead from the blood.

There are poison control centers in every state, most with an 800 number to call for emergency information in case of an accidental poisoning. Many local emergency departments have access to a toxicology database that advises emergency care workers on the signs, symptoms, and treatment for many household products, industrial products, and medications. Medical control should be contacted once the primary survey is completed to receive further instruction on handling a particular substance. Medical control will advise you whether or not to induce vomiting or administer activated charcoal, depending upon your local protocol and the ingested substance. Many products should not be vomited by the child because they are caustic and can do further damage if treated in that manner. All individuals should be aware of the problem of poisoning and prevent poisonings in the home by following a few guidelines as stated in Healthy Highlight 23–1.

Assessment and treatment for specific substances commonly seen in pre-hospital emergency care are discussed in Chapter 15.

HEALTHY HIGHLIGHT 23–1

Preventing Poisonings in Children

Medication Safety:

- Store all medications—prescription and nonprescription—in a locked cabinet, far from children's reach.
- Never leave vitamin bottles, aspirin bottles, or other medications on the kitchen table, countertops, bedside tables, or dresser tops. Small children may decide to emulate adults and help themselves.
- Don't ever tell a child that medicine is "candy."
- Take special precautions when you have houseguests. Be sure their medications are far from reach, preferably locked in one of their bags.
- Don't keep aspirin or other medicines in a pocketbook; children may find them when searching for gum or a toy.
- Child-resistant packaging does not mean childproof packaging. Don't rely on packaging to protect your children.
- Never administer medication to a child in the dark: you may give the wrong dosage or even the wrong medication.
- After taking or administering medication, be sure to reattach the safety cap, and store the medication away safely.

(continues)

HEALTHY HIGHLIGHT 23-1 *(continued)*

Preventing Poisonings in Children

Chemical Safety:

- Store household cleaning products and aerosol sprays in a high cabinet far from reach. Don't keep any cleaning supplies under the sink, including dishwasher detergent and dishwashing liquids.
- Never put cleaning products in old soda bottles or containers that were once used for food.
- When cleaning or using household chemicals, never leave the bottles unattended if there is a small child present.
- Never put roach powders or rat poison on the floors of your home.
- Keep hazardous automotive and gardening products in a securely locked area in your garage.
- Don't leave alcoholic drinks where children can reach them. Take special care during parties—guests may not be conscious of where they've left their drinks. Clean up promptly after the party.
- Keep bottles of alcohol in a locked cabinet far from children's reach.
- Keep mouthwash out of the reach of children. Many brands of mouthwash contain substantial amounts of alcohol.

Lead Paint:

- If you have an older home, have the paint tested for lead.
- If an older house underwent major renovation, the soil around the home may also need to be tested for lead.
- Have your child tested for lead after his or her second birthday.
- Do not use cribs, bassinets, highchairs, painted toys, or toy chests made before 1978; these may have a finish that contains dangerously high levels of lead.

Other Toxic Items:

- Never leave cosmetics and toiletries within easy reach of children. Be especially cautious with perfume, hair dye, hair spray, nail and shoe polish, and nail polish remover.
- Learn all the names of the plants in your house, and remove any that could be toxic.
- Discard used button-cell batteries safely, and store any unused ones far from children's reach (alkaline substances are poisonous).

SUMMARY

Childhood is a time for rapid growth and development—physically, emotionally, and intellectually. Some childhood diseases can interfere with normal growth and development, but most are acute illnesses that are common among young people. The most common diseases in children are infectious respiratory illnesses. Following a regularly scheduled immunization program can prevent many of the infectious diseases of children. Individuals with congenital disorders, premature infants, and children in low socioeconomic households are at highest risk for contracting one of the common childhood diseases. Trauma affects children of all ages, races, and socioeconomic status, and is one of the leading causes of disability and death in children.

REVIEW QUESTIONS

Short Answer

1. What are the most common diseases affecting children?

2. What are the common signs and symptoms of these diseases?

3. What are the signs and symptoms of otitis media?

4. Tuberculosis is found in which body system?

5. What is the difference between anorexia nervosa and bulimia?

6. What are the four types of child abuse?

7. How do children contract HIV?

8. What is the most common type of cancer diagnosed in children?

9. What is a mandated reporter?

10. At what age are children at greatest risk for ingesting a poisonous substance?

CASE STUDY

You respond to a call at 1:00 A.M. for an 18-month-old male child who is having difficulty breathing. According to the parents, he "had a cold" recently and has been warm but they do not have a thermometer to measure his temperature. You find the child in his father's arms appearing sick and pale. The toddler does not make eye contact with you and is using his accessory muscles to breathe. When he coughs, it sounds like a seal barking. What signs would indicate impending respiratory failure? How would you manage this patient? What do you think is the most likely cause for his illness?

BIBLIOGRAPHY

American Heart Association. (1997). Chapter 2: Recognition of respiratory failure and shock. *Pediatric Advanced Life Support.*

Anemia alert. (1997). *Parents, 72*(9), 43–45.

Bar-Or, O. (1998). Physical activity, genetic, and nutritional considerations in childhood weight management. *Medicine and Science in Sports and Exercise, 30*(1), 2–10.

Bouchard, C. (1997). Obesity in adulthood—the importance of childhood and parental obesity. *The New England Journal of Medicine, 337*, 926–927.

Byrne, J. (1998). Genetic disease in offspring of long-term survivors of childhood and adolescent cancer. *American Journal of Human Genetics, 62*(1), 45–52.

Centers for Disease Control and Prevention. (1997). Classification System for HIV Infection in Children Under 13, *Mortality and Morbidity Weekly Report, April 24, 1987, 36*(15), 225–230, 235–236. *http://www.cdc.gov/epo/mmwr/preview/mmwrhtml/00033741.htm*

Childhood Leukemia Center. (1998). *http://www.patientcenters.com/leukemia/leukfaq.html*

Davis, H. P. (1997). Childhood idiopathic thrombocytopenic purpura. *Lancet, 350*, 1252–1253.

Day, M. (1997). Born wheezers. *New Scientist, 156*, 14.

Diagnosing childhood cancer. (1997). *American Family Physician, 56*, 2127.

Dibenedetto, S.P. (1997). Residual clones in childhood leukemia. *The New England Journal of Medicine, 337*, 50–51.

FDA to require pediatric data prior to approvals. (1997). *Public Health Reports, 112*(6), 449.

Gausche, M., Lewis, R. J., Stratton, S. J., Haynes, B. E., Gunter, C. S., Goodrich, S. M., Poore, P. D., McCollough, M. D., Henderson, D. P., Pratt, F. D., & Seidel, J. S. (2000). Effect of out-of-hospital pediatric endotracheal intubation on survival and neurological outcome: a controlled clinical trial. *Journal of the American Medical Association*, 283(6), 783–790.

Goldman, L. R. (1997). Information, the key to preventing childhood lead poisoning. *Journal of Environmental Health, 59*(5), 45–46.

Inlen, L. J. (1997). Infection and childhood leukemia near nuclear sites. *Lancet, 349*, 1702.

Kher, U. (1998). Roaches cause asthma. *Discover, 19*(1), 58.

Lanphear, B. P. (1998). Environmental exposures to lead and urban children's blood lead levels. *Environmental Research Section A, 76*(2), 120–130.

MacKenzie, D. (1997). Vaccine failure. *New Scientist, 156*, 5.

Magrath, I. (1997). Limiting therapy for limited childhood non-Hodgkin's lymphoma. *The New England Journal of Medicine, 337*, 1304–1306.

McCarthy, M. (1997). Shorter treatment proposed for non-Hodgkin's lymphoma. *Lancet, 350*, 1373.

McGill, H. C. (1997). Childhood nutrition and adult cardiovascular disease. *Nutrition Reviews, 55*(1) pt. 2, S2–S11.

Mirza, N. M. (1997). Risk factors for diarrheal duration. *American Journal of Epidemiology, 146*, 776–785.

National Center for Health Statistics. (2001). *http://www.cdc.gov/nchswww/fastats/*

Platts-Mills, T. A. (1997). Rise in asthma cases. *Science 278*, 1001.

Salladay, S. A. (1997). Pediatric AIDS patient: Waiting for pain relief. *Nursing, 97 27*(2), 20–21.

Sears, M. R. (1997). Epidemiology of childhood asthma. *Lancet, 350*, 1015–1020.

Seppa, N. (1997). Smoke hurts kids' cholesterol status. *Science News, 152*, 223.

Smyth, A. (1997). Rickets and childhood pneumonia. *Lancet, 350*, 811.

Stoddard, J. J. (1997). Maternal smoking and medical expenditures for childhood respiratory illness. *American Journal of Public Health, 87*(2), 205–209.

Tips and timesavers for pediatric patient care. (1997). *Nursing 97, 27*(11), 51–53.

The dark side of immunizations? (1997). *Science News, 152, 332–333.*

The far-out flu. (1998). *Working Mother, 21*(2), 80.

Vaccine tracker. (1997). *Parents, 72*(11), 55.

Wallace, S. J. (1997). First tonic-clonic seizures in childhood. *Lancet, 349*, 1009–1012.

Wiant, C. J. (1997). Protecting the children. *Journal of Environmental Health, 60*(12), 37.

Glossary

abdominocentesis (ab-DOM-ih-no-sen-**TEE**-sis) paracentesis of the abdomen; a procedure in which a puncture is made into the abdominal cavity to withdraw fluid.

abortion the spontaneous or induced termination of a pregnancy.

abrasion a scraping away of skin surface.

abruptio placenta premature separation of the placenta from the wall of the uterus.

abscess a localized collection of pus.

absorption route of entry by which a poison is taken into the skin.

achlorhydria (a-klor-HIGH-dree-ah) absence of hydrochloric acid.

acid a substance that donates hydrogen ions.

acid-base balance the homeostasis of hydrogen ion concentration in body fluids.

acid-base buffer system a solution containing two or more chemical compounds that prevents marked changes in hydrogen ion concentration when either an acid or a base is added to a solution.

acidosis the state of the body when the number of free hydrogen ions increases to the point that the pH value becomes less than 7.35.

acute (a-CUTE) a disease that is short term.

addiction a physical and or psychological dependence on a substance.

Addison's disease hypoadrenalism; an uncommon undersecretion of hormones by the adrenal cortex.

adenoma (AD-eh-NO-ma; adeno = gland, oma = tumor) a tumor of glandular tissue.

adhesion (ad-HE-zhun) part of tissue that clings to the surface of adjoining organs as normal fibrous scar tissue develops in an operative site, resulting in a fibrous band.

affect outward expression of emotions.

afterload the amount of force the ventricle must overcome in order to provide blood flow through the circulatory system.

agonal respirations an abnormal respiratory pattern consisting of slow, shallow, irregular and, sometimes, gasping respirations.

AIDS acquired immunodeficiency syndrome.

albumin (al-BYOU-men) a blood protein distributed throughout the body; responsible for osmotic pressure of the blood.

alburninuria (al-BYOU-mih-**NEW**-ree-ah; albumin = a blood protein, uria = urine) albumin in the urine; usually albumin but may also be globulin; usually indicative of a disease process.

alkalemia blood that is alkalotic.

alkalosis the state of the body when the number of free hydrogen ions decreases to the point that the pH value becomes greater than 7.45.

alleles matched pairs of genes; the term used to refer to the product when the chromosomes (one from each parent) pair up during fertilization of the egg, the genes on the chromosomes align.

allergen the environmental substance that causes a reaction.

allergy the state when the immune response is too intense or hypersensitive to an environmental substance.

alopecia (AL-oh-**PEE**-shee-ah; in Greek, meaning fox mange, which caused hair loss) a partial or complete hair loss usually from the head.

amnesia (am-NEE-zee-ah) loss of memory.

amylase an enzyme; often elevated in pancreatic disorders.

anaerobic (an = without, aerobic = air) living without oxygen.

analgesia the absence of pain sensation.

anaphylaxis (AN-ah-fih-**LACK**-sis) an immediate and extreme allergic reaction characterized by contraction of smooth muscle and dilation of capillaries leading to severe respiratory distress or failure.

anaplastic (AN-ah-**PLAST**-ic) abnormal tissue, the more undifferentiated tissue.

androgens hormones secreted by the adrenal cortex responsible for male characteristics.

anemia (ah-NEE-me-ah; an = without, emia = blood) a condition of low numbers of red blood cells in the blood.

angiogenesis (AN-jee-oh-**JEN**-eh-sis; angio =vessel, genesis = formation) new growth of blood vessels.

angiography (AN-jee-**OG**-rah-fee; angio = vessel, graphy = procedure to record) a radiographic study of blood vessels after injection of fluorescein dye.

angioplasty (AN-jee-oh-**PLAS**-tee; angio = vessel, plasty = surgical repair) a procedure that involves passing a catheter into the artery, inflating a balloon on the catheter to push the plaque against the vessel wall thus widening the lumen of the vessel.

anomaly (ah-NOM-ah-lee) any abnormality.

anorexia nervosa (AN-oh-**RECK**-see-ah; an = without, orexia = appetite) a disorder of self-imposed starvation resulting from a distorted body image.

anoxia (ah-NOCK-see-ah) no oxygen.

antibody(ies) immunoglobulins that develop in response to an antigen; also called immune bodies, proteins that the body produces to react to and render the antigen harmless.

anticholinergic toxidrome agents that bind to acetylcholine and block action of the neurotransmitter on the autonomic nervous system.

antigen(s) (AN-tih-jens) a cell marker that induces a state of sensitivity after coming in contact with an antibody; any substance that causes the body some type of harm thus setting off this specific reaction.

antipyretics (anti = against, pyretic = fever) a class of medications given to reduce an elevated temperature.

anuria (ah-NEW-ree-ah; an = without, uria = urine) no urine output.

apnea (ap-NEE-ah; a = without, pnea = breathing) the condition of not breathing; a term used to describe the absence of respirations for a period of time.

apoptosis process of programmed cellular suicide.

arterial blood gas (ABG) the laboratory test that measures the amounts of oxygen and carbon dioxide and the level of acidity of arterial blood.

articular relating to a joint surface.

articular fracture one that involves a joint surface.

ascites (ah-SIGH-teez) fluid in the abdomen (peritoneal cavity).

asymptomatic (a = without, symptomatic = symptoms) not displaying symptoms.

atresia the congenital absence or closure of a normal opening or lumen in the body; it may occur in a variety of areas.

atrophy (AT-tro-fee) a decrease in cell size, which leads to a decrease in the size of the tissue and organ.

audiometry (AW-dee-**OM**-eh-tree; audio = sound, metry = measure) the basic test used to measure hearing.

aura symptom occurring at the onset of a partial epileptic seizure or migraine headache; it may include tingling of the fingers, ringing in the ears, and visual disturbances.

auscultation (AWS-kul-**TAY**-shun) using a stethoscope to listen to body cavities and organs.

autodigestion autolysis or digestion of self or one's own cells.

autoimmunity or **autoimmune** the state when the immune response attacks its own self.

autolysis process of self digestion.

autosome (auto = self, some = body) a chromosome other than a sex chromosome; they determine body function.

avulsion skin pulled or torn away.

avulsion fracture one where there is a separation of a small bone fragment from the bone where a tendon or ligament is attached.

bacteria a one-celled microorganism that may be aerobic or anaerobic and free-living, saprophytic, parasitic, or pathogenic.

base a substance that accepts hydrogen ions.

Bence Jones protein a special protein found in the blood and urine indicative of multiple myeloma.

benign (beh-NINE) having a limited growth, noncancerous.

bimanual examination (bi = two, manual = handed) an examination in which the physician places one hand on the abdomen and inserts fingers of the other hand into the vagina in order to feel the female organs between the two hands.

biopsy (BYE-op-see) removing a small piece of tissue for microscopic examination.

Biot's respiration an abnormal respiratory pattern with an irregular rate, and volume with intermittent periods of apnea.

bleeding time a test to determine the length of bleeding time or time it takes the blood to clot.

blood urea nitrogen (BUN) a test to determine the level of urea nitrogen or waste in the blood.

bloody show cervical secretion of blood stained mucous.

Boyle's law the pressure of a gas multiplied by its volume is equal to a constant number.

bradypnea a respiratory rate slower than normal.

Braxton Hicks contractions irregular, intermittent contractions felt by the pregnant woman toward the end of pregnancy.

bronchoscopy (brong-KOS-koh-pee; broncho = bronchus or lung passageways, oscopy = procedure to look into) a diagnostic or surgical procedure in which a scope is passed through the mouth into the bronchus.

bronchospasm (BRONG-ko-**SPA**-zm) muscular constriction of the bronchi of the respiratory tract.

buccal smear a test for evaluating chromosomes; this test is performed by obtaining squamous epithelial cells from the buccal cavity, staining the cell, and microscopically observing for X chromosomes called Barr bodies.

bulimia (byou-LIM-ee-ah) an eating disorder characterized by episodes of binge eating (an intake of approximately 50,000 calories in one to two hours) followed by activities to negate the calorie intake or purging.

cachexia (ca-KACK-see-ah) a term used to describe any individual who has an ill, thin, wasted appearance.

cancer a malignant tumor.

caput medusae tortuous, unsightly varicosities spreading from the umbilicus outward across the front of the abdomen.

carcinogen (kar-SIN-oh-jen) cancer causing agent or substance.

carcinogenesis (KAR-sin-oh-**JEN**-eh-sis) cancer development.

carcinoma (KAR-sih-**NO**-mah) the most common type of malignant neoplasm arising from epithelial tissue.

carcinoma in situ atypical cells residing in the epithelial layer of tissue, not having broken through the basement membrane and invading other local tissues.

cardiac catheterization (KATH-eh-ter-eye-**ZAY**-shun) an invasive procedure used to sample the blood in the chambers of the heart to determine the amount of oxygen content and blood pressure in the chambers.

cardiac output the amount of blood the heart pumps out of the left ventricle every minute.

cardiac palpitations an unusually strong, rapid, or irregular heart rate that is so abnormal the individual is aware or "can feel" it.

cardiogenic shock inability of the heart to pump enough blood to maintain blood pressure.

carotid endarterectomy (END-ar-ter-**ECK**-toh-me; endo = inside, arter = artery, ectomy = excision of) surgical intervention to remove plaque in the carotid arteries to improve blood flow and reduce the risk of a thrombus.

catarrhal (ka-TAR-all) inflammation of mucous membranes of head and mouth with increased mucus flow.

catheterization (KATH-er-ter-eye-**ZAY**-shun) a sterile procedure consisting of passing a soft catheter through the urethra and into the bladder for the purpose of (1) instilling or pouring fluids or medication into the bladder or (2) removing urine.

causal risk factor a risk factor that directly contributes to the development of a disease.

cauterization (KAW-ter-eye-**ZAY**-shun) the electrical burning of tissue to stop bleeding; used most frequently during surgery to stop bleeding from vessels.

cellulitis (SELL-you-LYE-tis) inflammation of connective tissue.

central neurogenic hyperventilation an abnormal respiratory pattern in which volume and rate are increased.

cephalalgia (SEF-ah-**LAL**-jee-ah; cephal = head, algia = pain) headache.

cephalopelvic disproportion inability of the fetal head to fit through the mother's pelvis.

cerumen (se-ROO-men) ear wax.

cervicitis (SER-vih-SIGH-tis) inflammation of the cervix.

chancre (SHANG-ker) a painless, highly contagious lesion occurring in the primary stage of syphilis.

chemotaxis the movement of cells or organisms in response to chemicals.

chemotherapy utilizing pharmacologic therapy in the treatment of cancer.

Cheyne-Stokes respiration an abnormal respiratory pattern in which the ventilation rate gradually increases, peaks than gradually decreases.

cholecystectomy (KOH-lee-sis-**TECK**-toh-me; chole = gall or bile, cyst = bladder, ectomy = removal) surgical removal of the gallbladder.

cholinergic toxidrome agents that alter the action of acetylcholine.

chorea (ko-REE-ah) a constant, jerky uncontrollable movement.

chronic a disease that persists for a long time.

chronotropism the rate of myocardial contraction.

circadian rhythm a normal 24 hour cycle of biological rhythms including sleep, metabolism, and glandular secretions.

cirrhosis a chronic, irreversible, degenerative disease of the liver.

clean catch a term used to describe a clean urine collection method involving cleansing the urethal area prior to urinating and catching the voided urine specimen.

closed or simple fracture a fracture that does not break through the skin.

clubbing a condition affecting the distal portion of the finger; characterized by soft tissue enlargement and an abnormal curvature of the nail.

colicky pain a sharp and stabbing or a dull and aching pain that comes and goes in waves.

Colle's fracture a fracture of the lower end of the radius with displacement of the fragment.

colloid protein or non-diffusible substance.

comminuted fracture one in which there are more than two ends or fragments.

co-morbidity chronic conditions that affect the complication rate or mortality rate of a given disease.

compensated shock a state of decreased blood volume for which the body is able to maintain an adequate blood pressure.

complete blood count (CBC) a laboratory test that identifies the number of red blood cells (RBCs), white blood cells (WBCs), and platelets per cubic millimeter.

complete fracture the fracture is completely through the bone.

complication the onset of a second disease or disorder in an individual that is already affected with a disease.

compound (open) fracture a fracture involving the bone puncturing through the skin or an object puncturing the skin making an opening through the skin to the fracture site.

compression fracture one in which the bone appears to be mashed down.

compulsion a repetitive act the affected individual is unable to resist performing.

Computerized Axial Tomography imaging by a cross-sectional plane of the body; also called computed tomography or CT.

conduction heat loss dissipation of heat between two objects that are in contact with one another.

congenital (kon-JEN-ih-tahl) present at birth; usually concerning a congenital anomaly or an abnormality present at birth.

contusion (kon-TOO-zhun) a large bruise.

convection heat loss dissipation of heat caused by air currents flowing over a warmer object.

convulsion an abnormal muscle contraction; a violent spasm or jerking of the face, trunk, or extremities.

corticosteroids (KORT-ti-ko-**STEHR**-oyds) powerful anti-inflammatory hormones.

cortisol hydrocortisone; a steroid hormone secreted by the adrenal cortex.

costovertebral angle tenderness tenderness to percussion along the flank at the angle of the lower ribs, suggestive of kidney inflammation.

creatinine one of the two most common nitrogenous waste products that are normally filtered from the blood, the final product of creatine catabolism.

crowning visual of the head from the birth canal.

crystalloids electrolyte solutions with the potential to form crystals.

culture and sensitivity a test to identify a pathogen and the type of treatment needed.

curative something that corrects or cures the disease or condition.

cyanosis (SIGH-ah-**NO**-sis; cyano = blue, osis = condition) a bluish condition of the skin caused by lack of oxygen in the blood.

cystogram (cysto = bladder, gram = picture) an X-ray picture of the bladder that helps determine the shape and function of the bladder.

cystoscopy (sis-TOS-koh-pee; cysto = bladder, scopy = procedure to look) an invasive procedure to look into the urethra and bladder using a lighted scope.

cytology (SIGH-**TOL**-oh-jee; cyto = cell, logy = study) the examination or study of cells.

cytoplasm the liquid inside the cell.

cytotoxic (cyto = cell, toxic = killing) something that kills cells.

Dalton's law the pressure of a gas that is made up of a mixture of several gasses is the same as the sum of the individual gas pressures if each gas occupies the same volume.

dead space areas in the respiratory system where gas exchange dose not occur.

débridement (day-breed-MON) a process of washing or cutting away necrotic tissue and foreign material.

decompensated shock a state of decreased blood volume for which the body is unable to maintain an adequate blood pressure.

decompression a release of pressure.

defecate to have a bowel movement.

degenerative diseases related to aging, or destruction of tissue, functions, and use.

dehiscence (dee-HISS-ens) separation of tissue margins.

delirium tremens (DTs) (dee-LIR-ee-um TREE-mens) a serious form of delirium caused by alcoholic withdrawal after a period of sustained intoxication that can be life-threatening.

delusions false beliefs that are firmly adhered too although it is not shared by others.

dementia (dee-MEN-she-ah) a loss of mental ability due to the loss of neurons or brain cells.

densitometry measurement of bone thickness.

dependency a psychological craving for a substance that may or may not be accompanied by a physical need.

diabetic retinopathy (DYE-ah-**BET**-ick RET-ih-**NOP**-ah-thee; retino = retina, opathy = disease) disease of the retina of the eye often resulting in blindness; caused by degeneration from diabetes mellitus.

diagnosis (DIE-ag-KNOW-sis) the identification or naming of a disease.

diapedesis (DYE-ah-pe-**DEE**-sis) passage of blood, or its formed elements, through the intact walls of blood vessels.

diastolic (dye-as-TOL-ick) relating to cardiac diastole; the process of the heart resting as the chambers refill with blood.

differential a detailed white blood cell count identifying the number of each type of leukocyte.

differential diagnosis a list of possible conditions that may be responsible for a particular disease or disorder.

differentiation the process of individual specialization of cells.

diffusion continual movement of molecules in a solution or a gas.

digital rectal examination a manual exam in which the physician feels the prostate for abnormal enlargement (hypertrophy or hyperplasia) and tumors.

dilatation and curettage (**KYOU**-reh-TAHZH) **or D&C** a procedure that involves a dilation of the cervix (dilatation) and scraping (curettage) of the uterine endometrial tissue; a D&C is commonly performed for abnormal uterine bleeding and following a spontaneous abortion.

discectomy surgery to remove a vertebral disc.

disease a change in structure or function within the body that is considered to be abnormal or any change from normal.

disorder a derangement or abnormality of function.

displaced fracture one in which fragments are out of position.

dominant in control.

Doppler a device that may be placed over arteries to magnify the sound of blood flow.

dormant state of being inactive.

Dowagers's hump abnormal curvature in upper thoracic spine.

dromotropism the speed of conduction of the electric impulse along the myocardial conduction system.

dry drowning a condition in which laryngospasm closes the lower airways.

dysentery an acute inflammation of the colon or colitis.

dysmenorrhea (DIS-men-oh-**REE**-ah; dys = painful, menorrhea = menses) pain with menstrual periods.

dyspareunia (DIS-pa-**ROO**-nee-ah) painful sexual intercourse.

dysphagia (dis-FAY-jee-ah; dys = difficulty, phagia = swallowing) difficulty swallowing.

dysphasia (dis-FAY-zee-ah; dys = difficulty, phasia = speaking) difficulty speaking.

dysplasia (dis-PLAY-zee-ah) an alteration in size, shape, and organization of cells.

dyspnea (disp-NEE-ah; dys = difficult, pnea = breathing) difficulty breathing.

dystocia long, difficult, or abnormal labor.

dysuria (dis-YOU-ree-ah; dys = difficult or painful, uria = urine) difficulty or pain with urination.

ecchymoses (ECH-ih-**MOH**-ses) large areas of bruising or hemorrhage.

eclampsia (eh-KLAMP-see-ah) a condition of pregnancy characterized by all the symptoms of toxemia or preeclampsia plus the symptoms of convulsions.

ectopic (eck-TOP-ick) out of normal place.

ectopic pregnancy implantation of a fertilized ovum outside the uterus.

edema swelling.

effacement thinning of the cervix.

electrocardiogram (ECG) (ee-LECK-troh-**KAR**-dee-oh-GRAM; electro = electrical, cardio = heart, gram = picture) the graphic drawing produced by an electrocardiograph; a machine that receives electrical information and draws heart action.

electrochemical gradient sum of all the diffusion forces acting on the membrane, from either a concentration gradient or an electrical or pressure gradient.

electrolyte a compound that when dissolved in water or another solvent forms or dissociates into ions.

electromyography (EMG) (ee-LECK-troh-my-o-grah-fee) a diagnostic test in which a small needle is inserted into muscle tissue and the electrical activity is recorded.

embolus (EM-boh-lus) material floating in the blood that may stick in a vessel and occlude or stop blood flow leading to ischemia or death of the organs supplied by that vessel.

empyema (EM-pye-**EE**-mah) an accumulation of pus in a body cavity.

encapsulated enclosed in a capsule.

encephalopathy (en-SEF-ah-**LOP**-ah-thee; encephalo = brain, opathy = disease) any disease or disorder of the brain.

endarterectomy (END-ar-ter-**ECK**-toh-me; endo = inside, arter = artery, ectomy = excision) a surgical procedure involving opening an artery and cleaning out the plaque.

endometritis (EN-doh-me-**TRY**-tis) inflammation of the uterus lining.

endotoxin a component of the cell wall that is antigenic in humans causing an inflammatory response against bacteria.

engagement when the widest diameter of the fetal presenting part enters the inlet to the true pelvis.

enteral relating to the small intestine.

epicanthus a vertical fold of skin across the medial canthus of the eye giving the eyes an Oriental appearance.

epidural hematoma (EP-ih-**DOO**-ral; epi = above, dural = dura, outer meninges) blood collecting between the skull and the dura mater.

epistaxis nose bleed.

erythema (ER-ih-**THEE**-mah) skin redness.

erythrocytopenia (erythrocyte = red cell, penia = decrease) a deficiency of red blood cells.

erythrocytosis (erythrocyte = red cell, osis = condition) a condition of increased red blood cells.

esophageal varices (eh-**SOF**-ah-JEE-al **VAYR**-ih-seez) varicosities (varicose veins) of the esophagus.

estimated date of confinement (EDC) due date.

estrogens hormones responsible for female characteristics.

etiology (ET-tee-**OL**-oh-jee) the study of cause or the cause of a disease.

eukaryotic cells that contain organelles in a membrane.

evaporation heat loss dissipation of heat when energy from a warm object causes liquid on the surface to dissipate into the air.

exacerbation (x-AS-er-**BAY**-shun) a time when symptoms flare up or become worse.

exocrine glands glands that excrete through a duct.

exophthalmos (ECK-sof-**THAL**-mos) abnormal protrusion of the eyeballs.

expiratory reserve the volume of air that can be exhaled during forced exhalation.

exsanguination loss of circulating blood volume.

extracapsular fracture a fracture outside or not involving the joint capsule.

extrinsic pathway a pathway in the coagulation system to activate clot formation.

exudate (ECKS-you-dayt) fluid that has seeped out of tissue or capillaries because of injury or inflammation.

fatal inevitable or causing death.

febrile seizure caused by a sudden rise or fall in body temperature.

femoral neck fracture a fracture involving the neck of the femur.

fetal attitude the relationship of fetal body parts to one another.

fetal lie the relationship of the head to foot axis of the fetus to the cephalocaudal axis of the mother.

fetal presentation determined by fetal lie and the part of the fetus that enters the pelvis first.

fever condition in which the body temperature is above 100 degrees Fahrenheit.

fibrillation (FIH-brih-**LAY**-shun) a heart rhythm that is wild and uncoordinated; a cardiac arrhythmia.

fibrinolysis the process of dissolving old clots after tissue heals.

filtration the movement of fluid through a semipermeable membrane from an area of higher hydrostatic pressure to an area of lower hydrostatic pressure.

FiO_2 the fraction of inspired air that consists of oxygen.

fissure a crack, split, or ulcer-like sore; a groove or slit.

fistula (FIS-tyou-lah) a tract that connects two organs or cavities to each other or to the surface of the skin.

fontanelles membranous areas where the sutures meet.

forced expiratory volume in one second (FEV_1) the volume of air that is forcibly exhaled over a period of one second after full inhalation.

frequency how often the individual is urinating.

frostbite a condition in which there is local tissue damage as a result of exposure to decreased temperatures.

frostnip superficial frostbite.

frozen section a technique that enables a pathologist to make a rapid determination of a tumor condition, either malignant or benign.

fulminant (FULL-ma-nant) occurring suddenly, rapidly, and intensely.

functional reserve capacity the amount of air remaining in the lungs after a normal exhalation.

fundus top of the uterus.

fungi forms of yeast and molds; microscopic plant-like organisms.

gangrene (GANG-green) a condition occurring when saprophytic (dead tissue loving) bacteria become involved in necrotic tissue.

genes the units on the chromosome that carry DNA information.

genotype the genetic pattern of the individual.

germ cells sex cells.

glucagon a hormone secreted by the alpha cells in the islets of Langerhans in the pancreas; responsible for elevating blood glucose concentration.

glucocorticoids a group of steroids of the adrenal cortex that affects metabolism such as causing glycogen storage and causing an anti-inflammatory effect.

glycogen (GLYE-ko-jen) the form that extra sugar is stored in, primarily in the liver.

glycosuria (GLYE-koh-**SOO**-ree-ah; glyco = glycogen or sugar, uria = urine) the "spilling" of sugar in the urine; a common symptom of diabetes mellitus.

goiter (GOI-ter) noticeable protrusion of the thyroid gland.

grading determining the degree of differentiation of cells through microscopic examination.

grand mal a term applied to seizures that are the type most often thought of as epilepsy; these seizures are characterized by convulsions, loss of consciousness, urinary and fecal incontinence, and tongue biting.

gravida total number of times pregnant.

greenstick fracture a common incomplete fracture that occurs in children; it appears to have broken partially like a sap-filled green stick.

gumma (GUM-mah) a characteristic soft gummy lesion caused by bacteria that invade organs throughout the body; found in the tertiary stage of syphilis.

gynecomastia (GUY-ne-koh-**MAS**-tee-ah) abnormal breast enlargement.

hallucinations (hah-LOO-sih-**NAY**-shun) a false sensation of sight, touch, sound, or feel.

hallucinogen a substance that produces a distortion of reality to the extent that the person ingesting the substance believes the distortion to be real.

hallucinosis a state of constant hallucinations.

heat cramps muscle spasms secondary to the loss of electrolytes from exposure to heat.

heat exhaustion a reaction to heat, marked by prostration, weakness, and collapse, caused by severe dehydration and loss of electrolytes.

heat stroke a life-threatening emergency in which body temperature increases to dangerous levels and the body loses the ability to compensate after exposure to heat.

HELLP syndrome pregnancy-induced hypertension (PIH) with liver damage.

helminths intestinal parasites; also called worms; nematodes, cestodes, and trematodes.

hemarthrosis (hem = blood, arthro = joint, osis = condition) bleeding into joints.

hematemesis (HEM-ah-**TEM**-eh-sis; hema = blood, emesis = vomiting) the act of vomiting blood.

hematochezia (HEM-at-toe-**KEE**-zee-ah) bright red blood in the feces.

hematocrit (he-MAT-oh-krit) a measurement of the amount of red cell mass as a proportion of whole blood.

hematoma (HEM-ah-**TOH**-mah) a large tumor or swelling filled with blood also called a bruise or contusion.

hematuria (HEM-ah-**TOO**-ree-ah; hema = blood, uria = urine) blood in the urine.

hemiparesis (HEM-ee-**PAR**-ee-sis; hemi = one half, paresis = paralysis) weakness or paralysis affecting one side of the body.

hemoglobin (Hgb) a measurement of the amount of hemoglobin or oxygen carrying potential available in the blood.

hemolytic (HE-moh-**LIT**-ick) destruction of red blood cells.

hemolyzed broken down cells.

hemoptysis (he-MOP-tih-sis; hemo = blood, ptysis = saliva) coughing up blood.

hemothorax (hemo = blood, thorax = chest) blood in the chest cavity.

Henry's law the amount of a gas that is dissolved in a liquid is proportional to the pressure of the gas.

hepatomegaly (HEP-ah-toh-**MEG**-ah-lee) enlarged liver.

heterozygous (hetero = different, zygo = yoked or paired) having different paired genes.

hirsutism (HER-soot-izm) abnormal hair on the face and body of the female.

histamine a substance that causes local arterioles, venules, and capillaries to dilate resulting in an increase in blood flow to the area; it is released in response to injury or irritation.

holistic medicine the concept considering the whole person rather than just the physical being.

homeostasis (HOME-ee-oh-**STAY**-sis) the state of sameness or normalcy of the internal environment that the body strives to maintain.

homozygous (homo = one, zygo = yoked or paired) having identical genes.

hydrocarbons products manufactured from petroleum products such as gasoline and pesticides.

hydrophobia (hydro = water, phobia = fear) fear of the water.

hydrostatic pressure force a liquid exerts on the sides of the container that holds it.

hypercalcemia an increase in the extracellular level of calcium.

hyperchloremia an increase in the extracellular level of chloride.

hyperemesis gravidarum excessive vomiting during pregnancy.

hyperemia (HIGH-per-**EE**-me-ah; hyper = increased, emia = blood) an increased blood flow in response to a release of histamine.

hyperglycemia (HIGH-per-glye-**SEE**-me-ah; hyper = excessive, glyc = glycogen or glucose, emia = blood) high blood sugar level.

hyperkalemia an increase in the extracellular level of potassium.

hypermagnesemia an increase in the extracellular level of magnesium.

hypernatremia excess in the extracellular level of sodium.

hyperphosphatemia an increase in the extracellular level of phosphorus.

hyperplasia (HIGH-per-**PLAY**-zee-ah) an increase in cell number; overgrowth in response to some type of stimulus.

hypersensitivity a condition in which there is an excessive response by the body to the stimulus of a foreign body.

hyperthermia an increase in core body temperature.

hypertonic a solution that has more solutes in proportion to the volume of water.

hypertrophy (HIGH-**PER**-tro-fee) an increase in the size of the cell leading to an increase in tissue and organ size.

hyperventilation an increased tidal volume above normal ranges.

hypoadrenal shock a type of vasogenic shock in which the adrenal glands are unable to respond to traumatic stressors.

hypocalcemia a decrease in the extracellular level of calcium.

hypochloremia a decrease in the extracellular level of chloride.

hypoglycemia (HIGH-poh-gly-**SEE**-me-ah; hypo = decreased, glyc = glucose, emia = blood) a low blood sugar level.

hypokalemia a decrease in the extracellular level of potassium.

hypomagnesemia a decrease in the extracellular level of magnesium.

hyponatremia deficit in extracellular level of sodium.

hypophosphatemia a decrease in the extracellular level of phosphorus.

hypothermia (hypo = low, thermia = heat or temperature) a significantly low body temperature.

hypotonic a solution that has fewer solutes in proportion to the volume of water .

hypoventilation a decreased tidal volume below normal ranges.

hypovolemic shock a disorder in which the volume of blood in the body is decreased.

hypoxemia (high-**POX**-SEE-me-ah; hypo = not enough, ox = oxygen, emia = blood) not enough oxygen in the circulating blood.

hypoxia (HIGH-**POX**-see-ah) not enough oxygen in tissues.

hypoxic ventilatory response (HVR) a normal physiologic response to hypoxia.

iatrogenic (eye-AT-roh-**JEN**-ick; iatro = medicine, physician, genic = rising from) a problem arising because of or related to a prescribed treatment.

idiopathic (ID-ee-oh-**PATH**-ick) an unknown cause of disease.

ileus (ILL-ee-us) absence of peristalsis.

immersion foot a condition in which tissue damage results from chronic exposure to a moist environment; also called trench foot.

immunodeficiency the state when the immune response is unable to defend the body because of a decrease or absence of leukocytes, primarily lymphocytes.

impacted fracture one that has a bone end forced over the other end.

impotent (IM-poh-tent) inability in the male to achieve or maintain a penile erection.

incidence rate the rate of new cases of disease over a period of time.

incision a laceration or cut with smooth even edges.

incompetent cervix dilation of the cervix in the second trimester of pregnancy.

incomplete fracture the bone is fractured but not in two.

incubation period the time between exposure to the disease and the presence of symptoms, which may last several days.

induration (IN-dur-**RAY**-shun) hardened tissue.

infarct (in-FARKT) necrosis of cells or tissues caused by ischemia.

infection (in-FECT-shun) invasion of microorganisms into the tissue causing cell or tissue injury thus leading to the inflammatory response.

inflammation (IN-flah-**MAY**-shun) a basic pathologic process of cytologic and chemical reactions that occur in the blood vessels and tissues in response to an injury or irritation; a protective immune response that is triggered by any type of injury or irritant.

ingestion route of entry by which a poison is taken in by mouth.

inhalation route of entry by which a poison is taken in via the nose and lungs.

injection route of entry by which a poison is taken through the skin and into the blood or subcutaneous tissues.

inotropism the strength of myocardial muscle contraction.

insensible fluid lost the fluid that is lost through perspiration and cannot be measured.

inspiratory capacity the volume of air inhaled during maximal inhalation.
inspiratory reserve the additional volume of air over normal tidal volume that can be inhaled.
inspiratory stridor (STRYE-dor) high-pitched sound during inspiration caused by blocked airways.
insulin a hormone secreted by the beta cells in the islets of Langerhans in the pancreas; responsible for glucose utilization.
intermittent claudication (KLAW-dih-**KAY**-shun) the condition of developing muscle cramps that are relieved with rest and increased with activity.
interphalangeal (inter = between, phalangeal = finger bones) usually referring to joints between the finger bones.
intertrochanteric fracture one that is in the trochanteric area of the femur.
intoxicated when the blood alcohol level reaches 0.10 percent or more.
intracapsular fractures a fracture inside the joint capsule.
intracranial pressure (ICP) pressure inside the skull.
intractable difficult to stop or control.
intravenous pyelogram (IVP) (IN-trah-**VEE**-nus **PYE**-eh-loh-GRAM) an X-ray picture taken after injecting dye into the individual's bloodstream; the dye accumulates in the urinary tract and improves the ability to identify obstructions, tumors, and deformities.
intrinsic factor a substance secreted by the stomach lining necessary for absorption of vitamin B12.
intrinsic pathway a pathway in the coagulation system to activate clot formation.
intussusception (IN-tus-sus-**SEP**-shun) the telescoping of one part of the intestine over the adjoining section.
invasion spreading into surrounding or local tissue.
involution the return of the reproductive organs to their size prior to pregnancy.
ischemia (iss-KEE-me-ah) hypoxia of cells or tissues caused by decreased blood flow.
islets of Langerhans specialized cells in the pancreas that act as an endocrine gland secreting hormones, primarily insulin.
isoimmune a high level of a specific antibody as a result of antigen stimulation from the red blood cells of another individual; isoimmunization may occur when an Rh negative person is treated with a transfusion of Rh positive blood.
isotonic a solution that has equal amounts of solutes in proportion to the volume of water.
Jacksonian seizure a partial seizure involving abnormal movement that starts in a very localized area and then spreads to other parts of the body as the electrical discharge spreads to and involves other areas of the brain.
jaundice yellow discoloration of the skin and mucous membranes as a result of obstruction of the bile ducts.
Kaposi's sarcoma (KAP-oh-seez sar-KOH-ma) blood vessel cancer that causes reddish-purple skin lesions.
karyotyping a method for identifying chromosomes; this process involves taking a picture of a cell during mitosis, arranging the chromosome pairs in order from largest to smallest and numbering them one to twenty-three.
keloid (KEE-loid) excessive collagen formation often resulting in a hard raised scar.
keratin a tough protein substance in nails, hair, and body tissues.
kernicterus neurological damage caused by severe jaundice.
ketoacidosis acidosis seen in diabetes mellitus caused by overproduction of ketone bodies.
ketones waste products produced when tissue cells burn fats and proteins.
kidneys-ureter-bladder (KUB) a common X-ray of the structures of the urinary tract to determine abnormalities.
Koplik's spots spots seen in the mouth in the early stage of measles; these spots are rather unique to measles and are often the definitive symptom that confirms the diagnosis.
Kussmaul's respirations an abnormal respiratory pattern consisting of deep, gasping respirations.
laceration a cut in the skin.
laminectomy surgery to cut away part of the vertebra to open the area around the spinal nerve.
laparoscopy (LAP-ah-**ROS**-ko-pee; laparo = abdomen, scopy = scope procedure) looking inside the abdominal cavity with a lighted scope; commonly used to view the female organs for abnormalities, diagnose endometriosis, and to perform a tubal ligation.
lesion (LEE-zhun) any discontinuity of tissue.
lethal something that kills.
leukemia (loo-KEE-me-ah; leuk = white, emia = blood) a progressive overgrowth of abnormal leukocytes; a malignant disease of the bone marrow.
leukocytopenia (leukocyte = white cell, penia = decrease) a decrease in white cell count.
leukocytosis (leuko = white, cyto = cell, osis = condition) an increase in white cell count.

leukorrhea (LOO-koh-**REE**-ah; leuk = white, orrhea = flow or discharge) a white, usually foul smelling, vaginal discharge.

lipids fats or fat-like substances.

lithotripsy (litho = stone, tripsy = breaking) a procedure for breaking kidney or gallbladder stones.

longitudinal fracture one that runs the length of the bone.

lumen (LOO-men) the inner open space or width of a tubular structure or anatomical part.

lymph a clear liquid similar to plasma containing many white cells.

lymphadenopathy (lim-FAD-eh-**NOP**-ah-thee; lymph = lymph, adeno = gland, opathy = disease) any disease of the lymph glands.

lymphangiography (lim-FAH-jee-**OG**-rah-fee; lymph = lymph, angio = vessel, ography = procedure) a radiographic procedure consisting of injecting a contrast dye and taking X-rays of lymphatic vessels.

lymphangiopathy (lim-FAN-jee-**OP**-ah-thee; lymph = lymph, angio = vessel, opathy = disease) a general term to describe any disease of the lymph vessels.

lymphedema (lymph = lymph, edema = swelling) an abnormal collection of lymph fluid usually observed in the extremities.

lymphocytes white blood cells formed in lymphatic tissue.

lymphocytopenia or **lymphopenia** a decrease in lymphocytes.

lymphocytosis increase in number of lymphocytes.

lymphomas (lim-FOH-maz) malignant neoplasms of blood-forming organs.

macrophage (macro = large, phage = eat) a monocyte that leaves the bloodstream and moves into the tissue and becomes phagocytic.

macrosomia excessive fetal growth.

Magnetic Resonance Imaging (MRI) a diagnostic radiological test using nuclear magnetic resonance technology.

malaise general ill feeling.

malignant (mah-LIG-nant) deadly or progressing to death, cancerous.

mania extreme elation or agitation.

mast cells also called tissue histocytes; found in all tissues of the body; play a major role in the inflammatory process.

mastitis inflammation of the breast.

mastoidectomy (MAS-toy-**DECK**-toh-me; ectomy = removal or excision) a procedure used to prevent complications and preserve hearing by removing the bony partitions forming the mastoid cells.

mechanisms of labor series of movements the fetus makes as it positions for delivery.

meiosis the process of reproduction of germ cells in which they divide before duplication.

melena (meh-LEE-nah) dark tarry stool caused by blood in feces.

menarche the first menstrual cycle.

menopause the stoppage of the menstrual cycle that occurs with aging.

metacarpophalangeal (meta = beyond, carpo = wrist, phalangeal = finger bones) referring to the metacarpus and the phalanges; specifically the articulations between them.

metaplasia (MET-ah-**PLAY**-zee-ah) a cellular adaptation in which the cell changes to another type of cell.

metastasis (meh-TAS-tah-sis) spreading to distant sites.

metastasize (meh-TAS-tah-sighz) move or spread.

metastatic (MET-ah-**STAT**-ic) moves from a site of origin to another secondary site in the body.

metatarsophalangeal (meta = between, tarso = foot, phalangeal = toe bones) referring to the metatarsus and the phalanges; specifically the articulations between them.

metritis inflammation of the uterus.

microcephaly (micro = small, cephal = brain) having an abnormally small head; usually associated with mental retardation.

mineralization a process that causes the characteristic hardness of bones.

mineralocorticoids one group of steroids of the adrenal cortex that influences sodium and potassium metabolism.

minute volume the volume of air that travels through the respiratory system during one minute of ventilation.

miscarriage spontaneous abortion.

mitosis the process of reproduction of cells in which the forty-six chromosomes duplicate and divide into two identical daughter cells each containing forty-six chromosomes.

mood emotion.

morbidity residual effects of a given disease.

mortality rate the rate at which people die from a particular disease.

motility ability to move.

multiparity (mul-TIP-ah-rah-tee) multiple births.

multiple organ dysfunction syndrome (MODS) damage or malfunction to more than one organ as a result of decreased perfusion or acute illness.

murmur an abnormal sound in the heart or vascular system.

MVAs motor vehicle accidents.

myelogram an X-ray picture taken after injecting dye into the spinal canal in order to reveal compression on the spinal cord or spinal nerves.

myringotomy (MIR-in-**GOT**-oh-me; myringo = eardrum, tomy = incision into) incision into the eardrum to remove fluid.

myxedema (MECK-seh-**DEE**-mah) advanced hypothyroidism in an adult.

necrosis (nee-CROW-sis) cellular death.

neoplasia (nee-oh-PLAY-zee-ah) the development of a new type of cell with an uncontrolled growth pattern.

neoplasms (new growths) an increase in cell number leading to an increase in tissue size, commonly called tumors.

nephrectomy (neh-FREC-toh-me; nephr = kidney, ectomy = excision or removal) the surgical removal of the kidney.

neurogenic shock a state of decreased blood volume as a result of an increase in the size of the vessels in the body.

neuromuscular junction the interface between the nerve and muscle.

neutopenia a decrease in neutrophils.

nits lice eggs.

non-causal risk factor a risk factor that does not directly cause a disease but increases the risk of development of disease.

non-displaced fracture one in which the fragments are still in correct position.

nosocomial (NOS-oh-**KOH**-me-al) a disease acquired from the hospital environment.

nuchal cord umbilical cord around the neck.

nuchal rigidity a stiffness in the neck that resists bending the neck forward or sideways.

oblique fracture a fracture that runs in a transverse pattern.

obsession repetition of a thought or emotion.

obstructive disease a pathological process that obstructs the flow of air out of the lung.

occult blood hidden blood; unable to see except under microscopic examination.

oliguria (OL-ih-**GOO**-ree-ah; olig = scanty or few, uria = urine) a decrease in urine output.

oncology (ong-KOL-oh-jee) the study of tumors.

oophoritis (OH-of-oh-**RYE**-tis) inflammation of the ovary.

open (compound) fracture a fracture involving the bone puncturing through the skin or an object puncturing the skin making an opening through the skin to the fracture site.

ophthalmoscope (aft-THAL-moh-skope; ophthalm = eye, scope = instrument used to look) the instrument used for a basic examination of the eye.

orchitis (or-KYE-tis) inflammation of a testis.

organ rejection when the body recognizes an organ (after a transplant) as foreign and attacks it leading to organ death.

organelle the structures within the cell.

organic related to an organ or physical component.

organophosphates insecticides.

ORIF (Open-Reduction Internal Fixation) surgical opening over a fracture site and internally fixing the fracture with plates, screws, or pins.

orthopnea (or-THOP-nee-ah; ortho = straight, pnea = breathing) the condition in which an individual has difficulty breathing in a lying down position or is able to breathe with less difficulty when standing or sitting "straight" up.

osmolality a measurement of the total concentration of dissolved particles per kilogram of water.

osmolarity the concentration of solutes per liter of cellular fluid.

osmole the unit of measure of osmotic pressure.

osmosis passage of a solvent from an area of lesser concentration to an area of greater concentration.

osmotic pressure force created when two solutions of different concentrations are separated by a selectively permeable membrane.

otalgia (oh-TAL-gee-ah; oto = ear, algia = pain) ear pain.

otoscope (OH-toh-skope; oto = ear, scope = instrument to look) the instrument used to examine the ear.

ova and parasite (O&P) an examination of a stool specimen for the presence of adult parasites or their eggs (ova).

palliative (PAL-ee-ay-tiv) something that is directed toward relief of symptoms but does not cure.

palmar erythema (ER-ih-**THEE**-mah) unusual redness of the palms of the hands.

palpation feeling lightly or by pressing firmly on internal organs or structures.

pancytopenia (pan = all, cyto = cell, penia = decrease) severe decrease or total absence of erythrocytes, leukocytes, and thrombocytes.

Pap test also called Papanicolaou test; a screening for cancer utilizing and examination of cells scraped from the cervical area.

para total number of deliveries.

paradoxical respiration movement of a flail segment opposite the rest of the chest during normal respiration.

paralytic obstruction a decrease or absence of peristalsis that causes intestinal blockage.

paraplegia (PAR-ah-**PLEE**-jee-ah; para = beyond or two like parts, plegia = paralysis) a loss of movement and feeling in the trunk and both legs.

parenteral (pah-REN-ter-al) a delivery route for fluid or medications that may include subcutaneous, intramuscular, or intravenous administration.

paresthesia (PAR-es-**THEE**-see-ah) abnormal sensation, burning, tingling, or numbness.

paronychia (PAR-oh-NICK-ee-ah) an infection of the skin around the nail.

parotid glands the salivary glands located just in front of the ears.

paroxysmal (PAR-ock-**SIZ**-mal) spasm or convulsion.

partial seizure a seizure in which the abnormal discharge is localized to a small portion of the brain.

patency openness.

patent open.

pathogenesis (PATH-oh-**JEN**-ah-sis; patho = disease, genesis = arising) a description of how a particular disease progresses.

pathogens (PATH-oh-jens) microorganisms or agents that cause disease.

pathologic (path-oh-LODGE-ick) caused by a pathogen or a disease.

pathologic fracture (path-oh-LODGE-ick) a fracture caused by weakness from another disease.

pathologist (pah-THOL-oh-jist; patho = disease, logist = one who studies) one who studies disease.

pathology (pah-THOL-oh-jee; patho = disease, ology = study) the study of disease.

pathophysiology the study of how and why a disease develops and progresses.

percussion (per-KUSH-un) tapping over various body areas to produce a vibrating sound.

percussion note a sound made upon percussion of the lungs used to detect lung abnormalities.

perforation an abnormal opening in an organ or tissue.

peristalsis the contraction of muscles along the gastrointestinal tract to move food and fluid.

peritonitis (PER-ih-toe-**NIGH**-tis) an inflammation of the peritoneum.

peritonsillar abscess an abscess that forms around the tonsil; it can occur up to several weeks after an infection.

permeability capability of a substance, molecule, or ion to diffuse through a membrane.

petechiae (pee-TEE-kee-ee) small hemorrhages in the skin.

petit mal a term applied to a type of seizure; these seizures consist of a brief change in the level of consciousness without convulsions; the involved individual may show symptoms of blank staring, blinking, and/or twitching of the eyes or mouth.

phenotype the physical expression of a genetic trait such as eye, hair, and skin color.

photophobia (photo = light, phobia = fear) an abnormal fear of light.

piloerection elevation of the small body hairs to provide a layer of insulation between the environment and the skin.

placenta previa implantation in the lower uterine segment with the placenta lying over the cervical os.

pneumocystis carinii (NEW-moh-**SIS**-tis kah-RYE-nee-eye) an opportunistic infection of the lung that occurs in patients with immunocompromised states, for example, those with acquired immune deficiency syndrome.

pneumonia a protozoan infection of the lungs commonly occurring in immunodeficient individuals.

portal hypertension increased pressure in the portal system frequently seen in cirrhosis.

Pott's fracture fracture of the lower part of the fibula and tibia, with outward displacement of the foot.

precipitate birth birth occurring suddenly and unexpectedly.

precipitate labor labor lasting less than 3 hours from the onset of contractions to birth.

predisposing factors also known as risk factors, make a person more susceptible to disease.

preeclampsia (PREE-ee-**KLAMP**-see-ah) the development of hypertension with proteinuria and/or edema caused by pregnancy; also called toxemia.

preload the pressure on the heart chamber exerted by the volume of blood returning to the heart.

presenting part the part of the fetus in contact with the cervix.

presyncope incomplete loss of consciousness.

prevalence rate the number of people who have a certain disease at any given point of time.

prevalent occurring more often.

preventive something that reduces risk.

primary union also called healing by first intention; involves approximating the edges of the wound.

primigravid (PRE-mih-**GRAV**-id; primi = first, gravid = pregnancy) the term used to describe a female who is pregnant with her first child.

productive cough coughing up sputum or excessive mucus.

prognosis (prawg-KNOW-sis) the predicted or expected outcome of the disease.

prokaryotic cells that do not contain organelles in a cell membrane.

prolapsed cord the umbilical cord lying below the presenting part of the fetus.

prone positioned face down on the stomach.

prophylactic (pro-fil-LACK-tic) something that works to prevent a disease or injury.

proteinuria protein in the urine; specific protein, albumin, may be identified resulting in albuminuria.

protoplasm a solution of carbohydrates, proteins, lipids, nucleic acids, and inorganic salts surrounded by a limiting cell membrane.

protozoa a parasite of the phylum Protozoa; a single-celled microscopic member of the animal kingdom.

pruritus (proo-RYE-tus) itching.

puerperal (pyou-ER-pier-al) relating to childbirth.

pulse deficit a difference between the apical and the peripheral pulse.

pulse pressure the difference between the systolic and diastolic blood pressure.

pulsus alternans a regular alternation in amplitude of the pulse.

pulsus paradoxus a condition seen with pericardial tamponade characteristic of a decrease in systolic blood pressure greater than 10 mm Hg upon inspiration.

purulent (PURR-you-lent) loaded with dead and dying neutrophils, tissue debris, and pyogenic (pus-forming) bacteria.

pus white or yellow exudate caused by death of numerous neutrophils mixed with exudate or blood fluid.

pustule (PUS-tyoul) a small pus filled lesion.

pylonidal cyst (PYE-loh-**NIGH**-dal) a particular type of sebaceous cyst found in the midline of the sacral area.

pyloromyotomy (pyloro = pyloric, myo = muscle, otomy = cut into) a surgical procedure that involves incising and suturing the pyloric sphincter muscle.

pyoderma (PYE-oh-**DER**-mah) inflammatory, purulent dermatitis.

pyrogens byproducts released by bacterial destruction and tissue damage.

pyuria (pye-YOU-ree-ah; py = pus, uria = urine) pus in the urine.

quadriplegia (KWAD-rih-**PLEE**-jee-ah; quadri = four, plegia = paralysis) the loss of movement and feeling in the trunk and all four extremities with the accompanying loss of bowel, bladder, and sexual function.

radiation the process of using light, short-waves, ultraviolet or X-rays, or any other rays.

radiation heat loss dissipation of heat from a warm object through heat waves into the surrounding air.

radical cystectomy (radical = a treatment that seeks to cure, aggressive, not palliative or conservative, sis-TECT-toh-me, cyst = bladder, ectomy = excision or removal) the removal of the entire bladder usually done as treatment for cancer of the bladder.

radiologic relating to medical imaging using X-rays, ionizing radiation, nuclear magnetic resonance, or ultrasound.

receptor structures along the cell membrane that help the cell communicate with other cells.

recessive lacking control; weak.

Reed-Sternberg cell a large connective tissue cell found in lymphatic tissue indicative of Hodgkin's disease.

referred pain pain that is located in one area but caused by a disease process in another area.

remission a time when symptoms are diminished or temporarily resolved.

residual volume amount of air in the lings after exhalation.

restrictive disease a pathological process that decreases the flow of air into the lungs.

retropharyngeal abscess an abscess that forms in the soft tissue posterior or behind the pharynx between the oral cavity and the spine.

rhinitis (RYE-**NIGH**-tis) inflammation of the nasal mucous membrane.

rhinorrhea (rhino = nose, orrhea = run through) a runny nose.

rickettsiae (Ric-KET-see-ah) microscopic organisms that are intermediate between bacteria and viruses. They live in the host and are spread by lice, fleas, ticks, and mites.

RPR (Rapid Plasma Reagin) a blood test for syphilis.

salpingitis (SAL-pin-**JIGH**-tis; salping = fallopian tube, itis = inflammation) inflammation of the fallopian tube.

sarcoma (sar-KOR-mah) a malignant neoplasm arising from connective tissue.

scar skin lesion resulting from fibrous connective tissue repair.

sciatica pain along the sciatic nerve often radiating down the leg and caused by pressure on the spinal nerve.

sebum oil produced by the sebaceous glands.

secondary union also called healing by secondary intention; the same process as primary union but involves a larger degree of tissue damage and more inflammation to resolve.

seizure a sudden onset or attack, but it is commonly used to indicate a convulsive seizure as occurs in epilespy.

self antigen the body's own antigen.

semipermeable selectively permeable.

sepsis infection/toxicity.

septic shock poor tissue perfusion as a result of sepsis (infection).

septicemia (SEP-tih-**SEE**-me-ah; septic = dirty, contaminated, emia = blood) a systemic disease caused by the spread of microorganisms in the blood; also called "blood poisoning."

serotonin syndrome a rare and life-threatening complication of antidepressant use.

signs observable or measurable factors used to determine a diagnosis.

simple (closed) fracture a fracture that does not break through the skin.

sinus a tract or opening to the surface of the body formed by a large ruptured abscess.

skin turgor the normal resiliency of the skin.

solubility the degree to which a substance is able to be dissolved in a solution.

solute substance dissolved in a solution.

solvent liquid that contains a substance in a solution.

somatic related to the body.

somatic pain pain that originates form the soft tissue or muscles in the body.

spasms uncontrolled muscle contractions.

spider angiomas telangiectasis or small dilated vessels in the skin; commonly seen on the face and chest of individuals with cirrhosis of the liver.

spinal stenosis (stenosis = narrowing) the condition of narrowing of nerve root openings in the spinal column.

spiral fracture a fracture that twists around the bone.

splenomegaly (SPLEE-no-**MEG**-ah-lee) enlargement of the spleen.

sputum (SPYOU-tum) fluid or secretions coughed up from the lungs.

staging determining the degree of spread of a malignant tumor.

Starling's law the relationship between contractibility of cardiac muscle and the amount of stretch placed in that muscle.

status asthmaticus (AZTH-**MAH**-ti-kus) a severe asthma attack that lasts for several days.

status epilepticus a life-threatening event; a state of continued convulsive seizure with no recovery of consciousness; it is a medical emergency.

stellate fracture a fracture that forms a star-like pattern.

sterility inability to impregnate a female related to sperm quality or quantity.

stool fecal matter; feces; bowel movement (BM).

strangulated hernia herniated portions of the intestine that twist and cut off the blood supply to the organ.

strep throat an acute form of pharyngitis caused by streptococcus.

streptococcal (**STREHP**-toh-KAHK-al) relating to the organism streptococcus; an anaerobic, gram-positive bacteria.

stress fracture related to too much weight or pressure.

striae (stretch marks) on the skin.

stricture a narrowing.

subcapital fracture a fracture below (sub) the head (caput) of the femur.

subcutaneous emphysema a bubbly, crinkly feeling in the skin as a result of air leaking out of the lung into the subcutaneous fat.

subdural hematoma (SUB-**DOO**-ral) blood collecting between the outer (dura mater) layer and the middle (arachnoid) layer of the meninges.

supine (SUE-pine) positioned on the back.

suppurative (SUP-you-**RAY**-tive) formation of pus.

sutures thin fibrous membranes covering the bones of the skull.

sympathomimetic toxidrome agents that heighten the sympathetic nervous system.

symptoms what patients report as their problem or problems.

syncope a transient loss of consciousness.

syndrome (SIN-drome) a group of symptoms that may be caused by a specific disease but may also be caused by several interrelated problems.

systemic inflammatory response syndrome (SIRS) a condition in which the body's normal inflammatory response to infection or other stress is out of control.

systolic (sis-TALL-ick) relating to cardiac systole; the process of cardiac contraction (heartbeat) when blood is ejected into the systemic circulation.

tachycardia (TACH-ee-**KAR**-dee-ah; tachy = rapid, cardia = heart rate) a rapid heart rate; usually a rate over 100 beats per minute.

tachypnea (TACK-ihp-**NEE**-ah; tachy = rapid, pnea = breathing) a severely increased respiratory rate.

tetany (TET-ah-nee) hyperirritability of muscles causing a spasm-like condition; usually the result of a lack of calcium.
therapeutic range the blood level of the medication that has been found to be beneficial to most patients.
thermogenesis the process of heat production.
thermolysis the dissipation of heat from the body.
thermoreceptors areas in the body responsive to heat and cold.
thrombocytopenia (THROM-boh-SIGH-toh-**PEE**-nee-ah; thrombocyte = platelet, penia = decrease) a decrease in platelets leading to a coagulation problem.
thrombocytosis (THROM-boh-sigh-**TOH**-sis; thrombocyte = platelet, osis = condition of) an increase in platelets.
thrombophlebitis formation of a clot in an inflamed vein.
thrombus (THROM-bus) a blood clot attached to a vein or artery.
thyroid storm a sudden life-threatening exacerbation of all symptoms of hyperthyroidism.
tidal volume the volume of air inhaled and exhaled in one breath.
tinnitus (tin-EYE-tus) ringing in the ears.
tolerance the ability to endure a larger amount of a substance without an adverse effect or the need for a larger amount or dose of the drug to have the same effect.
tonometry (toh-NOM-eh-tree; tono = tone or pressure, metry = measurement) a procedure to measure the pressure inside the eye.
tophi small whitish nodules of uric acid.
topical placed on the skin.
total lung capacity the total amount of air that can be held in the lung.
toxidrome a collection of signs and symptoms associated with groups of similar toxic agents; short for toxic syndrome.
TPN total parenteral nutrition intravenously giving a special solution that meets the total nutritional needs of the individual.
transurethral resection (TUR) (trans = through, urethral = uretha; resection = partial excision) a surgical procedure that may be performed to remove a tumor, visualize a structure, or take a piece of tissue for biopsy; a cystoscope is passed through the urinary meatus and the urethra for this procedure.
transverse fracture one that runs across or at a 90 degree angle.
trauma (TRAW-mah) a physical or mental injury.
traumatic shock a form of vasogenic shock that involves significant blood loss and fluid shifts.
trench foot a condition in which tissue damage results from chronic exposure to a moist environment; also called immersion foot.
trichomonas (TRICK-oh-MOH-nas) a parasitic protozoan that commonly infects the vagina and causes trichomoniasis.
tumor "swelling" or growth, originally used in the description of the swelling related to inflammation.
tympanoplasty (TIM-pah-no-**PLAS**-tee; tympano = eardrum, plasty = surgical correction) surgery to repair the tympanic membrane.
tympanostomy (TIM-pan-**OSS**-toh-me; tympano = eardrum, ostomy = new opening) a procedure in which tubes, commonly called PE tubes or pediatric ear tubes, are placed through the tympanic membrane to prevent the accumulation of fluid.
ulcer a crater-like lesion in the skin or mucous membranes.
urea a common nitrogenous waste product that is normally filtered from the blood.
uremia (you-REE-me-ah; ur = urine, emia = blood) a toxic condition of the blood caused by high levels of waste products.
urgency the severe need to urinate.
urinalysis (YOU-rih-**NAL**-ih-sis; urine analysis) a laboratory urine test for pH, specific gravity, protein, glucose or sugar, and blood; it also includes a microscopic examination to determine the presence of bacteria, crystals, and casts.
urine culture and sensitivity (C & S) a laboratory analysis that determines the type of bacteria present and the most effective antibiotic to prescribe for treatment.
urticaria (UR-tih-**KAR**-ree-ah) an allergic reaction resulting in a skin eruption of wheals that causes intense itching.
vasogenic shock a state of decreased blood volume as a result of inflammation which acts to increase the size of the vessels.
vasopressin anti-diuretic hormone (ADH) secreted by the posterior portion of the pituitary gland.
VDRL (Venereal Disease Research Laboratory) a blood test to screen for syphilis.
vermiform (VER-my-form) worm-like.
vertigo (VER-tih-go) dizziness.
vesicles (VES-ih-kuls) blister-like eruptions on the skin.
virulent (VIR-u-lent; infectious) difficult to kill; able to produce disease.

viruses a large group of infectious agents; they are much smaller than bacteria and must be viewed with an electron microscope. They can pass through fine filters that would retain most bacteria.

visceral pain pain that originates from the organs.

viscous (VIS-cuss) thick.

vital capacity the maximum volume of air that can be exhaled after maximum inspiration.

volvulus (VOL-view-lus) the bowel twisted upon itself.

wet drowning a condition in which the lungs completely fill with fluid interrupting the oxygen diffusion across the alveoli.

wheal(s) round, slightly reddened, spot(s) on the skin, usually accompanied by intense itching; also called urticarial lesion(s) or hives; caused by an allergic reaction to something such as food or medication.

wheezing a whistling, musical, or raspy sound during breathing usually indicative of partially blocked respiratory passages.

withdrawal the unpleasant physical and psychologic effects resulting from stopping the use of the substance after an individual is addicted.

working diagnosis the most likely reason for a particular disease or disorder used to guide further testing and evaluation.

xerosis (zee-ROE-sis) dry skin.

Index

A
abdominocentesis, 257
ABO incompatibility, 414
abortion, 408–409
abrasions, 334, 351–352
abruptio placenta, 410–411
abscesses, 52
  central nervous system, 161–162
  peritonsillar, 246
  pulmonary, 117
  retropharyngeal, 246
  skin, 330
absorption, 286
abuse, 376
  child, 449
  sexual, 449
  substances, 291–293, 376–379, 415
acetaminophen, 301–302
achlorhydria, 247
acid, 69
acid-base balance, 69
  disturbances, 78–82
  regulators, 69–70
acid-base buffer system, 69
acidosis, 69
  metabolic, 80–81
  respiratory, 79, 80
acute diseases, 5, 6
acute mountain sickness (AMS), 368–369
addiction, 376
adenocarcinoma, 279
adenoma, 210
adhesions, 56, 250
adult respiratory distress syndrome (ARDS), 118
affective disorders, 380–381
afterload, 132
aging, 25
agonal respirations, 110
AIDS (acquired immunodeficiency syndrome), 25, 231–233, 398
  childhood, 443
  transmission, 232–233
albumin, 257
albuminuria, 271
alcohol, 40, 291, 295
alcoholism, 376
alkalemia, 287
alkalosis, 69
  metabolic, 81–82
  respiratory, 79, 80
alleles, 17
allergens, 25, 223
allergies, 25, 112, 223, 224–226
alopecia, 334
altered mental status, 171
altitude emergencies, 366–369
Alzheimer's disease, 170, 379–380
amenorrhea, 394
American Cancer Society, 8, 32, 39, 40, 41, 42
American College of Surgeons, 95
American Heart Association, 134, 447
amnesia, 173
amphetamines, 378
amylase, 259
amyotrophic lateral sclerosis (ALS), 167–168
anaerobic wounds, 192
analgesia, 289
analgesics, 112, 300–302
anaphylaxis, 98, 226
anaplastic, 38
anatomy
  cardiovascular system, 128–132
  cell, 15–16
  ear, 343–345
  endocrine system, 206–209
  eye, 342–343
  female reproductive system, 390–391
  gastrointestinal system, 240–242
  hematologic system, 310–312
  immune system, 220–221
  lymphatic system, 221–223
  male reproductive system, 391
  musculoskeletal system, 184–185
  neurological system, 156–159
  renal/urologic system, 270–271
  respiratory system, 106–109
  skin, 326–327
androgens, 209
anemia, 312, 315–316
aneurysm, 138–139
angina pectoris, 139–140
angiogenesis, 35
angiography, 346
angioplasty, 139
angulated fractures, 193
anomaly, 19
anorexia nervosa, 375–376
anoxia, 25
anterior cord syndrome, 176
antibodies, 24, 48, 51
anticholinergic toxidrome, 288, 289
antigens, 24, 48, 223
antipyretics, 112
anuria, 271

anxiety disorders, 382–383
aplastic anemia, 316
apnea, 109
apoptosis, 16
appendicitis, 250
arterial blood gases (ABGs), 78–79, 85, 112
arterial gas embolism (AGE), 366
arteriosclerosis, 136–138
arthritis, 190, 227–228
articular cartilage, 190
ascites, 257
asphyxia, traumatic, 123
assessment, 8–9
asthma, 114, 224–225, 446
astigmatism, 347
asymptomatic, 246
atelectasis, 115–116
atherosclerosis, 136–138
atresia, 262
atrial septal defect, 149
atrophy, 26
attention-deficit hyperactivity disorder (ADHD), 375
audiometry, 346
aura, 165
auscultation, 8, 133
autism, 375
autodigestion, 259
autoimmune disorders, 223, 226–229
autoimmunity, 25
autolysis, 16
autonomic hyperreflexia, 178
autosomes, 16
avulsion fractures, 193
avulsions, 335

B

bacteria, 48, 56–57, 443
bacterial infections, 56–57, 329–330, 443–444
basal cell carcinoma, 333
base, 69
behavior diseases/disorders, 373–386
  diagnostic tests, 374
  older adult, 385
  signs/symptoms, 374
  trauma, 384–385
  types, 374–284
Bell's palsy, 167
Bence Jones protein, 318
benign tumors, 23, 32, 34–35
β-adrenergic blockers, 297–298
bimanual examination, 392
biopsy, 38, 42–43
Biot's respiration, 110
bipolar disorder, 381
bleeding time, 314
blood transfusion, 85–88
blood transfusion reaction, 229
blood urea nitrogen (BUN) test, 272
bloody show, 416
blunt cardiac injury (BCI), 148
blunt trauma, 334–335
body fluid, 64
  assessment, 82–85
  compartments, 64–65
  distribution, 65
  disturbances, 70–71
  during labor, 417
  factors affecting, 70
  imbalances, childhood, 447–448
  management, 85–88
  movement, 65–68
  regulators, 68–69
body water, 64
Boyle's law, 364, 367
bradypnea, 110
Braxton Hicks contractions, 416
bronchiectasis, 115
bronchitis, 114, 115
bronchoscopy, 112
bronchospasm, 224
Brown-Sequard syndrome, 177–178
bulimia, 375–376
burns, 335–336
bursitis, 199

C

cachexia, 24, 35, 44
caffeine, 377
calcium channel blockers, 298
cancer, 23
  bladder, 279–280
  causes, 38–40
  development, 36–37
  diagnosis, 42–43
  frequency, 41–42
  grading/staging, 37–38
  kidney, 279
  lung, 118
  lymphoma, 235
  metastasis, 37
  prevention, 40–41
  signs/symptoms, 43–44
  skin, 332–334
  treatment, 44
candidiasis, 330–331, 444–445
caput medusae, 256

carbon monoxide, 294–295
carbuncles, 330
carcinogenesis, 38
carcinogens, 36, 38–39
carcinoma, 33
carcinoma in situ, 37
cardiac catheterization, 133
cardiac glycosides, 297
cardiac output, 132
cardiac palpitations, 132
cardiogenic shock, 96
cardiovascular system, 127–151
  aging and, 151
  anatomy/physiology, 128–132
  developmental diseases/disorders, 149–150
  diagnostic tests, 133–134
  diseases, 120–121, 134–147, 413
  during labor, 417
  during pregnancy, 407
  newborn, 431
  postpartum, 432–433
  signs/symptoms, 132–133
  trauma, 147–149
carditis, 144
carotid endarterectomy, 165, 170
cataracts, 348–349
catarrhal stage, 443
catheterization, 272
cauda equina syndrome, 178
causal risk factor, 8
caustic agents, 293
cauterization, 174
CAUTION, 42
cellular environment, 14–21
  adaption, 26–27
  anatomy, 15–16
  death of cell, 27–28
  genetics, 16–20
  injury, 25–26
  reproduction, 16–20
  tissue types, 20–21
cellulitis, 52–53, 330
Centers for Disease Control and Prevention, 7, 56
central cord syndrome, 176
central nervous system (CNS), 156–158
central neurogenic hyperventilation (CNH), 110
cephalalgia, 165–166
cephalopelvic disproportion (CPD), 427
cerebral palsy (CP), 178
cerebrovascular accident (CVA), 163–165
cerumen, 343
cervicitis, 395
chancres, 399
chemicals, household, 293–294
chemotaxis, 51
chemotherapy, 43
Cheyne-Stokes respiration, 110
child abuse, 449
childhood diseases/disorders, 439–451
  cardiovascular, 448
  digestive, 447–448
  eye/ear, 448–449
  hematologic, 448
  infectious, 440–445
  musculoskeletal, 448
  neurologic, 448
  respiratory, 445–447
  trauma, 449–450
Childhood Leukemia Center, 448
chlamydial infection, 400
cholecystectomy, 258
cholecystitis, 258
cholelithiasis, 258–259
cholinergic toxidrome, 288–289
chorea, 168
chromosomes, 16–17
chronic diseases, 5, 6
chronic obstructive pulmonary disease (COPD), 114–115
chronotropism, 129
circadian rhythms, 381
cirrhosis, 255–258
clean catch, 271
cleft lip/palate, 262
closed fractures, 193
clubbing, 110
coarctation, 149
cocaine, 291–292, 377
cold emergencies, 360–363
colds, 112, 443
colicky pain, 271
Colle's fractures, 194
colloids, 68, 85
comminuted fractures, 193
co-morbidity, 9
compartment syndrome, 197–198
compensated shock, 95
complete blood count (CBC), 313
complete fractures, 193
complications, 9
compound fractures, 193
compression fractures, 188
compulsion, 382
computerized axial tomography (CT scan), 186
conduction heat loss, 361
congenital defects, 19

congestive heart failure (CHF), 143–144
conjunctival hemorrhage, 352
conjunctivitis, 348
contact dermatitis, 332
contusions, 335
  brain, 173
  pulmonary, 123
convection heat loss, 361
conversion disorder, 383
convulsions, 166
corneal abrasion, 351–352
coronary artery disease, 139
cor pulmonale, 121
corticosteroids, 226
cortisol, 209
costovertebral angle (CVA) tenderness, 271
creatinine, 272
creatinine clearance test, 272
Crohn's disease, 248
croup, 114, 446
crowning, 422
cruciate ligament tears, 199
crush injury, 197
crystalloids, 85
culture and sensitivity test, 59
curative treatment, 44
Cushing's syndrome, 211–212
cyanosis, 109, 133
cystic fibrosis, 124
cystitis, 274, 279
cystogram, 272
cystoscopy, 272
cysts, 332, 396
cytology, 42
cytoplasm, 15
cytotoxic, 231

D

Dalton's law, 365, 367
dead space, 108
death, 25–28
débridement, 55
decompensated shock, 95
decompression, 176
decompression illness, 366
decubitus ulcers, 336–337
deep vein thrombosis (DVT), 147, 435
defecation, 243
degenerative diseases, 25
degenerative joint disease, 190
dehiscence, 55
delirium, 379
delirium tremens (DTs), 257, 291, 376
delivery. *See* labor/delivery
delusional disorders, 380
delusions, 375
dementia, 169–170, 379
densitometry, 188
dental caries, 245
dependency, 376
depressants, 377–378
depression, 374, 380–381, 385
diabetes
  gestational (GDM), 214, 412
  mellitus, 212–214, 229, 412–413
diabetic retinopathy, 213
diapedesis, 50
diastolic pressure, 132
differential, 313
differential diagnosis, 8–9
differentiation, 34, 35
diffuse axonal injury (DAI), 172–173
diffusion, 67, 68
digital rectal examination, 393
dilation, 422
diptheria, 444
discectomy, 199
diseases, 4
  cardiovascular system, 120–121, 134–147, 413
  causes, 21–25
  childhood, 439–451
  ears, 349–351
  endocrine system, 209–215
  eyes, 346–349
  female reproductive system, 394–396, 397–401
  gastrointestinal (GI) system, 244–259, 447–448
  hematologic system, 315–319, 448
  immune system, 224–233, 332
  lymphatic system, 233–235
  male reproductive system, 397–401
  musculoskeletal system, 186–193
  neurological system, 161–171, 448
  renal/urologic system, 272–280
  respiratory system, 112–121, 445–447
  skin, 329–334
dislocations, 196–197
disorders, 4
displaced fractures, 193
disseminated intravascular coagulation (DIC), 319, 411, 435–436
dissociative disorders, 381–382
Diver's Alert Network (DAN), 364
diverticulosis/diverticulitis, 253
diving emergencies, 364–366
dominant genes, 18
doppler devices, 133
dormancy, 444
Dowager's hump, 188

dromotropism, 129
drowning, 364
Drug Abuse Warning Network, 291
dry drowning, 364
dysentery, 253
dysmenorrhea, 394, 395
dyspareunia, 395
dysphagia, 163
dysphasia, 163
dysplasia, 26, 37
dyspnea, 109, 132, 315
dysrhythmias, 144–147
dystocia, 425–427
dystonia, 167
dysuria, 271, 397

E

ears
  aging and, 353–354
  anatomy/physiology, 343–345
  diagnostic tests, 346
  diseases, 349–351
  signs/symptoms, 345
  trauma, 353
ecchymosis, 148, 313
eclampsia, 411, 412
ectopic areas, 395
ectopic pregnancy, 409
eczema, 332
edema, 71, 83
  high altitude cerebral (HACE), 369
  high altitude pulmonary (HAPE), 369
  pulmonary, 120–121
effacement, 416, 422
electrocardiograms, 133
electrochemical gradient, 67
electrolytes, 65, 66
  disturbances, 71–78
  during labor, 417
electromyography (EMG), 186
embolus, 137
emphysema, 115
empyema, 52, 119–120
encapsulated, 23
encephalitis, 161
encephalopathy, 448
endarterectomy, 138
endocrine system, 205–215
  aging effect on, 215
  anatomy/physiology, 206–209
  diagnostic tests, 209
  diseases, 209–215
  postpartum, 432
  signs/symptoms, 209
  trauma, 215
endometriosis, 394–395
endometritis, 395
endotoxin, 98
engagement, 416
enteral administration, 24
environment, 6–7
environmental diseases/disorders, 357–370
  altitude emergencies, 366–369
  cold emergencies, 360–363
  heat emergencies, 358–360
  water emergencies, 363–366
epididymitis, 397
epidural hematoma, 173
epiglottis, 113
epistaxis, 113, 313
erysipelas, 330
erythema, 327
erythroblastosis fetalis, 229–230
erythrocytopenia, 312
erythrocytosis, 313
esophageal varices, 246–247, 256
esophagitis, reflux, 246
estimated date of confinement (EDC), 406
estrogen, 209
etiology, 5–6
eukaryotic cells, 14
evaporation heat loss, 361
exacerbation, 9, 248, 329
exocrine glands, 124
exophthalmos, 210
expiratory reserve, 108
exsanguination, 148
extracapsular fractures, 193
extrinsic factors, 96
extrinsic pathway, 311
exudates, 50, 51–52, 444
eyes
  aging and, 353–354
  anatomy/physiology, 342–343
  diagnostic tests, 345–346
  diseases, 346–349
  signs/symptoms, 345
  trauma, 351–353

F

fatal disease, 9
febrile seizures, 166
female reproductive system
  aging and, 401
  anatomy/physiology, 390–391
  diagnostic tests, 392–393
  diseases, 394–396, 397–401
  during pregnancy, 407

female reproductive system *(continued)*
  postpartum, 431–432
  signs/symptoms, 391–392
  trauma, 401
femoral neck fractures, 193
fetal attitude, 418
fetal lie, 418
fetal presentation, 418
fever, 359–360
fibrinolysis, 312
fibroid tumors, 396
filtration, 67
FiO_2, 109
fistula, 52
flail chest, 121
fluid, body. *See* body fluid
fluid volume deficit (FVD), 71, 82
fluid volume excess (FVE), 71, 82
folic acid deficiency anemia, 315
fontanelles, 418
food poisoning, 302–303
forced expiratory volume in one second (FEV_1), 108
fractures
  complications, 194
  orbital, 352
  rib, 121
  skull, 171–172, 353
  sternal, 121
  treatment, 194
  types, 193–194
frequency, 271
frostbite, 363
frostnip, 363
frozen section, 43
fulminant, 255
functional reserve capacity, 108
fundus, 420
fungal infections, 58, 330–331, 444–445
fungi, 56, 58
furuncles, 330

G

gangrene, 28
gastritis, 247
gastroenteritis, 248
gastrointestinal (GI) system, 69, 239–264
  aging and, 263–264
  anatomy/physiology, 240–242
  assessment, 243–244, 260
  developmental/genetic disorders, 260–263
  diseases/disorders, 244–259, 447–448
  during labor, 417
  during pregnancy, 407
  pain evaluation, 260
  postpartum, 432
  signs/symptoms, 242–243
  trauma, 259–260
genes, 17
genital herpes, 398–399
genital warts, 400–401
genotypes, 18
germ cells, 16
Glasgow Coma Scale (GCS), 175–176
glaucoma, 349
globe, ruptured, 352
glomerulonephritis, 274–275
glucagon, 209
glucocorticoids, 209
glycogen, 212
glycosuria, 212
goiter, 210
gonorrhea, 399
gout, 190–191
grading, cancer, 37–38
grand mal seizures, 166
gravida, 406
great vessel injury, 149
greenstick fractures, 193
grief, 384–385
Guillain-Barré, syndrome, 168
gumma, 400
gynecomastia, 257

H

hair, diseases of, 334
hallucinations, 376
hallucinogenic toxidrome, 288, 290
hallucinogens, 290, 378
hallucinosis, 290
hand washing technique, 6
hay fever, 112
headaches, 165–166
heat cramps, 360
heat emergencies, 358–360
heat exhaustion, 360
heat stroke, 360
HELLP syndrome, 412
helminths, 56, 58
hemarthrosis, 318
hematemesis, 242, 319
hematochezia, 243
hematocrit (Hct), 314
hematologic system, 309–320
  aging and, 319–320
  anatomy/physiology, 310–312
  developmental/genetic disorders, 319

diagnostic tests, 313–315
diseases, 315–319, 448
signs/symptoms, 312–313
trauma, 319
hematomas, 32
epidural, 173
subdural, 173
hematuria, 271, 319
hemiparesis, 163
hemoglobin (Hgb), 314
hemolytic anemias, 223, 316
hemolyzed, 315
hemophilia, 318–319
hemoptysis, 109
hemorrhage, 148
conjunctival, 352
postpartum, 433–434
hemorrhagic anemia, 316
hemorrhoids, 253–254
hemothorax, 122–123, 148
Henry's law, 365, 367
hepatitis, 254–255, 398
hepatomegaly, 254
heredity of patient, 7–8, 21–22
hernias
hiatal, 246
inguinal, 248–250
strangulated, 249
herniated nucleus pulposus (HNP), 198–199
herpes, 329, 398–399
heterozygous, 18
hiatal hernias, 246
high altitude cerebral edema (HACE), 369
high altitude pulmonary edema (HAPE), 369
Hirschsprung's disease, 263
hirsutism, 334
histamine, 49
Hodgkin's disease, 317–318
holistic medicine, 10
homeostasis, 4, 64
homozygous, 18
hordeolum, 348
hormones, 39
Huntington's chorea, 168
hydrocarbons, 295
hydronephrosis, 275
hydrophobia, 163
hydrostatic pressure, 67
hydrothorax, 119
hyperadrenalism, 211–212
hypercalcemia, 75, 78
hyperchloremia, 78
hyperemesis gravidarum, 408
hyperemia, 49–50
hyperglycemia, 212, 214
hyperkalemia, 74, 77
hypermagnesemia, 75–76, 78
hypernatremia, 72–73, 77
hyperopia, 347
hyperphosphatemia, 76–77, 78
hyperplasias, 22–23, 26, 35–36
hypersensitivity, 223
hypersensitivity disorders, 224–226
hypertension, 134–136
chronic, 413
portal, 256
pregnancy-induced (PIH), 411–412
hyperthermia, 358
hyperthyroidism, 210
hypertonic solutions, 84, 86
hypertrophy, 26
hyperventilation, 80, 110
hyphema, 352
hypnotics, 299–300
hypoadrenalism, 212
hypoadrenal shock, 98
hypocalcemia, 74, 78
hypochloremia, 78
hypochondriasis, 383
hypoglycemia, 212, 214–215
hypokalemia, 73, 77
hypomagnesemia, 75, 78
hyponatremia, 72, 77
hypophosphatemia, 76, 78
hypothermia, 176, 358, 361–363
hypothyroidism, 210–211
hypotonic solutions, 84, 86
hypoventilation, 110
hypovolemia, 316
hypovolemic shock, 92–96
hypoxemia, 79, 109
hypoxia, 25, 115
hypoxic ventilatory response (HVR), 367

I

iatrogenic, 6
idiopathic, 6
ileus, 250
immersion foot, 363
immune system, 219–236
aging and, 235
anatomy/physiology, 220–221
defense mechanisms, 48
diagnostic tests, 223–224
diseases, 224–233, 332
during labor, 417

immune system *(continued)*
- signs/symptoms, 223
- trauma, 235

immunity, impaired, 24–25
immunodeficiency, 25
immunodeficiency disorders, 223, 231–233
impacted fractures, 193
impetigo, 329–330, 444
incidence rate, 8
incisions, 335
incomplete fractures, 193
incubation period, 440
induration, 59
infants
- care of, 428–429
- physiological changes, 430–431

infarcts, 27
infections, 22, 56–59
- ear, 349–351
- puerperal, 434–435
- tests, 58–59
- types, 56–58

infectious diseases
- childhood, 440–445
- intergumentary system, 329–331
- neurological system, 161–163

inflammation, 22, 48, 49
- chronic, 51
- exudates, 51–52
- eye, 347–348
- lesions, 52–53
- process, 49–51

influenza, 114, 443
ingestion, 285
inguinal hernias, 248–250
inhalants, 379
inhalation, 285
injection, 285–286
inotropism, 129
insect bites, 303
insensible fluid loss, 68–69, 95
inspiratory capacity, 108
inspiratory reserve, 108
inspiratory stridor, 446
insulin, 209
integumentary system, 68–69, 325–337
- aging and, 337
- anatomy/physiology, 326–327
- diagnostic tests, 327–329
- diseases, 329–334
- during labor, 417
- signs/symptoms, 327
- trauma, 334–337

intermittent claudication, 138
International Liaison Committee on Resuscitation (ILCOR), 143
interphalangeal joints, 190
intertrochanteric fractures, 193
intoxication, 376
intracapsular fractures, 193
intracranial pressure (ICP), 174–175
intravenous pyelogram (IVP), 272
intrinsic factor, 96, 241
intrinsic pathway, 311
intussusception, 250
invasion, 32–33, 37
involution, 431
iron deficiency anemia, 315
iron toxicity, 296
irritable bowel syndrome (IBS), 252–253
ischemia, 27, 133
islets of Langerhans, 212
isoimmune disorders, 223, 229–230
isotonic solutions, 84, 86

J

Jacksonian seizures, 166
jaundice, 243
Journal of the American Association, 447

K

Kaposi's sarcoma, 232, 334
keloids, 55
keratin, 327
kernicterus, 414
ketoacidosis, 212
ketones, 212
kidneys. *See* renal/urologic system
kidneys-ureter-bladder (KUB), 272
Koplik's spots, 441
Kussmaul's respirations, 110
kyphosis, 187

L

labor/delivery, 405–436. *See also* pregnancy
- complications, 423–428
- infant care, 428–429
- obstetric history, 406–407
- onset, 415–416
- physiology of normal, 415–423
- postpartum care/complications, 428–436
- preterm, 415, 424–425
- stages, 421–423

labyrinthitis, 351
lacerations, 335
laminectomy, 199

laparoscopy, 392
laryngitis, 113
lead toxicity, 296
lesions, 51, 52–53, 327
  abnormal pigmented, 334
  types, 328
lethal disease, 9
leukemia, 32, 33, 313, 317, 448
leukocytopenia, 313
leukocytosis, 58, 313
leukorrhea, 396
lice, 331, 445
lifestyle of patient, 7, 40, 70
lipids, 213
lithium, 299
lithotripsy, 276
longitudinal fractures, 193
lordosis, 187
low back pain (LBP), 198–199
lumen, 132
lungs, 69, 114–118
Lyme disease, 330
lymph, 222
lymphadenitis, 234
lymphadenopathy, 234
lymphangiography, 224
lymphangiopathy, 234
lymphangitis, 234
lymphatic system, 219–236
  anatomy/physiology, 221–223
  diagnostic tests, 223–224
  diseases, 233–235
  signs/symptoms, 223
lymphedema, 234–235
lymphocytes, 220, 223
lymphocytopenia, 223
lymphocytosis, 223
lymphomas, 33, 235, 317–318
lymphopenia, 313

M

macrophages, 51
macrosomia, 413, 426
magnetic resonance imaging (MRI), 186
malabsorption syndrome, 248
malaise, 58, 248, 440
male reproductive system
  aging and, 401
  anatomy/physiology, 391
  diagnostic tests, 393–394
  diseases, 397–401
  signs/symptoms, 392
  trauma, 401
malignant melanoma, 333–334
malignant tumors, 23, 32, 34–35. *See also* cancer
malingering, 383
mania, 381
MAO inhibitors, 299
marijuana, 292–293, 376–377
mast cells, 49
mastitis, 434
mastoidectomy, 351
mastoiditis, 350–351
measles, 329, 440–441
mechanisms of labor, 423
medication precautions, 57
medications, toxicology of, 297–302
meiosis, 16
melanoma, malignant, 333–334
melena, 243
menarche, 391
Ménière's disease, 351
meningitis, 161
meniscus, torn, 199
menopause, 391
menorrhagia, 394
menstrual cycle, 394
mental retardation, 375
mercury exposure, 296–297
metacarpophalangeal joints, 190
metaplasia, 26, 38
metastasis, 32, 37
metastasize, 23
metastatic cancers, 23
metatarsophalangeal joints, 190–191
metritis, 434
metrorrhagia, 394
mineralocorticoids, 209
minute volume, 108
miscarriage, 408
mitosis, 16
mononucleosis, 235, 317, 443
mood disorders, 380–381
morbidity, 9, 28
mortality rate, 8
mothers
  care of, 429–430
  postpartum changes, 431–433
  postpartum complications, 433–436
motility, 242
multiple myeloma, 318
multiple organ dysfunction syndrome (MODS), 98
multiple sclerosis (MS), 168
mumps, 441–442
Munchausen syndrome/Munchausen by proxy, 383–384

murmurs, 144
muscular dystrophy (MD), 191, 200
musculoskeletal system, 183–201
  aging and, 201
  anatomy/physiology, 184–185
  diagnostic tests, 186
  diseases, 186–193
  during labor, 417
  during pregnancy, 407
  genetic/developmental disorders, 200–201
  postpartum, 433
  signs/symptoms, 185–186
  trauma, 193–200
mushrooms, 293
MVC (motor vehicle crash), 22
myasthenia gravis, 191, 228–229
myelogram, 199
myocardial infarction, 140–143
myopia, 347
myringotomy, 350
myxedema, 211

N

nails, diseases of, 334
narcotic analgesics, 300
narcotics, 292, 378–379
National Center for Health Statistics, 364, 449
necrosis, 27
neoplasia, 26
neoplasms, 22–23, 31–45. *See also* cancer
  benign, 23, 32, 34–35
  brain, 171
  classifications, 32–33
  hyperplasias and, 35–36
  malignant, 23, 35, 36–37
  musculoskeletal, 192–193
nephrectomy, 279
neurogenic bladder, 280
neurogenic shock, 96–97
neurological system, 155–179
  aging and, 179
  anatomy/physiology, 156–159
  diagnostic tests, 160–161
  diseases, 161–171, 448
  genetic/developmental disorders, 178–179
  during labor, 417
  postpartum, 433
  signs/symptoms, 159–160
  trauma, 171–178
neuromuscular junction, 295
neutropenia, 313
nicotine, 377
nitrogen narcosis, 366
nits, 445
nocturia, 271
non-causal risk factor, 8
non-displaced fractures, 185
Non-Hodgkin's lymphoma (NHL), 318
non-steroidal anti-inflammatory drugs (NSAIDs), 300–301
nosocomial, 6
nuchal cord, 427
nuchal rigidity, 161
nutrition, 23–24
nystagmus, 349

O

oblique fractures, 193
obsession, 382
obsessive-compulsive disorder (OCD), 382–383
obstructive disease, 108
occult blood, 244
oliguria, 271
oncology, 23
oophoritis, 395, 434
open fractures, 193
ophthalmoscope, 345
opioid toxidrome, 288, 289–290
opportunistic infections, 56
orchitis, 397, 442
organelles, 14
organic mental disorders, 379–380
organophosphates, 295
organ rejection, 25, 230–231
ORIF, 194
orthopnea, 109
osmolality, 83–84
osmolarity, 84
osmosis, 67, 68
osmotic pressure, 67
osteoarthritis, 190
osteogenesis imperfecta, 200–201
osteomyelitis, 189
osteoporosis, 188–189
otalgia, 350
otitis externa, 350
otitis media, 349–350, 444
otoscope, 346
ova and parasite (O&P), 244
ovarian cysts, 396

P

pain disorder, 383
painless bleeding, 410
palliative treatment, 10, 44
pallor, 313, 315

palmar erythema, 257
palpation, 8
pancreatitis, 259
pancytopenia, 316
panic disorder, 382
Pap test, 41
para, 406
paradoxical respiration, 121
paralytic obstruction, 250
paraplegia, 176
parasitic diseases, 331, 445
parenteral administration, 24, 85
paresthesia, 168
Parkinson's disease, 168–169
paronychia, 334
parotid glands, 441
paroxysmal stage, 443
partial seizures, 166
patency, 133, 446
patent ductus arteriosus, 149
pathogens, 5
pathologic fractures, 5, 193
pathologists, 4
pathology, 4–5
pathophysiology, 5
pediculosis, 331, 445
pelvic inflammatory disease (PID), 395–396
peptic ulcers, 247–248
percussion, 8
percussion notes, 111
perforation, 242
pericardial tamponade, 148
peripheral nervous system (PNS), 158–159
peripheral neuropathy, 169
peripheral vascular disease (PVD), 138
peristalsis, 240
peritonitis, 243
peritonsillar abscesses, 246
permeability, 65
pernicious anemia, 316
personality disorders, 384
pertussis, 443
petechiae, 148, 313
petit mal seizures, 166
pharyngitis, 113, 245–246
phenotypes, 18
phobia disorder, 382
photophobia, 352
physiology. *See* anatomy
piloerection, 358
pilonidal cysts, 332
placenta previa, 409–410
plaque, 136
pleural effusion, 119
pleurisy/pleuritis, 118
pneumocystis carinii, 232
pneumonia, 116–117, 446
pneumothorax, 119, 122–123
Poison Control Center, 293, 300
poisoning, 450–451
poliomyelitis, 162, 442
polycythemia, 317
polyuria, 271
portal hypertension, 256
postpartum hemorrhage, 433–434
post-traumatic stress disorder (PTSD), 383
Pott's fractures, 194
precipitate birth, 427
precipitate labor, 427
predisposing factors, 6–8
preeclampsia, 411–412
pregnancy. *See also* labor/delivery
  disorders, 407–415
  high-risk, 408
  multiple, 414–415
  physiology of normal, 407
  trauma, 436
pregnancy-induced hypertension (PIH), 411–412
preload, 132
premature rupture of membranes (PROM), 425
presbyopia, 347
presenting part, 418
presyncope, 167
prevalence, 6
prevalence rate, 8
preventive measures, 10, 40–41
primary union, 54
productive cough, 109
progesterone, 209
prognosis, 9
prokaryotic cells, 14
prolapsed cord, 427–428
prone position, 446
prophylactic antibiotics, 227
prostatitis, 397
proteinuria, 271
protoplasm, 14
protozoa, 56, 58
pruritus, 271, 327, 350
psychosis, 380
puerperal infection, 434–435
pulmonary abscess, 117
pulmonary contusion, 123
pulmonary edema, 120–121
pulmonary over-pressure accidents, 366
pulmonary thromboembolism (PTE), 120

pulse deficit, 133
pulse pressure, 95
pulsus alternans, 133
pulsus paradoxus, 110–111, 133
purpura, 148, 319
purulent exudate, 52
purulent fluid, 350
pus, 51
pustules, 330
pyelitis, 274
pyelonephritis, 274
pyloric stenosis, 262–263
pyloromyotomy, 263
pyoderma, 444
pyrogens, 52, 360
pyuria, 271, 397

Q

quadriplegia, 176

R

rabies, 162–163
radiation, 36, 39
radiation heat loss, 361
radical cystectomy, 279
radiologic examinations, 186
rales, 111
rape, 401
rebound tenderness, 243
receptors, 15
recessive genes, 18
Reed-Sternberg cell, 317
referred pain, 260
reflux esophagitis, 246
regeneration, tissue, 53
remission, 9, 248
renal calculi, 275–276
renal failure, 276–279
renal/urologic system, 69, 70, 269–281
  aging and, 280
  anatomy/physiology, 270–271
  diagnostic tests, 271–272
  diseases, 272–280
  during labor, 417
  during pregnancy, 407
  postpartum, 433
  signs/symptoms, 271
  trauma, 280
reproductive system. *See* female reproductive system; male reproductive system
residual volume, 108
respiratory failure, 446–447
respiratory system, 105–124
  aging and, 124
  anatomy/physiology, 106–109
  developmental/genetic disorders, 123–124
  diagnostic tests, 111–112
  diseases, 112–121, 445–447
  during labor, 417
  during pregnancy, 407
  newborn, 430–431
  signs/symptoms, 109–111
  trauma, 121–123
restrictive disease, 108
retinal detachment, 352–353
retropharyngeal abscesses, 246
Reye's syndrome, 448
rhabdomyolysis, 192
rheumatic fever, 226–227
rheumatoid arthritis, 190, 227–228
Rh incompatibility, 414
rhinitis, 112, 443
rhinorrhea, 112
rhonchi, 111
RICE, 196
rickettsiae, 56, 58
risk factors, 8
rotator cuff, torn, 199
routes of entry, 284–286
RPR (Rapid Plasma Reagin), 392
rubella, 441

S

salicylates, 301
salpingitis, 395, 434
sarcoma, 33
scabies, 331
scars, 53
schizophrenia, 380
sciatica, 198
scoliosis, 187–188
seasonal affective disorder (SAD), 381
sebaceous cysts, 332
sebum, 326
secondary union, 54–55
sedatives, 299–300, 377–378
seizures, 166
self-antigens, 226
semipermeable, 65
sepsis, 98
septicemia, 58, 243, 396
septic shock, 98
serotonin syndrome, 298–299
sexually transmitted diseases (STD), 397–401
shin splints, 200
shock, 91–100
  age-related differences, 100
  assessment, 99–100